Primary Care Medicine
Recommendations

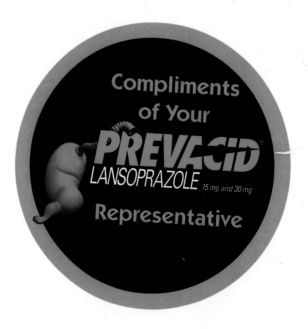

Primary Care Medicine Recommendations

ALLAN H. GOROLL, M.D.

Physician, Massachusetts General Hospital
Associate Professor of Medicine
Harvard Medical School
Boston, Massachusetts

ALBERT G. MULLEY, JR., M.D., M.P.P.

Chief, General Internal Medicine Unit
Massachusetts General Hospital
Harvard Medical School
Boston, Massachusetts

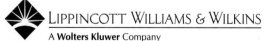

LIPPINCOTT WILLIAMS & WILKINS
A **Wolters Kluwer** Company

Philadelphia • Baltimore • New York • London
Buenos Aires • Hong Kong • Sydney • Tokyo

Acquisitions Editor: Richard Winters
Developmental Editors: Delois Patterson and Elizabeth Willingham, Silverchair Science + Communications
Supervising Editor: Mary Ann McLaughlin
Production Editor: Elizabeth Willingham, Silverchair Science + Communications
Manufacturing Manager: Benjamin Rivera
Cover Designer: Patricia Gast
Compositor: Silverchair Science + Communications
Printer: Victor Graphics

ISBN 0-7817-3352-9

Care has been taken to confirm the accuracy of the information presented and to describe generally accepted practices. However, the authors, editors, and publisher are not responsible for errors or omissions or for any consequences from application of the information in this book and make no warranty, expressed or implied, with respect to the currency, completeness, or accuracy of the contents of the publication. Application of this information in a particular situation remains the professional responsibility of the practitioner.

The authors, editors, and publisher have exerted every effort to ensure that drug selection and dosage set forth in this text are in accordance with current recommendations and practice at the time of publication. However, in view of ongoing research, changes in government regulations, and the constant flow of information relating to drug therapy and drug reactions, the reader is urged to check the package insert for each drug for any change in indications and dosage and for added warnings and precautions. This is particularly important when the recommended agent is a new or infrequently employed drug.

Some drugs and medical devices presented in this publication have Food and Drug Administration (FDA) clearance for limited use in restricted research settings. It is the responsibility of health care providers to ascertain the FDA status of each drug or device planned for use in their clinical practice.

10 9 8 7 6 5 4 3 2 1

To Richard Winters,
consummate medical publishing professional,
valued colleague, and friend

Contents

Preface

Primary Care Medicine Recommendations was derived to be both a pocket handbook and a PDA application from the fourth edition of our textbook *Primary Care Medicine* (PCM). It is designed as a portable decision tool and provides detailed specific recommendations for the screening, workup, and management of more than 200 unique clinical problems seen in the outpatient setting. The recommendations have been organized, written, and formatted for the pocket handbook and PDA platform so that they are easily readable and readily accessible wherever and whenever you need them.

The rationale and evidence for each of these recommendations is contained in the textual material and annotated bibliographies of the source textbook (PCM), which should be read by students and residents so that you develop an understanding of the material rather than just know a "right" answer. The goal is to provide you with recommendations that represent the latest and best approaches to your patients' problems.

For over two decades, our goal has been to make PCM the most useful, reliable, and cost-effective source of primary care information. With the advent of Internet and PDA technology, we have the opportunity to expand our efforts and make the information even more accessible. We hope you find *Primary Care Medicine Recommendations* a uniquely useful tool in the care of your patients.

Allan H. Goroll, M.D.
Albert G. Mulley, Jr., M.D., M.P.P.

Acknowledgments

This work represents our abstracting of material presented in the parent work *Primary Care Medicine*, 4th edition. Thus, we are indebted to and recognize the many contributors to that textbook whose work forms the basis for the recommendations in this book (see the table of contents and contributors' list in *Primary Care Medicine*, 4th edition, for a complete listing of authors, their chapter contributions, and their affiliations). Presented here in summary by section:

- *Principles of Primary Care*: John D. Stoeckle; Edward T. Ryan
- *Systemic Problems*: Harvey B. Simon, Stephen L. Boswell
- *Cardiovascular Problems*: Katherine K. Treadway, Harvey B. Simon, Mason W. Freeman, Gale S. Haydock, David C. Brewster, Richard R. Liberthson
- *Pulmonary Problems*: Harvey B. Simon, Benjamin Davis, John D. Stoeckle, William A. Kormos, Nancy A. Rigotti
- *Gastrointestinal Problems*: Michael J. Barry, Lawrence S. Friedman, Jules L. Dienstag, James M. Richter
- *Hematologic and Oncologic Problems*: Elaine M. Hylek, Robert A. Hughes, Thomas Delaney, Linda A. King, J. Andrew Billings, Eric L. Krakauer
- *Endocrinologic Problems*: Samuel R. Nussbaum
- *Gynecologic Problems*: Nancy J. Gagliano, Susan Oliverio
- *Genitourinary Problems*: Benjamin Davis, Harvey B. Simon, Michael J. Barry, John D. Goodson, Leslie S.-T. Fang
- *Musculoskeletal Problems*: Jesse B. Jupiter, David Ring, Robert J. Boyd, Samuel R. Nussbaum
- *Neurologic Problems*: Amy A. Pruitt, M. Cornelia Cremens, Michael A. Jenike
- *Dermatologic Problems*: Arthur J. Sober, William V.R. Shellow, Alice Y. Liu, Ellie J.C. Goldstein, Eric Kortz, Charles J. McCabe
- *Ophthalmologic Problems*: Claudia U. Richter, Roger F. Steinert, David A. Greenberg, Elizabeth S. Gould
- *ENT Problems*: John P. Kelly, A. Julianna Gulya, William R. Wilson, William A. Kormos
- *Psychiatric/Behavioral Problems*: John J. Worthington III, Scott L. Rauch, William E. Minichiello, Eleanor Z. Hanna, Linda Shafer, Arthur J. Barsky III, Jeffrey B. Weilberg, Carolyn J. Crimmins-Hintlian, Nancy A. Rigotti, Patrick L. Lillard, Todd E. Gorman
- *Allied Fields*: Ernie-Paul Barrette, Lawrence J. Ronan

Finally, we are indebted to the editorial excellence, professionalism, and dedication of the publishing professionals that make up the Lippincott Williams & Wilkins team, especially Richard Winters, as well as Elizabeth Willingham, Nancy J. Winemiller, and Thane Kerner of Silverchair Science + Communications. We are most grateful for their commitment to this project.

Principles of Primary Care

MANAGEMENT

- Organize PCP practice to provide coordinated, comprehensive, and personal care, available on first contact and continuous basis. Tasks of primary care include
  1. Medical Dx and Rx
  2. Psychological Dx and Rx
  3. Personal support of patients of all backgrounds, in all stages of illness
  4. Communication of information about Dx, Rx, prevention, and prognosis
  5. Maintenance of patients with chronic illness
  6. Prevention of disability and disease through detection, education, behavioral change, and preventive Rx
- PCP's recognition of and response to patients' emotional reactions to illness is critical determinant of quality of primary care. Equally important is eliciting and addressing patient expectations and requests. Patients' expectations often play major part in their seeking care and complying with Rx, and in determining health outcomes. Requests are specific and concrete helping actions and behaviors that are identified by patients. Attention to requests can make practice more efficient and more effective.
- When patients confront serious illness, elicit their beliefs about that illness. Confirmation or corrections of patients' attributions with PCP's clinical or scientific explanations of illness provide labels, names, and models so that patient feels illness can be understood and controlled, regardless of its technical Rx.
- To gain patients' full cooperation in Rx, it is important to learn about patient's views of Rx and any self-treatment. By making clinical decision a "shared" process, PCP fosters partnership that enhances compliance and outcomes.
- Attention to patient's social network can be critical to understanding symptoms and in fashioning realistic strategies for prevention and Rx.

BIBLIOGRAPHY

- For the current annotated bibliography on the practice of primary care, see the print edition of *Primary Care Medicine*, 4th edition, Chapter 1, or www.LWWmedicine.com.

Diagnostic Tests

MANAGEMENT

- Diagnostic tests have several uses:
  1. To make Dx in patient known to be sick
  2. To provide prognostic information for patient with known disease
  3. To identify person with subclinical disease or at risk for subsequent development of disease
  4. To monitor ongoing Rx
- In each case objective is not simply to classify or "label," but to reduce M&M and increase satisfaction and sense of well-being.
- Dx process is inherently uncertain; uncertainty can be expressed by probabilities. Probability of any particular disease being present, as test results are being interpreted, depends on both its probability of being present before testing and the validity of information provided by test results.
- *Sensitivity* is probability that test result will be positive when person tested actually has disease. Perfectly sensitive test can rule out disease if result is negative.
- *Specificity* is probability that test result will be negative when person tested actually does not have disease. Perfectly specific test can rule in disease if result is positive.
- When test results are known, probabilities of disease or its absence in light of these results are most relevant to PCPs and patients. Predictive value positive is probability of disease with positive test. (Probability that disease is absent despite positive test can be thought of as probability of false alarm.) Predictive value negative is probability of no disease with a negative test. (The probability that disease is present despite negative test can be thought of as probability of false reassurance.) All of these probabilities are determined by probability of disease before test was ordered and sensitivity and specificity of test.
- Importance of pretest probability of disease in individual patient (or prevalence of disease in population of such patients) for determining predictive values of test is often not fully appreciated and may lead to disappointment in clinical performance of test.
- Probabilities of disease can also be revised using pretest odds of disease and likelihood ratios. If p is probability of disease, ratio of p to $(1 - p)$, or $p/(1 - p)$ is odds favoring that disease being present and $(1 - p)/p$ is odds against that disease.
- Pretest odds of disease multiplied by positive likelihood ratio produces posttest odds of disease after positive test result. Positive likelihood ratio is probability of positive result (or result within specified range) given presence of disease divided by probability of that result given absence of disease. Positive likelihood ratio is therefore ratio of sensitivity to false-positive rate (i.e., 1 − specificity).
- Negative likelihood ratio is ratio of false-negative rate (i.e., 1 − sensitivity) to specificity. Pretest odds of disease multiplied by negative like-

lihood ratio produces posttest odds of disease after a negative test result.

- Published test evaluations often provide optimistic estimates of information provided by test in question. PCPs can avoid being mislead by paying attention to common problems in study design, including
  - unrealistic expectations about predictive values because of higher disease prevalence in study population than in practice;
  - unrealistic estimates of sensitivity and specificity because of overlap in test being evaluated and test(s) used to define presence of disease;
  - unrealistic estimates of sensitivity when population with disease in study has more severe and more easily detectable disease than those in practice;
  - unrealistic estimates of specificity when population without disease in study is too well and more free of disease that might be confused with disease in question than those in practice;
  - unrealistic estimates of clinical value of test when study authors do not consider how much new information is provided by test in question when compared with that provided by other tests.
- Sensitive tests or less stringent criteria for disease and resulting low false-negative rate should be favored when effective Rx for condition exists and cost of lost opportunity is great. High specificity or more stringent criteria for disease and resulting low false-positive rate are most important when positive result does not significantly influence Rx or outcome and may be burden for patient.

BIBLIOGRAPHY

- For the current annotated bibliography on diagnostic tests, see the print edition of *Primary Care Medicine*, 4th edition, Chapter 2, or www.LWWmedicine.com.

SCREENING AND/OR PREVENTION

CRITERIA FOR SCREENING

- Characteristics of the disease
  - Significant effect on quality or length of life
  - Prevalence sufficiently high to justify costs
  - Acceptable Rx available
  - Asymptomatic period during which detection and Rx significantly reduce M&M
  - Rx in asymptomatic phase yields better therapeutic result than does Rx delayed until symptoms appear
- Characteristics of test
  - Sufficiently sensitive to detect disease during asymptomatic period
  - Sufficiently specific to provide acceptable predictive value positive
  - Acceptable to patients
- Characteristics of population screened
  - Sufficiently high disease prevalence
  - Accessibility compliance with subsequent diagnostic tests and necessary Rx

CONDITIONS THAT WARRANT PERIODIC EVALUATION IN ALL PATIENTS OF APPROPRIATE AGE AND GENDER

- HTN: see Hypertension
- Hyperlipidemia: see Hypercholesterolemia
- Smoking: see Smoking Cessation
- Colon cancer: see Colorectal Cancer
- Breast cancer: see Breast Cancer
- Cervical cancer: see Cervical Cancer
- Alcoholism: see Alcohol Abuse

CONDITIONS THAT WARRANT PERIODIC EVALUATION IN SELECTED PATIENTS

- Rubella susceptibility
  - Risk factors: anticipated pregnancy and risk group membership; occupation (health care worker); see Immunization
- HIV infection
  - Risk factors: anticipated pregnancy and risk group membership; blood transfusion 1978–1985; see HIV-1 Infection
- Endocarditis susceptibility
  - Risk factors: valvular heart disease; see Bacterial Endocarditis
- Rheumatic fever susceptibility
  - Risk factors: rheumatic fever Hx; see Rheumatic Fever
- TB (PPD reactivity)
  - Risk factors: occupational exposure; see Tuberculosis

- Occupational lung disease
  - Risk factors: occupational exposure; see Occupational and Environmental Respiratory Disease
- Susceptibility to HBV
  - Risk factors: male homosexual; exposure; occupation (health care worker); see Viral Hepatitis
- Anemia
  - Risk factors: pregnancy; see Anemia
- Sickle cell trait
  - Risk factors: African-American of childbearing age
  - Genetic counseling must be acceptable; see Sickle Cell Disease
- Thyroid cancer
  - Risk factors: radiation of head and neck; see Thyroid Nodules and Thyroid Cancer
- Diabetes
  - Risk factors: pregnancy; family Hx of DM; obesity; Hx of gestational diabetes; see Diabetes Mellitus
- Endometrial cancer
  - Risk factors: exogenous estrogens; see Endometrial Cancer
- Vaginal cancer
  - Risk factors: *in utero* diethylstilbestrol exposure; see Vaginal Cancer
- Syphilis
  - Risk factors: male homosexual; pregnancy; other STDs; see Syphilis
- Chlamydial genitourinary infection
  - Risk factors: other STDs; women of childbearing age; see Chlamydial Infection
- Bacteriuria
  - Risk factors: pregnancy; kidney stones; see Urinary Tract Infection
- Lower urinary tract cancer
  - Risk factors: occupational exposure to aromatic amines (e.g., dyestuffs, leather tanning, rubber); see Bladder Cancer
- Testicular cancer
  - Risk factors: cryptorchidism; see Scrotal Pain, Masses, and Swelling; Testicular Cancer
- Osteoporosis
  - Risk factors: early menopause; see Osteoporosis
- Cerebrovascular disease
  - Risk factors: advanced age, TIA Hx; see Transient Ischemic Attack and Asymptomatic Carotid Bruit
- Skin cancer
  - Risk factors: fair skin, sun exposure; family Hx; see Skin Cancer
- Glaucoma
  - Risk factors: family Hx; advanced age; see Glaucoma
- Oral cancer
  - Risk factors: alcohol; tobacco; see Oral Cancer
- Decreased hearing
  - Risk factors: advanced age; excessive ncise; see Hearing Loss

BIBLIOGRAPHY

■ For the current annotated bibliography on health maintenance and the role of screening, see the print edition of *Primary Care Medicine*, 4th edition, Chapter 3, or www.LWWmedicine.com.

MANAGEMENT

- Doctor–patient dialogues about future implications of illness or risk factor are often momentous for patients. Few tasks of primary care are more important. Information about uncertain future must be communicated with clarity, compassion, and appreciation for uniqueness of each patient's needs.
- Patients vary significantly in desire for information about future. PCP should elicit and honor these preferences. Also helpful to let patient know that they should be prepared to express their preferences for having or not having information to specialists and other clinicians involved in care.
- To avoid being misled and misleading patients, PCPs must understand biases that can be introduced when suboptimal methods are used to gather information to help predict future.
- Some problems are specific to case-control studies that compare rates of "exposure" to risk factors among those with disease or outcome and those without same disease or outcome. These rates are used to produce an odds ratio, which is estimate of relative risk of disease or outcome with risk factor compared to risk without risk factor. In order for odds ratio to be accurate estimate of relative risk, disease or outcome in question must be rare.
- Accuracy of retrospective case-control method or of retrospective cohort studies requires that similar degrees of scrutiny be applied to Hx of cases and controls.
- Perhaps most important bias for PCPs to recognize in studies of prognosis has been termed referral filter bias. It occurs frequently as result of fact that patients in many published reports have been described because they have been referred to academic centers and they are often different from those seen in primary care settings.
- Communicating risk and prognosis can be difficult. Important source of confusion is distinction between relative and absolute risk. Effect of risk factors is usually expressed as relative risk or risk ratio, and effects of interventions are usually expressed as relative risk reductions. When absolute risks are low, this approach can give an unrealistic view of potential harms and benefits. Another way of conveying implications of risk factor is to cite risk attributable to risk factor or risk reduction attributable to an intervention. Attributable risk is difference between incidence among exposed people and incidence among those who are not exposed.
- Another approach to summarizing this kind of data is to cite number of patients one would need to treat to have desired effect in single patient.
- Proportion of people with particular condition who eventually die of that disease is the case fatality rate. Some indication of duration of survival may be included by describing survival at point in time after Dx (e.g., 5-yr survival rate). Simple rates have advantage of being

easy to remember and communicate. However, valuable information is lost when prognosis, the distribution of uncertain events over time, is summarized by single rate. More complete picture of prognosis is captured in survival curve.

■ Sometimes, proportion of people who experience events, rather than proportion who are event-free, is plotted on vertical axis. Such cumulative incidence curves convey same information. More complete picture presented by survival curve, including attention to low annual incidence of recurrence in near term, may be more helpful to patient.

■ Different people respond differently to same risk. A 1% risk for stroke during 5- or 10-yr period may be threatening to some but inconsequential to others. This can be explained by very real competing risks that different people face because of other medical conditions or the environment in which they live. Similarly, different people have different attitudes about trade-offs between present or near future and distant future. Putting up with side effects or inconvenience now for some possible benefit in future makes good sense to some but little sense to others. Again, competing risks explain some of these differences.

BIBLIOGRAPHY

■ For the current annotated bibliography on risk and prognosis, see the print edition of *Primary Care Medicine*, 4th edition, Chapter 4, or www.LWWmedicine.com.

Choosing Treatment Options

MANAGEMENT

- Randomized-control clinical trials provide best evidence regarding Rx effectiveness. When multiple trials have been performed, overviews, or meta-analyses, of these trials provide most comprehensive understanding of issues. Unfortunately, randomized-control studies are relatively rare for many common illnesses and their Rx.
- Even when randomized trials are performed, uncertainty remains about effectiveness of Rx for specific patients, which reflects methods used in clinical trials to measure isolated effects of experimental Rx.
- PCP must be concerned both about internal validity of trial as test of effectiveness or efficacy of intervention for specified population under controlled circumstances and about its external validity: the extent to which results are applicable to different patients seen in practice.
- Because of relative scarcity of randomized-control trials, PCPs must often rely on quasi-experimental clinical trials or observational studies without comparisons. However, great caution must be used in applying conclusions of observational studies to patient care. Differences in patient characteristics among alternative Rx groups may lead to erroneous conclusions about Rx effectiveness.
- There is ample evidence demonstrating that patients' expectations regarding effectiveness of Rx has profound influence on Rx outcome. It is not at all unusual for patients receiving inactive agents (placebos) or sham surgical procedures to report an improvement in symptoms. There are also examples of studies in which patients who have sufficiently high expectations to comply faithfully with prescribed regimen do better than patients who do not. These "compliance effects" occur regardless of whether regimen includes active agent or actual procedure.
- Even if probabilities of outcomes contingent on alternative Rx choices can be estimated precisely, there is still much work to be done to ensure wise Rx choice for particular patient. Different patients have different responses to same health outcomes. They also can also view very differently the same level of risk or same trade-offs over time. The right choice, therefore, requires careful communication between PCP and patient about what possible outcomes will mean for that patient's quality of life over foreseeable future.

BIBLIOGRAPHY

- For the current annotated bibliography on choosing treatment options, see the print edition of *Primary Care Medicine*, 4th edition, Chapter 5, or www.LWWmedicine.com.

MANAGEMENT

SUMMARY OF RECOMMENDATIONS FOR ROUTINE ADULT IMMUNIZATIONS

Influenza

- For whom recommended
  - Adults aged ≥65.
  - People aged 6 mos–65 yrs with medical problems such as heart disease, lung disease, diabetes mellitus (DM), renal dysfunction, hemoglobinopathies, and immunosuppression; people living in long-term care facilities.
  - People aged ≤6 mos working or living with at-risk people.
  - All health care workers and those who provide key community services.
  - Healthy pregnant women who will be in second or third trimesters during influenza season.
  - Pregnant women who have underlying medical conditions should be vaccinated before flu season, regardless of state of pregnancy.
  - Anyone who wishes to reduce likelihood of becoming ill with influenza.
  - Persons traveling to areas in which influenza activity exists or among people from areas of world in which there is current influenza activity.
- Contraindications and precautions (mild illness not a contraindication)
  - Previous anaphylactic reaction to this vaccine, to any of its components, or to eggs.
  - Moderate or severe acute illness.
- Schedule
  - Given every year.
  - In temperate northern hemisphere, October–November is optimal time to receive annual flu shot to maximize protection, but vaccine may be given any time during influenza season (typically December–March) or at other times when risk of influenza exists.
  - May be given with all other vaccines but at separate site.
- Route of administration
  - IM

Pneumococcal Pneumonia

- For whom recommended
  - People aged 2–65 who have chronic illness or other risk factors, including chronic cardiac or pulmonary diseases, chronic liver disease, alcoholism, DM, and CSF leaks; and persons living in special environments or social settings (including Alaska natives and certain American Indian populations). Those at highest risk of fatal pneumococcal infection are persons with anatomic or functional asplenia (including sickle cell disease); immunocompromised persons, including those with HIV infection, leukemia, lymphoma, Hodgkin's disease,

multiple myeloma, generalized malignancy, chronic renal failure, or nephrotic syndrome; those receiving immunosuppressive chemotherapy (including corticosteroids); and those who have received an organ or bone marrow transplant.

- Contraindications and precautions (mild illness not a contraindication)
  - Previous anaphylactic reaction to this vaccine, to any of its components, or to eggs.
  - Moderate or severe acute illness.
- Schedule
  - Routinely given as 1-time dose; administer if previous vaccination Hx unknown.
  - One-time revaccination is recommended 5 yrs later for people at highest risk of fatal pneumococcal infection or rapid antibody loss (e.g., renal disease) and for people aged >65 if first dose was given before age 65 and ≥5 yrs have elapsed since previous dose.
  - May be given with all other vaccines but at separate site.
- Route of administration
  - IM or SQ

Hepatitis B

- For whom recommended
  - High-risk adults, including household contacts and sex partners of HbsAg-positive persons; users of illicit injectable drugs; heterosexuals with >1 sex partner in 6 mos; men who have sex with men; people with recently diagnosed STDs; patients in hemodialysis units and patients with renal disease that may result in dialysis; recipients of certain blood products; health care workers and public safety workers who are exposed to blood; clients and staff of institutions for developmentally disabled; inmates of long-term correctional facilities; certain international travelers. (Note: Prior serologic testing may be recommended depending on specific level of risk or likelihood of previous exposure.)
  - All adolescents.
  - Note: In 1997, NIH Consensus Development Conference, a panel of national experts, recommended that hepatitis B vaccination be given to all persons infected with HCV.
  - *Editor's note: Perform serologic screening for people who have emigrated from endemic areas. When HbsAg-positive persons are identified, offer them appropriate disease management. In addition, screen their household members and intimate contacts and, if found susceptible, vaccinate.*
- Contraindications and precautions (mild illness not a contraindication)
  - Previous anaphylactic reaction to this vaccine, to any of its components, or to eggs.
  - Moderate or severe acute illness.
- Schedule
  - 3 doses needed on 0-, 1-, 6-mos schedule.
  - Alternate timing options for vaccination include 0, 2, 4 mos; 0, 1, 4 mos.
  - There must be 4 wks between doses 1 and 2, and 8 wks between doses 2 and 3. Overall, there must be ≥4 mos between doses 1 and 3.
  - Schedule for those who have fallen behind: if series is delayed between doses, do not start series over. Continue from where you left off.
  - May be given with all other vaccines but at separate site.

■ Routes of administration
  • IM
■ Other comments
  • Brands may be used interchangeably.

Hepatitis A

■ For whom recommended
  • People who travel outside U.S. (except for northern and western Europe, New Zealand, Australia, Canada, and Japan).
  • People with chronic liver disease, including people with HCV infection, people with hepatitis B who have chronic liver disease, illicit drug users, men who have sex with men, people with clotting factor disorders, people who work with HAV in experimental lab settings (this does not refer to routine medical labs), and food handlers when health authorities or private employers determine vaccination to be cost-effective.
  • Note: Prevaccination testing is likely to be cost-effective for persons aged >40 as well as for younger persons in certain groups with high prevalence of HAV infection.
■ Contraindications and precautions (mild illness not a contraindication)
  • Previous anaphylactic reaction to this vaccine, to any of its components, or to eggs.
  • Moderate or severe acute illness.
  • Safety during pregnancy undetermined, so weigh benefits against potential risk.
■ Schedule
  • 2 doses needed.
  • Minimum interval between doses 1 and 2 is 6 mos.
  • If dose 2 is delayed, do not repeat dose 1. Just give dose 2.
  • May be given with all other vaccines but at separate site.
■ Route of administration
  • IM
■ Other comments
  • Brands may be used interchangeably.

Tetanus-diphtheria

■ For whom recommended
  • All adolescents and adults.
  • After primary series has been completed, booster dose is recommended q10yrs. Make sure patients have received primary series of 3 doses.
  • Booster dose as early as 5 yrs later may be needed for wound management, so consult ACIP recommendations.
■ Contraindications and precautions (mild illness not a contraindication)
  • Previous anaphylactic reaction to this vaccine, to any of its components, or to eggs.
  • Moderate or severe acute illness.
■ Route of administration
  • IM

Measles, Mumps, Rubella (MMR)

■ For whom recommended

- Adults born in 1957 or later who are aged ≥18 (including those born outside U.S.) should receive at least 1 dose of MMR if there is no serologic proof of immunity or documentation of dose given on or after first birthday.
- Adults in high-risk groups, such as health care workers, students entering colleges and other educational institutions after high school, and international travelers, should receive 2 doses.
- All women of childbearing age (i.e., adolescent girls and premenopausal adult women) who do not have acceptable evidence of rubella immunity or vaccination.
- Note: Adults born before 1957 are usually considered immune, but proof of immunity may be desirable for health care workers.

■ Contraindications and precautions (mild illness not a contraindication)

- Previous anaphylactic reaction to this vaccine or to any of its components. (Anaphylactic reaction to eggs is no longer contraindication to MMR.)
- Pregnancy or possibility of pregnancy within 3 mos.
- HIV positivity is *not* a contraindication to MMR except for those who are severely immunocompromised.
- Immunocompromise caused by cancer, leukemia, lymphoma, and immunosuppressive drug Rx, including high-dose steroids or radiation Rx.
- If blood products or immune globulin (IG) have been administered during past 11 mos, consult ACIP recommendations regarding time to wait before vaccinating.
- Moderate or severe acute illness.
- Note: MMR is *not* contraindicated if PPD test has been done recently. PPD should be delayed for 4–6 wks after MMR has been given.

■ Schedule

- 1 or 2 doses needed.
- If dose 2 is recommended, give it no sooner than 4 wks after dose 1.
- May be given with all other vaccines but at separate site.
- If varicella vaccine and MMR (or other live viral vaccines such as yellow fever vaccine) are needed and are not administered on same day, space them ≥4 wks apart.

■ Route of administration

- SQ

Varicella (Chickenpox)

■ For whom recommended

- All susceptible adults and adolescents. Make special efforts to vaccinate susceptible persons who have close contact with persons at high risk for serious complications (e.g., health care workers and family contacts of immunocompromised persons) and susceptible persons who are at high risk of exposure (e.g., teachers of young children, day care employees, residents and staff in institutional settings such as colleges and correctional institutions, military personnel, adolescents and adults living with children, nonpregnant women of childbearing age, and international travelers who do not have evidence of immunity).
- Note: Assume immunity in people with reliable Hx of chickenpox (e.g., self-report or parental report of disease). For adults without reliable Hx, serologic testing may be cost-effective because most adults with negative or uncertain Hx of varicella are immune.

- Contraindications and precautions (mild illness not a contraindication)
  - Previous anaphylactic reaction to this vaccine or to any of its components.
  - Pregnancy or possibility of pregnancy within 1 mo (manufacturer recommends 3 mos).
  - Immunocompromise caused by malignancies and primary or acquired cellular immunodeficiency, including HIV/AIDS. Note: For those on high-dose immunosuppressive Rx, consult ACIP recommendations regarding delay time.
  - If blood products or IG have been administered during past 5 mos, consult ACIP recommendations regarding time to wait before vaccinating.
  - Moderate or severe acute illness.
  - Note: Manufacturer recommends that salicylates be avoided for 6 wks after administration of varicella vaccine because of theoretical risk of Reye's syndrome.
- Schedule
  - 2 doses needed.
  - Dose 2 is given 4–8 wks after dose 1.
  - May be given with all other vaccines but at separate site.
  - If varicella vaccine and MMR (or other live viral vaccines such as yellow fever vaccine) are needed and are not administered on same day, space them ≤4 wks apart.
  - If dose 2 is delayed, do not repeat dose 1. Just give dose 2.
- Route of administration
  - SQ

Polio (IPV)

- For whom recommended
  - Not routinely recommended for persons aged ≥18.
  - Note: Adults living in the U.S. who never received or completed primary series of polio vaccine need not be vaccinated unless they intend to travel to areas where exposure to wild-type virus is likely. Previously vaccinated adults should receive 1 booster dose if traveling to polio-endemic areas.
- Contraindications and precautions (mild illness not a contraindication)
  - Refer to ACIP recommendations (below).
- Schedule
  - Refer to ACIP recommendations regarding unique situations, schedules, and dosing information.
  - May be given with all other vaccines but at separate site.
- Route of administration
  - Give IM or SQ

Lyme Disease

- For whom recommended
  - Consider for persons aged 15–70 who reside, work, or play in areas of high or moderate risk and who engage in activities that result in frequent or prolonged exposure to tick-infested habitat.
  - Persons with Hx of previous uncomplicated Lyme disease who are at continued high risk for Lyme disease (see preceding description).
  - See ACIP statement for definition of high and moderate risk.

- Contraindications and precautions (mild illness not a contraindication)
  - Previous anaphylactic reaction to this vaccine or to any of its components.
  - Pregnancy.
  - Moderate or severe acute illness.
  - Rx-resistant Lyme arthritis.
  - There are not enough data to recommend Lyme disease vaccine to persons with these conditions: immunodeficiency, diseases associated with joint swelling (including RA) or diffuse muscular pain, chronic health conditions resulting from Lyme disease.
- Schedule
  - 3 doses needed. Give at intervals of 0, 1, and 12 mos. Schedule dose 1 (given in yr 1) and dose 3 (given in yr 2) to be given several wks before tick season. See ACIP statement for details.
  - Safety of administering Lyme disease vaccine with other vaccines has not been established.
  - ACIP says if it must be administered concurrently with other vaccines, give it at separate site.
- Route of administration
  - IM

Adapted from the Advisory Committee on Immunization Practices by the Immunization Action Coalition *ad hoc* team (August 1999), with additions.

INDICATIONS FOR VACCINATION DURING PREGNANCY

- Delay pregnancy for 3 mos following MMR, yellow fever, or varicella vaccines. (ACIP recommends ≥1-mo delay after varicella vaccine; manufacturer recommends 3-mo delay.)
- Live virus vaccine:
  - MMR (live attenuated)
    - Contraindicated. May give immunoglobulin for exposure.
  - Yellow fever (live attenuated)
    - Contraindicated except if exposure to yellow fever virus is unavoidable.
  - Poliomyelitis [trivalent live attenuated oral polio vaccine (OPV)]
    - Persons at substantial risk of exposure. ACIP has recommended use in outbreak. Many would use inactivated polio virus (IPV) (see below).
  - Varicella (live attenuated)
    - Contraindicated. If exposure and susceptible, give varicella zoster IG.
- Inactivated virus vaccines:
  - Hepatitis A (killed virus)
    - Data on safety in pregnancy are unavailable. Should weigh theoretical risk of vaccination against risk of disease.
  - Hepatitis B (recombinant-produced purified HBsAg)
    - Pregnancy is not a contraindication. Preexposure and postexposure prophylaxis can be administered if indicated.
  - Influenza (inactivated type A and B virus vaccines)
    - Women who will be in second or third trimester during flu season. All high-risk pregnant women.
  - Japanese encephalitis (killed virus)
    - Should reflect actual risks of disease and probable benefits of vaccine.

- Poliomyelitis [killed virus (IPV)]
  - May be preferred over OPV because of risk of vaccine-associated paralysis.
- Rabies (killed virus)
  - Substantial risk of exposure. Pregnancy is not contraindication for postexposure prophylaxis.
■ Live bacterial vaccines:
  - Typhoid (Ty21a; live bacterial)
    - Avoid on theoretical grounds (see below)
  - TB (BCG; live bacterial)
    - Contraindicated
■ Inactivated bacterial vaccines:
  - Typhoid (heat/phenol-inactivated)
    - Avoid because of systemic reactions and febrile responses (see below).
  - Plague (killed bacterial)
    - Selective vaccination of exposed persons.
  - Meningococcal (polysaccharide)
    - Only in unusual outbreak situations or high-risk persons.
  - Pneumococcal (polysaccharide)
    - Only for high-risk persons.
  - *H. influenzae* type b conjugate (polysaccharide-protein)
    - Only for high-risk persons.
  - Typhoid (Vi capsular polysaccharide vaccine; polysaccharide)
    - Use if indicated. Preferred over Ty21a and heat/phenol-inactivated vaccine in pregnancy.
■ Toxoids:
  - Tetanus-diphtheria (combined tetanus-diphtheria toxoids, adult formulation)
    - Safe. Indication: lack of primary series, or no booster within past 10 yrs.
■ IGs, pooled or hyperimmune (IG or specific globulin preparations)
  - Exposure or anticipated unavoidable exposure to measles, hepatitis A, hepatitis B, rabies, tetanus, or varicella.

Adapted from Centers for Disease Control and Prevention, *Health Information for International Travel 1996–1997*, DHHS, Atlanta, GA, with additions.

SUMMARY OF ACIP RECOMMENDATIONS ON IMMUNIZATION OF IMMUNOCOMPROMISED PERSONS

Tetanus-diphtheria

■ Recommended
  - Routine (not immunocompromised)
  - HIV infection/AIDS
  - Severely immunocompromised (non–HIV related)
  - After solid organ transplant on chronic immunosuppressive Rx (anecdotal reports of organ transplant rejection after vaccination with tetanus, diphtheria)
  - Asplenia
  - Renal failure
  - DM
  - Alcoholism and alcoholic cirrhosis

MMR

■ Recommended/considered
  • HIV infection/AIDS (avoid if severely immunocompromised)
■ Use if indicated
  • Routine (not immunocompromised)
  • Asplenia
  • Renal failure
  • DM
  • Alcoholism and alcoholic cirrhosis
■ Contraindicated
  • Severely immunocompromised (non–HIV related)
  • After solid organ transplant on chronic immunosuppressive Rx

Hepatitis B

■ Recommended
  • Renal failure (Patients with renal failure on dialysis should have their anti-HBs response tested after vaccination, and those found not to respond should be revaccinated.)
■ Use if indicated
  • Routine (not immunocompromised)
  • HIV infection/AIDS
  • Severely immunocompromised (non–HIV related)
  • After solid organ transplant on chronic immunosuppressive Rx
  • Asplenia
  • DM
  • Alcoholism and alcoholic cirrhosis

H. influenzae Type B

■ Recommended
  • Asplenia
■ Considered
  • HIV infection/AIDS (In some areas, HIV-infected individuals may have higher incidence of infection with _H. influenzae_ b; not routinely recommended.)
  • Severely immunocompromised (non–HIV related)
  • After solid organ transplant on chronic immunosuppressive Rx
■ Use if indicated
  • Renal failure
  • DM
  • Alcoholism and alcoholic cirrhosis
■ Not recommended
  • Routine (not immunocompromised)

Pneumococcal Pneumonia

■ Recommended
  • Routine (not immunocompromised; if aged ≥65 or high risk)
  • HIV infection/AIDS
  • Severely immunocompromised (non–HIV related)
  • After solid organ transplant on chronic immunosuppressive Rx
  • Asplenia
  • Renal failure
  • DM

• Alcoholism and alcoholic cirrhosis

Meningococcal Disease

■ Recommended
  • Asplenia
■ Use if indicated
  • Routine (not immunocompromised)
  • HIV infection/AIDS
  • Severely immunocompromised (non–HIV related)
  • After solid organ transplant on chronic immunosuppressive Rx
  • Renal failure
  • DM
  • Alcoholism and alcoholic cirrhosis

Influenza

■ Recommended
  • Routine (not immunocompromised; if aged ≥65 or high risk)
  • HIV infection/AIDS
  • Severely immunocompromised (non–HIV related)
  • After solid organ transplant on chronic immunosuppressive Rx
  • Asplenia
  • Renal failure
  • DM
  • Alcoholism and alcoholic cirrhosis

Live Vaccines

BCG

■ Use if indicated
  • Not immunocompromised
  • Asplenia (generally avoid)
  • Renal failure (generally avoid)
  • DM (generally avoid)
  • Alcoholism and alcoholic cirrhosis (generally avoid)
■ Contraindicated
  • HIV infection/AIDS
  • Severely immunocompromised (non–HIV related)
  • After solid organ transplant or long-term immunosuppressive Rx

OPV

■ Use if indicated
  • Not immunocompromised (generally avoid)
  • Asplenia (generally avoid)
  • Renal failure (generally avoid)
  • DM (generally avoid)
  • Alcoholism and alcoholic cirrhosis (generally avoid)
■ Contraindicated
  • HIV infection/AIDS
  • Severely immunocompromised (non–HIV related)
  • After solid organ transplant or long-term immunosuppressive Rx

Varicella

■ Use if indicated
  • Not immunocompromised
  • Asplenia (generally avoid)

- Renal failure (generally avoid)
- DM (generally avoid)
- Alcoholism and alcoholic cirrhosis (generally avoid)

■ Contraindicated

- HIV infection/AIDS (If asymptomatic HIV infection, probably safe. Avoid if severely immunocompromised.)
- Severely immunocompromised (non–HIV related)
- After solid organ transplant or long-term immunosuppressive Rx

Typhoid, Ty21a (Vi Capsular Polysaccharide Vaccine Preferred)

■ Use if indicated

- Not immunocompromised
- Asplenia (generally avoid)
- Renal failure (generally avoid)
- DM (generally avoid)
- Alcoholism and alcoholic cirrhosis (generally avoid)

■ Contraindicated

- HIV infection/AIDS (If asymptomatic HIV infection, probably safe. Avoid if severely immunocompromised.)
- Severely immunocompromised (non–HIV related)
- After solid organ transplant or long-term immunosuppressive Rx

Yellow Fever

■ Use if indicated

- Not immunocompromised
- Asplenia (generally avoid)
- Renal failure (generally avoid)
- DM (generally avoid)
- Alcoholism and alcoholic cirrhosis (generally avoid)

■ Contraindicated

- HIV infection/AIDS (If asymptomatic HIV infection, probably safe. Avoid if severely immunocompromised.)
- Severely immunocompromised (non–HIV related)
- After solid organ transplant or long-term immunosuppressive Rx

Killed or Inactivated Vaccines

IPV

■ Use if indicated

- Not immunocompromised
- HIV infection/AIDS
- Severely immunocompromised (non–HIV related)
- After solid organ transplant or long-term immunosuppressive Rx
- Asplenia (generally avoid)
- Renal failure (generally avoid)
- DM (generally avoid)
- Alcoholism and alcoholic cirrhosis (generally avoid)

Cholera

■ Use if indicated

- Not immunocompromised
- HIV infection/AIDS
- Severely immunocompromised (non–HIV related)
- After solid organ transplant or long-term immunosuppressive Rx

- Asplenia (generally avoid)
- Renal failure (generally avoid)
- DM (generally avoid)
- Alcoholism and alcoholic cirrhosis (generally avoid)

Hepatitis A
- Use if indicated
  - Not immunocompromised
  - HIV infection/AIDS
  - Severely immunocompromised (non–HIV related)
  - After solid organ transplant or long-term immunosuppressive Rx
  - Asplenia (generally avoid)
  - Renal failure (generally avoid)
  - DM (generally avoid)
  - Alcoholism and alcoholic cirrhosis (generally avoid)

Typhoid (Nonliving; Vi Capsular Polysaccharide Vaccine Preferred)
- Use if indicated
  - Not immunocompromised
  - HIV infection/AIDS
  - Severely immunocompromised (non–HIV related)
  - After solid organ transplant or long-term immunosuppressive Rx
  - Asplenia (generally avoid)
  - Renal failure (generally avoid)
  - DM (generally avoid)
  - Alcoholism and alcoholic cirrhosis (generally avoid)

Rabies
- Use if indicated
  - Not immunocompromised
  - HIV infection/AIDS
  - Severely immunocompromised (non–HIV related)
  - After solid organ transplant or long-term immunosuppressive Rx
  - Asplenia (generally avoid)
  - Renal failure (generally avoid)
  - DM (generally avoid)
  - Alcoholism and alcoholic cirrhosis (generally avoid)

Japanese Encephalitis
- Use if indicated
  - Not immunocompromised
  - HIV infection/AIDS
  - Severely immunocompromised (non–HIV related)
  - After solid organ transplant or long-term immunosuppressive Rx
  - Asplenia (generally avoid)
  - Renal failure (generally avoid)
  - DM (generally avoid)
  - Alcoholism and alcoholic cirrhosis (generally avoid)

Adapted with permission from MMWR Morb Mortal Wkly Rep 1993;42(RR-4):1, with additions.

WOUND MANAGEMENT AFTER EXPOSURE: TETANUS

- Patients with ≥3 previous tetanus toxoid doses
  - Give tetanus-diphtheria toxoids (adsorbed) for clean, minor wounds only if >10 yrs since last dose.

- For other wounds (such as, but not limited to, wounds contaminated with dust, feces, soil, and saliva; puncture wounds; convulsions; wounds resulting from missiles, crushing, burns, frostbite), give tetanus-diphtheria if >5 yrs since last dose.
- Patients with <3 or unknown number of prior tetanus toxoid doses
  - Give tetanus-diphtheria for clean, minor wounds.
  - Give tetanus-diphtheria and tetanus IG (250 U IM) for other wounds.

Adapted with permission from MMWR Morb Mortal Wkly Rep 1991;40(RR-10):1; and from *Tetanus and Diphtheria Toxoids 7/28/98* at www.cdc.gov/nip.

RABIES IMMUNIZATION

Preexposure Immunization

- Consists of 3 doses of human diploid cell vaccine (HDCV), purified chick embryo cell culture (PCEC), or rabies vaccine adsorbed (RVA), 1 mL, IM (i.e., deltoid area), 1 each on days 0, 7, and 21 or 28. Only HDCV may be administered ID (0.1 mL ID on days 0, 7, and 21 or 28). If traveler will be taking chloroquine or mefloquine for malaria chemoprophylaxis, complete 3-dose series before antimalarials begin. If this is impossible, use IM dose/route. Administration of routine booster doses of vaccine depends on exposure risk category as noted below. Preexposure immunization of immunosuppressed persons not recommended.
- Continuous risk (virus present continuously, often in high concentrations; specific exposures likely to go unrecognized; bite, nonbite, or aerosol exposure)
  - Criteria for preexposure immunization in typical populations: rabies research lab workers [judgment of relative risk and extra monitoring of vaccination status of lab workers is responsibility of lab supervisor (see U.S. Department of Health and Human Service's *Biosafety in Microbiological and Biomedical Laboratories*, 1984)]; rabies biologics production workers.
  - Preexposure regimen: primary course; serologic testing q6mos; booster vaccination if antibody titer is below acceptable level [preexposure booster immunization consists of 1 dose HDCV, PCEC, or RVA, 1 mL/dose, IM (deltoid area); or HDCV, 0.1 mL ID (deltoid)]. Minimum acceptable antibody level is complete virus neutralization at 1:5 serum dilution by rapid fluorescent focus inhibition test. Administer booster dose if titer falls below this level.
- Frequent risk
  - Criteria for preexposure immunization in typical populations: rabies diagnostic lab workers [judgment of relative risk and extra monitoring of vaccination status of lab workers is responsibility of lab supervisor (see U.S. Department of Health and Human Service's *Biosafety in Microbiological and Biomedical Laboratories*, 1984)]; spelunkers; veterinarians and staff; animal control and wildlife workers in rabies-epizootic areas.
  - Preexposure regimen: primary course; serologic testing q6mos; booster vaccination if antibody titer is below acceptable level. [Preexposure booster immunization consists of 1 dose HDCV, PCEC, or RVA, 1 mL/dose, IM (deltoid area); or HDCV, 0.1 mL ID (deltoid)]. Minimum acceptable antibody level is complete virus neutralization at 1:5 serum dilution by rapid fluorescent focus inhibition test. Administer booster dose if titer falls below this level.

- Infrequent risk (greater than that of population at large; exposure nearly always episodic with source recognized; bite or nonbite exposure).
  - Criteria for preexposure immunization in typical populations: veterinarians and animal control and wildlife workers in areas with low rabies rates; veterinary students; travelers visiting areas in which rabies is enzootic and immediate access to appropriate medical care, including biologics, is limited.
  - Preexposure regimen: primary course; no serologic testing or booster vaccination.
- Rare risk (population at large; exposure always episodic, with source recognized; bite or nonbite exposure; rabies research lab workers).
  - Criteria for preexposure immunization in typical populations: U.S. population at large, including individuals in rabies-epizootic areas.
  - Preexposure regimen: no preexposure immunization necessary.

Postexposure Immunization

- Rx should begin with immediate thorough cleansing of all wounds with soap and water.
- Persons not previously immunized: rabies IG, 20 IU/kg body weight, infiltrated at bite site (if possible), remainder IM; 5 doses of HDCV, PCEC, or RVA, 1 mL IM (i.e., deltoid area), 1 each on days 0, 3, 7, 14, and 28.
- Persons previously immunized (preexposure immunization with HDCV, PCEC, or RVA; prior postexposure prophylaxis with HDCV, PCEC, or RVA; or persons previously immunized with any other type of rabies vaccine + documented Hx of positive antibody response to prior vaccination): 2 doses of HDCV, PCEC, or RVA, 1 mL, IM (i.e., deltoid area), 1 each on days 0 and 3. Do not administer rabies IG.
- Adapted from Centers for Disease Control and Prevention, *Health Information for International Travel 1999-2000*, DHHS, Atlanta, GA.

BIBLIOGRAPHY

- For the current annotated bibliography on immunization, see the print edition of *Primary Care Medicine*, 4th edition, Chapter 6, or www.LWWmedicine.com.

Systemic Problems

Chronic Fatigue

DIFFERENTIAL DIAGNOSIS

- Psychological
  - Depression
  - Anxiety
  - Somatization disorder
- Pharmacologic
  - Hypnotics
  - Antihypertensives
  - Antidepressants
  - Tranquilizers
  - Drug abuse and drug withdrawal
- Endocrine-metabolic
  - Hypothyroidism
  - DM
  - Apathetic hyperthyroidism of the elderly
  - Pituitary insufficiency
  - Hyperparathyroidism or hypercalcemia of any origin
  - Addison's disease
  - Chronic renal failure
  - Hepatocellular failure
- Neoplastic-hematologic
  - Occult malignancy (e.g., pancreatic cancer)
  - Severe anemia
- Infectious
  - Endocarditis
  - TB
  - Mononucleosis
  - Hepatitis
  - Parasitic disease
  - HIV infection
  - CMV infection
- Cardiopulmonary
  - Chronic CHF
  - COPD
- Connective tissue disease-immune hyperreactivity
  - Rheumatoid disease
  - CFS
- Disturbed sleep
  - Sleep apnea
  - Esophageal reflux
  - Allergic rhinitis
  - Psychological etiologies (see above)

WORKUP

HISTORY

- Obtain thorough description of fatigue to be sure patient is not confusing focal neuromuscular disease with generalized lassitude; elicit patient concerns.
- Conduct detailed Hx, including comprehensive review of systems; include checks for substance abuse, depression, sleep disturbances, and use of hypnotic medications.

PHYSICAL EXAM

- Perform complete PE and specifically address etiologies suggested by Hx and of concern to patient.

LAB STUDIES

- Confine lab evaluation to testing leading diagnoses suggested by Hx and PE, but when Hx and PE are unrevealing, obtain serum creatinine, calcium, albumin, glucose, transaminase, and TSH determinations.
- Consider tests that address patient concerns, but avoid those that have no diagnostic value, such as antibodies to *Candida* and EBV.

MANAGEMENT

CHRONIC FATIGUE SYNDROME

- Because there is no test diagnostic of CFS, base Dx on clinical criteria and the ruling out of other etiologies.
- Establish strong patient-doctor alliance by taking patient's complaints and perception of disability seriously and by providing detailed explanation about CFS (including what is known and unknown about causation, prognosis, and Rx). Specifically address patient concerns.
- Consider instituting program of cognitive behavioral Rx that combines patient ed with goal setting and gradual exposure to activities the patient currently avoids because of fatigue.

BIBLIOGRAPHY

- For the current annotated bibliography on chronic fatigue, see the print edition of *Primary Care Medicine*, 4th edition, Chapter 8, or www.LWWmedicine.com.

Fever

DIFFERENTIAL DIAGNOSIS

CAUSES OF FEVER OF UNKNOWN ORIGIN

- "The big three"
  - Infections: 20–40%
    - Systemic
      - TB (miliary)
      - Infective endocarditis (subacute)
      - Miscellaneous: CMV infection, toxoplasmosis, brucellosis, psittacosis, gonococcemia, chronic meningococcemia, disseminated mycoses
    - Localized
      - Hepatic infections (liver abscess, cholangitis)
      - Other visceral infections (pancreatic, tubo-ovarian, pericholecystic abscesses, empyema of gallbladder)
      - Intraperitoneal infections (subhepatic, subphrenic, paracolic, appendiceal, pelvic, and other abscesses)
      - UTIs (pyelonephritis, renal carbuncle, perinephric abscess, prostatic abscess)
  - Neoplasms: 7–20%. Especially lymphomas, leukemias, renal cell carcinoma, atrial myomas, and cancer metastatic to bone or liver.
  - Collagen-vascular and other multisystem disease: 15–25%. Including TA and juvenile RA, as well as SLE, RA, polyarteritis nodosa, Wegener's granulomatosis, mixed connective tissue disease, sarcoidosis.
- Less common causes: 5–15%
  - Noninfectious granulomatous diseases (e.g., granulomatous hepatitis)
  - Inflammatory bowel disease
  - Pulmonary embolization
  - Drug fever
  - Factitious fever
  - Hepatic cirrhosis with active hepatocellular necrosis
  - Miscellaneous uncommon diseases (familial Mediterranean fever, Whipple's disease)
  - Undiagnosed

Modified from Jacoby GA, Swartz MN. Fever of unknown origin. N Engl J Med 1973;289:1407, with permission.

WORKUP

GENERAL STRATEGY

- If illness is insidious in onset and only slowly progressive, or if patient is nontoxic and clinically stable, proceed with deliberate ambulatory workup, using serial clinical observations and time as key Dx tools.
- If patient is compromised or is acutely ill and toxic, hospitalize and consider aggressive approach to Dx and Rx.

- In fever of unknown origin (FUO) patient who is not deteriorating, consider using time as Dx tool; halt workup for period of clinical observation followed by repeat Hx and PE.
- In high-risk patients (e.g., HIV infection with low CD4 count, cancer with neutropenia) with unexplained fever, consider opportunistic infection and
  - careful Hx and PE
  - blood cultures for bacteria, fungi, and mycobacteria
  - liver and bone marrow biopsies with cultures if blood cultures are negative, but suspicion of mycobacterial and fungal infections persists
  - serum cryptococcal antigen testing for suspected disseminated infection
- In cancer patients, consider chest and abdominal CT scans with contrast and lymph node biopsy.

Febrile Patients Who Require Special Attention

- Vulnerable hosts
  - Age (very young or very old)
  - Corticosteroid or immunosuppressive Rx
  - Serious underlying diseases (neutropenia, sickle cell anemia, DM, cirrhosis, advanced COPD, renal failure, malignancies, AIDS)
  - Implanted prosthetic devices (heart valves, joint prostheses)
  - IV drug abuse
- Toxic patients
  - Rigors, prostration, extreme pyrexia
  - Hypotension, oliguria
  - CNS abnormalities
  - Cardiorespiratory compromise
  - New significant cardiac murmurs
  - Petechial eruption
  - Marked leukocytosis or leukopenia

HISTORY

- Stress (1) host factors, (2) epidemiology, (3) symptomatology, especially for localization, and (4) drug Hx.

PHYSICAL EXAM

- Concentrate on areas suggested by patient's presenting symptoms, but perform detailed exam when site of infection is unclear. Do not overlook genitorectal exam.

LAB STUDIES

- In acute fever, limit to studies that confirm clinical suspicion or guide Rx (e.g., culturing).
- With persistent FUO, consider more extensive testing. Although testing must be individualized, potentially helpful studies include
  - CBC, differential, ESR, urinalysis;
  - radiologic studies (kidneys, ureters, bladder; upright abdominal plain films; abdominal ultrasound; abdominal or chest CT; bone films; radionuclide bone scanning; MRI);
  - blood chemistries, including blood sugar, LFTs, amylase;
  - exam of body fluids, especially if meningitis or abnormal fluid collection is suspected. Send fluid for culture, stains, sugar and protein determinations;

- immunologic studies, particularly serology for HIV, rheumatic fever, and other streptococcal infections, infectious mononucleosis, and *Salmonella*; also TB skin testing and ANA and RF determinations.
- In workup of obscure fevers, freeze and save "acute phase serum" for later comparison with "convalescent serum."

MANAGEMENT

- In acutely ill toxic patient who requires admission, begin broad antibiotic coverage even before establishing Dx. Obtain cultures of blood, urine, and other pertinent fluids before Rx.
- In nontoxic patient with acute febrile illness and in most persons with true FUO, avoid blind therapeutic trials (especially of antibiotics) for Dx; halt all nonessential medications; consider
  - empiric IV antibiotics only in limited situations (e.g., suspected culture-negative endocarditis or occult TB);
  - empiric salicylates or steroids only for suspected noninfectious inflammatory disease.
- Always conduct empiric trials with specific end point or time limit, carefully planned observations, and patient consent.

BIBLIOGRAPHY

- For the current annotated bibliography on fever, see the print edition of *Primary Care Medicine*, 4th edition, Chapter 11, or www.LWWmedicine.com.

SCREENING AND/OR PREVENTION

GENERAL APPROACH

- Whenever possible, conduct HIV-1 testing anonymously.
- Provide patient ed on HIV-1 transmission and risk reduction as part of every screening effort.

PATIENT SELECTION

- Screen CDC-designated high-risk patients, including
  - persons with STDs.
  - IV drug users, sexually active gay and bisexual men, hemophiliacs, prostitutes, and persons who received transfusions 1978–1985.
  - sexual partners of high-risk persons and of those with known HIV infection.
  - persons who consider themselves at high risk or request test.
  - women at increased risk who are of childbearing age or pregnant.
  - individuals with clinical or lab findings suggesting HIV.
  - patients with TB.
  - recipients and sources of blood and body fluid exposures.
  - health care workers who perform exposure-prone invasive procedures.
  - patients aged 15–55 who are admitted to hospital with seroprevalence rate of ≥1% or where AIDS patients = >1 in 1,000 discharges.
  - donors of blood, semen, and organs.
- Rescreen q6–12mos high-risk patients with negative test results who continue high-risk behavior.
- Rescreen at 6 mos those with indeterminate result on initial screening.

TEST SELECTION AND INTERPRETATION

- Screen with enzyme immunoassay test, e.g., ELISA assay.
- Confirm positive ELISA result with Western blot testing.
- Interpret test results by taking into account pretest probability, sensitivity, and specificity of testing methods, and timing of testing in relation to time of possible infection.
- If initial Western blot result is indeterminate, repeat in 6 mos.
- Counsel low-risk donors and low-risk persons who desire to know their HIV-1 status about possibility of false-positive result, especially about indeterminate Western blot result after positive ELISA result.

WORKUP

CONFIRMING DIAGNOSIS OF HIV-1 INFECTION

- Check for persistent HIV-1 antibody positivity; screen with ELISA test; confirm with Western blot analysis.
- Attempt direct detection of virus by viral culture, PCR assay, branched-chain DNA assay, or p24 antigen) if clinical suspicion is high but standard

serologic screening test results are normal (e.g., early phase of infection or patient too debilitated immunologically to produce antibodies).

CONFIRMING DIAGNOSIS OF AIDS

- Check CD4+ T-lymphocyte count for level <200/mm^3.
- Evaluate for presence of AIDS-indicator disease, clinically and by histologic or cytologic study, culturing, serologic study, neuroimaging, or endoscopy.
- Review for pulmonary TB, recurrent pneumonia, and invasive cervical cancer in patients with lab evidence of HIV-1 infection and absence of another reason for immune impairment.

FURTHER TESTING OF SEROPOSITIVE PATIENTS

Tests to Determine Whom to Treat, When to Treat, and Response to Therapy

- All patients
  - CBC, differential, platelets (as needed)
  - Chemistry (as needed)
  - CD4+ T-cell count (q3–4mos)
  - HIV RNA (viral load) (q1–4mos)
  - Rapid plasma reagent or VDRL (yearly)
  - Toxoplasma IgG (as indicated)
  - Varicella IgG (baseline only)
  - CMV IgG (baseline only)
  - HAA (baseline only)
  - HBsAg (baseline and as indicated)
  - HBsAb and/or HBcAb (baseline)
  - Anti-HCV (baseline and as indicated)
  - CXR (as indicated)
- All patients without written documentation of positive serology
  - HIV serology (baseline only)
- Patients without Hx of PPD positivity, TB Rx or prophylaxis
  - PPD (yearly for those at high risk)
- Nonwhite patients
  - G-6-PD (baseline only)
- All women
  - Pap smear (yearly)
- Check CD4-cell count and CD4 percentage.
- Determine viral load by plasma HIV-1 RNA assay.
- Repeat these determinations q3–4mos.
- Obtain CBC; if you detect anemia, measure serum iron, ferritin, folate, and vitamin B$_{12}$. Periodically check vitamin B$_{12}$ levels.
- Check baseline serum chemistries (electrolytes, BUN, creatinine, transaminase, alkaline phosphatase) before Rx (facilitates identifying drug toxicities and comorbid conditions).
- Perform serologic testing for syphilis; if positive, order FTA absorption test to exclude false-positive.

- Assess immune status with *T. gondii* immunoglobulin G serology and CMV serology.
- Plant intermediate-strength PPD TB skin test (routine anergy testing not necessary).
- Screen for hepatitis B and C (see Hepatitis).
- Consider testing for G-6-PD deficiency before Rx with oxidant drugs (e.g., dapsone, primaquine, sulfonamides).
- Perform baseline pelvic exam with Pap smear; repeat at least annually in asymptomatic women.

MANAGEMENT

IMMUNIZATION

- Administer as early as possible:
  - Pneumococcal polysaccharide vaccine
  - Influenza vaccine (yearly)
  - Hepatitis B vaccine (if not already antibody-positive)
  - Tetanus-diphtheria booster

Vaccine Indications and Schedule

- Pneumovax: all patients without Hx of vaccination; consider repeat after 5–6 yrs
- Hepatitis A vaccine: all patients negative for HAA, especially those with chronic hepatitis B and hepatitis C infections; 1 series only
- Hepatitis B vaccine: Patients negative for HBsAb or HBcAb; 1 series only
- Tetanus booster: patients without tetanus booster in ≥10 yrs; q10yrs
- Flu vaccine: all patients as clinically appropriate; yearly

INITIAL ANTIRETROVIRAL THERAPY

- Initiate Rx in any patient who exhibits
  - signs or symptoms of HIV-1 infection;
  - absolute CD4-cell count <500/mL (some argue for <250/mL); or
  - plasma HIV-1 RNA concentration (viral load >10,000 copies/mL).
- Consider antiretroviral Rx for patients with lab evidence of primary infection, including detectable HIV RNA in plasma together with negative or indeterminate result of HIV antibody test.
- Choose from clinical trial regimen for acute infection or from options available for treating established infection (see below).
- Maintain antiretroviral Rx indefinitely pending availability of further information.
- Match strength of antiretroviral program to plasma HIV-1 RNA concentration.
- For patients with very high plasma HIV-1 RNA concentrations (>100,000 copies/mL), begin triple-drug regimen involving 2 nucleoside reverse transcriptase inhibitors (NRTIs) and either a non-nucleoside reverse transcriptase inhibitor (NNRTI) or a protease inhibitor (PI) (see below).

- In tailoring antiretroviral therapy to individuals, consider overlapping toxicities, pharmacokinetic interactions, absence of cross-resistance, and drug sequencing that preserves future antiretroviral options.

Recommended Antiretroviral Agents for Treatment of Established HIV Infection

Preferred

- PI or NNRTI
  - Indinavir
  - Nelfinavir
  - Ritonavir
  - Saquinavir-SGC
  - Ritonavir + saquinavir-SGC
  - Efavirenz
- NRTI
  - Zidovudine + didanosine
  - D4T + didanosine
  - Zidovudine + zalcitabine
  - Zidovudine + 3TC
  - D4T + 3TC
  - Didanosine + 3TC

Alternative

- Nevirapine or delavirdine + 2 NRTIs (see above)
- Abacavir + zidovudine + 3TC

Not Generally Recommended

- 2 NRTIs
- Saquinavir-HGC + 2 NRTIs

Not Recommended

- D4T + zidovudine
- Zalcitabine + didanosine
- Zalcitabine + D4T
- Zalcitabine + 3TC

SUBSEQUENT ANTIRETROVIRAL THERAPY

Antiretroviral Options for Patients Unresponsive to Therapy

- Prior: 2 NRTIs + nelfinavir
  - New: 2 new NRTIs + 1: ritonavir; or indinavir; or saquinavir + ritonavir; or NNRTI + ritonavir; or NNRTI + indinavir; or amprenavir
- Prior: 2 NRTIs + ritonavir
  - New: 2 new NRTIs + 1: saquinavir + ritonavir; nelfinavir + NNRTI; or nelfinavir + saquinavir; or APV
- Prior: 2 NRTIs + indinavir
  - New: 2 new NRTIs + 1: saquinavir + ritonavir; nelfinavir + NNRTI; or nelfinavir + saquinavir; or amprenavir
- Prior: 2 NRTIs + saquinavir
  - New: 2 new NRTIs + 1: ritonavir + saquinavir; or NNRTI + indinavir
- Prior: 2 NRTIs + NNRTI
  - New: 2 new NRTIs + 1 PI

- Prior: 2 NRTIs
  - New: 2 new NRTIs + 1 PI; or 2 new NRTIs + ritonavir + saquinavir; or 1 new NRTI + 1 NNRTI + 1 PI; or 2 PIs + NNRTI
- Prior: 1 NRTI
  - New: 2 new NRTIs + 1 PI; or 2 new NRTIs + NNRTI; or 1 new NRTI + 1 NNRTI + PI
- Change antiretroviral if viral load significantly increases or desired reduction is not achieved, if CD4-cell count decreases significantly, or if clinical progression occurs.
- If new regimen fails to achieve 3- to 6-fold reduction in viral load by 4 wks, or <10-fold reduction by 8 wks, consider change in Rx.
- If regimen achieves 4- and 8-wk goals but fails to suppress viral load to undetectable levels by 4–6 mos, reevaluate regimen.
- When considering change in antiretrovirals, distinguish between drug failure and drug toxicity.
- For drug toxicity, substitute ≥1 antiretroviral of same potency and from same class of agents as agent suspected of causing toxicity.
- In case of drug failure, perform detailed review of current and past antiretroviral agents.
- *S*eek agents with as little overlapping resistance as possible. In 3-drug regimen, use at least 2 and preferably 3 new agents.
- As patient becomes more "drug-experienced," rely extensively on plasma viral load and CD4-cell count to inform drug choices.
- Consider viral genotyping or phenotyping to guide drug choices in initial Rx or Rx failure; also consider viral resistance testing.

POSTEXPOSURE PROPHYLAXIS

- For high-risk occupational exposure, consider postexposure antiretroviral Rx.
- Individualize decision, taking into account severity of exposure, very low risk for seroconversion, inability to provide absolute protection, high incidence of drug side effects, and need for frequent monitoring.
- Follow current consensus recommendations.
  - For needlestick, consider 2 NRTIs (1 from group A, 1 from group B for 1 mo + a PI for very-high-risk exposure).
  - For high-risk sexual exposures, no guidelines currently available.
  - For preventing perinatal transmission, consider zidovudine and/or nevirapine during pregnancy; both decrease likelihood of HIV-1 transmission significantly in perinatal setting.

OPPORTUNISTIC INFECTION: PROPHYLAXIS AND TREATMENT

P. carinii Pneumonia

Prophylaxis
- Initiate if CD4-cell counts <200 (or <14% of total lymphocytes) or Hx of oropharyngeal candidiasis.
- Prescribe TMP-SMX (1 DS tab/day), or dapsone (50–100 mg/day); TMP-SMX SS qd is also effective and may be better tolerated.

- Consider aerosolized pentamidine (300 mg q4wks via Respirgard II nebulizer) or atovaquone (1,500 mg/day) if sulfa-allergic.
- Use caution with nebulizer Rx if TB suspected.

Suspected P. carinii *Pneumonia*

- For new respiratory symptoms in those with CD4-cell count <200, obtain CXR, arterial blood gases, and induced sputum for Gram's stain, routine culture, mycobacterial stain and culture, fungal wet preparation and culture, and immunofluorescent stain for *P. carinii*.
- If CXR shows bilateral interstitial infiltrate and sputum Gram's stain is not diagnostic, treat presumptively for *P. carinii* pneumonia pending immunofluorescent stains.
- If patient appears clinically stable, is not in respiratory distress, and is not hypoxemic (PaO_2 >70 mm Hg), treat as outpatient with careful follow-up. **Choose among**
  - TMP-SMX (2 DS tab q8h × 3 wks), or
  - dapsone (100 mg/day in average-sized adult) + TMP (15 mg/kg/day q8h), or
  - atovaquone (750 mg bid × 3 wks), or
  - clindamycin (300–450 mg q8h) + primaquine (15 mg/day) for patients unable to tolerate dapsone/TMP or TMP-SMX due to G-6-PD deficiency.
- If patient is in respiratory distress or has significant alveolar-arterial gradient (>30 mm Hg), consider hospitalization for IV antibiotics and systemic corticosteroid Rx.

Tuberculosis Prophylaxis and Treatment

- For HIV-1 patients with PPD showing 5 mm of induration or anergic individuals with Hx of PPD positivity, choose among
  - INH, 300 mg/day, + 50 mg pyridoxine × 9 mos
  - INH (900 mg), pyridoxine (100 mg) 2 × wk for 9 mos
  - rifampin (600 mg) + pyrazinamide (20 mg/kg) qd × 12 mos
- For anergic HIV-infected patients with Hx of PPD positivity, consider course of INH.
- For active TB, see Tuberculosis.

M. avium Complex (MAC) Prophylaxis and Treatment

- Initiate prophylaxis for those with CD4-cell counts <50/mm^3. Start clarithromycin (500 mg/day) and azithromycin (1,200 mg/wk).
- Treat MAC infection with multidrug regimen:
  - Clarithromycin (500 mg q12h) and ethambutol (15 mg/kg/day) ± rifabutin (300 mg/day)
  - Azithromycin substituted for clarithromycin (500–600 mg/day)

Toxoplasmosis Prophylaxis

- Begin TMP-SMX (1 SS tab/day or 1 DS tab 3 × wk) or
- Dapsone (50 mg/d) + pyrimethamine (50 mg/wk) and folinic acid (25 mg/wk).
- For those with CD4-cell counts <100/mm^3 and seropositivity for *T. gondii*, consider dapsone (200 mg/wk) + pyrimethamine (75 mg/wk) + folinic acid (25 mg/wk).
- Instruct seronegative patients to cook meat thoroughly and wash hands carefully after contact with raw meat.

- Instruct cat owners to wear gloves while cleaning litter boxes and wash hands carefully afterward.
- Encourage HIV-positive gardeners to wear gloves while gardening.
- Hospitalize for signs of encephalitis.

Candida **Prophylaxis and Treatment**

- For oral candidiasis, do not routinely use prophylaxis, but consider long-term maintenance Rx to stem recurrent infections. **Choose among**
  - clotrimazole troche (10-mg held in mouth 15–30 mins tid)
  - chlorhexidine gluconate for significant gingivitis and periodontitis
  - nystatin oral pastilles (200,000 U tid) or nystatin suspension (100,000 U/mL, swish-and-swallow 15 mL 6 × day)
- For esophageal candidiasis, fluconazole (200 mg/day × 2–3 wks) or itraconazole (100–200 mg bid, or a 100- to 200-mg oral suspension qd). Reserve amphotericin B ± flucytosine for unresponsive infections.
- For vulvovaginal candidiasis prophylaxis, choose among
  - intravaginal miconazole suppository (200 mg × 3 days or 2% cream × 7 days)
  - clotrimazole (1% cream x 7–14 days, 100 mg/day × 7 days, 100-mg tab bid × 3 days, or 500 mg taken once)
  - fluconazole (150-mg tab PO once)
- For vulvovaginal candidiasis maintenance Rx to prevent frequent relapse,
  - ketoconazole (100 mg/day)
  - fluconazole (50–100 mg/day or 200 mg/wk).

Cytomegalovirus Treatment

- Treat CMV retinitis with 1 of these parenteral programs:
  - Foscarnet (60 mg/kg IV q8h or 90 mg/kg q12h × 14–21 days), superior for patients with normal renal function.
  - Ganciclovir (5 mg/kg IV bid × 14–21 days), preferred for impaired renal function; monitor granulocyte counts. Consider alternating or combining with foscarnet to reduce toxicity; intraocular release device (Vitrasert) for local Rx.
  - Cidofovir (5 mg/kg IV qwk × 2 wks, followed by 5 mg/kg IV q2wks ± 2 g probenecid 3 hrs before each dose and 1 g PO at 2 and 8 hrs after each dose).
  - Fomivirsen (330 mg by intravitreal injection on days 1 and 15, then monthly); not first-line Rx.
- Treat extraocular disease with ganciclovir and foscarnet at doses similar to those used for ocular disease. Give for 3–6 wks at outset; use maintenance Rx if there is relapse.

COUNSELING

- Assist patients in understanding and accepting changes in sense of self and in life plans and goals.
- Educate regarding Rx; focus on what patients can do rather than on what is out of their control.
- Give accurate positive information on current estimates of prognosis; do not destroy hope; screen for suicidality (see Depression).

- Review safe sex measures to prevent transmission of HIV-1 and other STDs.
- Help patient develop additional supports, make use of community resources.
- When appropriate, provide opportunity to discuss death and dying; reach common understanding of patient's wishes.

INDICATIONS FOR ADMISSION AND CONSULTATION

- Admit for signs or symptoms of significant pulmonary, CNS, or disseminated infection (especially severe *P. carinii* pneumonia, TB, atypical mycobacterial infection, syphilis, toxoplasmosis, histoplasmosis, coccidioidomycosis, cryptococcosis, or CMV).
- Initiate Rx of such patients in the hospital, even though outpatient Rx may be possible later.
- Immediately hospitalize suicidal patients and obtain urgent psychiatric consultation.
- Attempt hospice care at home in late phases of illness; try to minimize hospital admissions except as needed for comfort.

BIBLIOGRAPHY

- For the current annotated bibliography on HIV-1 infection, see the print edition of *Primary Care Medicine*, 4th edition, Chapters 7 and 13, or www.LWWmedicine.com.

Lymphadenopathy

DIFFERENTIAL DIAGNOSIS

IMPORTANT CAUSES OF LYMPHADENOPATHY

- Generalized
  - Infections
    - Mononucleosis
    - AIDS
    - AIDS-related complex
    - Toxoplasmosis
    - Secondary syphilis
  - Hypersensitivity reactions
    - Serum sickness
    - Phenytoin and other drugs
    - Vasculitis (systemic lupus erythematosus, rheumatoid arthritis)
  - Metabolic disease
    - Hyperthyroidism
    - Lipidoses
  - Neoplasia
    - Leukemia
    - Hodgkin's disease (advanced stages)
    - Non-Hodgkin's lymphoma
- Localized
  - Anterior auricular
    - Viral conjunctivitis
    - Trachoma, posterior auricular
    - Rubella
    - Scalp infection
  - Submandibular or cervical (unilateral)
    - Buccal cavity infection
    - Pharyngitis (can be bilateral)
    - Nasopharyngeal tumor
    - Thyroid malignancy
  - Cervical bilateral
    - Mononucleosis
    - Sarcoidosis
    - Toxoplasmosis
    - Pharyngitis
  - Supraclavicular, right
    - Pulmonary malignancy
    - Mediastinal malignancy
    - Esophageal malignancy
  - Supraclavicular, left
    - Intra-abdominal malignancy
    - Renal malignancy
    - Testicular or ovarian malignancy
  - Axillary
    - Breast malignancy or infection
    - Upper extremity infection

- Epitrochlear
  - Syphilis (bilateral)
  - Hand infection (unilateral)
- Inguinal
  - Syphilis
  - Genital herpes
  - Lymphogranuloma venereum
  - Chancroid
  - Lower extremity or local infection
- Any region
  - Cat-scratch fever
  - Hodgkin's disease
  - Non-Hodgkin's lymphoma
  - Leukemia
  - Metastatic cancer
  - Sarcoidosis
  - Granulomatous infections
- Hilar adenopathy, bilateral
  - Sarcoidosis
  - Fungal infection (histoplasmosis, coccidioidomycosis)
  - Lymphoma
  - Bronchogenic carcinoma
  - TB
- Hilar adenopathy, unilateral
  - Lymphoma
  - Bronchogenic carcinoma
  - TB
  - Sarcoidosis

WORKUP

HISTORY AND PHYSICAL EXAM

■ Address the following:
  - Is palpable mass indeed a lymph node?
  - Is lymphadenopathy acute or chronic?
  - What is character of enlarged node?
  - Is adenopathy localized or generalized?
  - Are there associated systemic or localizing symptoms or signs?
  - Are there unusual epidemiologic clues?

LAB STUDIES

■ In determining extent of adenopathy, consider CXR and abdominal and chest CT.

■ For localized adenopathy, obtain CBC with differential and consider throat culture (adding Thayer-Martin plate if gonococcal infection is possible), urethral or cervical cultures and smears, blood cultures; consider lymph node biopsy and bone marrow biopsy (see below).

■ For hilar adenopathy detected by CXR, perform TB skin test and angiotensin-converting enzyme determination. Consider skin tests for coccidioidomycosis and tularemia if patient at risk. If all results negative and patient is white, consider bronchoscopy and/or mediastinoscopy to rule out lymphoma.

- For generalized adenopathy, obtain CBC with differential, and consider heterophile, serologic test for syphilis, acute and later-phase sera for antibody titers against viruses, fungi, and toxoplasmosis; also serologic testing for brucellosis and immunologic testing (e.g., ANA, RF).

Lymph Node Biopsy

- Consider lymph node biopsy only when simpler approaches have failed to reveal Dx and clinical suspicion of therapeutically important cause remains (e.g., TB, lymphoma, cancer, sarcoidosis, cat-scratch disease).
- Refer any patient suspected of harboring malignancy for consult with oncologist or oncologic surgeon regarding need for biopsy and best approach.
- If patient appears otherwise well and devoid of evidence for malignancy, consider watchful waiting for spontaneous regression before proceeding to biopsy. Obtaining consultation can confirm reasonableness of approach.
- If undiagnosed adenopathy persists during period of wks–mos, especially if nodes are enlarging or if patient manifests symptoms or signs suggesting serious underlying disease (e.g., weight loss, night sweats, nodes >2 cm, abnormal CXR), proceed to node biopsy. Consider
  - careful node selection (enlarged supraclavicular nodes have highest diagnostic yield); avoid inguinal or axillary nodes if possible because their frequent reactive hyperplasia may hinder interpretation;
  - excisional biopsy with submission of material for appropriate smears, stains, and cultures in addition to histologic study;
  - needle aspiration in cases of fluctuant nodes, which may be due to infectious process.
- If pathologic study reveals reactive hyperplasia or is nondiagnostic, follow patient carefully, as up to 25% may eventually exhibit illness responsible for lymphadenopathy, most often lymphoma.

BIBLIOGRAPHY

- For the current annotated bibliography on lymphadenopathy, see the print edition of *Primary Care Medicine*, 4th edition, Chapter 12, or www.LWWmedicine.com.

Overweight and Obesity

DIFFERENTIAL DIAGNOSIS

IMPORTANT CAUSES OF OBESITY

- Primary
  - Psychological factors
    - Depression
    - Anxiety
    - Frustration
  - Biologic factors
    - Reduced thermogenesis
    - Increased fat cell mass
    - Autonomic dysfunction
    - Altered hypothalamic set point
    - Single large daily meal taken before bedtime
    - Decreased energy expenditure
    - Drugs (e.g., tricyclic antidepressants, oral contraceptives, cortico-steroids, phenothiazines)
  - Genetic influences
    - Familial obesity
  - Social and occupational factors
    - Lower socioeconomic class
    - Social/occupational situation
- Secondary
  - Endocrine disease
    - Hypothyroidism
    - Stein-Leventhal syndrome
    - Cushing's syndrome
  - Neurologic disease
    - Hypothalamic injury (e.g., trauma, encephalitis, craniopharyngioma)

WORKUP

HISTORY

- Check Hx for etiologic factors ranging from familial propensity and early age of onset to dietary excess, physical inactivity, and underlying medical and psychological conditions.
- Review major cardiovascular risk factors and symptoms of end-organ damage to determine absolute risk of cardiovascular M&M.

PHYSICAL EXAM

- Estimate body fat content by calculating BMI (body weight in kg divided by square of height in m).
- Determine fat distribution by measuring waist circumference at narrowest area above umbilicus.

- Check for signs of end-organ damage from cardiovascular risk factors (e.g., DM, HTN).
- Check for evidence of valvular cardiac injury by auscultation (and cardiac ultrasonography if valvular injury suspected by exam) any patients who have previously been prescribed fenfluramine or dexfenfluramine.

LAB STUDIES

- Use lab testing only to check etiologic hypotheses suggested by Hx and PE or to screen for cardiovascular risk factors (e.g., hypercholesterolemia, DM).
- At end of assessment, provide patient with estimate of disease risk posed by excessive weight and assessment of factors contributing to it.

MANAGEMENT

- Identify and treat specifically any etiologic factors.
- Prescribe comprehensive approach to weight management that includes low-fat diet, dietary counseling, behavior modification, and exercise (see Exercise).
- Avoid and discourage gimmicky food programs and appetite suppressants until safe and effective agents become available.
- Individualize changes in eating and exercise patterns; make them gradual to maximize potential for long-term compliance.
- Recommend weight loss group to those who seek benefit of group support; suggest one that is under professional supervision.
- Advise dietitian-supervised weight management program for patients who continually go from one fad diet to another. Warn against diets based on unsubstantiated medical claims, which may have popular appeal but are ineffective for long-term weight control.
- Restrict use of very-low-calorie diets to patients >30–40% above ideal weight; require medical supervision.
- Consider pharmacologic intervention only for persons at very high risk for cardiovascular, metabolic, or orthopedic morbidity and only after weighing risks of such Rx (most available appetite suppressants are catecholaminergic stimulants—e.g., phenylpropanolamine), which should not be used in persons with heart disease.
- Consider referral for surgical Rx only for patients with life-threatening obesity unresponsive to other measures.

BIBLIOGRAPHY

- For the current annotated bibliography on overweight and obesity, see the print edition of *Primary Care Medicine*, 4th edition, Chapters 10 and 233, or www.LWWmedicine.com.

Weight Loss

DIFFERENTIAL DIAGNOSIS

IMPORTANT CAUSES OF WEIGHT LOSS

- Decreased intake
  - HIV infection, AIDS
  - Depression, bereavement
  - Anxiety
  - Poor dentition, loss of taste
  - Esophageal disease
  - GI disease worsened by food (e.g., peptic ulcer)
  - Drugs (e.g., digitalis excess, quinidine, amphetamines, NSAIDs, anti-tumor agents)
  - Hypercalcemia
  - Alcoholism
  - Prodrome of viral hepatitis
  - Hypokalemia
  - Uremia
  - Malignancy
  - Chronic CHF
  - Chronic inflammatory disease
  - Anorexia nervosa
  - Social isolation, poverty
  - Dementia
- Impaired absorption
  - Cholestasis
  - Pancreatic insufficiency
  - Postgastrectomy
  - Small-bowel disease
  - Parasitic infection (e.g., giardiasis)
  - Blind loop syndrome
  - Drugs (e.g., cholestyramine, cathartics)
  - AIDS
- Increased nutrient loss
  - Uncontrolled DM
  - Persistent diarrhea
  - Recurrent vomiting
  - Drainage from fistulous tract
- Excess demand
  - Hyperthyroidism
  - Fever
  - Malignancy
  - Emotional states (e.g., manic disease)
  - Amphetamine abuse

WORKUP

HISTORY AND PHYSICAL EXAM

- Document that weight loss has indeed occurred and determine its extent and duration.
- Assess underlying mechanism by obtaining details of daily food intake (including calorie count) and inquiring into any appetite disturbance, dysphagia, odynophagia, steatorrhea, diarrhea, vomiting, polyuria, or symptoms of hypermetabolic state.
- Conduct rest of Hx and PE according to suspected underlying mechanism (decreased intake, impaired absorption, increased nutrient loss, excessive demand).
- Pay particular attention to detection of depression (see Depression), a key cause of "idiopathic" weight loss.

LAB STUDIES

- Target any lab investigation to suspected underlying mechanism.
- Omit lab testing (especially for occult malignancy) if probability of serious medical illness is low after detailed Hx and PE; screening lab studies add little to assessment in such circumstances.
- For suspected decreased intake manifested by markedly reduced appetite accompanied by nausea, obtain serum calcium, potassium, creatinine, transaminase, and amylase determinations.
- For suspected impaired absorption, obtain stool for gross and microscopic exam and guaiac testing; qualitative stool fat and, if necessary, 72-hr stool collection for quantitative stool fat (<8 g/day rules out malabsorption); serum carotene. Use D-xylose test to distinguish pancreatic dysfunction from small-bowel disease, secretin stimulation test to assess pancreatic exocrine function; consider small-bowel biopsy if sprue is a consideration, and stool for O&P for giardiasis.
- For suspected nutrient loss, check urine for glycosuria.
- For suspected excess demand, check TSH. In febrile HIV patient with adequate caloric intake, weight loss likely represents excessive demand; cultures of blood and stool for AFB and of blood and urine for CMV required.

BIBLIOGRAPHY

- For the current annotated bibliography on weight loss, see the print edition of *Primary Care Medicine*, 4th edition, Chapter 9, or www.LWWmedicine.com.

Cardiovascular Problems

Aortic Regurgitation

MANAGEMENT

- Assess severity with initial cardiac ultrasound (U/S) exam including Doppler, and follow patients with evidence of severe regurgitation with serial U/S exams in addition to regular office assessments.
- Avoid activity restrictions in young asymptomatic patients with mild regurgitation.
- Treat asymptomatic patients with moderately severe disease with afterload reduction (e.g., lisinopril, 10 mg bid).
- Refer for consideration of surgery patients, even asymptomatic ones, with worsening LV function (e.g., ECG showing LV hypertrophy with strain pattern, increasing cardiomegaly on chest film, falling ejection fraction, and increasing LV end-systolic dimension on U/S exam). Patients with declining left ventricle have increased risk of VT and increased 5-yr mortality rate. Early identification of high-risk patients is suggested in hopes of correcting aortic regurgitation before irreversible myocardial decompensation develops, which may have already started when symptoms occur.
- In absence of significant LV dysfunction, treat onset of mild symptoms of pulmonary congestion (dyspnea on climbing >1 flight of stairs) medically with digitalization, mild diuretic (50–100 mg hydrochlorothiazide), or afterload reduction (e.g., lisinopril, 10 mg bid), but close clinical follow-up and frequent serial U/S exams are essential to prevent inappropriate delay of surgery.
- Proceed to prompt cardiac referral if progression of disease is suspected based on developing dyspnea after climbing <1 flight of stairs or worsening LV function on follow-up U/S exam.
- Patients with dyspnea prompted by minimal exertion, orthopnea, or paroxysmal nocturnal dyspnea require prompt referral for surgery because life expectancy is <1 yr without surgery. Medical Rx with digitalis and diuretics may provide some temporary symptomatic relief but medical Rx must not be used in place of valve surgery at this stage of illness.
- See also Valvular Heart Disease.

BIBLIOGRAPHY

- For the current annotated bibliography on aortic regurgitation, see the print edition of *Primary Care Medicine*, 4th edition, Chapter 33, or www.LWWmedicine.com.

Aortic Stenosis

MANAGEMENT

- Follow patients with aortic sclerosis expectantly; unless there is progressive valve calcification, such persons are not at increased risk from valvular disease, but sclerosis is marker of increased atherosclerotic risk, which should be addressed.
- Do not restrict activity in asymptomatic patients with mild aortic stenosis.
- Advise young asymptomatic patients with evidence of tight stenosis against heavy physical exertion (e.g., competitive sports) and refer to cardiologist for consideration of catheterization and valvuloplasty or valve replacement. Cardiac catheterization is needed.
- Refer young patients with tight aortic stenosis to cardiologist for consideration of transcatheter aortic balloon valvuloplasty. Results in appropriately selected young patients are comparable to those of surgical valvuloplasty. In the elderly, especially those with fibrotic, calcified valves and associated aortic incompetence, balloon valvuloplasty is appropriate only as palliative measure in those unfit for surgery.
- Obtain prompt cardiac and cardiac surgical consultations if angina, effort syncope, or CHF develop. These are signs of critical stenosis and predict poor prognosis without definitive Rx. Such patients are at risk for sudden death. Medical Rx is no substitute.
- Treat CHF symptomatically on temporary basis by prescribing digitalis and moderate diuretic program [e.g., cautious use of furosemide, 20–40 mg/day (see Congestive Heart Failure)]. Such Rx may help reduce pulmonary congestion and sustain cardiac output temporarily, but keep in mind need for high diastolic filling pressure; overzealous diuretic Rx can cause precipitous fall in cardiac output; afterload reduction may also be dangerous in severe aortic stenosis.
- Treat angina symptomatically but cautiously with nitrates pending surgery (see Stable Angina); beta blockers are contraindicated due to negative inotropic effects. Coronary angiography is required at time of cardiac catheterization to determine whether there is coexisting significant CAD and need for bypass procedure at time of valve replacement.
- Do not deny surgery to the elderly, even patients in their 80s, if they are otherwise reasonable surgical candidates and demonstrate adequate ejection fraction, even in setting of severe aortic stenosis. Advanced age is not absolute contraindication to valve replacement. Survival from surgery is predominantly function of patient's myocardial reserve.
- Provide careful follow-up exams of patients with calcific aortic stenosis, even when disease appears hemodynamically insignificant and patient is asymptomatic because calcification of aortic valve can progress rapidly over few yrs.
- See also Valvular Heart Disease.

BIBLIOGRAPHY

■ For the current annotated bibliography on aortic stenosis, see the print edition of *Primary Care Medicine*, 4th edition, Chapter 33, or www.LWWmedicine.com.

Arterial Insufficiency

WORKUP

HISTORY

Overall Strategy

- Check for triad of (1) cramp or ache in calf or thigh muscles brought on by exercise, (2) relieved within 2–5 mins by simply stopping, and (3) ability to walk same distance again once discomfort ceases.
- Use location of discomfort to localize occlusive process.
- Consider other Dx if pain differs from classic triad.
- Check for rest pain in feet, improved by dependency (sign of advanced ischemic disease).
- Inquire into leg ulceration and historic clues suggesting nonischemic etiology, such as trauma, skin disease, and venous insufficiency.
- Note any erectile dysfunction.
- Identify any atherosclerotic risk factors for arteriosclerosis (e.g., family Hx, smoking, DM, HTN, lipid disorders).
- Note any Hx or symptoms of atherosclerotic disease elsewhere.

Differentiating True Claudication from Pseudoclaudication

- True claudication
  - Cramping, tightness, tiredness, aching
  - Located in buttock, hip, thigh, calf, foot
  - Exercise-induced
  - Distance to pain same each time
  - Does not occur with standing
  - Relieved when walking stops
- Pseudoclaudication
  - Cramping, tightness, tiredness, aching, tingling, weakness, clumsiness
  - Located in buttock, hip, thigh, calf, foot
  - Walking distance to pain variable
  - Occurs with standing
  - Is relieved with sitting or position change

PHYSICAL EXAM

- Palpate peripheral pulses, including femoral, popliteal, posterior tibial, and dorsalis pedis pulses; check abdominal aorta as well.
- Note edema or marked obesity that may hinder palpation.
- Note abnormally prominent pulsations suggesting aneurysmal disease.
- Auscultate aortic and groin regions for bruits; exercise patient at bedside to intensify suspected femoral bruits.
- Check for abnormal pallor on leg elevation, rubor on dependency, and prolonged capillary filling time (especially when 1 leg is compared with the other).
- Note any temp differences, skin atrophy, and skin ulcers.

- Rule out nonvascular causes of exertional lower extremity pain by careful spine, hip, knee, and neurologic exams.

LAB STUDIES

- Omit vascular lab studies in patients with clinically mild to moderate disease free of limb-threatening ischemia or unacceptable activity limitations.
- Investigate potential atherosclerotic risk factors (e.g., hyperlipidemia, HTN, smoking, hyperhomocysteinemia, and DM).
- In patients with premature atherosclerotic disease but no evident precipitants, obtain serum homocysteine level after overnight methionine loading.
- Obtain noninvasive vascular lab studies if Dx or degree of impairment is uncertain or if disease is clinically severe enough to warrant consideration of surgery.
- Refer to vascular lab for segmental BP measurements, pulse-volume recordings, and Doppler ultrasound (U/S).
  - Use segmental pressures to screen for further evaluation and to gauge severity. Review ankle/brachial ratio or index (ratio of SBP in posterior tibial-dorsalis pedis arteries divided by that in brachial artery).
  - Consider pulse-volume recordings for assessment of distal vascular disease, especially in patients with stiff vessels (e.g., diabetics). Be sure treadmill exercise is part of test to maximize sensitivity.
  - Order duplex U/S when more precise anatomic and flow data are needed. Adding color-flow enhancement (triplex scanning) improves test performance.
- Consider contrast arteriography for precise anatomic definition only when contemplating surgery.
- Consider MRA as noninvasive alternative to contrast angiography, especially in those with risk of dye-induced acute renal failure or allergic reaction.

MANAGEMENT

SMOKING CESSATION

- Insist on total smoking cessation to limit disease progression and prevent reocclusion after interventional Rx.
- Firmly tell patients that they must stop smoking completely. Smoking as few as 5 cigarettes/day can compromise limb. Be unequivocal, because patients often interpret half-hearted advice as only suggestion (see Smoking Cessation).

EXERCISE

- Encourage patients to exercise regularly; in patients with claudication, best exercise is daily walking.
- Advise patients to walk to point of discomfort, stop briefly, and resume.
- Recommend ≥30 mins/day of relatively continuous walking. Weekly group sessions can be extremely useful.
- Suggest using exercise bicycle as alternative mode of exercise.

- Emphasize that pain does not indicate harm or damage to leg, and exercise helps rather than aggravates condition.
- Consider patient's cardiac status in design of exercise program (see Cardiovascular Rehabilitation; Exercise).

ELEVATING HEAD OF BED

- Advise patients with advanced ischemia and nocturnal rest pain to raise head of bed on 6- to 8-in. blocks so that feet and legs are slightly dependent, aiding blood flow enough to allow more comfortable sleep.

FOOT CARE

- Emphasize importance of attention to foot care and regular inspection for signs of ulceration, skin necrosis, and infection, especially in diabetic patients who may have concurrent peripheral neuropathy and sensory loss.
- Urge patient to call at first sign of difficulty; delay can lead to limb loss if gangrene or osteomyelitis ensues.
- Be sure patient is taught essentials of foot care:
  - Inspecting. Inspect feet daily for scratches, cuts, fissures, blisters, or other lesions, particularly around nail beds, between toes, and on heels.
  - Washing. Wash feet daily with mild soap and lukewarm (never hot) water. Rinse thoroughly and dry gently but completely, particularly between toes. Avoid excessive soaking, which leads to maceration.
  - Moisturizing. Apply moisturizing cream such as lanolin or Eucerin lotion to foot and heel but not between toes. A light film, rubbed in well, will prevent drying and cracking of skin, which is often genesis of lesions, particularly on heel. Do not apply cream thickly or allow it to "cake" on foot.
  - Preventing lesions. Patients may place small amount of lambast or dry cotton or gauze between toes to prevent lesions, which may occur if toes rub together, particularly if orthopedic deformities of toes are present.
  - Drying. Apply antifungal powder such as nystatin between toes if excessive moisture or maceration is problematic.
  - Choosing footwear. Properly fitting shoes with ample forefoot space are essential. Special shoes are rarely necessary.
  - Cutting nails. Cut nails with extreme care, in good light, and only if vision is normal. Cut nails straight across and even with end of toe, never close to skin or into corner of nail bed. Arrange regular podiatric Rx if patients cannot cut nails themselves or if any abnormality of nails or corns or calluses are present.
  - Avoiding trauma. Never use adhesive tape on skin (paper tape is better) or strong antiseptic solution. Avoid heating pads, hot packs, heat lamps, and scalding hot water. Never walk barefoot.

WEIGHT REDUCTION

- Encourage patients to lose weight if necessary (see Overweight and Obesity).

ATHEROSCLEROTIC RISK FACTOR REDUCTION

- Take aggressive measures to control major atherosclerotic risk factors [e.g., HTN (see Hypertension), hyperlipidemia (see Hypercholesterolemia), and smoking]. Aggressive control can halt disease progression and may promote plaque regression. It also lowers associated cardio-vascular M&M (see Cardiovascular Rehabilitation; Stable Angina).

- In patients with premature disease, test for homocysteine elevation and treat with folate and vitamins B_6 and B_{12} if positive (see Cardio-vascular Rehabilitation).

MEDICATIONS

- Consider daily aspirin Rx for its generally beneficial effects on cardio-vascular risk (see Cardiovascular Rehabilitation).
- Consider short course (≤3 mos) of cilostazol if symptoms interfere with ability to exercise; avoid long-term use and use in persons with heart failure or ventricular dysrhythmias.

REVASCULARIZATION

- Consider revascularization if claudication pain is disabling and refrac-tory to full trial of comprehensive medical Rx.
- Obtain Doppler U/S study to screen potential candidates for revascular-ization. Refer for consideration of angioplasty (PTA) those with claudi-cation attributable to focal proximal disease by noninvasive study.
- Refer for consideration of bypass surgery only those unresponsive to medical Rx, who have disease that appears amenable to surgery but not to PTA, and are so significantly disabled by claudication that liveli-hood or lifestyle is intolerably compromised by inability to walk dis-tances. Final decision requires angiography.
- Consider surgery with some urgency for patients with more severe dis-ease and those with rest pain, nonhealing ulcers, or early gangrene who have jeopardized limb.
- Conduct preoperative stress testing to identify patients with high car-diac risk who might need further cardiac evaluation and possibly car-diac revascularization before peripheral vascular surgery.

BIBLIOGRAPHY

- For the current annotated bibliography on arterial insufficiency, see the print edition of *Primary Care Medicine*, 4th edition, Chapters 23 and 34, or www.LWWmedicine.com.

Asymptomatic Systolic Murmur

DIFFERENTIAL DIAGNOSIS

- Innocent murmurs
- Physiologic murmurs
  - Exercise or emotion
  - Fever
  - Anemia
  - Hyperthyroidism
  - Conditions with large stroke volumes: atrial septal defect, aortic regurgitation, bradycardia
  - Pregnancy
- Aortic murmurs
  - Aortic stenosis
  - Hypertrophic cardiomyopathy
  - Sub- and supravalvular fixed stenoses
- Pulmonic murmurs
  - Pulmonic stenosis
- Mitral regurgitation murmurs
  - Rheumatic mitral insufficiency
  - Mitral valve prolapse
  - Congenital mitral valve disease
  - Rupture of chordae tendineae
  - Papillary muscle dysfunction
  - Left atrial myxoma
  - Dilated mitral valve ring
- Tricuspid regurgitation murmurs
  - Rheumatic tricuspid insufficiency
  - Dilated tricuspid valve ring
- Ventricular septal defect (VSD)

WORKUP

PHYSICAL EXAM AND LAB STUDIES

- Determine whether systolic murmur is regurgitant or ejection in quality by attention to its location, quality, and timing.
- Differentiate right-sided from left-sided pathology by observing response of murmur to inspiration.
- If murmur is ejection in quality, distinguish between innocent/physiologic murmurs and those due to structural heart disease.
- For left-sided ejection murmurs, distinguish between aortic stenosis and hypertrophic cardiomyopathy.
- If aortic stenosis is suspected, estimate clinical severity by PE and obtain Doppler cardiac ultrasound (U/S) in persons with PE findings suggestive of hemodynamically significant disease.

- Follow patients with calcific aortic stenosis closely, and repeat U/S exam periodically.
- If you find PE evidence of hypertrophic cardiomyopathy (idiopathic hypertrophic subaortic stenosis), confirm with Doppler cardiac U/S.
- For holosystolic murmurs, differentiate by PE between arteriovenous valve regurgitation and VSD; if arteriovenous valve regurgitation suspected, determine whether murmur is mitral or pulmonic. Obtain Doppler U/S if clinical evidence of hemodynamically significant regurgitation.
- For late systolic murmurs, differentiate between MVP and valve regurgitation due to papillary muscle dysfunction. If hemodynamically significant MVP suspected, confirm with Doppler U/S.
- Refer for cardiac consultation any patient with severe aortic stenosis or other hemodynamically significant lesion with poor prognosis (e.g., hypertrophic cardiomyopathy, mitral regurgitation with falling ejection fraction).
- Provide detailed reassurance to patients with harmless lesions to minimize demand for unnecessary testing, and make clear to patients with hemodynamically significant disease the need for close follow-up.

BIBLIOGRAPHY

- For the current annotated bibliography on asymptomatic systolic murmur, see the print edition of *Primary Care Medicine*, 4th edition, Chapter 21, or www.LWWmedicine.com.

Atrial Fibrillation

DIFFERENTIAL DIAGNOSIS

IMPORTANT CAUSES OF ATRIAL FIBRILLATION

- Paroxysmal AF
  - "Lone" fibrillation
  - Acute ischemia
  - Alcohol intoxication and early alcoholic cardiomyopathy
  - Sick sinus syndrome
  - WPW syndrome
  - Acute pulmonary embolization
  - Acute pericarditis
  - Acute pulmonary decompensation
  - Acute heart failure
  - Any cause of chronic atrial fibrillation
- Sustained AF
  - Advanced rheumatic mitral valve disease
  - Chronic CHF
  - Advanced aortic valve disease
  - Advanced hypertensive heart disease
  - CAD
  - Advanced cardiomyopathy
  - Congenital heart disease
  - Apathetic hyperthyroidism of the elderly
  - Sick sinus syndrome
  - "Lone" fibrillation
  - Constrictive pericarditis
  - Digitalis toxicity (rarely)

WORKUP

GENERAL STRATEGY

- Base Dx of AF on characteristic ECG findings (irregularly irregular ventricular response and AF waves, best seen in leads V1–V3, and the augmented voltage unipolar left foot lead).
- If ventricular response rate is too rapid to reveal atrial activity, consider vagal maneuvers and gentle carotid sinus massage (provided there is no evidence of carotid artery disease) to slow rate and uncover any hidden fibrillatory or P waves.
- Perform workup for etiology on outpatient basis if patient is tolerating rhythm well and there is no evidence of failure, ischemia, or embolization.

HISTORY

- Review for etiologic clues:
  - In younger patients, prior Hx of such episodes, excess intake of stimulants and alcohol, emotional stress, fever, heart murmur, and chest pain.

- In older patients, preexisting heart disease, HTN, chest pain, dyspnea, cough, calf pain, leg edema, fever, light-headedness, near-syncope, loss of consciousness, weight loss, depression, Hx of heart murmur or rheumatic fever, and any prior attacks of palpitations.
- Take careful drug Hx with emphasis on alcohol abuse (see Alcohol Abuse).
- Note any Hx of recurrent attacks dating from young adulthood (WPW syndrome), marked weight loss, concurrent depression, apathy (apathetic hyperthyroidism), or episodes of altered consciousness (sick sinus syndrome).

PHYSICAL EXAM

- Check for hemodynamic state and etiologic clues (see above).
- Note apical pulse rate, BP, respiratory rate, jugular venous pulse, any apathetic appearance, marked weight loss, cyanosis, goiter, wheezes, friction rub, heart murmur (especially mitral), calf tenderness, asymmetric leg edema, and any signs of alcohol intoxication.

LAB STUDIES

- Check:
  - ECG for ventricular response rate (rate >200 bpm or widening of QRS due to delta waves suggests WPW syndrome), pattern of fibrillatory waves (coarse ones = marked left atrial enlargement; fine ones = atherosclerotic and hypertensive heart diseases).
  - ECG for evidence of LV hypertrophy, and ST and T waves for evidence of ischemia, strain, digitalis effect, and pericarditis (see Chest Pain).
  - ECG after return to sinus rhythm for a shortened PR interval, delta waves, and sinus node dysfunction.
  - 24-hour Holter monitor for the episodes of bradycardia and tachycardia (sick sinus syndrome).
  - CXR for heart failure, cardiomegaly, and intrapulmonary pathology.
  - Echocardiogram for evaluating suspected valvular, congenital, cardiomyopathic, and pericardial forms of heart disease.
  - TSH in the elderly with otherwise unexplained AF.

MANAGEMENT

RATE CONTROL

- Admit for consideration of urgent cardioversion any patient with evidence of hemodynamic compromise (i.e., acute or worsening CHF, ischemia, or acute embolization) or very rapid ventricular response rate (>150 bpm).
- Begin Rx for rate control if ventricular response rate at rest is >85 bpm or >110 bpm after mild exercise. Unless there is concurrent heart failure, start with modest dose of a beta blocker (e.g., atenolol, 25 mg/day) or a calcium channel blocker (e.g., diltiazem, 30 mg qid, switching to sustained-release formulation once effective dose is established). In setting of LV systolic dysfunction, consider digoxin or very cautious low-dose beta blocker use, and avoid calcium channel blockers (see Congestive Heart Failure).
- In WPW syndrome and other preexcitation syndromes, refer for consideration of EPS and ablative Rx; do not treat with digoxin or calcium channel

blockers because of their tendency to enhance conduction through accessory pathways. Young patients with brief and infrequent bouts of AF due to WPW syndrome need not be treated if episodes are well tolerated hemodynamically and ventricular response rate is <150 bpm.

■ In sick sinus syndrome, use considerable caution in initiating rate-control Rx because such patients are especially susceptible to symptomatic bradycardia; if marked bradycardia occurs on initiation of such Rx, refer for consideration of pacemaker implantation.

■ If rate control is difficult to achieve, recheck for failure, ischemia, fever, hypovolemia, hypoxia, recurrent pulmonary embolization, hyperthyroidism, and WPW syndrome. Direct Rx at underlying condition.

■ Hospitalize and cardiovert if AF is not well tolerated hemodynamically.

■ Advise patients with paroxysms of AF from whatever cause to use alcohol in moderation and avoid bouts of acute intoxication, because such bouts increase vulnerability for AF.

STROKE PROPHYLAXIS

Immediate Cardioversion vs Initial Anticoagulation

■ For patients with underlying heart disease and AF duration <48 hrs, consider immediate referral for elective cardioversion (either pharmacologic or electrical); precardioversion warfarin anticoagulation is unnecessary so long as cardioversion occurs within 48 hrs of onset.

■ For all patients with underlying heart disease and AF of unknown duration or duration >48 hrs, begin PO anticoagulant Rx with warfarin as early as possible, unless serious contraindication to warfarin Rx (see Anticoagulant Therapy).

■ Prescribe adjustable-dose warfarin program that achieves PT INR 2–3.

Elective Cardioversion

■ For those at high risk for systemic embolization (e.g., prior embolization or stroke, systolic dysfunction, clinical CHF, significant left atrial mural thrombus, or female sex + age >75), consider elective cardioversion.

■ Also consider for elective cardioversion those with exercise intolerance or fatigue due to AF, intolerable symptomatic palpitations, or inability to take long-term PO anticoagulation.

■ Screen out those with high probability of unresponsiveness or relapse (e.g., AF duration >1 yr, marked left atrial enlargement, rheumatic etiology).

■ Before elective cardioversion in persons with AF duration >48 hrs, prescribe 3–4 wks of adjusted-dose warfarin anticoagulation (to achieve PT INR 2–3).

■ If desirable to proceed directly to elective cardioversion without waiting 3–4 wks for oral anticoagulation, use TEE to enhance determination of stroke risk.

■ If no thrombus is detected by TEE in left atrium or left atrial appendage, then reasonable to proceed directly to cardioversion.

■ After cardioversion, preceded by warfarin or not, prescribe adjusted-dose warfarin for ≥4 wks after restoration of sinus rhythm.

■ After cardioversion in those with high risk of AF recurrence (e.g., marked left atrial enlargement, advanced age, high amount of energy required for cardioversion), consider chronic adjusted-dose warfarin prophylaxis, especially if patient has clinical features conferring high stroke risk.

- Alternatively, consider chronic antiarrhythmic Rx with low-dose amiodarone (e.g., 100–200 mg/day); monitor liver function tests and TSH level q6mos.
- Refer those with frequent recurrences of AF that occur despite antiarrhythmic Rx for consideration of interventional approaches (e.g., atrial ablation, pacing, or defibrillator placement), especially if recurrences are not well tolerated hemodynamically.

Chronic Anticoagulation

- For those with clinical characteristics that make them poor candidates for elective cardioversion (e.g., AF duration >1 yr, advanced rheumatic valvular disease, marked left atrial enlargement), consider long-term adjusted-dose warfarin anticoagulation, especially if they have clinical features predictive of high stroke risk.
- For AF patients with low to moderate risk of embolic stroke (i.e., no CHF or significant systolic dysfunction, no previous thromboembolism, SBP <160 mm Hg, and age <75), consider chronic aspirin Rx (e.g., 325 mg/day). Those with concurrent atherosclerotic risk factors are likely to benefit most.
- Consider chronic aspirin Rx for those who cannot take or refuse PO anticoagulation.

BIBLIOGRAPHY

- For the current annotated bibliography on atrial fibrillation, see the print edition of *Primary Care Medicine*, 4th edition, the appendix to Chapter 25 and Chapter 28, or www.LWWmedicine.com.

Bacterial Endocarditis

SCREENING AND/OR PREVENTION

- Strongly consider endocarditis prophylaxis even though effectiveness is difficult to demonstrate definitively.
- Always refer to latest consensus recommendations, which are updated regularly.
- Estimate degree of endocarditis risk by considering type of heart abnormality present and likelihood that event or procedure will produce bacteremia.

CARDIAC RISK FACTORS

- High risk: prosthetic heart valve(s), Hx of endocarditis
- Moderate risk: rheumatic or other acquired valvular disease, congenital heart disease (excluding ASD of secundum type), IHSS
- Probable moderate risk: MVP, undiagnosed murmurs

BACTEREMIA RISK FOR PROCEDURES AND EVENTS (% INSTANCES OF BACTEREMIA)

Common Procedures and Events

- Dental extraction (75)
- Periodontal surgery (50)
- Tooth brushing, flossing, or irrigation in presence of gingivitis (50); normal gingiva (20)
- Bronchoscopy
  - Rigid (15)
  - Flexible (<1)
- Colonoscopy (10)
- Sigmoidoscopy (5)
- Barium enema (10)
- Liver biopsy (5)
- Transurethral resection of prostate
  - Infected urine (50)
  - Sterile urine (10)

Other Procedures and Events Associated with Bacteremia

- Tonsillectomy and/or adenoidectomy
- Surgical operations that involve respiratory mucosa
- Sclerotherapy for esophageal varices
- Esophageal stricture dilation
- Endoscopic retrograde cholangiography with biliary obstruction
- Biliary tract surgery
- Surgical operations that involve intestinal mucosa
- Prostatic surgery

- Cystoscopy
- Urethral dilation

CURRENT CONSENSUS RECOMMENDATIONS

For Dental, Oral, Respiratory Tract, or Esophageal Procedures

- Amoxicillin 1 hr before procedure; if unable to take PO then 2 g IM or IV, within 30 mins before procedure.
- If penicillin-allergic, then clindamycin, 600 mg PO, 1 hr before procedure; or cephalexin or cefadroxil, 2 g PO, 1 hr before procedure (avoid cephalosporins if immediate-type hypersensitivity to penicillins); or azithromycin or clarithromycin, 500 mg PO, 1 hr before procedure.
- If penicillin-allergic and cannot take oral Rx, then clindamycin, 600 mg IV, within 30 mins before procedure; or cefazolin, 1 g IV, within 30 mins before procedure.

For Genitourinary and GI (Excluding Esophageal) Procedures

High-Risk Patients

- Ampicillin, 2 g IM or IV + gentamicin, 1.5 mg/kg (not >120 mg), within 30 mins before procedure; 6 hrs later, ampicillin, 1 g IM/IV, or amoxicillin, 1 g PO.
- If penicillin-allergic, then vancomycin, 1 g IV over 1–2 hrs + gentamicin, 1.5 mg/kg IV/IM (not >120 mg); complete injection/infusion within 30 mins before procedure.

Moderate-Risk Patients

- Amoxicillin, 2 g PO, 1 hr before procedure, or ampicillin, 2 g IM/IV, within 30 mins before procedure.
- If penicillin-allergic, then vancomycin, 1 g IV over 1–2 hrs; complete infusion within 30 mins before procedure.

PATIENT EDUCATION

- Urge all patients with identifiable risk to maintain high level of oral health to minimize potential for recurrent bacteremia.
- Advise patients who take continuous rheumatic fever prophylaxis that their Rx does not protect them from endocarditis.

BIBLIOGRAPHY

- For the current annotated bibliography on bacterial endocarditis, see the print edition of *Primary Care Medicine*, 4th edition, Chapter 16, or www.LWWmedicine.com.

Cardiovascular Rehabilitation

MANAGEMENT

PHASE I (INPATIENT INITIAL REHABILITATION; FIRST WK)

- Prevent physical deconditioning by initiating program of low-level activity, patient ed on coronary risk factors, and counseling to limit psychological disability.
- Before discharge and in absence of complications, consider submax exercise testing (5 METS) to determine prognosis.

PHASE II (OUTPATIENT EARLY CONVALESCENCE/ PHYSICAL TRAINING; 3–6 WKS AFTER DISCHARGE)

- Combine exercise program that enhances patient's physical conditioning with dietary modification and aggressive Rx of risk factors (see below) to encourage lifelong adherence to good health habits.
- Continue low-level exercise program (walking/stationary biking); monitor exercise peak heart rate, which should not exceed predischarge submax exercise test level or level associated with any abnormalities on stress testing.
- Continue educating patient and family about coronary risk factors.

PHASE III (LATE CONVALESCENCE/PHYSICAL TRAINING)

- Increase patient's level of physical conditioning based on max exercise test performed 3–6 wks after discharge to document patient's heart rate and BP when exercising and to screen for latent myocardial ischemia and ventricular dysrhythmias.
- Expand exercise training modalities to establish balanced program with long-term patient appeal; upper extremity conditioning may be added.
- Emphasize diet that lowers serum total cholesterol and LDL levels and raises HDL level.
- Recommend achievement as close to ideal body weight as possible.
- Attend to HTN control (see Hypertension) and smoking cessation (see Smoking Cessation).
- Address any psychological stress and depression (see Anxiety; Depression).
- Provide detailed patient ed regarding effects of Rx on prognosis.

PHASE IV (MAINTENANCE/FOLLOW-UP)

- Encourage lifelong adherence to healthy habits established during phase III. Follow up at 6- to 12-mo intervals.
- Check BP, pulse, and serum lipids, and consider repeat max exercise tolerance test to provide patient feedback and indicate areas that may require lifestyle change to minimize coronary risk.

- Initiate additional medical Rx proven to reduce cardiovascular risk:
  - Low-dose aspirin
  - Beta-blockade
  - ACE inhibitors
- Consider supplemental measures of potential efficacy:
  - Homocysteine reduction by supplementation with folic acid and vitamins B_6 and B_{12}.
- Avoid prescribing supplementary measures of little proven efficacy:
  - Hormone replacement therapy
  - Vitamin E
  - Beta carotene
  - Vitamin C
- Consider revascularization (see Stable Angina).
- Refer patients with high-risk disease (moderate to severe angina; large amount of myocardium at risk; suspected 3-vessel, left-main, or left-main-equivalent disease; reduced ejection fraction).
- Consider angioplasty for lower-risk patients who achieve insufficient symptomatic control with max medical Rx alone; however, emphasize there is as yet no proved mortality benefit.

BIBLIOGRAPHY

- For the current annotated bibliography on cardiovascular rehabilitation, see the print edition of *Primary Care Medicine*, 4th edition, Chapter 31, or www.LWWmedicine.com.

Chest Pain

DIFFERENTIAL DIAGNOSIS

- Chest wall
  - Muscular disorders
    - Muscle spasm (precordial-catch syndrome)
    - Pleurodynia
    - Muscle strain
  - Skeletal disorders
    - Costochondritis (Tietze's syndrome)
    - Rib fracture
    - Metastatic disease of bone
    - Cervical or thoracic spine disease
  - Neurologic disorders
    - Herpes zoster infection or postherpetic pain
    - Nerve root compression
- Cardiopulmonary
  - Cardiac disorders
    - Pericarditis
    - Myocardial ischemia
    - Mitral valve prolapse
  - Pleuropulmonary disorders
    - Pleurisy of any origin
    - Pneumothorax
    - Pulmonary embolization with infarction
    - Pneumonitis
    - Bronchospasm
- Aortic
  - Dissecting aortic aneurysm
- GI
  - Esophageal disorders
    - Reflux
    - Spasm
  - Others
    - Cholecystitis
    - Peptic ulcer disease
    - Pancreatitis
    - Splenic flexure gas
- Psychogenic
  - Anxiety (± hyperventilation)
  - Cardiac neurosis
  - Malingering
  - Depression

WORKUP

HISTORY

- Identify high-risk chest pain patient who requires immediate hospitalization by performing triage Hx focusing on evidence for acute coronary syndrome, significant pulmonary embolization, aortic dissection, and acute cardiopulmonary compromise. Avoid common biases based on patient age, gender, and race.
- If story is strongly suggestive, admit by ambulance; minimize delay.

PHYSICAL EXAM AND LAB STUDIES

- If initial Hx is not strongly indicative of 1 of these etiologies, evaluate promptly in the office with more detailed Hx and careful PE, supplemented where appropriate by ECG and CXR.
- Formulate initial differential Dx from these data; include pretest estimate of myocardial ischemia, pulmonary embolization, and aortic dissection, because immediate decision making and optimal locus and approach to further workup of these conditions heavily depends on such probability estimates.
- Select appropriate testing strategy based on pretest probability for condition in question.

For Suspected Coronary Artery Disease

- Low pretest probability: explain why chest pain is unlikely to be of cardiac origin and consider obtaining resting ECG if it will help reassure patient.
- Intermediate pretest probability: if presentation is suggestive of unstable angina, proceed to immediate hospitalization and ER triage protocols. If presentation is of "stable" (i.e., noncrescendo) chest pain, proceed to nonemergent stress testing. Obtain either exercise ECG (if resting ECG normal) or exercise echocardiography; both are reasonably cost effective. If other noninvasive modalities (e.g., radionuclide stress testing) are available locally at lower cost or with enhanced sensitivity and specificity, their use may also be cost effective and should be considered.
- High pretest probability: if presentation is very suggestive of unstable angina, proceed to immediate hospitalization and ER triage protocols. For those with ECG changes on arrival in ER, immediate angiography without prior noninvasive testing appears to be more cost-effective diagnostic approach. For those whose presentation is indicative of stable angina, proceed to nonemergent stress testing to determine amount of myocardium at risk (see Stress Testing).
- To minimize delay in hospitalization, teach high-risk patient and family symptoms of acute coronary syndromes and instruct them to call 911 immediately if symptoms occur.
- Reduce requests for unnecessary testing by eliciting patient concerns about chest pain, performing detailed Hx and PE, obtaining ECG, and addressing concerns by careful review of clinical findings.
- Omit routine use of esophageal studies in assessment of chest pain in patients who rule out for coronary disease.

For Suspected Pulmonary Embolization

- Low pretest probability: screen by ordering sensitive, noninvasive test such as D-dimer assay or V/Q scan; selection dependent on availability and local expertise. Nondiagnostic V/Q scan or D-dimer level >0.5 µg/dL necessitate additional testing, with serial venous ultrasound (U/S) a reasonable choice.

■ Intermediate pretest probability: begin with V/Q scan. Normal V/Q scan rules out Dx; nondiagnostic V/Q result does not and should be followed by D-dimer or serial U/S, which, if negative, rules out embolism.

■ High pretest probability: admit to hospital and begin anticoagulation, pending results of testing. Start with V/Q scan, followed by U/S if result is indeterminate. If U/S is positive, Dx is confirmed; if negative or equivocal, angiography is indicated because noninvasive testing is insufficiently sensitive to rule out embolization in patient with high pretest probability.

BIBLIOGRAPHY

■ For the current annotated bibliography on chest pain, see the print edition of *Primary Care Medicine*, 4th edition, Chapter 20, or www.LWWmedicine.com.

Congestive Heart Failure

WORKUP

- Identify etiology of CHF (e.g., dysrhythmia, HTN, valvular disease, ischemia, cardiomyopathy) and any precipitating factors (e.g., fever, anemia, AF, infection, salt excess); treat these specifically if amenable to Rx rather than relying solely on symptomatic measures to ameliorate CHF (see also the workup section in Dyspnea).
- Identify underlying pathophysiology, particularly degree of systolic or diastolic dysfunction, to help tailor program to patient's pathophysiology.

MANAGEMENT

MILD DISEASE (NYHA CLASS I)

- Initiate no-added-salt diet (4 g sodium) but do not restrict water intake unless dilutional hyponatremia ensues.
- Begin diuretics if evidence of volume overload or pulmonary venous congestion. If symptoms are mild, begin with thiazide (e.g., hydrochlorothiazide, 50–100 mg/day).
- If thiazides do not suffice, switch to loop diuretic (e.g., furosemide, 20–40 mg qd–bid). Be alert for very brisk diuresis in patients who have never received loop diuretics. Exercise particular caution with use of potent diuretics in situations that require high filling pressure (e.g., critical aortic stenosis).
- In initial stages of loop diuretic use, divide daily dose to minimize inconvenience of large diuresis in the morning or evening that might interfere with activity. Avoid giving evening dose if sleep is being interrupted by nocturia.
- If patient does not respond adequately to divided loop diuretic dose, try combining daily dose into 1 administration before increasing total daily dose.

MILD TO MODERATE DISEASE (NYHA CLASS II–III)

- If moderate doses of diuretic Rx do not relieve congestive symptoms, add ACE inhibitor, starting at low dose to minimize risks of hypotension and hypoperfusion (e.g., 6.25 mg captopril tid or 5 mg lisinopril/day).
- Monitor BP, potassium, BUN, and creatinine, and decrease diuretic dose if BP falls or prerenal azotemia develops.
- Gradually advance ACE inhibitor Rx to improve exercise tolerance and relieve congestive symptoms while continuing to monitor BP, potassium, and renal function. If tolerated, advance to doses associated with best outcomes (e.g., captopril, 50 mg tid; lisinopril, 10–20 mg/day).

MODERATE TO SEVERE DISEASE (NYHA CLASS III–IV)

- In patients with moderate to severe CHF due to worsening systolic dysfunction (low ejection fraction, S_3, LV dilation), add digitalis preparation to program of loop diuretic and ACE inhibitor.

- Use digoxin as digitalis preparation of choice, except in severe renal failure, when digitoxin or markedly reduced doses of digoxin are indicated.
- If candidate for digitalis is relatively stable, begin Rx with PO maintenance dose (e.g., digoxin, 0.25 mg/day), checking serum level in 1 wk and making any needed dose adjustments based on clinical response and serum level.
- If digitalis candidate has worsening CHF but does not require immediate hospitalization, start digitalis Rx with loading dose of 1–1.25 mg of digoxin PO in 4 divided doses/24 hrs. Dose is then adjusted as above.
- If volume overload persists, advance loop diuretic to full doses (e.g., furosemide, 80–120 mg/day) given once daily to achieve max effect; add thiazide or metolazone (if there is azotemia) if additional diuresis desired. Monitor and halt advancement of diuretic program if prerenal azotemia becomes marked.
- Be sure full doses of ACE inhibitor are prescribed and taken (e.g., captopril, 50 mg tid; lisinopril, 10–20 mg/day).
- For patients unable to tolerate ACE inhibitor because of irritating dry cough, consider switching to angiotensin II antagonist (e.g., losartan, 50 mg/day).

REFRACTORY DISEASE: ADJUNCTIVE PROGRAMS, HOSPITALIZATION, AND TRANSPLANTATION

- Consider adding low-dose spironolactone (25 mg/day) in persons with severe disease who are still unacceptably symptomatic. Cease potassium supplementation and monitor potassium levels closely; use with extreme caution, if at all, in setting of worsening renal function (creatinine >2.5 mg/dL).
- Consider adding low-dose beta blocker Rx (e.g., carvedilol, 3.25 mg/day; or sustained-release metoprolol, 12.5–25 mg/day) for patients with moderate disease and suboptimal response to standard Rx.
- Obtain cardiac consultation to facilitate case selection and initiation of beta blocker Rx.
- In most instances, resting heart rate should be >70–80 bpm and SBP >100–110 mm Hg.
- Titrate beta blocker dose slowly upward to achieve resting heart rate 50–60 bpm.
- Monitor patient closely for fluid retention and clinical worsening, especially in first 2 mos of Rx; adjust diuretic dose upward if necessary.
- Consider hospitalization for patients with severe refractory disease for full review of disease status, precipitants, aggravating factors, compliance, and initiation of any adjunctive therapies.
- Also admit for markedly worsening CHF, suspected digitalis toxicity, or inadequate support and supervision at home.
- Refer for consideration of transplantation relatively young patients with end-stage myocardial disease, but preserved renal, hepatic, pulmonary, and neurologic function.

MONITORING AND ADJUSTING THERAPY

- Advise patient and family to check weight regularly, measuring before breakfast and calling if unexplained weight gain of >2–3 lbs since last reading.

- Monitor potassium, BUN, and creatinine regularly and, in persons taking digitalis, follow serum digoxin level. Avoid having serum digoxin measured <6 hrs after last dose, because of transient increase in serum level after PO dose.
- Monitor serum potassium particularly closely in those taking digitalis + potent diuretics or ACE inhibitor + potassium-sparing diuretic or potassium supplementation. Correct any potassium abnormality promptly to minimize risk of serious dysrhythmia.
- If prerenal azotemia develops or worsens, adjust diuretic program.
- For those taking digoxin, obtain serum digoxin level and reduce dose until level is available to guide further administration, or estimate required dose from available nomograms.
- Monitor heart rate and rhythm; if cardiac dysrhythmia noted, investigate and treat promptly, especially in persons taking digitalis who manifest paroxysmal atrial tachycardia with block, ventricular irritability (especially bigeminy), junctional tachycardia, or severe bradycardia.
- Use PO potassium supplements and potassium-sparing diuretics with extreme caution, if at all, in patients taking ACE inhibitors, and only if serum potassium falls to <3.5 mg/dL. If potassium-sparing diuretic is used, stop chronic PO potassium supplementation.
- Monitor serum magnesium in patients taking digitalis and in those with refractory hypokalemia. Diuretic-induced hypomagnesemia is common and may impair potassium repletion; it also enhances sensitivity to toxic effects of digitalis.

ADDITIONAL MEASURES AND PRECAUTIONS

- Initiate PO anticoagulant Rx for CHF patients if prolonged bed rest, AF, or severe congestive cardiomyopathy ensue (see Anticoagulant Therapy).
- Avoid, if possible, large doses and combinations of cardiac drugs with negative inotropic effects, such as verapamil, disopyramide, and beta blockers. If beneficial, use smallest dose possible and prescribe in conjunction with cardiac consultation.
- Consider discontinuing calcium channel blockers in patients with chronic CHF, especially those with ejection fractions <0.3. Of available calcium channel blockers, only amlodipine is not associated with increased risk of worsening failure, life-threatening dysrhythmias, and sudden death. Obtain cardiac consultation if continued use is essential.
- Provide patient and family with thorough instruction on purpose and proper use of medications prescribed for CHF.
- Advise bed rest for exacerbations of CHF, but discourage major reorganization of patient's lifestyle unless symptoms are severe and refractory. Gentle exercise may actually improve exercise tolerance once exacerbation has cleared.

BIBLIOGRAPHY

- For the current annotated bibliography on congestive heart failure, see the print edition of *Primary Care Medicine*, 4th edition, Chapter 32, or www.LWWmedicine.com.

Deep Vein Thrombophlebitis

DIFFERENTIAL DIAGNOSIS

CAUSES OF "IDIOPATHIC" DVT

- Hereditary causes
  - Factor V Leiden mutation
  - Deficiency in protein S or C or antithrombin III
  - Homocysteinemia
  - Prothrombin gene mutation
- Acquired causes
  - Adenocarcinoma
  - Antiphospholipid antibodies

WORKUP

- Evaluate patient for DVT (see Leg Edema for Hx, PE, and lab studies).
- If initial evaluation unrevealing but clinical suspicion remains high, repeat Doppler ultrasound (U/S) testing q3–4d over next 10–14 days to rule out DVT above knee.
- In cases of DVT without obvious precipitant, especially recurrent disease, consider hereditary and acquired causes; check for family Hx of DVT and conditions associated with acquired hypercoagulability (occult malignancy, SLE); also consider testing for factor V Leiden, prothrombin gene mutation, hyperhomocysteinemia, and deficiencies in proteins S and C and antithrombin III if results will influence management (see below).

MANAGEMENT

FOR DVT ABOVE KNEE

- Hospitalize to start IV heparin Rx and begin oral anticoagulation with warfarin.
- Consider early discharge for uncomplicated DVT when there is supportive home environment in which fixed, weight-adjusted dose of low-molecular-weight heparin (LMWH) can be administered SQ bid (e.g., dalteparin, 100 units/kg SQ bid or enoxaparin, 1 mg/kg SQ bid).
- Continue LMWH and warfarin until PT (measured by INR) has been in therapeutic range (INR 2–3) for about 3 days, monitor platelet counts and PT INR on days 3 and 7, then stop LMWH.
- Continue warfarin Rx for prophylaxis of recurrent DVT.
- Prescribe 3-mo course for uncomplicated DVT with clear-cut, self-limited precipitant.
- Consider substantially longer or even indefinite course of oral anticoagulation for patients with initial episode of idiopathic disease or with known major risk factor for persistent hypercoagulability (e.g., circulating lupus anticoagulant).

- Weigh risk of long-term anticoagulation (3–5%/yr) with that of recurrent DVT (10%/yr).
- Prescribe long-term anticoagulation in patients with idiopathic disease, especially if there is recurrence, persistent lupus anticoagulant, concurrent cancer, or if degree of thrombosis was severe or complicated by pulmonary embolization.
- Aim for INR of 2–3.
- Refer to vascular specialist for consideration of thrombolytic Rx (streptokinase, tPA) patients with acute proximal DVT extending into iliofemoral system; must treat within 3 days of symptom onset for best results.

FOR DVT BELOW KNEE

- Follow expectantly with serial evaluation for evidence of propagation above knee.
- Keep closest tabs on patients with multiple DVT risk factors.
- Repeat Doppler U/S or plethysmography if suspicion of propagation.
- Hold off anticoagulation as long as no evidence of clot at or above popliteal fossa, because risk of embolization is very low.

BIBLIOGRAPHY

- For the current annotated bibliography on deep vein thrombophlebitis, see the print edition of *Primary Care Medicine*, 4th edition, Chapter 35, or at www.LWWmedicine.com.

Exercise

SCREENING AND/OR PREVENTION

- Encourage all persons to engage regularly in physical activity that provides aerobic exercise.
- Help individual choose medically appropriate activity that is enjoyable and readily incorporated into daily living.
- For those uninterested in structured training, design program of lifestyle change that provides regular aerobic activity (e.g., walking more, riding less; taking stairs instead of elevators).
- For those interested in formal fitness program, screen for underlying cardiopulmonary disease by careful Hx and PE.

WORKUP

HISTORY

- Obtain detailed personal Hx regarding chest pain, palpitations, dyspnea, undue fatigue, light-headedness, syncope, and claudication.
- Review health habits for previous exercise patterns, smoking, diet, and use of oral contraceptives.
- Note family Hx for CHD, peripheral vascular disease, HTN, stroke, DM, and sudden death or exercise-related syncope.

PHYSICAL EXAM

- Record height and weight and calculate BMI or measure percent body fat (see Overweight and Obesity).
- Measure BP at rest, supine, and standing.
- Check heart rate and BP after mild exercise (stair climbing or sit-ups).
- Examine chest for rales, wheezes, and rhonchi, and heart for cardiomegaly, gallops, murmurs, and rhythm disturbances.
- Palpate abdomen and peripheral pulses to exclude abdominal aortic aneurysm and atherosclerotic disease.
- Assess muscles and joints to exclude significant pathology and to determine whether patient requires specific flexibility or strengthening exercises.

LAB STUDIES

- Check glucose, lipid profile, serum hemoglobin, and creatinine.
- For patients aged >40 (especially those with cardiac risk factors or family Hx of heart disease), obtain resting ECG and check for ischemia, LV hypertrophy, and disturbances of rate and rhythm.
- Also obtain ECG in young persons who are going to engage in competitive athletics and who have Hx of heart murmur, palpitations, dyspnea, undue fatigue, syncope, light-headedness, or family Hx of sudden death, premature heart disease, or dysrhythmias.

- Perform exercise stress test if Hx, PE, or screening lab studies suggest underlying heart disease or reveal important cardiac risk factors.
- Consider stress testing in men aged >50 and women aged >60 who are considering vigorous exercise programs, even if they are asymptomatic and apparently healthy, because heart disease is so prevalent in our society.
- In addition to stress testing, consider Holter monitoring in persons with Hx of palpitations or symptoms of light-headedness.
- Order echocardiogram if there is heart murmur or clinical suspicion of hypertrophic cardiomyopathy (e.g., family Hx of early syncope or sudden death).
- Consider forced expiratory volume, vital capacity, and arterial blood gases in patients with suspected pulmonary disease.

RISK STRATIFICATION

- Classify each patient based on medical screening, and assign into 1 of 3 categories: (1) No restrictions/no supervision: healthy; (2) Some restrictions/some supervision: stable, controlled cardiopulmonary disease; (3) Marked restrictions/marked supervision: controlled severe cardiopulmonary disease.
- Exclude from exercise program patients with severe uncontrolled cardiopulmonary disease, ventricular or aortic aneurysm, or hemodynamically significant aortic stenosis.
- Refer exercise candidates in categories 2 and 3 to specialized exercise rehabilitation program that can provide medical supervision and emergency Rx.

MANAGEMENT

- For persons medically appropriate for fitness training, prescribe aerobic exercise 3 × wk. Start with 5 mins for warm-up, 10–12 mins for exercise, and 5 mins for cool-down. As rule of thumb, beginners should plan to exercise aerobically for 10–12 mins at pace sufficient to increase heart rate to 60–80% of max without producing breathlessness.
- Design program so patient attains optimal fitness goals very slowly and gradually. Intensity target should be at comfortable level (e.g., "talking" pace: intensity sufficient to feel one is working hard while still able to talk without feeling dyspneic).
- Increase intensity gently and duration gradually (e.g., by 10%/wk). Avoid too much too soon. Set starting point and rate of progression according to health, age, and fitness of participant.
- For those who desire maximum cardiopulmonary fitness, set goal of exercising continuously for 15–60 mins, performing aerobic exercises strenuous enough to raise heart rate to 80% of max [max rate in bpm $\doteq$ (220 – age) × 0.8]. Equal degrees of fitness can be attained through less intense exercise sustained over longer periods or through more vigorous effort for shorter periods.
- Consider program of moderate exercise for those who desire near-maximum reduction in risk of coronary disease without achieving maximum cardiopulmonary fitness [e.g., recommend for middle-aged women a program of walking at moderate pace (20 mins/mi) for ≥3 hrs/wk]. One

need not prescribe vigorous exercise to maximize coronary risk reduction. Encourage those who have been previously inactive to begin program of moderate exercise, with walking an excellent and practical suggestion.

- For persons engaged in fitness training, recommend minimum 3 sessions/wk to develop and maintain fitness; recommend 5 sessions/wk for those interested in maximum benefit.
- For those who prefer routine of daily activity, recommend alternating easier and harder workouts to prevent injuries and allow muscles to recover.
- Review cardiac warning signs (chest pressure, dizziness, light-headedness, dyspnea, palpitations, unusual fatigue, nausea, diaphoresis). Teach all exercisers to stop activity immediately if symptoms develop and call for assistance.

BIBLIOGRAPHY

- For the current annotated bibliography on exercise, see the print edition of *Primary Care Medicine*, 4th edition, Chapter 18, or www.LWWmedicine.com.

Hypercholesterolemia

SCREENING AND/OR PREVENTION

- Perform fasting lipid profile (total cholesterol, HDL cholesterol, triglycerides, and LDL cholesterol) q5yrs on all adults aged >20.
- Screen more frequently those at increased risk of CHD events, especially persons with known CHD, smoking, diabetes mellitus (DM), HTN, family Hx of premature CHD, or symptomatic noncoronary atheromatous disease.
- If patient is not at high risk for CHD and screening opportunity is nonfasting, limit screening to determinations of total cholesterol and HDL cholesterol.
- If nonfasting total cholesterol >200 mg/dL or HDL cholesterol <40 mg/dL, have patient return for full fasting lipid profile.

WORKUP

CORONARY HEART DISEASE RISK ASSESSMENT AND STRATIFICATION

- Perform risk assessment and stratification for CHD event by reviewing major independent CHD event risk factors if total cholesterol >200 mg/dL, LDL cholesterol >100 mg/dL, or triglycerides >200 mg/dL.
- Identify those at highest risk (10-yr CHD risk >20%) by checking for established CHD (see Coronary Heart Disease) and established "CHD equivalents" [i.e., DM (see Diabetes Mellitus) and clinically evident noncoronary atheromatous disease (see Deep Vein Thrombophlebitis; Superficial Thrombophlebitis; Varicose Veins; Venous Insufficiency)].
- Identify those at slightly lesser risk (10-yr risk 10–20%) by checking for multiple (2+) independent CHD risk factors (smoking, HTN + family Hx of premature CHD, low HDL cholesterol, age >45 in men and >55 in women).
- Identify those with still elevated but lesser 10-yr risk (<10%) by noting presence of 1–2 CHD risk factors.
- Refine risk assessment for these latter 2 groups by referring to table of Framingham Risk Scores (see Chapter 27 in *Primary Care Medicine*, 4th edition).
- Review also for lifestyle and emerging CHD risk factors (abdominal obesity, inactivity, high-fat diet, homocystinemia, glucose intolerance, subclinical atheromatous disease, prothrombic factors); use presence of these risk factors to modulate risk stratification and Rx aggressiveness.
- Note those patients with "metabolic syndrome" (constellation of major, lifestyle, and emerging risk factors, such as obesity, insulin resistance, HTN, low HDL cholesterol, high triglycerides).

MANAGEMENT

OVERALL APPROACH

- Use estimate of total CHD risk (performed by reviewing nonhyperlipidemic CHD risk factors and refined by reference to Framingham Risk Scores; see *Primary Care Medicine*, 4th edition) to guide how aggressively to treat cholesterol abnormalities (especially when to initiate pharmacologic Rx and how low a goal to set for LDL cholesterol).
- Refine approach by attention to LDL cholesterol level and modify if there are abnormalities in HDL cholesterol and/or triglycerides.
- Aggressively treat all concurrent major CHD risk factors (see Diabetes Mellitus; Hypertension; Smoking Cessation, Overweight and Obesity). Do not focus solely on hyperlipidemia.
- Give priority to lifestyle modifications [diet and exercise (see Exercise)], especially if patient has evidence of metabolic syndrome (HTN, insulin resistance, obesity, low HDL cholesterol, elevated triglycerides).
- Treat postmenopausal women same way as men with similar CHD risk; do not substitute hormone replacement Rx (HRT) for standard medical Rx.

TREATMENT OF ELEVATED LDL CHOLESTEROL

CHD 10-Yr Risk >20% (Established CHD, DM, or Other Clinical Atherosclerotic Disease) and LDL Cholesterol >130 mg/dL

- Aggressively treat all other CHD risk factors.
- Carefully initiate exercise program (see Cardiovascular Rehabilitation).
- Prescribe dietary restriction of total fat intake ≤20% of calories, substituting polyunsaturated and monounsaturated fats for saturated fat, partially hydrogenated unsaturated fat, and cholesterol.
- Offer highly motivated individuals option of avoiding or limiting lifelong medication by strict adherence to phase II or III dietary programs (see Chapter 27 in *Primary Care Medicine,* 4th edition), achieving LDL reductions of 40–80 mg/dL.
- Initiate LDL-lowering pharmacologic Rx at same time as lifestyle measures if LDL cholesterol much >130 mg/dL.
- Begin with statin preparation and match choice of statin with degree of LDL cholesterol reduction desired (e.g., atorvastatin or simvastatin if 30–40% reduction needed; choose lowest cost statin if <25% reduction needed).
- Consider niacin (average effective dose, 1.5–3 g/day) as alternative if LDL elevation is accompanied by low HDL (<40 mg/dL).
- Do not substitute HRT for statin Rx in postmenopausal women with hypercholesterolemia.
- Consider adding second agent for those who do not respond to diet + max doses of single agent. Bile resins (e.g., cholestyramine or colestipol, 1–2 scoops bid) are well suited to combination programs.

- Avoid combinations of statin + gemfibrozil because of increased risk of rhabdomyolysis, and of statin + full doses of niacin because of increased risk of myositis (lower niacin doses may be considered when HDL cholesterol levels remain unacceptably low; monitor muscle enzymes regularly).
- Aim for LDL cholesterol <100 mg/dL.

CHD 10-Yr Risk >20% (Established CHD, DM, or Other Clinically Evident Atherosclerotic Disease) and LDL Cholesterol 100–129 mg/dL

- Same as for high-risk patients with LDL >130 mg/dL, except delay onset of statin Rx by a few months if patient willing to undertake major lifestyle changes to achieve goal.
- Aim for LDL cholesterol of <100 mg/dL.
- If HDL cholesterol is low or triglycerides are elevated, consider use of nonstatin agent (e.g., niacin or fibric acid derivative) to correct lipid profile.

CHD 10-Yr Risk 10–20% (e.g., 2+ CHD Risk Factors) and LDL Cholesterol >130 mg/dL

- Begin with diet and exercise programs as above.
- Treat as for higher risk patients (see above) except delay onset of statin Rx for 3 mos to observe effect of lifestyle modifications.
- If LDL cholesterol remains >130 mg/dL, begin statin Rx as above.
- Aim for LDL cholesterol of <130mg/dL.

CHD 10-Yr Risk <10% (e.g., 2 CHD Risk Factors) and LDL Cholesterol >130

- Begin with several mos of lifestyle modifications.
- In patients with large intakes of saturated fat and cholesterol, emphasize phase I diet (see Chapter 27 in *Primary Care Medicine*, 4th edition) to achieve total cholesterol reduction of 20–40 mg/dL.
- Moderately increase polyunsaturated fatty acids, but not >10% of total calories.
- Consider more aggressive dietary fat restriction (phase II diet) in those who do not respond adequately.
- Aim for LDL cholesterol of <130 mg/dL.
- Consider initiation of statin Rx if, despite lifestyle modifications, LDL cholesterol remains >160 mg/dL.
- Aim for LDL cholesterol Rx goal of < 130 mg/dL.

CHD 10-Yr Risk <10% (0–1 Risk Factors) and LDL Cholesterol >160 mg/dL

- Initiate phase I diet and exercise program (see Exercise).
- Aim for LDL cholesterol <160.
- If after 6 months, LDL not <160 mg/dL, begin statin Rx if LDL remains >190 mg/dL. Statin Rx optional if LDL cholesterol 160–189.

- Consider familial hypercholesterolemia in young persons with LDL cholesterol >190 mg/dL and positive family Hx. Treat such persons aggressively. Two-drug regimen may be necessary.

Low HDL Cholesterol (<40 mg/dL)

- Prescribe nonpharmacologic measures that can increase HDL, including aerobic exercise, smoking cessation, and weight loss if obese.
- Prescribe phase I diet, in which saturated fat, cholesterol, and partially hydrogenated vegetable oils are restricted and replaced by monounsaturated and polyunsaturated fats.
- In those with multiple cardiac risk factors and low HDL cholesterol, consider statin Rx for middle-aged and elderly persons and niacin for younger persons.
- Always take into account HDL cholesterol level when designing pharmacologic program for persons with LDL elevation.

Elevated Triglycerides (Fasting Triglycerides >200 mg/dL)

- Emphasize lifestyle changes (diet and exercise), especially if there is evidence of metabolic syndrome (obesity, insulin resistance, HTN, low HDL cholesterol).
- Consider pharmacologic Rx in persons with elevated triglycerides in setting of low HDL (<40 mg/dL), as latter may rise substantially with use of triglyceride-lowering drugs.
- Consider gemfibrozil (600 mg bid) or fenofibrate (67–201 mg/day) if lifestyle modifications unsuccessful, especially if multiple CHD risk factors present.
- Avoid using gemfibrozil + statin due to increased risk of rhabdomyolysis.
- Aim for triglyceride level <150 mg/dL.
- Also consider triglyceride-lowering agent to reduce risk of pancreatitis in persons with very high triglyceride levels (>500 mg/dL).

PATIENT EDUCATION

- Fully explain condition and rationale for Rx to ensure compliance; emphasize importance of dietary modification, exercise, and compliance with any drug program that might be necessary.
- Customize patient ed and Rx programs to needs and capabilities of patient.
- Address patient concerns, especially those regarding long-term use of lipid-lowering medications or dietary modifications. Enlist dietitian if there are concerns or questions regarding dietary changes.

INDICATION FOR REFERRAL

- Consider for referral to lipid specialist patients with high-risk lipid profiles who do not respond to diet + 1–2 first-line drugs, those with extremes of any lipoprotein level, or family Hx of premature CHD (age ≤55).

BIBLIOGRAPHY

■ For the current annotated bibliography on hypercholesterolemia, see the print edition of *Primary Care Medicine*, 4th edition, Chapters 15 and 27, or www.LWWmedicine.com.

SCREENING AND/OR PREVENTION

- Screen all adults regularly for HTN by measuring BP at every health encounter.
- Pay particular attention to checking for BP elevation in persons with DM, heart failure, coronary disease, or renal disease, because HTN can markedly worsen prognosis, and Rx can greatly improve it.

MEASURING BP

- Have patient rest for 5 mins before taking measurement.
- Take BP in both arms with patient seated comfortably with back and arm supported.
- Take ≥2 readings, separated by 2 mins, and repeat if readings differ by >5 mm Hg.
- Have patient refrain from smoking or drinking caffeinated beverage at least 30 mins before determination.
- Note if patient is cold, anxious, has full bladder, or has recently exercised, smoked, or had caffeine.
- Place cuff as high on arm as possible and support arm positioned at heart level.
- Be sure width of cuff's inflatable bladder is >two-thirds arm width and its length >two-thirds arm circumference.
- Auscultate using stethoscope bell for its superior transmission of low-pitched sounds.
- Determine SBP as point at which sound is first heard (Korotkoff 1).
- Determine DBP as point at which sound disappears (Korotkoff 5) rather than when it changes in quality (Korotkoff 4).
- Average 2 successive measurements in each arm.
- Confirm HTN Dx by taking multiple determinations over several visits.

DIFFERENTIAL DIAGNOSIS

- Primary or essential disease: 90–95%
- Secondary disease: 5–10%
  - Renal failure
  - Renovascular disease
  - Primary hyperaldosteronism
  - Drugs
  - Pheochromocytoma
  - Cushing's syndrome

WORKUP

HISTORY

- Elicit date of onset, last previously normal BP, level at onset, any medications taken, and response to Rx.

- Note such clues to secondary disease as sudden onset at extremes of age, very high pressure, no family Hx, refractoriness to Rx, and rapid and severe course.
- Check for contributing factors, such as prior renal disease, salt and alcohol excess, and recent weight gain.
- Inquire into cardiovascular risk factors.
- Review Hx for evidence of atherosclerotic disease (e.g., prior MI, stroke, symptoms of angina, CHF, claudication, transient ischemic attack).
- Inquire into cocaine, alcohol, and amphetamine use.
- Review medication list for oral contraceptives, corticosteroids, thyroid hormone, sympathomimetics, decongestants, and NSAIDs.
- Check for symptoms suggesting secondary HTN (e.g., hirsutism, easy bruising, paroxysms of palpitations and sweats, weakness, muscle cramps, leg claudication).

PHYSICAL EXAM

- Confirm Dx with determinations on ≥2 separate office visits; if in doubt, supplement with home or work-site determinations (see Screening in this topic).
- Check for signs of secondary disease and target organ injury.
- In the elderly, also measure pressure standing to detect any postural changes.
- Note any auscultatory gap (loss and reappearance of Korotkoff sounds), which correlates with arterial stiffness and carotid atherosclerosis (predictors of prognosis).

Classify Degree of BP Elevation

- Classification of BP for adults aged ≥18 (mm Hg; based on average of ≥2 readings taken at each of ≥2 visits after initial screening)
  - Normal
    - Systolic: <130
    - Diastolic: <85
  - High normal
    - Systolic: 130–139
    - Diastolic: 85–89
  - HTN
    - Stage 1 (mild)
      - Systolic: 140–159
      - Diastolic: 90–99
    - Stage 2 (moderate)
      - Systolic: 160–179
      - Diastolic: 100–109
    - Stage 3 (severe)
      - Systolic: ≥180–209
      - Diastolic: ≥110–119
    - Stage 4 (malignant)
      - Systolic: >210
      - Diastolic: >120
- Measure weight and pulse.
- Note skin for stigmata of Cushing's syndrome, chronic renal failure, or neurofibromatosis.

- Check fundi for arteriolar narrowing, increased vascular tortuosity, arteriovenous nicking, and hemorrhages; thyroid for enlargement or nodularity; carotid pulses for bruits or diminution of pulse; lungs for signs of heart failure; and heart for LV heave, S_4, and S_3.
- Examine abdomen for masses and bruits, and perform neurologic exam for focal deficits.
- Check peripheral vasculature for pulses, bruits, and abnormalities in bilateral arm and leg pressure measurements.
- Simultaneously palpate radial and femoral pulses.

LAB STUDIES

- Obtain CBC, urinalysis, BUN, creatinine, potassium, calcium (with albumin), fasting blood sugar, total and HDL cholesterol, and ECG.
- Avoid more extensive lab testing, except in presence of clinical evidence for secondary etiology.

Primary vs Secondary Hypertension: Specific Screening Protocols

- Cause: coarctation
  - Screen: arm and leg BP, CXR
  - Confirm: echocardiography or CT
- Cause: Cushing's syndrome
  - Screen: Cushingoid appearance; 1-mg dexamethasone suppression test
- Cause: drug-induced syndrome
  - Screen: Hx: amphetamines, oral contraceptives, estrogens, corticosteroids, licorice, thyroid hormone
- Cause: increased intracranial pressure
  - Screen: neurologic exam
- Cause: pheochromocytoma
  - Screen: Hx of paroxysmal HTN, headache, perspiration, palpitations or fixed DBP ≥130 mm Hg; 24-hour urinary metanephrine or vanillylmandelic acid
  - Confirm: catecholamine levels, angiography, CT
- Cause: primary aldosteronism (Conn's or idiopathic)
  - Screen:serum potassium;serum aldosterone: plasma renin ratio ≥50:1
  - Confirm: inhibition and stimulation of aldosterone and renin secretion
- Cause: renal disease
  - Screen: Hx of congenital disease, DM, proteinuria, pyelonephritis, obstruction; urinalysis; BUN or creatinine
  - Confirm: creatinine clearance, IV pyelogram, ultrasound, biopsy
- Cause: renovascular disease
  - Screen: clinical prediction rule, captopril renal scan and/or MRA.
  - Confirm: angiography and differential renal vein renins

RISK STRATIFICATION

- Incorporate findings of severity, cardiovascular risk, and target-organ damage into risk profile to guide Rx.
- Consider use of JNCI VI risk groups:
  - A (no additional risk): no cardiovascular risk factors; no clinical cardiovascular disease or target-organ damage

- B (moderate additional risk): ≥1 risk factor, not including DM, clinical cardiovascular disease, or target-organ disease
- C (marked additional risk): clinical cardiovascular disease or target-organ disease or DM, ± other risk factors

MANAGEMENT

FOR ALL PATIENTS

- Prescribe no-added-salt diet (3–4 g/day) low in saturated fat and rich in fruits, vegetables, and low-fat dairy products.
- Consider greater sodium restriction in persons likely to have volume-overload HTN (e.g., African-Americans, the elderly, persons with nocturia or leg edema).
- Advise weight reduction (especially if >15% above ideal weight).
- Limit alcohol intake to 1 oz/day.
- Insist on complete smoking cessation (see Smoking Cessation).
- Prescribe exercise program (see Exercise).

FOR PATIENTS WITH STAGE 1 HYPERTENSION + NO ADDITIONAL CARDIOVASCULAR RISK FACTORS; NO SIGNS OF TARGET-ORGAN DISEASE

- Institute full nonpharmacologic measures.
- Repeat BP determinations regularly over next 6 mos.
- If improvement noted (DBP <90; SBP <140), continue nonpharmacologic measures and monitor BP q3mos.
- If no improvement after 6–12 mos of nonpharmacologic Rx or if it fails to lower BP (DBP <90; SBP <140), add first-line antihypertensive agent (see below) to nonpharmacologic program.

FOR PATIENTS WITH STAGE 1 HTN + ADDITIONAL CARDIOVASCULAR RISK FACTORS OR SIGNS OF TARGET-ORGAN DISEASE

- Immediately institute full nonpharmacologic program.
- Repeat BP determinations regularly over 3 mos.
- If BP not normalized after 3 mos, add first-line antihypertensive agent (see below) to nonpharmacologic program.

FOR PATIENTS WITH STAGE 2 HTN, ESPECIALLY IF ACCOMPANIED BY CARDIOVASCULAR RISK FACTORS OR TARGET-ORGAN DAMAGE

- Immediately institute full nonpharmacologic program.
- If BP not normalized after 1–2 mos, add first-line antihypertensive agent (see below) to nonpharmacologic program and advance pharmacologic program as needed.
- Monitor BP closely.

FOR PATIENTS WITH STAGE 3 HTN

- Immediately institute full doses of first-line agent (see below) and consider early use of second first-line agent if necessary.

- If BP improved but not normalized within 1 wk, add second first-line agent.
- If no response to initial first-line agent within a few days, begin second first-line agent from different class at full doses and consider adding second drug at same time.
- Prescribe full nonpharmacologic program.
- Follow closely.

FOR PATIENTS WITH STAGE 4 HTN

- Consider emergency hospitalization, especially if evidence of acute target-organ injury (e.g., papilledema, retinal hemorrhages, heart failure, altered mental status).
- Give patients with similarly elevated BP but no evidence of target-organ involvement PO labetalol in the office to acutely reduce BP, start them on 2- or 3-drug regimen, and follow up in a few days.

INITIATION AND ADVANCEMENT OF PHARMACOLOGIC THERAPY

- Begin pharmacologic Rx with first-line agent, preferably diuretic, beta blocker, or ACE inhibitor.
- Choose agent based on consideration of patient's overall clinical situation and likely underlying pathophysiology.
- Start with modest dose unless clinical situation requires institution of full doses immediately.
- If BP does not improve within 1 mo of initiating drug Rx, increase dose and recheck in 4 wks.
- If no response despite increasing dose, switch to a first-line drug from different class.
- If only partial response, choice is to either increase dose further or add low dose of another first-line drug from different class (e.g., add hydrochlorothiazide, 12.5–25 mg/day, or a beta blocker).
- Once BP normalizes, recheck at 3- to 6-mo intervals.
- If 2-drug regimen using 2 first-line agents from different classes insufficient, select third drug from new class. Particularly effective 3-drug regimen is ACE inhibitor, thiazide diuretic, and beta blocker.
- Consider sustained-release formulation if likely to increase compliance and reduce cost of daily dose.

FIRST-LINE AGENTS: RECOMMENDATIONS FOR USE

Thiazides

- Consider for almost all patients, but especially useful in those likely to have volume-overload HTN; provides effective low-cost Rx and enhances antihypertensive effects of beta blockers, calcium channel blockers, and ACE inhibitors.
- Limit doses to modest amounts (e.g., 12.5–25 mg/day hydrochlorothiazide) to minimize adverse metabolic effects, particularly in patients with marked hypercholesterolemia, poorly controlled DM, symptomatic gout, cardiac arrhythmias, or severe underlying coronary disease.
- For monotherapy, use no more than moderate doses (e.g., 25–50 mg/day hydrochlorothiazide).

- Regularly monitor serum potassium in persons with underlying heart disease.

Beta Blockers

- Consider for most patients and preferred in those with concurrent CAD or high cardiovascular risk; not as effective or well tolerated in the elderly; among most cost-effective.
- Choose relatively cardioselective preparation (e.g., atenolol, metoprolol) to minimize adverse systemic effects.
- Prescribe generic formulations to minimize expense.
- Use with caution in patients with bronchospasm or nonischemic heart failure.
- Add small dose of thiazide if fluid retention develops or if enhanced BP control desired.

ACE Inhibitors

- Consider for most patients; preferred agent for those with DM or heart failure; useful choice in those with volume-overload HTN, underlying sexual dysfunction, depression, or intolerance to CNS effects of other antihypertensive agents. May be used alone or with diuretic or beta blocker, which enhances their effectiveness; contraindicated in pregnancy and bilateral renal artery stenosis.
- Monitor renal function and serum potassium, especially in those with underlying renal dysfunction.
- Consider generic formulations to minimize expense.

Calcium Channel Blockers

- Until more data on safety and efficacy are available, use with caution and not as preferred class for HTN.
- Consider as alternative to thiazides and ACE inhibitors in patients with volume-overload HTN and DM.
- Avoid use of short-acting preparations because of concerns about increased risk of MI and cardiac sudden death.
- Use cautiously in patients with conduction defects, especially if already taking beta blockers.
- Avoid if possible in patients bothered by peripheral edema; short-acting agents contraindicated in heart failure.
- If use unavoidable, consider agent with least known adverse peripheral vascular and cardiovascular effects (e.g., amlodipine).
- Prescribe sustained-release preparation to minimize cost and cardiac risk and switch from short-acting preparation to long-acting preparation if patient already taking calcium channel blocker.
- Obtain cardiac consultation regarding use in persons with known CAD.

BIBLIOGRAPHY

- For the current annotated bibliography on Hypertension, see the print edition of *Primary Care Medicine*, 4th edition, Chapters 14, 19, and 26, or www.LWWmedicine.com.

Leg Edema

DIFFERENTIAL DIAGNOSIS

IMPORTANT CAUSES OF LEG EDEMA

- Unilateral or asymmetric swelling
  - Increased hydrostatic pressure
    - Deep vein thrombophlebitis
    - Venous insufficiency
    - Popliteal (Baker's) cyst
  - Increased capillary permeability
    - Cellulitis
    - Trauma
    - Lymphatic obstruction (local)
- Bilateral swelling
  - Decreased oncotic pressure
    - Malnutrition
    - Hepatocellular failure
    - Nephrotic syndrome
    - Protein-losing enteropathy
  - Increased hydrostatic pressure
    - CHF
    - Renal failure
    - Use of salt-retaining drugs (e.g., corticosteroids, estrogens)
    - Venous insufficiency
    - Pulmonary HTN
    - Premenstrual state
    - Pregnancy
  - Increased capillary permeability
    - Systemic vasculitis
    - Idiopathic edema
    - Allergic reactions
    - Lymphatic obstruction (retroperitoneal or generalized)

WORKUP

HISTORY AND PHYSICAL EXAM

For Unilateral or Markedly Asymmetric Leg Edema

- Review Hx for risk factors for DVT [e.g., active malignancy, recent paralysis or plaster casting, prolonged immobilization, recent major surgery (especially of hip or knee), current estrogen use, family Hx of DVT].
- Check PE for key signs of DVT (e.g., difference in calf circumferences >3 cm, tenderness along deep veins, palpable cord, pitting edema of entire leg, prominence of collateral superficial veins).
- Estimate pretest probability of DVT based on Hx and PE.

For Bilateral Leg Edema

- Review Hx for symptoms of venous insufficiency, CHF, and chronic pulmonary disease, especially sleep apnea. Also check for Hx of renal or hepatic disease, malnutrition, and use of nifedipine, NSAIDs, and corti-costeroids.

LAB STUDIES

For Unilateral or Markedly Asymmetric Leg Edema

■ Obtain compression Doppler venous ultrasound (U/S) or plethysmography of involved limb in all patients. If negative result is obtained but clinical suspicion persists, repeat within 3–5 days.

■ Use combination of pretest probability and test results to determine need for further testing. When pretest probability is intermediate and initial noninvasive study is negative, either repeat noninvasive study q3d for up to 2 wks or obtain D-dimer determination; if these are unavailable, proceed directly to venography.

For Bilateral Leg Edema

■ Check serum albumin; if normal and no other etiology evident, obtain cardiac U/S for detection of subclinical CHF and pulmonary HTN.

BIBLIOGRAPHY

■ For the current annotated bibliography on leg edema, see the print edition of *Primary Care Medicine*, 4th edition, Chapter 22, or www.LWWmedicine.com.

Mitral Regurgitation

MANAGEMENT

- Do not restrict activity of asymptomatic young patients.
- Treat onset of fatigue or dyspnea with gentle diuretic program (e.g., 50–100 mg/day hydrochlorothiazide) in conjunction with no-added-salt diet. Modest diuretic program that adequately controls symptoms may suffice for yrs in patients with mild to moderate mitral regurgitation and is not indication for surgery.
- Obtain prompt cardiac consultation for consideration of valve replacement if there is increase in dyspnea that requires escalation of diuretic Rx. Progressive deterioration in clinical status and increasing heart size suggest presence of myocardial decompensation. At this stage, medical Rx is no substitute for valve surgery. Even refractory CHF due to mitral regurgitation is not contraindication to surgery, although risk is increased.
- Before surgery, consider ACE inhibitor Rx (e.g., captopril, 25–50 mg tid; see Congestive Heart Failure) to lessen symptoms; inhibitor Rx can diminish magnitude of regurgitant flow by decreasing afterload. Use of vasodilators can also benefit inoperable patient.
- Refer patients with incapacitating dyspnea and pulmonary congestion thought to be caused by papillary muscle dysfunction to cardiologist for catheterization to determine whether valve replacement will be beneficial. Valve reconstruction is increasingly frequent option in mitral regurgitation, obviating need for artificial valve and its attendant risks in many cases.
- Treat any coexisting coronary disease (see Stable Angina).
- For patients with MVP
  - Initiate endocarditis prophylaxis if regurgitant heart murmur is readily audible or there is ultrasound (U/S) evidence of clinically significant lesion (see Bacterial Endocarditis).
  - Omit salt restriction and diuretics unless dyspnea is present (magnitude of regurgitation usually insignificant and rarely progressive); however, follow those with dilated left ventricle and marked regurgitation with serial cardiac U/S for early detection of LV dysfunction, a sign of poor prognosis and indication for consideration of repair.
  - Consider Rx for malignant ventricular dysrhythmias (see Ventricular Irritability) only for rare patients with Hx of syncope or ventricular tachycardia or family Hx of sudden death; those with isolated palpitations do not need Rx.
  - Omit prophylaxis for systemic embolization in absence of concurrent risk factors.
- Follow patients with calcification of mitral valve annulus for development of heart block. Regurgitant flow is usually small; consequently, dyspnea and pulmonary congestion are not major problems.
- Start chronic oral anticoagulation in mitral regurgitation with AF, especially when accompanied by marked left atrial and LV enlargement.
- See also Valvular Heart Disease.

BIBLIOGRAPHY

■ For the current annotated bibliography on mitral regurgitation, see the print edition of *Primary Care Medicine*, 4th edition, Chapter 33, or www.LWWmedicine.com.

Mitral Stenosis

MANAGEMENT

- Inform asymptomatic patients with mild to moderate stenosis that they need not restrict activity.
- Advise those with evidence of tight stenosis, even if relatively asymptomatic, of risk of precipitating symptoms by extreme exertion or pregnancy.
- Start mild diuretic program (e.g., hydrochlorothiazide, 50–100 mg/day) for patients with mild dyspnea that occurs only on exertion, and advise them to follow no-added-salt diet.
- Omit digitalis unless there is AF.
- Counsel patients to avoid situations that could precipitate hemodynamic deterioration and symptoms (e.g., extremely vigorous exertion, emotional upset).
- Start chronic warfarin oral anticoagulation, particularly with onset of AF (see Atrial Fibrillation).
- Obtain cardiologic consultation when there is evidence of developing tight mitral stenosis (e.g., worsening dyspnea inadequately controlled by mild diuretic program and salt restriction, short S_2-opening snap interval, prolonged diastolic murmur, left atrial enlargement and upper zone redistribution on CXR, narrowed valve orifice and reduced flow on ultrasound). Surgery or balloon angioplasty may be indicated, even if few symptoms are reported.
- Consider early cardiac referral of young patients with evidence of isolated tight mitral stenosis with pliable noncalcified valve, even before symptoms are disabling, because early interventional Rx (transcatheter or surgical valvotomy) can be performed. Both procedures provide lasting hemodynamic improvement; catheter valvulotomy may obviate need for surgical mitral commissurotomy.
- Follow older patients with fibrotic valves (absent opening snap, heavy valve calcification, and limited motion) more expectantly. Their only option is valve replacement surgery, which need not be advised until symptoms are more disabling. However, do not delay surgery until symptoms occur at rest or on minimal exertion because operative risk and long-term mortality increase substantially. Walk with patient down corridor or up stairs to help both you and patient determine that time for surgery has arrived.
- Obtain cardiac consultation for consideration of catheterization when contemplating surgery, when there is question of mixed mitral disease or involvement of multiple valves, or when symptoms are disproportionate to objective evidence of disease.
- See also Valvular Heart Disease.

BIBLIOGRAPHY

- For the current annotated bibliography on mitral stenosis, see the print edition of *Primary Care Medicine*, 4th edition, Chapter 33, or www.LWWmedicine.com.

Palpitations

DIFFERENTIAL DIAGNOSIS

- Isolated single palpitations
  - Premature atrial or ventricular beats
  - Beat after blocked beat
  - Beat after compensatory pause
- Paroxysmal episodes with abrupt onset and resolution (rate usually rapid)
  - Rhythm irregular
    - Paroxysmal AF
    - Paroxysmal atrial tachycardia with variable block
    - Frequent atrial or ventricular premature beats
    - Multifocal atrial tachycardia
  - Rhythm regular
    - Supraventricular tachycardias with constant block 1:1 conduction
- Paroxysmal episodes with less abrupt onset or resolution (rhythm usually regular, rate rapid)
  - Exertion
  - Emotion
  - Drug side effect (e.g., sympathomimetics, theophylline compounds)
  - Stimulant use (coffee, tea, tobacco)
  - Insulin reaction
  - Pheochromocytoma
- Persistent palpitations at rest with regular rhythm (rate normal, slow, or rapid)
  - Aortic or mitral regurgitation
  - Large ventricular septal defect
  - Bradycardia
  - Severe anemia
  - Hyperthyroidism (may also cause AF)
  - Pregnancy
  - Fever
  - Marked volume depletion
  - Anxiety neurosis

WORKUP

HISTORY

- Elicit complete description of patient's palpitations; fluttering, stopping, or beating irregularly are predictive of arrhythmia; any isolated thumping or flip-flopping suggests atrial or ventricular premature beat.
- Include its mode of onset, frequency, rate, rhythm, duration, termination, associated symptoms, and precipitants and alleviating factors (especially relation of onset to exertion).

- Identify precipitants such as emotional upset, stimulant intake, fever, pregnancy, volume depletion, severe anemia, insulin reaction, hyperthyroidism.
- Note correlation or lack thereof between symptoms and Holter monitoring results (see below).
- Note any pounding in neck indicative of arterioventricular dissociation.
- Inquire into concurrent dyspnea, chest pain, light-headedness, near-syncope, and syncope. Include checking for symptoms of panic and somatization disorders (see Anxiety; Somatization Disorders).
- Review use of cardiotonic drugs and those associated with QT prolongation: antiarrhythmics, terfenadine, astemizole, macrolide antibiotics, ketoconazole, itraconazole, phenothiazines, and tricyclic antidepressants.
- Review use of OTC decongestants and diet pills as well as ephedra-containing supplements and alcohol abuse.
- Check family Hx for early-onset syncope or sudden death.

PHYSICAL EXAM

- Check BP for elevation, marked postural change, and widened pulse pressure.
- Note apical pulse for rate and rhythm disturbances; do not rely on peripheral pulse.
- Conduct detailed PE focusing on possible etiologies (see above) (e.g., skin for pallor and signs of hyperthyroidism; eyes for exophthalmos; neck for goiter; carotid pulse for abnormal upstroke; jugular venous pulse for distention and cannon A waves; chest for rales, rhonchi, wheezes, and dullness; heart for heaves, thrills, clicks, murmurs, rubs, and S_3; and extremities for edema and calf tenderness); and conduct mental status exam for manifestations of anxiety, depression, panic disorder, and substance abuse (see Alcohol Abuse; Anxiety; Depression; Somatization Disorders; Substance Abuse).
- Note response to modest exercise.

LAB STUDIES

- If patient manifests persistent hyperkinetic state, check CBC and TSH; if paroxysmal, consider testing for pheochromocytoma (see Hypertension) and hypoglycemia (see Hypoglycemia).
- For patients with suspected heart disease, check serum potassium, calcium, magnesium, and, if taking digitalis preparations, serum cardiac glycoside level.
- Direct most of the remainder of testing toward identifying rhythm disturbance and detecting underlying heart disease.
- Obtain resting ECG and check for axis shift, short PR interval (<0.12 s), and abnormal P-wave morphology, including signs of atrial enlargement, QRS widening, increase in QRS voltage, prominent septal Q waves, prolonged QT interval, delta waves, and ST- and T-wave changes.
- If you note dysrhythmia, obtain 2-min rhythm strip to better characterize rhythm disturbance.
- Proceed with ambulatory ECG monitoring in patients with evidence of underlying heart disease but no cause for admission (i.e., no syncope, near-syncope, heart failure, or angina associated with palpitations).

- Unless patient has daily symptoms, use event recorder with 2-wk monitoring period rather than Holter monitoring to maximize cost-effectiveness.
- Consider stress testing those who report palpitations occurring during or immediately after exercise. To ensure patient safety, rule out hemodynamically significant aortic stenosis, hypertrophic cardiomyopathy, and QT prolongation before proceeding with exercise testing.
- Obtain echocardiography in patients with suspected valvular or cardiomyopathic disease.
- Consider EPS in patients with palpitations leading to syncope or near-syncope, especially when occurring in context of underlying organic heart disease.

MANAGEMENT

- For patients with underlying heart disease, treat etiologically.
- For patients without underlying heart disease who find symptoms intolerable, consider simple symptomatic measures:
  - For bothersome atrial or ventricular premature beats, begin beta blocker (e.g., atenolol or metoprolol, 25–50 mg/day).
  - For idiopathic chronic ventricular bigeminy causing fatigue or exertional near-syncope because of slow effective heart rate, consider radioablation if no response to beta-blockade.
  - Stop all nonessential palpitation-causing drugs and limit caffeinated beverages to <2–3 cups/day.

BIBLIOGRAPHY

- For the current annotated bibliography on palpitations, see the print edition of *Primary Care Medicine*, 4th edition, Chapter 25, or www.LWWmedicine.com.

Rheumatic Fever

SCREENING AND/OR PREVENTION

SECONDARY PREVENTION

- Prevention of rheumatic fever recurrences depends on continuous streptococcal prophylaxis of patients at risk.
- Base duration of prophylaxis on risk incurred by patient.
- For all patients with rheumatic fever, prescribe prophylactic antibiotic Rx until age 25 or for 5 yrs after an attack of rheumatic fever (whichever is longer).
- In those with ≥2 previous attacks of rheumatic fever or with rheumatic heart disease, continue Rx until age 40 or for 10 yrs after last episode.
- Continue antibiotic prophylaxis indefinitely in patients with rheumatic heart disease at high risk of strep exposure.

Antibiotic Regimens

- Prescribe parenteral penicillin [penicillin G benzathine (1,200,000 U IM q3–4wks)] in patients with high risk of both rheumatic recurrence after strep infection (Hx of recurrent rheumatic fever) and continued strep exposure. Provides most effective prophylaxis and is recommended in high-risk patients.
- Consider oral regimen in patients at lower risk (e.g., no recurrence of rheumatic fever, little strep exposure risk). Prescribe sulfadiazine, 1 g/day PO; or penicillin G, 250 mg PO bid; or erythromycin, 250 mg PO bid (in patients allergic to both penicillin and sulfa drugs).

PRIMARY PREVENTION

- Test for group A beta-hemolytic strep infection in patients with sore throat and risk factors or suggestive clinical features (see Pharyngitis).
- Treat those who test positive (see Pharyngitis).

BIBLIOGRAPHY

- For the current annotated bibliography on rheumatic fever, see the print edition of *Primary Care Medicine*, 4th edition, Chapter 17, or www.LWWmedicine.com.

Stable Angina

MANAGEMENT

FOR ALL PATIENTS (INCLUDING THOSE UNDERGOING REVASCULARIZATION)

- Identify and aggressively treat all major CHD risk factors (see Diabetes Mellitus; Hypercholesterolemia; Hypertension; Smoking Cessation).
- Check for and correct any concurrent precipitating or aggravating factors, such as CHF, severe anemia, hyperthyroidism, COPD, and valvular heart disease.
- Use risk categorization to guide further program design.
- Determine prognosis and degree of CHD risk by
  - ascertaining amount of myocardium at risk through stress testing (see Stress Testing), and
  - assessing LV function through echocardiography or radionuclide scanning (see Congestive Heart Failure; Stress Testing).
- Screen for and treat psychosocial factors that can adversely effect outcomes, including anxiety (see Anxiety), depression (see Depression), situational stress, and social isolation.
- Begin low-dose enteric-coated aspirin (81 mg/day).
- Initiate ACE inhibitor Rx if patient has reduced ejection fraction (<0.4) (see Congestive Heart Failure); consider also for CHD patients with preserved LV function and multiple CHD risk factors (e.g., DM, HTN).
- Thoroughly review with patient and family rationale and proper use of Rx.
- Encourage monitoring response to Rx.
- Counsel on allowable activity, encouraging exercise as tolerated and helping avoid self-imposed unnecessary limits on activity.
- Begin gentle exercise program (e.g., walking 20 mins, 3 × wk) and more intensive program for highly motivated; obtain exercise stress test first (see Cardiovascular Rehabilitation).
- Promptly admit and obtain cardiac consultation for any patient with unstable angina or markedly worsening LV dysfunction.

LOW-RISK PATIENTS (MILD TO MODERATE ANGINA, NORMAL EJECTION FRACTION, SMALL AMOUNT OF MYOCARDIUM AT RISK, PROBABLE SINGLE-VESSEL DISEASE)

- Prescribe prn TNG, 0.4 mg, for symptomatic relief of anginal episodes.
- Instruct patient to rest at time of pain and take second and third TNG if pain does not resolve within 5 mins of each dose.
- Advise maintaining fresh supply of TNG and discarding any bottle that has been open for >6 mos or any tablets that fail to cause sublingual burning or head throbbing.
- Prescribe prophylactic sublingual TNG before inciting activity if angina is stable, predictable, and short-lived.

- Begin beta-blockade with generic formulation of long-acting cardiose-lective agent (e.g., atenolol, 25–50 mg/day; or metoprolol, 25 mg bid); adjust dose to ensure adequate beta-blockade (heart rate <60 bpm at rest; <100 bpm with vigorous exertion).
- If beta-blockade must be terminated, do so only in tapering fashion over 1–2 wks; have patient reduce activity during this time.
- If anginal control is insufficient with above measures but patient responds well to TNG, add long-acting nitrate to program (e.g., isosor-bide dinitrate, beginning with 5 mg tid and advancing slowly over 1–2 wks in increments of 5 mg/dose); dose in asymmetric fashion (8 A.M., 2 P.M., 8 P.M.) to minimize risk of nitrate tolerance.
- Consider trial of calcium channel blocker Rx (e.g., amlodipine, 5 mg/day) only if patient continues to be unacceptably symptomatic despite full doses of nitrates and beta blockers. Use only long-acting calcium channel blocker formulation. Monitor conduction and LV function, especially when using with beta blocker. With exception of amlodipine, do not use with underlying heart failure or clinically sig-nificant conduction system disease.
- Consider referral for angiography and possible revascularization only if patient continues to be unacceptably limited by angina despite full compliance with medical regimen + aggressive Rx of CHD risk factors.

MODERATE-RISK PATIENTS (MODERATE ANGINA, MODERATE AMOUNT OF MYOCARDIUM AT RISK, PROBABLE 2-VESSEL DISEASE, NORMAL EJECTION FRACTION)

- Give trial of full medical regimen as outlined for patients with low-risk disease.
- If medical Rx provides adequate control of symptoms, continue indefi-nitely in conjunction with very aggressive and comprehensive Rx of CHD risk factors and precipitants.
- If exercise tolerance and functional status remain impaired, refer for angiography and determination of candidacy for revascularization.
- If candidate for revascularization, assess patient's preference for PTCA vs CABG.

HIGH-RISK PATIENTS (MODERATE TO SEVERE ANGINA; LARGE AMOUNT OF MYOCARDIUM AT RISK; SUSPECTED 3-VESSEL, LEFT-MAIN, OR LEFT-MAIN-EQUIVALENT DISEASE; REDUCED EJECTION FRACTION)

- Refer immediately for angiography and consideration of CABG.
- Recommend CABG for those with left-main, left-main-equivalent, or 3-vessel disease, especially if complicated by LV dysfunction. (Some proximal LAD lesions might be suitable for PTCA + stenting.)

BIBLIOGRAPHY

- For the current annotated bibliography on stable angina, see the print edition of *Primary Care Medicine*, 4th edition, Chapter 30, or www.LWWmedicine.com.

Stress Testing

WORKUP

TEST SELECTION FOR CHD DIAGNOSIS AND PROGNOSIS

- ECG stress test remains cost-effective for CHD testing in patients with normal resting ECG.
- Although standard max ECG stress test is rather insensitive for identification of single-vessel disease, its sensitivity for high-risk CHD and correlation with prognosis are very high, approaching those of much more expensive radionuclide studies.
- Submax stress testing (up to 5 METS) shortly after acute MI provides important prognostic information.
- Even in setting of nonspecific resting ECG abnormalities, ECG stress test retains prognostic utility when using Duke treadmill score.
- Echocardiographic stress testing is another cost-effective option for CHD Dx. Sensitivity and specificity when performed by experts are similar to that for radionuclide scanning, and similar to more expensive scans, information is provided on LV function and regional perfusion.
- Consequently, ECG stress test should be initial stress study for detection of high-risk CHD in patients with normal resting ECG.
- In persons with abnormal resting ECG, inability to exercise, or in settings in which enhanced detection of lower-risk coronary disease is desirable, consider echocardiographic stress testing and stress radionuclide study, with echocardiographic study being more cost-effective.
- Because ECG, thallium, and stress echocardiography are only moderately sensitive and specific for CHD Dx in premenopausal women, a high degree of clinical suspicion and careful consideration of all clinical evidence are essential in CHD assessment of such women.

BIBLIOGRAPHY

- For the current annotated bibliography on stress testing, see the print edition of *Primary Care Medicine*, 4th edition, Chapter 36, or www.LWWmedicine.com.

Superficial Thrombophlebitis

WORKUP

- Differentiate from cellulitis and lymphangitis by palpating thrombosed vein and noting focal distribution of erythema and swelling along its course and lack of generalized edema.

MANAGEMENT

- Prescribe combination of local heat and compression with good elastic stocking.
- Consider aspirin or another NSAID to lessen inflammation.
- Avoid antibiotics; they have no role.
- Consider discontinuing estrogen-containing Rx (e.g., oral contraceptives, HRT).
- Recommend walking and avoiding prolonged sitting or standing.
- Consider anticoagulation if superficial phlebitis extends above knee, and surgical consultation for possible saphenous vein ligation if extension continues.

BIBLIOGRAPHY

- For the current annotated bibliography on superficial thrombophlebitis, see the print edition of *Primary Care Medicine*, 4th edition, Chapter 35, or www.LWWmedicine.com.

Syncope

DIFFERENTIAL DIAGNOSIS

IMPORTANT CAUSES OF SYNCOPE

- Cardiac
  - Arrhythmias (sick sinus syndrome, ventricular tachycardia, very rapid supraventricular tachycardia)
  - Heart block (Stokes-Adams attacks)
  - Aortic stenosis, severe
  - Asymmetric septal hypertrophy, severe
  - Primary pulmonary HTN
  - Atrial myxoma
  - Prolapsed mitral valve
- Vascular-reflex
  - Neurocardiogenic (vasovagal, vasodepressor)
  - Orthostatic HTN (ganglionic blocking agents, DM, old age, prolonged bed rest)
  - Carotid sinus hypersensitivity
  - Cerebral vascular disease, severe
  - Subclavian steal syndrome
  - Posttussive syncope
  - Valsalva syncope
  - Postmicturition syncope (emptying distended bladder)
  - Postprandial syncope
- Psychologic-neurologic
  - Seizures
  - Hysteria
  - Generalized anxiety disorder
  - Depression
  - Panic disorder
- Metabolic
  - Hyperventilation
  - Hypoxia
  - Hypoglycemia (rarely)

WORKUP

HISTORY AND PHYSICAL EXAM

- Begin evaluation with comprehensive Hx and focused PE emphasizing detection of underlying heart disease; obtain resting ECG.
- Base further test selection on pretest likelihood of underlying heart disease.

LAB STUDIES

For Intermediate to High Pretest Probability of Serious Underlying Heart Disease

■ Conduct initial evaluation in hospital and include Holter monitoring or EPS (if high suspicion of ventricular tachycardia), supplemented by stress testing and/or ECG.

For Low Pretest Probability of Serious Underlying Heart Disease

■ Conduct assessment in outpatient setting and include continuous-loop event monitoring (especially for persons with structurally normal hearts, Hx of palpitations, and frequent episodes), psychiatric testing (especially for younger persons with frequent episodes in absence of evidence for heart disease, for those with multiple somatic and psychiatric symptoms, and for those with no injury from syncopal episodes), and tilt-table testing [especially for persons with infrequent episodes who have no evidence of underlying heart disease and Hx suggesting neurocardiogenic (vasovagal) syncope or conversion reaction].

■ Also consider conducting initial evaluation on inpatient basis for persons suspected of having seizure disorder or stroke and for the frail elderly who sustain serious injury from first syncopal episode.

Adapted from the clinical guidelines proposed by Linzer M, Yang EH, Estes M III, et al. Diagnosing syncope. Part 1. Value of history, physical examination, and electrocardiography. Ann Intern Med 1997;126:989, with permission.

BIBLIOGRAPHY

■ For the current annotated bibliography on syncope, see the print edition of *Primary Care Medicine*, 4th edition, Chapter 24, or www.LWWmedicine.com.

Valvular Heart Disease

MANAGEMENT

- Monitor all patients by periodic assessment of exercise tolerance and hemodynamic state by careful review of Hx, cardiopulmonary exam, CXR, and cardiac ultrasound exam (including Doppler).
- Administer bacterial endocarditis prophylaxis to all patients with valvular heart disease (see Bacterial Endocarditis).
- Consider rheumatic fever prophylaxis for patients aged <35 with previous rheumatic fever (see Rheumatic Fever), particularly if they have frequent beta-streptococcal infections or exposure to young children.
- Immediately admit for cardioversion those patients with acute onset of rapid AF accompanied by acute hemodynamic compromise. Patients with slower rates who tolerate AF can often be treated on outpatient basis (see Atrial Fibrillation).
- Also admit promptly for IV anticoagulant Rx followed by long-term PO anticoagulant Rx (see Anticoagulant Therapy) patients with evidence of acute systemic embolization. Refer for consideration of need for valve replacement.
- See also Aortic Regurgitation; Aortic Stenosis; Mitral Regurgitation; Mitral Stenosis.

BIBLIOGRAPHY

- For the current annotated bibliography on valvular heart disease, see the print edition of *Primary Care Medicine*, 4th edition, Chapter 33, or www.LWWmedicine.com.

Varicose Veins

WORKUP

- Note extent and location of varicosities and any signs of deep venous disease (e.g., stasis skin changes, ulceration, edema).
- For varicosities appearing after trauma, check for bruit indicative of traumatic arteriovenous fistula.
- For severe varicosities occurring at young age, consider congenital arteriovenous malformation and listen for bruit.

MANAGEMENT

- Prescribe proper elastic support of medium weight and periodic daily extremity elevation.
- Specify below-knee stocking: best for compliance and stays up best.
- Recommend weight reduction.
- Advise against prolonged standing and wearing of constricting garments such as tight garters or panty girdles.
- Avoid recommending sclerotherapy except on occasion for small isolated varices or so-called spider veins.
- Consider surgical referral for persistently symptomatic veins if they are resistant to conservative Rx, cosmetically unacceptable, or the source of recurrent superficial thrombophlebitis.

BIBLIOGRAPHY

- For the current annotated bibliography on varicose veins, see the print edition of *Primary Care Medicine*, 4th edition, Chapter 35, or www.LWWmedicine.com.

Venous Insufficiency

WORKUP

- Assess for full range of causes of leg edema (see Leg Edema).
- Differentiate any accompanying leg ulcers from those due to arterial disease (see Arterial Insufficiency).

MANAGEMENT

- Recommend daily daytime use of knee-length heavyweight elastic support stockings. Have patient apply them qam and remove qhs.
- Advise periodic daytime leg elevation, and consider nocturnal leg elevation for severe edema.
- Institute mild diuretic program (e.g., hydrochlorothiazide, 25–50 mg/day) if nonpharmacologic measures insufficient.

BIBLIOGRAPHY

- For the current annotated bibliography on venous insufficiency, see the print edition of *Primary Care Medicine*, 4th edition, Chapter 35, or www.LWWmedicine.com.

Ventricular Irritability

WORKUP

GENERAL STRATEGY

- Focus workup on detection of principal independent determinants of prognosis: (1) underlying heart disease, and (2) LV failure.
- Assess complexity of ventricular ectopy (another determinant of prognosis) especially in patients with heart disease and LV failure. Ventricular tachycardia (VT) portends especially high risk of cardiac sudden death.

LAB STUDIES

- Patients with nonsustained ventricular tachycardia (NSVT) after recent MI and reduced ejection fraction should undergo EPS to test for inducible sustained VT, an indication for prophylaxis.
- Patients with syncope and clinical evidence suggesting cardiac etiology are also candidates for EPS to test for inducible sustained VT.

MANAGEMENT

- Principal goals are prevention of symptomatic sustained VT, cardiac arrest, and sudden death.
- Consider cardioverter-defibrillator implantation as Rx of choice in very-high-risk patients.
  - For primary prevention
    - In those with NSVT + inducible sustained VT in conjunction with underlying CHD and reduced ejection fraction (<0.4).
    - In those with an inherited condition posing high risk for life-threatening ventricular dysrhythmias (e.g., prolonged QT syndrome, hypertrophic cardiomyopathy), especially if accompanied by Hx of syncope or family Hx of sudden death or cardiac arrest at early age.
  - For secondary prevention
    - Hx of ventricular fibrillatory arrest and resuscitation without self-limited cause.
    - Hx of sustained VT with hemodynamic compromise in absence of self-limited cause.
    - Unexplained syncope + inducible sustained VT.
- Prescribe beta blocker Rx for all patients with malignant ventricular irritability due to underlying CAD, especially those who have had MI.
- Relegate antiarrhythmic drugs to second-line position because of proarrhythmic potential and failure in most instances to achieve significant reductions in sudden death and all-cause mortality; best results found with use of class III agents manifesting antiadrenergic activity (e.g., amiodarone).
- Consider amiodarone for high-risk patients who refuse or are not candidates for cardioverter-defibrillator implantation.

- Because drug Rx is fraught with many potentially adverse effects, undertake only in conjunction with cardiac consultation. EPS testing for ability to suppress inducible VT no longer recommended because results do not correlate with outcomes.
- Refer patients with symptomatic VT without structural heart disease for consideration of catheter radioablation.
- Note investigational combination strategies, such as cardioverter-defibrillator implantation + antiarrhythmic agent, and beta blocker use + antiarrhythmic agent.
- Promptly admit patients with underlying heart disease, LV dysfunction, and any evidence of sustained VT (very high risk of sudden death).
- Obtain immediate cardiac consultation, especially if evidence of hemodynamic compromise.
- Initiate Rx in inpatient setting, collaborating with cardiologist skilled in treating malignant ventricular arrhythmias.
- Consider outpatient assessment and initiation of Rx in asymptomatic persons with NSVT who show no hemodynamic compromise and no signs of underlying heart disease or heart failure, but prompt cardiac consultation is warranted.
- Monitor by checking for hemodynamic compromise (near-syncope, dyspnea, angina), number of shocks (in persons with defibrillators), ECG for QT interval prolongation and new dysrhythmias, and serum potassium, magnesium, creatinine, transaminase, and drug concentrations (especially if taking antiarrhythmic drugs).

BIBLIOGRAPHY

- For the current annotated bibliography on ventricular irritability, see the print edition of *Primary Care Medicine*, 4th edition, Chapter 29, or www.LWWmedicine.com.

Respiratory Problems

Asthma

WORKUP

- See Chronic Cough; Chronic Dyspnea.

MANAGEMENT

FOR ALL PATIENTS

- Before treating for asthma, always briefly consider other causes of bronchospasm and wheezing.
- Identify offending allergens and irritants; consider skin testing, especially if single allergen suspected (e.g., seasonal asthma), and desensitization if single allergen is discovered; design avoidance program for those with multiple allergens; emphasize smoking cessation for those who continue to smoke.
- Encourage active patient participation in management by providing parameters (such as changes in peak flow or symptoms) for self-initiated adjustments in Rx. Be sure patient is fully informed about medications, their side effects, and proper use.
- Teach proper use of handheld peak flowmeter, MDI, and spacer. Demonstrate and check MDI and peak flowmeter technique. Consider breath-activated inhalers for persons who cannot use MDIs.
- Provide written instructions for carrying out Rx programs for maintenance and exacerbation, with emphasis on what to do when. Keep it simple and customized to patient's capacity for compliance. Directly elicit and address patient concerns.
- Remind patients to avoid overreliance on short-acting bronchodilators for disease control and never to use antianxiety agents or sedatives in setting of exacerbation.
- Remember that severe exacerbation (peak flow <60% of predicted) can occur with any category of asthma and that prompt initiation of short course of prednisone (40–60 mg/day with rapid tapering to cessation in 5–10 days) should be considered if prompt response to bronchodilators and full doses of inhaled steroids does not occur.
- Administer trivalent influenza vaccine each fall at least 6 wks before start of flu season. Also administer pneumococcal vaccine (see Immunization).
- Arrange prompt ER care if signs of severe airway obstruction are present (e.g., peak flow reduced by 50%, pulsus paradoxus, forced expiratory volume in 1 second <1 L/s, use of accessory muscles of respiration).
- Consider referral for patients who require systemic steroids frequently or persistently.

MILD INTERMITTENT ASTHMA

- Prescribe inhaled semiselective β_2-agonist prn (e.g., 2–3 puffs albuterol, repeated in 20 mins if necessary) for episode of bronchospasm and a few mins before exercise or exposure to cold as prophylaxis for exercise- and cold-induced asthma. Avoid regular use.

- As alternative to albuterol for prophylaxis, consider trial of cromolyn or nedocromil (2 puffs inhaled a few mins before activity or cold exposure).
- If planned exercise or need for prophylactic protection against unexpected exercise is prolonged, prescribe long-acting β_2-agonist prn (e.g., 1–3 puffs salmeterol bid at least 30 mins before exercise) or leukotriene receptor antagonist (e.g., montelukast, 10 mg qam). Avoid regular use of salmeterol because it may decrease duration of protection.
- Teach patient self-management program, including proper MDI technique, importance of prn use only, and avoidance of environmental precipitants.
- Consider advancing to Rx of mild persistent asthma if patient requires >twice-weekly use of β_2-agonist Rx.

MILD PERSISTENT ASTHMA

- Add daily antiinflammatory Rx; begin low-dose inhaled glucocorticosteroids (e.g., beclomethasone, 2–4 puffs bid); to avoid corticosteroids, begin 4-wk trial of mast cell stabilizer (e.g., 2 puffs cromolyn or nedocromil bid–qid) or consider montelukast (10 mg qam).
- Teach patient how to perform periodic self-monitoring with peak flowmeter and how to make prompt adjustment in steroid dose with any decline in airflow.
- Continue Rx of acute symptoms with short-acting β_2-agonist prn. Any requirement for daily or increased dosing should lead to consideration of Rx for moderate persistent asthma.

MODERATE PERSISTENT ASTHMA

- Advance antiinflammatory program to intermediate-dose inhaled corticosteroids (e.g., 4–8 puffs beclomethasone bid).
- If nocturnal symptoms are problematic or limited steroid exposure desirable, continue low-dose inhaled steroid Rx and add long-acting β_2-agonist (e.g., 1–2 puffs salmeterol q12h) or methylxanthine (e.g., 300 mg/day extended-release theophylline qhs) to program. Never use long-acting bronchodilator in absence of corticosteroid Rx.
- Consider montelukast (10 mg qam) as another alternative for limiting steroid dose in persons with mild to moderate disease.
- Emphasize need for daily monitoring of peak flow and for increasing dose of inhaled steroid at first sign of decline.
- Continue use of short-acting β_2-agonist prn for Rx of acute symptoms; continued requirements for daily or increased dosing should lead to consideration of Rx for severe asthma.

SEVERE PERSISTENT ASTHMA

- Advance antiinflammatory program to high-dose inhaled corticosteroids (e.g., 4–6 puffs beclomethasone qid) and supplement with long-acting β_2-agonist (e.g., 2 puffs salmeterol q12h) or sustained-release theophylline (300 mg q12h, with regular monitoring of serum theophylline level).
- For acute severe exacerbations, supplement inhaled steroids with short course of high-dose systemic glucocorticosteroids (e.g., prednisone, started at 40–60 mg/day and tapered to full cessation within 5–10 days).

- Emphasize importance of regular daily monitoring of peak flow and prompt initiation of high-dose prednisone at first sign of markedly declining airway function. Have patient fill prednisone prescription and keep it for prompt initiation of Rx. Inform patient that delay in initiating steroid Rx and overreliance on short-acting bronchodilators can be dangerous.

- Continue use of short-acting β_2-agonist prn for Rx of acute symptoms and consider adding trial of inhaled ipratropium (e.g., 2 puffs prn) if β_2-agonist Rx alone insufficient for acute attack. Increase number of puffs of short-acting bronchodilator and monitor patient carefully if exacerbation is marked (e.g., peak flow <60% of predicted). Consider and start promptly a short course of systemic steroids if improvement is slow.

- Consider any persistent requirements for daily or increased dosing of bronchodilator Rx as indications to add daily systemic steroid Rx (e.g., 10–20 mg prednisone qam).

- Make repeated attempts to taper systemic steroids to lowest dose sufficient to prevent attacks and, if possible, discontinue systemic steroids; if discontinuation of systemic steroids is impossible, consider switching to alternate-day Rx (e.g., 10–20 mg qod). To facilitate tapering and maintain control, continue inhaled corticosteroid Rx at full doses in conjunction with long-acting bronchodilator program.

- Taper systemic steroids slowly if patient has been taking prednisone long enough to cause hypothalamic-pituitary-adrenal suppression (see Glucocorticoid Therapy).

- At times of stress and severe flares, be sure inhaled steroid Rx is at maximum doses and consider resuming full doses of systemic steroid Rx (e.g., prednisone, 40–60 mg/day) until episode passes.

- In refractory cases, check for and treat exacerbating factors, such as exposure to offending allergen, gastroesophageal reflux, sleep apnea, and allergic bronchopulmonary aspergillosis (suggested by eosinophil count >1,000/mL). Immunotherapy indicated if single responsible allergen is identified. Check for poor compliance with inhaled corticosteroid program and failure to monitor peak flows, which indicate need for more patient ed and counseling.

BIBLIOGRAPHY

- For the current annotated bibliography on asthma, see the print edition of *Primary Care Medicine*, 4th edition, Chapter 48, or www.LWWmedicine.com.

Bronchitis and Pneumonia

DIFFERENTIAL DIAGNOSIS

GENERAL CONSIDERATIONS

- When patients present with productive cough, dyspnea, and pleuritic chest pain, address these questions:
  - Is process limited to trachea and bronchi, or is pneumonia present?
  - Is diagnostic workup indicated or can empiric Rx begin?
  - Are antibiotics indicated and, if so, which ones?
  - Can you treat patient safely as outpatient or is hospitalization necessary?

COMMUNITY-ACQUIRED PNEUMONIA

- Bacterial
  - *S. pneumoniae*
  - *H. influenzae*
  - *Legionella* spp. (most often *L. pneumophila*)
  - *S. aureus*
  - *K. pneumoniae* (and other *Enterobacteriaceae*)
  - *M. catarrhalis*
  - *S. pyogenes*
  - Mixed aerobic/anaerobic organisms (aspiration)
- Nonbacterial
  - *M. pneumoniae*
  - *C. pneumoniae*
  - *C. psittaci*
  - *M. tuberculosis*
  - *C. burnetii* (Q fever)
- Viral (influenza virus, adenovirus)
  - *P. carinii*
- In most epidemiologic studies, *S. pneumoniae* is most common cause, followed by *H. influenzae*, influenza virus, and *Legionella*.
- "Classic" community-acquired pneumonia presents with sudden chill followed by fever, pleuritic pain, and productive cough.
- "Atypical pneumonia" syndrome, associated with mycoplasma or chlamydia infection, often begins with sore throat and headache followed by nonproductive cough and dyspnea.

INFECTIOUS ORGANISMS

Gram-Positive Organisms

- *S. pneumoniae* is agent infecting healthy young ambulatory patients but may affect all age groups. Is also responsible for acute exacerbations in patients with chronic bronchitis, but its role in acute bronchitis in healthy persons is unclear.
- *S. aureus* most commonly follows viral respiratory tract infection, particularly influenza.

Gram-Negative Organisms

- *H. influenzae* is common cause of bronchitis in adults with chronic lung disease. It is increasingly a cause of frank pneumonia, sometimes with bacteremia.

- *K. pneumoniae* typically produces pulmonary infection in debilitated patients, especially alcoholics, and klebsiella pneumonia is one of several gram-negative bacillary pneumonias seen commonly in ambulatory patients.

- *M. (Branhamella) catarrhalis* is gram-negative coccus that causes lower respiratory tract infection in some patients with COPD. DM, alcoholism, malignancy, and steroid use are other known risk factors.

- *B. pertussis*, gram-negative pleomorphic bacillus, is frequently overlooked cause of acute bronchitis that accounts for up to 25% of cases lasting ≥2 wks.

- *L. pneumophila*, aerobic, fastidious, small, gram-negative bacillus, is causative agent in 5–10% of all community-acquired pneumonia cases and in up to 30% of severe cases.

Mixed Flora

- Aspiration pneumonias are usually mixed infections caused by aerobic and anaerobic strep, *Bacteroides*, and *Fusobacterium*. Predisposing factors include alteration of consciousness (drugs, anesthesia, alcohol, head trauma) and diminution of gag reflex, which permits aspiration.

Nonbacterial Organisms

- *M. pneumoniae* is cell wall–deficient organism that accounts for 10–25% of community-acquired pneumonia cases. It is leading cause of atypical pneumonia syndrome (fever, dry cough, nonspecific infiltrate on CXR) and also cause of acute bronchitis in otherwise healthy adults.

- *C. pneumoniae* (TWAR) is obligate intracellular organism that causes atypical pneumonia or acute bronchitis. It accounts for 10–20% of community-acquired pneumonia cases, with higher rates in young adults.

Viruses

- Viruses are most common cause of acute bronchitis, accounting for >80% of all cases. Viral pneumonia resembles atypical pneumonia.

Other Infectious Agents

- Psittacosis is caused by member of *Chlamydia* group of obligate intracellular parasites transmitted from parrots or other birds (including pigeons and turkeys) to humans. Clinical features of psittacosis are indistinguishable from those of other nonbacterial pneumonias.

- Q fever, caused by *C. burnetii*, is unique among rickettsial infections in that pneumonia is prominent, no rash is associated, and spread is through inhalation of infected dust particles related to contact with cattle, sheep, goats, or infected animal hides or hide products. Clinical features of Q fever are similar to those of other nonbacterial pneumonias, except that hepatitis occurs in up to one-third of patients.

Fungi and Other Opportunistic Organisms

- Immunosuppressed patients are at heightened risk for community-acquired opportunistic infection (e.g., *Aspergillus*, *Candida*, or *Pneumocystis*; see HIV-1 Infection).

- HIV-positive patients also at increased risk for primary TB (see Tuberculosis).
- Some fungal infections may occur in immunocompetent hosts. Exposure to spore-containing dusts may lead to histoplasmosis (Midwest) or coccidioidomycosis (Southwest), characterized in initial phases by nonproductive cough, flulike illness, liver or splenic enlargement, alveolar infiltrates, and sometimes hilar adenopathy; CXR is often normal.

WORKUP

OVERALL STRATEGY

- First differentiate lower respiratory tract infection from other causes of cough (see Chronic Cough; Congestive Heart Failure; Hemoptysis; Sarcoidosis) and from URI (see Common Cold; Pharyngitis; Sinusitis).
- Predominant symptom of patient with lower respiratory tract infection is usually cough. Predominant symptom of nasal discharge, sore throat, or ear pain can direct workup away from lower respiratory tract.
- If lower tract infection suspected, focus on diagnosing pneumonia or bronchitis. You cannot reliably base distinction on any single element of Hx or PE.
- Search for specific cause is important if presentation is unusual, unique exposures are present, or patient is immunosuppressed.

HISTORY

- Hx most useful to determine additional comorbid conditions and identify unusual exposures or epidemiologic associations that may influence prognosis or clarify etiology.
- Advanced age, CHF, cerebrovascular disease, active malignancy, and renal or liver disease predict poorer outcome. Alcoholics have higher incidence of infection with gram-negative organisms, especially *K. pneumoniae*, and patients with chronic lung disease are often colonized with *H. influenzae* and *M. catarrhalis*.
- Consider nosocomial pathogens, including resistant organisms and *Pseudomonas*, in nursing home residents. HIV-positive patients are at risk for infection with several opportunistic pathogens, such as *P. carinii* and *M. tuberculosis*.
- Determine whether patients have close contact with birds (psittacosis), livestock (Q fever), or rabbits (tularemia). Patients residing in or traveling to southwestern U.S. (coccidioidomycosis) or Midwest (histoplasmosis) may acquire acute fungal pneumonia, which is usually self-limited without Rx except in immunocompromised hosts.
- Assess patients at high risk for TB exposure (immunosuppressed, homeless, exposed to known contact) for mycobacterial infection.

PHYSICAL EXAM

- No single PE finding can definitively diagnose pneumonia.
- PCP should focus on vital signs and pulmonary exam to assist Dx and prognosis. High fever (>104°F), hypothermia, tachypnea, and tachycardia are associated with increased 30-day mortality. Several studies

have demonstrated that entirely normal vital signs decreases probability of pneumonia to <1% in outpatients.

- Pulmonary exam often demonstrates crackles, although patients with bronchitis may have similar findings. Classic findings of lung consolidation (dullness to percussion, egophony, bronchial breath sounds) are more specific for pneumonia but are found in <25% of patients with CXR evidence of pneumonia.
- Some PE findings may have etiologic significance. Erythema multiforme is associated with mycoplasma pneumonia, and confusion is seen more often in legionella infection.

LAB STUDIES

- If pneumonia suspected, posteroanterior and lateral CXR confirms Dx.
- Value of routine sputum collection for Gram's stain and culture remains controversial. For patients with pneumonia, American Thoracic Society recommends empiric Rx without aggressive etiologic workup, but Infectious Disease Society of America advocates performing sputum Gram's stain and culture in all patients hospitalized with community-acquired pneumonia. Obtain sample from deep cough using nebulized saline solution if necessary, and be sure sample is interpreted by experienced observer.
- Blood cultures are positive in 10–15% of patients and may be only accurate method of identifying causative organisms. Draw blood from different sites for 2 sets of cultures before starting antibiotic Rx.
- Detection of legionella urinary antigen is accessible and rapid method for diagnosing legionnaires' disease. Perform legionella urinary antigen test in all patients with suspected legionellosis.

MANAGEMENT

OVERALL APPROACH

- You can manage many patients with community-acquired lower respiratory tract infections on outpatient basis provided that they are alert, reliable, have help available to them, and have no signs of serious compromise.
- Patients with bronchitis or pneumonia often ask for medication to relieve cough that prompted them to seek medical care. Suppression is not encouraged in patients with acute cough because cough reflex is important defense mechanism.
- Cough suppressants, which directly diminish cough reflex, include dextromethorphan and codeine. These medicines may provide temporary relief, especially when taken qhs (see Chronic Cough). Although tab form is equally effective, patients may prefer syrup for cough suppression.
- Initiate antibiotic Rx promptly when appropriate. Because most etiologic testing requires 24–48 hrs, Rx is usually empiric. Modify Rx in response to test results and patient's response to Rx. For most bacterial infections, continued Rx for 10–14 days is standard of care.
- Tailor Rx for lower respiratory tract infections to clinical syndrome and likely pathogens.

EMPIRIC THERAPY FOR LOWER RESPIRATORY TRACT INFECTIONS

- Acute bronchitis: doxycycline, erythromycin
- Acute exacerbation of chronic bronchitis: second-generation cephalosporin or second-generation macrolide (clarithromycin and azithromycin), TMP-SMX
- Community-acquired pneumonia
  - Healthy young adults: macrolide or doxycycline, newer fluoroquinolone (agents with adequate pneumococcal activity, including levofloxacin and sparfloxacin)
  - Elderly (age >60) or comorbid disease: second- or third-generation cephalosporin, or second-generation macrolide, β-lactam/β-lactamase inhibitor
  - Hospitalized patient: third-generation cephalosporin, macrolide, or both, or second-generation macrolide, newer fluoroquinolone

RECOMMENDATIONS FOR SPECIFIC PATHOGENS

- *S. pneumoniae*
  - Penicillin sensitive (MIC <0.1 μg/mL): penicillin or erythromycin
  - Intermediate penicillin resistance (MIC 0.1–1.0 μg/mL): parenteral penicillin or ceftriaxone
  - Highly penicillin resistant (MIC >2.0 μg/mL): vancomycin or newer fluoroquinolone
- *L. pneumoniae*: erythromycin or second-generation macrolide, newer fluoroquinolone
- *H. influenzae, M. catarrhalis*: second-generation cephalosporin or second-generation macrolide, TMP-SMX
- *C. pneumoniae, C. psittaci, M. pneumoniae*: doxycycline, erythromycin or second-generation macrolide, newer fluoroquinolone
- *S. aureus*: nafcillin or vancomycin (if methicillin-resistant), cefazolin
- *K. pneumoniae*: second- or third-generation cephalosporin or β-lactam/β-lactamase inhibitor, fluoroquinolone
- *S. pyogenes*: penicillin or cephalosporin, erythromycin
- *C. burnetii* (Q fever): doxycycline or chloramphenicol
- Mixed anaerobic/aerobic infection (aspiration): clindamycin or penicillin + metronidazole
- *B. pertussis*: erythromycin or second-generation macrolide, TMP-SMX
- Influenza A: amantadine or rimantadine

BRONCHITIS

- At least 8 randomized, placebo-controlled trials have failed to show benefit of empiric antibiotic Rx (doxycycline, TMP-SMX, or erythromycin) in healthy patients with acute bronchitis. Despite this, several studies have suggested that PCPs prescribe antibiotics for >60% of outpatients with acute cough and no underlying lung disease.
- One exception to this approach is patient with pertussis who is treated with 500 mg erythromycin qid for 7–14 days. Prophylactic Rx with same regimen (adjusted for weight in children) is recommended for household members and close contacts, especially unvaccinated infants. In erythromycin-intolerant patients, substi-

tute TMP-SMX or second-generation macrolide (e.g., azithromycin, clarithromycin).

■ Antibiotics are effective in relieving symptoms and preventing deterioration of lung function in patients with established chronic bronchitis. *S. pneumoniae*, *H. influenzae*, and *M. catarrhalis* are common pathogens in these patients. Second-generation β-lactam, such as cefuroxime, is Rx of choice. Alternatives include second-generation macrolide or TMP-SMX. Additional Rx depends on patient's condition and underlying lung function (see Chronic Obstructive Pulmonary Disease).

PNEUMONIA

■ Antibiotics are clearly indicated for Rx of community-acquired pneumonia, although no randomized trials have been completed. Direct initial Rx at most common pathogens, and classify patients by age, comorbidities, and severity of pneumonia.

■ In healthy adults <60 yrs, most common organisms are *S. pneumoniae*, *Mycoplasma*, *Chlamydia*, and *Legionella*. Erythromycin (500 mg qid), which is first-line Rx, adequately covers these organisms. Alternative agents include doxycycline (100 mg bid) or second-generation macrolides. Newer fluoroquinolones, such as levofloxacin, have adequate activity against pathogens and are well tolerated.

■ In older adults with comorbidity, *S. pneumoniae* remains most common cause of pneumonia, but *H. influenzae*, *M. catarrhalis*, and other gram-negative organisms are alternative possibilities. Therefore, recommended first-line Rx is second- or third-generation cephalosporin. Cefuroxime (although not officially approved for pneumonia) is common choice because it has adequate activity against common pathogens and is available in bid dosing. Alternatives include β-lactam/β-lactamase inhibitor combinations (e.g., amoxicillin/clavulanate), second-generation macrolides, and fluoroquinolones with adequate pneumococcal coverage.

■ For patients with severe pneumonia and inconclusive Gram's stain, first-line Rx is third-generation cephalosporin (e.g., 1 g/day ceftriaxone) + macrolide in dose sufficient for legionella infection (e.g., 1 g erythromycin qid). For patients in whom fluid overload is concern, divide erythromycin equally between oral and IV doses.

■ Approximately 25% of pneumococci in U.S. have intermediate penicillin resistance (MIC 0.1–1.0 µg/mL), and up to 10% are highly penicillin-resistant (MIC >2.0 µg/mL). These highly resistant organisms are often cross-resistant to multiple antibiotics, including TMP-SMX and erythromycin. Fortunately, parenteral penicillin appears to achieve adequate levels in tissues for effective Rx of pneumococci with intermediate resistance. For highly resistant organisms, alternative agents are recommended. Fluoroquinolone resistance has been very low in *S. pneumoniae*.

■ Repeating CXR at frequent intervals is wasteful if patient is progressing well clinically. Clearing of radiologic findings often lags far behind clinical resolution.

■ Base decision to hospitalize patients with community-acquired pneumonia on age, comorbid illness, and PE and lab findings. Quantitative risk estimation may be helpful in some cases.

Pneumonia Patient Outcomes Research Team Scoring

- Obtain risk score (total point score) for patient by summing patient age in yrs (age – 10 for female) and points for each applicable patient characteristic:
  - Demographic factors
    - Age
    - Male: (yrs)
    - Female: (yrs) – 10
    - Nursing home resident: +10
  - Comorbid illnesses
    - Neoplastic disease: +30
    - Liver disease: +20
    - CHF: +10
    - Cerebrovascular disease: +10
    - Renal disease: +10
  - PE findings
    - Altered mental status: +20
    - Respiratory rate >30/min: +20
    - SBP <90 mm Hg: +20
    - Temp <35°C or >40°C: +15
    - Pulse >125/min: +10
  - Lab findings
    - pH <7.35: +30
    - BUN >10.7 mmol/L: +20
    - Sodium <130 mEq/L: +20
    - Glucose >13.9 mmol/L: +10
    - Hematocrit <30%: +10
    - PO_2 <60 mm Hg (oxygen saturation <90% also considered abnormal): +10
    - Pleural effusion: +10

Adapted from Fine MJ, Auble TE, Yealy DM, et al. A prediction rule to identify low-risk patients with community-acquired pneumonia. N Engl J Med 1997;336:243, with permission.

BIBLIOGRAPHY

- For the current annotated bibliography on bronchitis and pneumonia, see the print edition of *Primary Care Medicine*, 4th edition, Chapter 52, or www.LWWmedicine.com.

Chronic Cough

DIFFERENTIAL DIAGNOSIS

GENERAL CONSIDERATIONS

- Physiologic function of cough is to remove foreign substances and mucus from respiratory tract. Cough involves deep inspiration, increasing lung volume, muscular contraction against closed glottis, and sudden opening of glottis. Keep function in mind when considering pharmacologic suppression of cough reflex.
- Causes of chronic cough differ in primary care and referral settings.
  - In primary care, asthma and postnasal drip are most common (20% each). Gastroesophageal reflux accounts for about 5%.
  - In referral setting, postnasal drip can account for 40%, asthma for about 25%, esophageal reflux for 20%, and chronic bronchitis for 5%.

COMMON CAUSES OF CHRONIC COUGH

- Environmental irritants
  - Cigarette smoking (cigar and pipe smoking to lesser degree)
  - Pollutants (sulfur dioxide, nitrous oxide, particulate matter)
  - Dusts (all agents capable of producing pneumoconioses)
  - Lack of humidity
- Lower respiratory tract problems
  - Lung cancer
  - Asthma (including variant asthma)
  - COPD (especially bronchitis)
  - Interstitial lung disease
  - CHF (chronic interstitial pulmonary edema)
  - Pneumonitis
  - Bronchiectasis
- Upper respiratory tract problems
  - Chronic rhinitis
  - Chronic sinusitis
  - Disease of external auditory canal
  - Pharyngitis
  - ACE inhibitors
- Extrinsic compressive lesions
  - Adenopathy
  - Malignancy
  - Aortic aneurysm
- Psychogenic factors
- GI problems
  - Reflux esophagitis

WORKUP

HISTORY

- Take thorough Hx to distinguish patients with serious causes of chronic cough (cancer, TB, heart failure) from those with more common treatable causes (asthma, esophageal reflux, postnasal drip).
- Among patients with chronic cough, approximately 70% have true-positive finding on Hx, 50% on PE, and 20% on lab exam.
- Ask about smoking, environmental and occupational exposures, and ACE inhibitor use.
- Review for previous allergies, asthma, sinusitis, recent respiratory infection, and TB exposure.

PHYSICAL EXAM

- Focus on upper respiratory tract, chest, and cardiovascular system.
- Examine skin for cyanosis and clubbing; pharynx for postnasal discharge, mucosal edema, and tonsillar enlargement; nose for polyps, discharge, and obstruction; sinuses for tenderness; and ears for impacted cerumen or otitis.
- Palpate trachea for position and neck for masses and adenopathy.
- Auscultate and percuss lungs (including apices) to detect wheezing, crackles, and signs of consolidation or effusion.
- During cardiac exam, evaluate jugular venous pulse for elevated systemic venous pressure, palpate for chamber enlargement, and listen for S_3 (signs of heart failure).

LAB STUDIES

- CXR is essential when Hx or PE suggests carcinoma, pneumonitis, TB, heart failure, or bronchiectasis. Test is overused and unnecessary in nonsmoker with persistent cough after recent URI and normal PE findings.
- Sinus films usually unnecessary when Hx positive for postnasal drip. There is poor correlation between appearance on films and symptoms considered typical of sinusitis.
- When CXR shows purulent sputum or infiltrate, try to obtain sputum for exam.
- When cause remains elusive despite Hx, PE, and CXR, consider postnasal drip syndrome, variant asthma, and gastroesophageal reflux. Starting empiric Rx with decongestants, bronchodilators, or H_2 antagonists is reasonable. Avoid empiric antibiotic Rx.

MANAGEMENT

- Most effective means of stopping cough is to identify and treat underlying cause (see Chronic Obstructive Pulmonary Disease; Heartburn and Reflux; Nasal Congestion and Discharge; Tuberculosis).
- Among smokers and those with passive exposure to cigarette smoke, cessation of smoking (or exposure) is key to symptom relief. Within 1 mo nearly 80% have stopped coughing and remaining 20% experience decrease.

- Patients may get symptomatic relief by maintaining appropriate humidity in surroundings and adequate hydration (≥1,500 mL fluid/day).
- Codeine is drug of choice for pharmacologic suppression of cough when indicated. Give in relatively small doses of 8–15 mg q3–4h prn. In many instances, qhs dose suffices. Liquid and tablet preparations are equally effective.
- Inhaled topically active corticosteroids and bronchodilators will decrease cough in patients with asthma. Patients with persistent cough after recent respiratory tract infection and no signs of pneumonitis may also benefit from short course of inhaled steroid Rx. Topical steroid Rx may also help in allergic rhinitis.
- Patients with suspected reflux should respond to course of antireflux Rx with antacids and H_2 blockers, although relief may take several wks.
- Follow expectantly patients with normal CXR and no risk factors for serious etiologic Dx. Bronchoscopy has low likelihood of positive study in this situation.

BIBLIOGRAPHY

- For the current annotated bibliography on chronic cough, see the print edition of *Primary Care Medicine*, 4th edition, Chapter 41, or www.LWWmedicine.com.

DIFFERENTIAL DIAGNOSIS

GENERAL CONSIDERATIONS

■ Patients experience shortness of breath when ventilatory demand exceeds actual or perceived capacity of lungs to respond. Underlying problems include altered chest wall mechanics, decreased lung compliance, airway obstruction, increased ventilatory requirements, or exogenous factors such as obesity.

CAUSES OF CHRONIC DYSPNEA

■ Cardiac
  • Congestive heart failure
  • Other causes of pulmonary venous congestion (mitral stenosis, mitral regurgitation)
■ Pulmonary
  • COPD
  • Pulmonary parenchymal disease (including interstitial diseases)
  • Pulmonary HTN
  • Severe kyphoscoliosis
  • Exogenous mechanical factors (ascites, massive obesity, large pleural effusion)
  • Chronic asthma
■ Psychological
  • Anxiety
■ Hematologic
  • Severe chronic anemia

WORKUP

HISTORY

■ Patient Hx leads to Dx in about 75% of cases, but differentiating cardiac and pulmonary causes of dyspnea can be difficult.
■ Hx of chronic cough, sputum production, recurrent respiratory infection, occupational exposure, or heavy smoking suggests lung disease rather than cardiac origin, but PE and lab studies needed for better differentiation (see below).
■ Multiple bodily complaints, Hx of emotional difficulties, absence of activity limitations, and lack of exacerbation on exercising, onset at rest, and sense of chest tightness or suffocation suggest psychogenic cause.
■ Precisely define degree of activity that causes dyspnea, estimate severity of disease, determine extent of disability, and detect changes over time.
■ Query patient about smoking, occupational exposure (see Occupational and Environmental Respiratory Disease), excessive salt intake, weight gain, and increasing sputum production.

- Ask patient about hemoptysis, which raises possibilities of bronchiectasis, endobronchial malignancy, embolization with infarction, and pneumonia.
- If embolization suspected, inquire about pleuritic chest pain, leg edema, and other symptoms of DVT (see Leg Edema), in addition to risk factors such as chronic venous insufficiency, inactivity, and, in young women, pregnancy or oral contraceptive use.
- Inquire about evidence of recurrent pulmonary embolization if you encounter pulmonary HTN.

PHYSICAL EXAM

- Check for tachycardia, tachypnea, fever, and HTN.
- Weight increase may be early sign of worsening CHF (see Congestive Heart Failure).
- Observe patient's respiratory efforts; carefully estimate work expended in breathing.
- Examine chest for increased A-P diameter (suggesting COPD) and deformity resulting from kyphoscoliosis or ankylosing spondylitis; percuss chest for dullness and hyperresonance; and auscultate for wheezes, crackles, and quality of breath sounds.
- Normal findings on lung exam do not rule out pulmonary pathology but do lessen its probability and likelihood that it is severe.
- Focus cardiac exam on signs of left-sided heart failure (see Congestive Heart Failure), detection of left-sided heart murmurs (see Asymptomatic Systolic Murmur; Valvular Heart Disease), and signs of pulmonary HTN and its consequences.
- Many signs of right-sided heart failure may be consequences of long-standing pulmonary disease and are not specific for cardiac etiology.
- Examine abdomen for ascites and hepatojugular reflux.
- Check legs for edema and other signs of phlebitis (see Bacterial Endocarditis; Stable Angina).
- Check patient's mental status for manifestations of anxiety disorder; note any excessive sighing.

LAB STUDIES

- Examine CXR for pulmonary venous redistribution, effusions, interstitial changes, hyperinflation, infiltrates, enlargement of pulmonary arteries (indicative of pulmonary HTN), cardiac chamber enlargement, and valve calcification.
- When infiltrate is present on CXR and patient is producing sputum, Gram's stain and culture are often informative, especially when patient is febrile or coughing more than usual. Ziehl-Neelsen stain for acid-fast bacilli and sputum culture for TB also important if infiltrate detected (see Tuberculosis).
- PCP can reliably perform simple pulmonary function tests in office. Forced expiratory volume in 1 second (FEV_1) and FVC are best for assessing obstructive and restrictive defects. FEV_1 to FVC ratio is markedly reduced in clinically important obstructive disease. In restrictive disease, ratio is close to 1, but FVC is significantly reduced.
- Patients with anxiety-induced dyspnea often benefit from reassurance afforded by CXR and pulmonary function testing. Anxiolytics are helpful only in patients with dyspnea as manifestation of severe anxiety disorder.

- Walk with patient up and down several flights of stairs to provide reassurance to anxious patients and to quantifying exercise tolerance in patients with cardiopulmonary disease.
- Consider treatable causes of pulmonary HTN when there are signs of right-sided heart strain on PE or ECG, or prominent pulmonary artery and hilar vessels on CXR.

MANAGEMENT

- Etiologic Dx is critical for patients with dyspnea, whether it is heart disease (see Congestive Heart Failure; Stable Angina; Valvular Heart Disease), lung disease (see Asthma; Bronchitis or Pneumonia; Chronic Obstructive Pulmonary Disease), mechanical factor such as massive obesity (see Overweight and Obesity), or anxiety disorder (see Anxiety). Explanation and prognostic information is central to care.
- Home oxygen Rx warranted if patient has condition causing chronic hypoxemia provided there is no evidence of carbon dioxide retention.
- Regular exercise can be therapeutic, and attention to changes in exercise tolerance is important aspect of monitoring for decompensation of underlying cardiopulmonary disease.

BIBLIOGRAPHY

- For the current annotated bibliography on chronic dyspnea, see the print edition of *Primary Care Medicine*, 4th edition, Chapter 40, or www.LWWmedicine.com.

Chronic Obstructive Pulmonary Disease

WORKUP

- See Chronic Dyspnea.

MANAGEMENT

BASIC MEASURES FOR ALL PATIENTS

- Review entire Rx program thoroughly with patient and family; encourage patient participation in setting goals and monitoring functional status.
- Insist on complete smoking cessation, and design comprehensive smoking cessation program (see Smoking Cessation).
- Advise patient to reduce exposure to known environmental irritants and allergens (see Asthma; Nasal Congestion and Discharge; Occupational and Environmental Respiratory Disease).
- Design, with patient participation, an exercise program; walking is probably best, although any aerobic exercise suffices. Begin with easily achieved activity level (e.g., half-maximal pace) and increase slowly in small increments. Frequency is 3–4 times/day, with duration of 5–15 mins.
- Administer to all patients with COPD (except those with known egg allergy) trivalent influenza vaccine (0.5 mL IM) each fall at least 6 wks before usual winter onset of flu season. Consider administering antiviral Rx to unvaccinated COPD patients during influenza epidemic (see Immunization).
- Administer pneumococcal vaccine to all COPD patients. Dose is 0.5 mL IM and can be given with influenza vaccine. Repeated administration after 5 yrs may be needed in elderly persons (see Immunization).
- Advise patients bothered by heavy sputum production to keep well hydrated and humidify indoor environment (particularly those living in centrally heated homes). Nebulized detergents and oral expectorants are of no proved benefit. Teach postural drainage techniques to patients bothered by difficulty raising sputum.
- Perform pulmonary function testing on all patients with peak flow rate <350 L/min, obvious bronchospasm, or dyspnea on exertion. Measure forced expiratory volume in 1 second (FEV_1) before and after inhalation of rapidly acting bronchodilator (e.g., albuterol) to determine candidacy for bronchodilator Rx.

STABLE DISEASE

Bronchodilator and Antiinflammatory Therapies

- Begin bronchodilator Rx in those with increase in FEV_1 >200 mL/s or >12% in response to bronchodilator inhalation. Also consider empiric trial of bronchodilator for those who are symptomatically dyspneic or show substantial reduction in expiratory flow rate (e.g., FEV_1 <1.5–2 L/s or FEV_1/FVC <0.5), even if they do not demonstrate response to single dose of albuterol (single-dose response does not necessarily predict response to continuous bronchodilator Rx).

- For patients with mild, intermittent symptoms, begin with MDI formulation of rapidly acting β_2-agonist (e.g., 1–2 puffs albuterol q4–6h prn). Carefully instruct patient in proper MDI use (see Asthma) and warn that dose should not be >12 puffs/24 hrs. Exert caution in prescribing for patients with heart disease because these agents are relatively cardioselective at low to moderate doses.

- For patients who require or are inadequately controlled by round-the-clock β-agonist Rx, begin MDI formulation of topically active, unabsorbed anticholinergic (e.g., 2–3 puffs ipratropium qid) and supplement with albuterol (1–4 puffs prn for acute flare, or 2 puffs qid). Instruct patients to avoid spraying ipratropium in eyes, especially if they have narrow-angle glaucoma. Sequencing and timing of combination inhaler Rx do not seem to matter.

- Judge response to bronchodilator Rx on basis of change in exercise tolerance and expiratory flow rates after about 4 wks of Rx.

- If patient demonstrates no response, halt inhaled bronchodilator Rx.

- If some bronchodilator response but control of symptoms inadequate, especially at night, consider adding sustained-release oral theophylline preparation before bed (e.g., 200–400 mg/day generic sustained-release theophylline qhs).

- Monitor symptoms closely for response after about 4 wks of Rx before deciding to continue Rx. Check serum theophylline level and adjust dose to achieve therapeutic range of 8–12 µg/mL. Do not prescribe for patients with cardiac arrhythmias, and prescribe with caution for persons with underlying CHD. Do not use anal suppository preparations.

- Consider initiation of empiric trial of glucocorticosteroids in persons who respond inadequately to bronchodilator Rx and remain symptomatic.

- For patients with stable COPD who fail to achieve adequate control of symptoms with bronchodilators, begin 2-wk trial of oral prednisone (40 mg/day) and check FEV_1 for objective improvement (>20%). If responsive, try switching to topically active inhaled corticosteroid MDI formulation (e.g., 2 puffs beclomethasone qid or 4 puffs bid), a qod prednisone program, or lowest effective dose of daily prednisone.

- After 6–8 wks, evaluate for sustained response; if no symptomatic or objective improvement, stop inhaled steroid Rx.

STABLE LATE-STAGE DISEASE

- For functionally limited patients with advanced disease, consider referral for comprehensive program of pulmonary rehabilitation that includes exercise training, breathing retraining, chest physiotherapy, psychosocial support, and patient ed. Emphasize elements that have proved most beneficial (i.e., exercise training and psychosocial support).

- Teach slow, relaxed, deep breathing to patients likely to hyperventilate when dyspneic; consider targeted inspiratory muscle training in patients with severe COPD; respiratory therapist may be of help in teaching effort.

- Be sure program includes detailed patient and family ed to help sustain benefit of rehabilitation program once completed.

- Begin long-term continuous oxygen Rx in chronically hypoxemic patients [resting PO_2 <55 mm Hg, or 56–59 mm Hg if evidence of concurrent right-sided heart failure or secondary polycythemia (hematocrit >55%) is present].

- Provide continuous administration for ≥18 hr/day. Administration for less time unlikely to improve long-term outcome and prognosis.
- Consider supplemental noncontinuous oxygen Rx during exertion to improve exercise capacity in nonhypoxemic patients only if they exhibit desaturation on pulse oximetry during exercise, or reduced diffusing capacity on routine pulmonary function testing; patient should demonstrate consistently better performance on oxygen than on air when both are administered in single-blind fashion.
- For patients with cor pulmonale, begin diuretic program (e.g., 20–40 mg/day furosemide) when peripheral edema develops; increase program prn to control fluid accumulation caused by systemic venous HTN.
- Phlebotomize patient with secondary erythrocytosis (hematocrit >55%) when acute decompensation (worsening of right-sided heart failure or hypoxemia) is present.
- Consider short-term trial of cardiac glycoside Rx (e.g., 0.25 mg/day digoxin) in patients with severe right-sided heart failure; treat for 2 wks and check for objective signs of improvement (e.g., decreased edema, lower jugular venous pressure, reduced heart size). Use with care in setting of hypoxemia, and check serum levels regularly. Monitor closely for evidence of digitalis toxicity (see Congestive Heart Failure).
- Refer for consideration of surgical Rx only nonsmoking, severely emphysematous patients who have incapacitating disease refractory to comprehensive program of maximal medical Rx and who could tolerate major thoracic surgical procedure.

ACUTE EXACERBATION

- Initiate intensive MDI bronchodilator Rx with rapidly acting β-agonist (e.g., 6–8 puffs albuterol immediately, repeated q30–60mins). Hospitalize if response inadequate (e.g., patient still manifests marked dyspnea and severe wheezing) or drug is poorly tolerated (e.g., palpitations, chest pain); if response is adequate, add 4–8 puffs ipratropium q6h, reduce albuterol to 2 puffs qid, and follow closely.
- Consider initiating empiric antibiotic Rx, but only for patients with new onset or marked increase of grossly purulent sputum in conjunction with other signs of infection (e.g., fever, elevated WBC count). Prescribe amoxicillin (500 mg tid) or TMP-SMX (1 DS tab bid); doxycycline (100 mg bid) is reasonable alternative for penicillin-allergic patients.
- Consider using broad-spectrum, penicillinase-resistant antibiotic (e.g., amoxicillin/clavulanate, later-generation cephalosporin, second-generation macrolide, or fluoroquinolone) only for patients with severe COPD who manifest signs of acute infection + risk factors for resistant organism (i.e., >4 exacerbations/yr, concurrent CHF, DM). Culturing sputum in such patients may help rationalize antibiotic choice.
- Consider 2-wk course of systemic corticosteroids (e.g., oral prednisone, starting at 40 mg/day) for those with severe exacerbation. Taper or if possible switch to qod or high-dose inhaled Rx as soon as possible (see Asthma; Glucocorticoid Therapy).

INDICATIONS FOR CONSULTATION

- Obtain pulmonary consultation when patient remains incapacitated despite comprehensive, fully implemented program of medical Rx. Sur-

gical consult is not recommended without prior recommendation of pulmonary specialist.
- Refer patients with known α_1-antitrypsin deficiency for consideration of augmentation Rx with α_1-antitrypsin only if they are nonsmokers, show signs of emphysema, are symptomatic, and have antitrypsin level <80 mg/dL.

BIBLIOGRAPHY

- For the current annotated bibliography on chronic obstructive pulmonary disease, see the print edition of *Primary Care Medicine*, 4th edition, Chapter 47, or www.LWWmedicine.com.

Clubbing

DIFFERENTIAL DIAGNOSIS

- Clubbing is enlargement and increased sponginess of nail beds of fingers and toes and reduction in angle created by nail and dorsum of distal phalanx. Sometimes accompanied by chronic subperiosteal osteitis, hypertrophic osteoarthropathy.
- With decline in incidence of chronic pulmonary infectious diseases (e.g., TB, lung abscess, and bronchiectasis), lung carcinoma has emerged as leading cause of hypertrophic osteoarthropathy.

WORKUP

OVERALL STRATEGY

- Begin with confirmation of characteristic physical findings: loss of angle made by nail and increase in ballotable characteristic of nail bed.
- Identify hypertrophic osteoarthropathy using radiography of long bones; typical changes are increase in periosteal thickness and new bone formation at distal ends.
- Once clubbing or hypertrophic osteoarthropathy confirmed, begin looking for cause.

HISTORY

- Before beginning search for serious illness, establish whether clubbing has been lifelong and is present in other family members (harmless familial variety).
- Cough, sputum production, hemoptysis, and dyspnea point to respiratory problem and may have already triggered evaluation of lungs (see Chronic Cough; Chronic Dyspnea; Hemoptysis).
- Question patient about Hx of heart murmur, exercise intolerance, prior liver disease, cramping lower abdominal pain, diarrhea, bloody stools, and joint problems.
- Assess risk factors related to development of lung cancer (see Lung Cancer).
- Ascertain exposure to TB (see Tuberculosis).

PHYSICAL EXAM

- Check for fever, tachypnea, tachycardia, cyanosis, tobacco stains, jugular venous distention, barrel chest, wheezes, rhonchi, rales (crackles), signs of consolidation or effusion, heart murmur, skin lesions of hepatocellular disease, and signs of cirrhosis.
- Palpate lymph nodes for enlargement, and check joints for hypertrophic changes and signs of inflammation.

LAB STUDIES

- Obtain CXR. Early pleural, pulmonary, or mediastinal neoplasm may be asymptomatic.

- CBC and exam of stool for occult blood may be helpful.
- Undertake further evaluation of liver, thyroid, heart, or bowel only if symptoms or PE suggest disease in these areas.
- Follow for development of pulmonary neoplasm patients with new-onset clubbing and long Hx of smoking; periodic exams including sputum cytology and CXR are appropriate.
- Differentiating osteoarthropathy from rheumatoid disease can be difficult.

MANAGEMENT

- No symptomatic Rx available for clubbing. Treat bone and joint discomfort due to hypertrophic osteoarthropathy with aspirin.
- Inform patient that clubbing can be harmless finding in addition to helpful guide to early Dx of disease.
- Strongly advise smoking cessation (see Smoking Cessation).

BIBLIOGRAPHY

- For the current annotated bibliography on clubbing, see the print edition of *Primary Care Medicine*, 4th edition, Chapter 45, or www.LWWmedicine.com.

Common Cold

MANAGEMENT

OVERALL APPROACH

- "Common cold" describes self-limited catarrhal illness caused by variety of respiratory viruses. PCP's task is to distinguish common cold from bacterial infections, allergic conditions, and epidemic diseases such as influenza. Once common cold diagnosed, reassure patient about its self-limited nature and give advice about symptomatic Rx. Avoid antibiotics, which are frequently prescribed inappropriately.
- Transmission can occur through virus-laden respiratory secretions that travel only a few ft. Most efficient transmission is direct mucous membrane contact with virus, usually on contaminated hands, with subsequent self-inoculation by touching nose or eyes.
- Prospective controlled studies suggest that psychological stress, especially chronic life stresses and poor social supports, can increase infection risk.
- If patient has typical influenza symptoms, consider further diagnostic testing using rapid testing. Otherwise, identifying specific virus causing common cold is impractical and unimportant.

SYMPTOMATIC THERAPY

- Sympathomimetics are mainstay of decongestant Rx; nasal sprays are good for short-term Rx, whereas oral preparations are better when Rx must continue >3–4 days. These agents can worsen symptomatic benign prostatic hypertrophy and glaucoma, and patients with these conditions should avoid them.
- Use of prescription second-generation, nonsedating antihistamine has no place in management of common cold because these agents have little anticholinergic activity and cold symptoms have no allergic pathophysiology.
- Ipratropium, a topically active anticholinergic now available as nasal spray, is being heavily promoted for relief of nasal symptoms of common cold. Trials have shown significant reduction in subjective and objective measures of rhinorrhea and sneezing compared to saline placebo. Side effects include increased nasal dryness and blood-tinged mucus in about 10–15% of subjects. It is expensive.
- Among analgesics, aspirin is least costly; other agents can be expensive. Acetaminophen has similar effects. Aspirin and acetaminophen have been shown to delay immune response in lab studies.
- Hydration helps loosen secretions and prevent upper airway obstruction and complications. Warm fluids can increase rate of mucus flow as can inhaled steam or use of dilute saline nasal spray.
- Cough suppressants, including narcotics such as codeine and non-narcotic agents such as dextromethorphan, are effective and useful symptomatically, especially in allowing patient to sleep uninterrupted by cough.
- Results of well-designed, controlled studies using zinc gluconate lozenges have been equally divided between showing efficacy and show-

ing no benefit. *Echinacea* extracts have gained widespread acceptance in Germany as Rx for common cold. Although many randomized trials have suggested reduction of symptoms, evidence remains inconclusive. In general, you should not recommend these combination preparations as first-line Rx.

- Amantadine and rimantadine are oral antiviral drugs effective only against influenza A. Rimantadine is more expensive but has fewer side effects, notably fewer CNS effects. Dosage for both drugs is 100 mg bid, except in the elderly, in whom decreased drug clearance allows for once-daily dosing. Discontinue after 3–5 days (or earlier if symptoms resolve) to decrease opportunity for drug resistance.

- Neuraminidase inhibitors zanamivir and oseltamivir are newly approved agents active against influenza A and influenza B and decreasing illness duration by 1.0–1.5 days if administered within 48 hrs of symptom onset. Zanamivir is administered by inhaler bid; oseltamivir is given as pill (75 mg) bid.

- Relief from cold symptoms and avoidance of complications are facilitated by rest, adequate fluid intake, aspirin, and perhaps steam inhalation. Taking cough suppressant qhs (e.g., 15 mg codeine sulfate) and using sympathomimetic nasal decongestant spray for several days (e.g., phenylephrine; see Sinusitis) may aid symptomatic management and are superior to expensive combination agents.

- Treat incapacitating rhinorrhea and sneezing not well controlled by first-generation antihistamines with short course of ipratropium nasal spray (2 sprays 0.06% solution in each nostril qid).

PATIENT EXPECTATIONS

- Explain role of antibiotic Rx in viral URI (i.e., only for complications such as otitis and sinusitis) in addition to risks of unnecessary antibiotic Rx (e.g., allergic reactions, alteration of bacterial flora, emergence of resistant strains). Unnecessary office visits and phone calls have been reduced 30–40% through well-designed patient ed.

- Proactive patient ed just before start of cold season may reduce unnecessary office visits, phone calls, and antibiotic requests. Zinc and *Echinacea* remain popular among patients, but efficacy has not been clearly demonstrated. Second-generation antihistamines and antibiotics are useless in uncomplicated viral URI.

BIBLIOGRAPHY

- For the current annotated bibliography on common cold, see the print edition of *Primary Care Medicine*, 4th edition, Chapter 50, or www.LWWmedicine.com.

Hemoptysis

DIFFERENTIAL DIAGNOSIS

GENERAL CONSIDERATIONS

- Most patients with hemoptysis have inconsequential lesions, but thorough evaluation is necessary because seriousness of underlying cause does not correlate with amount of blood coughed up.
- In most cases, blood-tinged sputum originates in upper respiratory tract. Detailed or elaborate evaluation is unnecessary when such source is evident.

IMPORTANT CAUSES OF HEMOPTYSIS

- Gross hemoptysis
  - TB (with cavitary disease)
  - Bronchiectasis
  - Bronchial adenoma
  - Bronchogenic carcinoma (uncommon)
  - Aspergilloma
  - Necrotizing pneumonia
  - Lung abscess
  - Pulmonary contusion
  - Arteriovenous malformation
  - Hereditary hemorrhagic telangiectasia
  - Bleeding disorder or excessive anticoagulant Rx
  - Mitral stenosis (with bronchial vessel rupture)
  - Immune alveolar disease
- Blood-streaked sputum
  - Any cause of gross hemoptysis
  - URI
  - Chronic bronchitis
  - Sarcoidosis
  - Bronchogenic carcinoma
  - TB
  - Pulmonary infarction
  - Pulmonary edema
  - Mitral stenosis
  - Idiopathic pulmonary hemosiderosis
  - Immune alveolar disease

WORKUP

HISTORY

- Concern about pulmonary neoplasm should be highest in older men with long Hx of heavy smoking or asbestos exposure.
- Presume reactivated TB in elderly patients with evidence of old disease on CXR.

- Adolescents with hemoptysis may have new infection resulting from recent TB exposure.
- Compromised host with previous cavitary disease is at risk for aspergilloma.
- Patient's description of hemoptysis-associated sputum helpful:
  - Pink sputum: pulmonary edematous fluid
  - Putrid sputum: lung abscess
  - Material resembling currant jelly: necrotizing pneumonia
  - Copious purulent sputum mixed with blood: bronchiectasis
  - Blood-streaked sputum: nonspecific
- Ask patient about previous episodes of bleeding, family Hx of hemoptysis, hematuria, concurrent pleuritic chest pain, known heart murmur or Hx of rheumatic fever, lymph node enlargement, blunt chest trauma, symptoms of heart failure (see Congestive Heart Failure), and anticoagulant drug use.
- Be certain that patient has no Hx of coexisting nasopharyngeal problem or source of GI bleeding that may be mistaken for true hemoptysis.

PHYSICAL EXAM

- Focus PE on detecting nonpulmonary sources of bleeding and evidence of chest and systemic disease.
- Check vital signs for fever and tachypnea, skin for ecchymoses and telangiectases, nails for clubbing [associated with neoplasm, bronchiectasis, lung abscess, and other severe pulmonary disorders (see Clubbing)], nodes for enlargement [suggestive of sarcoidosis, TB, and malignancy (see Lymphadenopathy; Sarcoidosis)], and neck for jugular venous distention (consistent with heart failure and severe mitral disease).
- Examine chest for bruits, signs of consolidation, wheezes, crackles, and chest wall contusion.

LAB STUDIES

- When no evident upper respiratory source, CXR is essential to assessment. Vast majority of patients with hemoptysis resulting from bronchogenic carcinoma have abnormal CXR.
- If sputum appears grossly purulent or patient is febrile, perform sputum Gram's stain. Acid-fast stain for tubercle bacilli is also essential for Dx and for rough assessment of contagion (see Tuberculosis).
- Sensitivity of acid-fast smear depends on technique and can be as low as 20% of culture-positive samples. Despite very high specificity of positive smear, predictive value may be as low as 50% when sputum specimens of low-risk patients are examined.
- Perform tuberculin skin test if patient's PPD reactivity status is unknown. About 7% of adults (25% of adults aged >50) have positive reactions (see Tuberculosis).
- Obtain sputum cytologies in all patients without clear Dx. Sensitivity is limited to 70%; specificity approaches 100% when interpreted by experienced cytopathologist.
- Do not view fiberoptic bronchoscopy as routine part of hemoptysis evaluation. Yield is extremely low in situations in which risk for malignancy is very low (e.g., nonsmokers aged <50 with normal CXR).

- Chest CT will better define suspect lesion seen on CXR. CT may be indicated for some patients with normal CXR and risk factors for parenchymal or endobronchial lesions.
- Cryptogenic hemoptysis (hemoptysis in patients with normal or nonlocalizing CXR and nondiagnostic findings on fiberoptic bronchoscopy) has favorable prognosis. Of these patients, >90% have resolution of hemoptysis by 6 mos. No cases of cancer, active TB, or other serious pathology are reported in most series.
- Patients with hemoptysis at increased risk for underlying malignancy (abnormal CXR, male sex, age >50, smoking Hx) are candidates for bronchoscopy.
- Hospitalize patients with brisk bleeding.

BIBLIOGRAPHY

- For the current annotated bibliography on hemoptysis, see the print edition of *Primary Care Medicine*, 4th edition, Chapter 42, or www.LWWmedicine.com.

Interstitial Lung Disease

DIFFERENTIAL DIAGNOSIS

CAUSES OF INTERSTITIAL LUNG DISEASE

- Pneumoconiosis
  - Silicosis
  - Asbestosis
  - Coal worker's pneumoconiosis
  - Berylliosis
  - Organic dusts (pigeons, turkey, duck, chicken, humidifier)
- Drugs
  - Chemotherapeutic agents (busulfan, bleomycin, methotrexate)
  - Antibiotics (nitrofurantoin, sulfonamides, isoniazid)
  - Gold
  - Amiodarone
  - Penicillamine
  - Lupus-like reactions (hydralazine, procainamide)
  - Radiation
- Connective tissue disease
  - SLE
  - RA
  - Scleroderma
  - Polymyositis
- Primary lung disease
  - Sarcoidosis
  - Histiocytosis X
  - Lymphangiomyomatosis
  - Lymphangiectatic carcinomatosis
  - Lipoidosis
- Alveolar filling disease
  - Diffuse alveolar bleeding (Goodpasture's syndrome, lupus, mitral stenosis, idiopathic pulmonary hemosiderosis)
  - Alveolar proteinosis
  - Alveolar cell carcinoma
  - Eosinophilic pneumonia
  - Lipoid pneumonia
- Other
  - Idiopathic pulmonary fibrosis
  - Bronchiolitis obliterans with organizing pneumonia
  - Lymphocytic interstitial pneumonia

WORKUP

HISTORY

- Focus Hx on duration of symptoms, speed of progression, and presence of fever, hemoptysis, pleuritic chest pain, and symptoms of extrathoracic disease (e.g., joint pain, lymphadenopathy, skin changes).

- Most conditions have chronic, progressive course, but acute onset with fever and rapidly progressive course suggests hypersensitivity pneumonitis.
- Fever, bothersome dry cough, and subacute course (2–10 wks) accompanied by patchy, bilateral air space process characterize bronchiolitis with obliterans organizing pneumonia, in which lymphocytic infiltrate and granulation tissue occupy distal airways and alveoli.
- Productive cough is rare, but its presence indicates fluid-filled alveoli (as in diffuse alveolar cell carcinoma). Hemoptysis suggests conditions that cause diffuse alveolar bleeding (e.g., Goodpasture's syndrome, lupus, severe mitral stenosis, idiopathic pulmonary hemosiderosis). Bleeding that originates from or occurs in context of upper airway disease is hallmark of Wegener's granulomatosis.
- Pleuritic pain indicates spread of inflammatory process to pleura, characteristic of connective tissue diseases and some drug-induced conditions. Sudden, severe pleuritic pain and acute dyspnea raise question of spontaneous pneumothorax, which occurs with many primary lung diseases (e.g., histiocytosis X, lymphangiomyomatosis).
- Extrapulmonary symptoms, especially if they predate lung findings, can be diagnostic.
- Polyarticular symptoms and skin changes characterize connective tissue/rheumatoid diseases and sarcoidosis; latter often associated with lymph gland enlargement. Patients with idiopathic pulmonary fibrosis may have arthralgias, but symptoms of joint inflammation are absent.
- Hx of renal disease, especially nephritis, can be clue for Goodpasture's syndrome and lupus, although in former, pulmonary disease usually predates renal involvement.
- Drug and occupational Hx are most important parts of assessment. Long-term use of chemotherapeutic agents (e.g., methotrexate, busulfan, bleomycin, cyclophosphamide) may result in interstitial lung changes, as may prolonged use of nitrofurantoin, gold, amiodarone, or penicillamine. Radiation Rx may trigger diffuse pneumonitis 6–12 wks after Rx, followed by fibrosis. Occupational exposures, including distant ones, to inorganic dusts (e.g., silicone, asbestos, talc, beryllium, and coal) deserve careful review. Query patients with hypersensitivity pneumonitis about occupational exposure to organic dusts. Also ask about nasal inhalation of cocaine, which has been reported as cause of hypersensitivity pneumonitis.
- Smoking Hx is always pertinent. Uncommon for lung disease to develop in nonsmoking patients with Goodpasture's syndrome.

PHYSICAL EXAM

- PE is particularly useful for signs of extrathoracic disease; pulmonary findings usually nonspecific.
- Check skin for signs of connective tissue disease (rheumatoid nodules, malar flush, changes of scleroderma) and sarcoidosis, and lymph nodes for sarcoid-related enlargement.
- For patients with hemoptysis, perform upper airway exam, including search for necrotizing changes in nasal passages and sinuses that typify Wegener's granulomatosis.

- Examine joints for evidence of inflammation (swelling, warmth, redness, effusion) indicative of rheumatoid disease but also occurring with sarcoidosis and Wegener's granulomatosis.

- Enlargement of liver and spleen are often features of sarcoidosis and occasional findings in advanced connective tissue disease and histiocytosis X.

- Pulmonary findings are typically nonspecific and may be grossly normal. Bilateral basilar rales are common in many forms of interstitial lung disease, especially drug-related, idiopathic, connective tissue, and pneumoconiosis varieties. In those conditions associated with alveolar filling, rales are likely to be "wet," whereas those without fluid in alveoli produce "dry" crackles (sometimes referred to as "Velcro" rales) on end inspiration.

- Check heart for mitral stenosis if patient has Hx of hemoptysis, and for signs of cor pulmonale and right-sided failure (right ventricular heave or S_3, increased intensity of S_2, jugular venous distention, peripheral edema) resulting from chronic hypoxemia-induced pulmonary HTN.

LAB STUDIES

Chest X-Ray

- Findings are usually nonspecific but can be helpful. No particular radiographic pattern is diagnostic, although several emerge as useful.

- Alveolar filling diseases tend to produce alveolar densities in ill-defined or "fluffy" nodular pattern; air bronchogram might ensue as involved alveoli become silhouetted by uninvolved airway. Development of this pattern in patient with previous interstitial disease suggests superimposed process, such as alveolar cell carcinoma or active inflammation.

- Frankly nodular infiltrates are seen with sarcoidosis and Wegener's granulomatosis; nodular infiltrates may occur with pneumoconioses and hypersensitivity pneumonitis.

- Radiographic findings outside lung parenchyma are important and worth noting. Concurrent appearance of pleural involvement suggests connective tissue disease, asbestosis, and occasionally sarcoidosis. Bilateral hilar adenopathy can be pathognomonic of sarcoidosis. Diffuse infiltrates, hilar adenopathy, and pneumothorax point to histiocytosis X. Thin rim of calcium in hilar nodes is characteristic of silicosis.

Pulmonary Function Tests

- Help confirm interstitial nature of disease (particularly when radiographic findings are minimal) and provide baseline for judging disease course.

- Forced expiratory volume in 1 second (FEV_1)/FVC ratio increases and demonstrates restrictive pattern secondary to steady reduction in FVC. Some interstitial conditions (e.g., lymphangiomyomatosis, histiocytosis X) can also cause airway obstruction and may reduce FEV_1.

- Diffusion capacity is typically reduced, although it may be preserved until late in course of illness, when mismatching of ventilation and perfusion becomes prominent.

- Arterial blood gases are initially normal, but with disease progression, hypoxemia, hypocarbia, and respiratory alkalosis ensue.

Other Tests

- Few routine noninvasive lab studies are of diagnostic value.

- Urinalysis can provide important evidence of glomerular injury (RBCs, casts, albuminuria) suggestive of connective tissue disease, Wegener's granulomatosis, and Goodpasture's syndrome.
- Order most other tests only when Hx, PE, and CXR indicate reasonable pretest probability of suspected condition.
- If connective tissue disease suspected, consider RF, ANA, and DNA binding studies (see Polyarticular Complaints) and urinalysis.
- Hypersensitivity pneumonitis, especially if drug-induced, may produce finding of 10–20% eosinophils on peripheral smear exam, but sensitivity is low (20%).
- ACE level is useful for gauging disease activity but lacks sensitivity for Dx of sarcoidosis.
- Measurement of precipitating antibodies is frequently ordered for suspected inhalation of potentially sensitizing organic dust, but test does not distinguish between etiologic role and exposure.
- Patients with suspected Goodpasture's syndrome are usually positive for antiglomerular basement membrane antibody. Patients with Wegener's granulomatosis test positive for antineutrophil cytoplasmic autoantibodies in only 60% of cases, but specificity is high (<95%).
- Fiberoptic bronchoscopy with bronchoalveolar lavage provides opportunity to sample cellular and fluid contents of distal airways (counts of total WBCs, macrophages, lymphocytes and lymphocyte subsets, neutrophils, and eosinophils; malignant cells; antibodies). Alterations in normal cellular profile may aid Dx, as can discovery of malignant cells. Because of considerable overlap among causes, findings are usually nonspecific. Lavage data sometimes help stage illness and predict response to Rx.
- Except for patients with connective tissue disease, pneumoconiosis, or drug- or radiation-induced disease, most patients with interstitial lung disease usually require tissue Dx. Morbidity of transbronchial biopsy is low, but it rarely establishes definitive tissue Dx.
- Most forms of interstitial disease that necessitate tissue Dx require more tissue than that obtained using transbronchial approach. When sarcoidosis, lymphangitic carcinomatosis, or alveolar filling disease suspected, transbronchial biopsy may suffice. In most other instances, open lung biopsy or, when experienced operator is available, video-assisted thoracic lung biopsy is required.

BIBLIOGRAPHY

- For the current annotated bibliography on interstitial lung disease, see the print edition of *Primary Care Medicine*, 4th edition, Chapter 51, or www.LWWmedicine.com.

Occupational and Environmental Respiratory Disease

SCREENING AND/OR PREVENTION

- Include occupational/environmental Hx as routine part of screening medical exam in all patients.
- Recommend testing when Hx suggests exposure (see below).
- Ultimate goal in prevention is to eliminate exposure by using rigorous engineering and environmental controls. Removal from job or home should be last resort.

WORKUP

LAB STUDIES

- Consider obtaining DLCO determination if pulmonary fibrosis is a concern, CXR if pneumoconiosis suspected, and prework and postwork spirometry supplemented by bronchial provocation testing if occupational asthma is possible.
- If Dx confirmed, inform patient and explain possible relation to occupational or environmental causes. Ascertaining patient understanding is important because of statutes of limitation associated with legal remedies, such as workers' compensation.

MANAGEMENT

- Work with patient, employer, and community if possible to develop reasonable approach to reducing or eliminating causal exposure.
- Inform employee and regulatory agencies, such as OSHA or EPA, of any serious or potentially life-threatening hazards to patient, co-workers, or other citizens to facilitate evaluation of workplace and environment and elimination of toxic exposure.
- Encourage patients to abstain from habits such as smoking that are toxic to lungs and exacerbate respiratory effects of workplace and environmental exposures.
- Institute appropriate medical surveillance for subsequent development of other exposure-related pulmonary disease, such as lung cancer.

BIBLIOGRAPHY

- For the current annotated bibliography on occupational and environmental respiratory disease, see the print edition of *Primary Care Medicine*, 4th edition, Chapter 39, or www.LWWmedicine.com.

Pleural Effusions

DIFFERENTIAL DIAGNOSIS

CAUSES OF PLEURAL EFFUSION

- Transudates
  - CHF
  - Hypoalbuminemia, severe
  - Salt-retention syndromes
  - Ascites secondary to cirrhosis
  - Early phases of sympathetic effusion
  - Neoplasm (on occasion)
  - Peritoneal dialysis
  - Postpartum
  - Cardiac bypass graft surgery
- Exudates
  - Neoplasms
    - Bronchogenic carcinoma
    - Breast cancer
    - Lymphoma
    - Mesothelioma
    - Meigs's syndrome
  - Infections
    - TB (and atypical mycobacteria in AIDS patients)
    - Bacterial pneumonia (including empyema)
    - Viral pneumonitis
    - Mycoplasmal pneumonia
    - Pneumocystis pneumonia
  - Pulmonary embolization
  - Connective tissue disease
    - RA
    - SLE
  - Intra-abdominal disease
    - Subphrenic abscess
    - Pancreatitis
  - Idiopathic

ETIOLOGIC DIAGNOSIS

- Begin by distinguishing transudates from exudates.
  - Effusion is transudative if 2 of these criteria are met:
    - Pleural fluid protein to serum protein ratio <0.5
    - Pleural fluid LDH to serum LDH ratio <0.6
    - Pleural fluid LDH < two-thirds ULN for serum LDH
  - Effusion is exudative if above ratios or levels exceeded.
- Most effusions due to CHF are bilateral, but there can be isolated right-sided effusions; isolated left-sided effusions due to CHF are rare.

- Transudative effusion associated with pulmonary embolus may result from localized interstitial edema. Effusions resulting from infarction are more likely to be bloody.
- Intra-abdominal diseases occasionally cause transudative effusions. Between 5% and 10% of patients with ascites due to cirrhosis develop right-sided pleural effusion; composition of effusion resembles that of ascitic fluid.
- Pleural effusions are common after coronary bypass graft surgery and do not imply serious pathology. Same holds for postpartum patients. Transudates may form in setting of pericardial disease, myxedema, and sarcoidosis; mechanism(s) unknown.
- Exudates result from inflammatory or infiltrative disease of pleura and its adjacent structures; damage occurs to capillary membranes, and protein-rich material accumulates in pleural space.
- Bronchogenic carcinoma is tumor most frequently associated with pleural effusion.
- Pleural effusions due to metastatic carcinoma are more likely to be bilateral than those due to bronchogenic carcinoma because they result from lymphatic obstruction or diffuse seeding of pleura. When effusions are due to seeding, cytologic exam of pleural fluid is positive in up to 90 percent of cases.
- Breast carcinoma is leading metastatic tumor producing pleural effusions, accounting for 25% percent of malignant effusions.
- About 5% of patients with pneumococcal pneumonia develop effusion, usually small and transient. Such effusions are parapneumonic, implying that bacteria need not have entered pleural space to cause effusion.
- Dx of empyema is reserved for cases in which organisms are recovered from pleural fluid by Gram's stain or culture.
- Empyema is rare but worrisome event seen in <1% of outpatient pneumococcal pneumonias, with most cases occurring due to delayed antibiotic Rx.

WORKUP

HISTORY

- Ask about fever, cough, sputum production, chest pain, dyspnea, edema, abdominal pain; Hx of malignant, hepatic, renal, or HIV; exposure to TB or asbestos; and symptoms of rheumatoid disease (see Polyarticular Complaints).
- Cough, fever, and sputum production with pleuritic chest pain suggest pneumonitis with pleural involvement. Pleuritic pain is also consistent with embolization, malignancy, and pleural inflammation with adjacent pericarditis due to connective tissue disease.
- Dyspnea may be induced by effusion alone, but symptom indicates CHF when accompanied by orthopnea and paroxysmal nocturnal dyspnea.
- Hx of peripheral edema raises possibilities of hypoalbuminemia, volume overload, and CHF. Hx of alcohol abuse, recent abdominal surgery, or abdominal pain or distention points to source below diaphragm.

PHYSICAL EXAM

- Assess for respiratory compromise and check vital signs for fever and weight change.
- Inspect integument for petechiae, purpura, spider angiomas, jaundice, clubbing (see Clubbing), manifestations of rheumatoid disease (see Polyarticular Complaints), and rashes.
- Check neck for jugular venous distention and tracheal deviation; lymph nodes for enlargement; breasts for masses; and extremities for edema, calf tenderness, and signs of joint inflammation.
- On lung exam, determine level of effusion and extent of involvement. Note any compression of adjacent lung, suggested by egophony and bronchial breath sounds heard above effusion. Pleural friction rub may be audible but usually lacking when there is considerable fluid accumulation.
- Check heart for S_3 indicative of pump failure, and 3-component friction rub suggestive of pericarditis.
- Examine abdomen for signs of ascites, organomegaly, focal tenderness, and peritonitis (see Abdominal Pain).
- Perform pelvic exam to rule out ovarian mass.

LAB STUDIES

- Perform CXR and pleural fluid analysis. Study CXR for pleural-based densities, infiltrates, signs of CHF (see Congestive Heart Failure), hilar adenopathy, coin lesions, and fluid loculation (detection of which requires lateral decubitus views).

Diagnostic Thoracentesis

- When etiology not readily evident from Hx, PE, and CXR, perform diagnostic thoracentesis (need not be performed on first visit). Follow with CXR afebrile patients with clinical evidence of CHF, postpartum women who are otherwise well, patients who have had bypass graft surgery, or young patients with small effusion in conjunction with viral or mycoplasmal pneumonia; if effusion does not clear with resolution of presumptive etiology, perform thoracentesis.
- Because pleural fluid rises in meniscus in which it contacts parietal pleura, pass thoracentesis needle into chest 1 interspace above upper border of effusion as determined by exam. Avoid injury to neurovascular bundle along inferior surface of rib by aiming needle just above rib's superior margin, accomplished by "walking" needle over anesthetized surface of rib.
- Minimize pneumothorax by withdrawing or changing needle position as soon as air bubbles begin to appear or visceral pleura contacts needle tip; onset of coughing is common at this stage.
- Low pleural fluid glucose level (<60 mg/dL) is associated with TB, other serious infections, and advanced pleural involvement with malignancy. Low pleural fluid pH (<7.30) has similar meaning. Very low glucose levels (<30 mg/dL) usually associated with effusion of rheumatoid arthritis.
- In about 15% of cases, etiology of exudative effusion is not evident after complete lab analysis of pleural fluid from initial thoracentesis. If suspicion of malignancy persists, repeat thoracentesis. Sensitivity approaches 90% with submission of fluid specimens from 3 separate pleural taps in patients with underlying malignancy.

- Pleural biopsy alone may be less sensitive than cytologic exam of pleural fluid in detecting malignancy, but tests are complementary, with sensitivity >90% when used together. Pleural biopsy is most useful in detecting TB, with sensitivity of 60–80%.

MANAGEMENT

- Manage pain in patients before establishing Dx. Pleuritic pain often responds to indomethacin, which is superior to narcotics because it does not suppress respiration.
- Remove fluid when effusion is compromising respiratory efforts. Remove ≤1 liter each time to avoid intravascular volume depletion on reequilibration.
- Malignant pleural effusions are notoriously difficult to treat in setting of advanced disease with marked pleural involvement (pleural fluid pH <7.30 and glucose <60 mg/dL). Comfort measures preferable to repeated attempts at sclerosing Rx under such circumstances [see Cancer (General)].

BIBLIOGRAPHY

- For the current annotated bibliography on pleural effusions, see the print edition of *Primary Care Medicine*, 4th edition, Chapter 43, or www.LWWmedicine.com.

Sarcoidosis

DIFFERENTIAL DIAGNOSIS

- Sarcoidosis is a granulomatous disease of unknown etiology. Early disease is reversible, either spontaneously or with corticosteroid Rx, but fibrosis that characterizes advanced chronic sarcoidosis is irreversible.
- Most common presentation is bilateral hilar adenopathy which occurs in 50% of patients and is often detected on routine CXR. About 25% present with bilateral hilar adenopathy and pulmonary infiltrates, and 15% present with infiltrates alone. Some patients exhibit cough, shortness of breath, wheezing, or chest discomfort, in addition to constitutional symptoms of fever, malaise, and fatigue.
- Biopsy confirmation of sarcoidosis may be unnecessary in HIV-negative asymptomatic patients with bilateral hilar adenopathy and negative PE findings (see Interstitial Lung Disease) or erythema nodosum or uveitis. Some clinicians prefer to obtain tissue Dx in all cases of sarcoidosis, including those with asymptomatic bilateral hilar adenopathy.

WORKUP

LAB STUDIES

- For tissue Dx of hilar adenopathy, mediastinoscopy is most direct approach. To document pulmonary sarcoid, fiberoptic bronchoscopy with transbronchial biopsy is favored (sensitivity, 60–80%).
- Serum levels of ACE are elevated in about 70% of patients with active sarcoidosis, but ACE determinations lack sensitivity and specificity for establishing sarcoidosis Dx. Same is true of scanning with gallium 67.

MANAGEMENT

- Reassure patients with clear lungs and asymptomatic hilar adenopathy that they have excellent prognosis. In one large series of untreated cases, complete remission occurred in >75% within 5 yrs. In 50% with untreated pulmonary parenchymal involvement, complete resolution occurred within 2 yrs.
- Rx goals include relief of symptoms and prevention of significant impairment of organ function.
- When instituting Rx, most authorities recommend starting with large daily doses of steroids (e.g., 40–60 mg prednisone) given for 6 wks–6 mos, then tapering and/or switching to qod Rx (e.g., 15–25 mg qod) if measures of disease activity indicate response. Improvement is usually evident by 2–3 wks.
- Steroid Rx most effective when instituted before development of pulmonary fibrosis, but there is no evidence that prophylactic Rx prevents fibrosis or is worth adverse effects of long-term steroid use (see Glucocorticoid Therapy).

- Counsel patients about side effects and risks. Inhaled steroids have not been proved effective.
- Because adrenal corticosteroids are indicated for active ocular disease, patients with sarcoid should have ophthalmologic exam. Topical steroids may be used, but systemic Rx is usually added.
- Steroid Rx is also indicated for significant or progressive involvement of any other organ, which may present as onset of hepatitis, facial nerve palsies, meningitis, myocardial conduction defects, hypercalcemia, or persistent constitutional symptoms (fever, fatigue).
- Methotrexate, chloroquine, and cyclosporine have been used, but effectiveness is not well documented.
- Neither CXR nor determination of lung volumes and confusion capacity is sensitive measure of disease activity. Nevertheless, best current approach to monitoring appears to be serial determinations of diffusion capacity and lung volumes + CXR, or serial determinations of ACE levels (if initial serum ACE level is elevated).
- Emphasize need for careful follow-up in asymptomatic patients (to detect development of functional abnormalities) and symptomatic patients (to document objective benefits of Rx).
- Instruct patients about early signs of important complications, such as red eyes, blurred vision, eye pain, and dyspnea on exertion.

BIBLIOGRAPHY

- For the current annotated bibliography on sarcoidosis, see the print edition of *Primary Care Medicine*, 4th edition, Chapter 51, or www.LWWmedicine.com.

Sleep Apnea

DIFFERENTIAL DIAGNOSIS

GENERAL CONSIDERATIONS

- Be aware of varied manifestations of sleep apnea so that you can begin timely workup and institute Rx before onset of potentially life-threatening consequences.
- Adverse cardiovascular consequences of sleep apnea are due to hypoxemia and increased pulmonary vascular resistance, which can lead to pulmonary HTN and cor pulmonale, particularly in persons with underlying COPD or morbid obesity. Compensatory increases in sympathetic tone contribute to systemic HTN, cardiac arrhythmias, and increased cardiovascular M&M. Sleep apnea is independent risk factor for HTN.
- Severe obstructive sleep apnea can also lead to hypercarbia and central suppression of respiration, as seen in persons with obesity-hypoventilation (pickwickian) syndrome.
- Dysmenorrhea and amenorrhea are consequences in women of reproductive age.
- Suppressive effects of alcohol and sedatives on neuromuscular function may explain their role in exacerbating obstructive sleep apnea.

RISK FACTORS

- Nuchal obesity
- Deviated septum
- Nasal polyps
- Enlarged uvula and soft palate
- Small chin with deep overbite
- Enlarged tonsils
- Hypertrophy of lateral pharyngeal musculature
- Hypothyroidism

WORKUP

OVERALL STRATEGY

- Obstructive sleep apnea may present as daytime tiredness, and PCP must differentiate from other causes of chronic fatigue (see Chronic Fatigue). In patients with interrupted sleep, other sleep disturbances deserve consideration (see Insomnia). In those with nighttime breathing difficulty, consider CHF (see Congestive Heart Failure), COPD (see Chronic Obstructive Pulmonary Disease), and other causes of snoring (see Snoring).

HISTORY

- High index of suspicion is appropriate when patient, obese or not, presents with symptoms of excessive daytime sleepiness, tiredness, or fatigue. Hx of very loud intermittent snoring, irregular respiratory activity with spells of gasping or choking that interrupt sleep, or witnessed episodes of apnea is strongly suggestive.

- Also worth noting are accidents, job performance difficulties, and personality changes or cognitive difficulties, especially if occurring in context of daytime sleepiness.
- Risk factors that help identify patients with obstructive sleep apnea include marked obesity (body mass index >28 kg/m^2), increasing age, obstructive upper airway abnormalities, regular use of sedatives or alcohol, and hypothyroidism.

PHYSICAL EXAM

- Check BP for elevation and integument for cyanosis, clubbing, or signs of hypothyroidism (see Hypothyroidism).
- Examine upper airway for overbite, high hard palate, other potentially obstructing nasopharyngeal lesions (e.g., nasal polyps, tonsillar hypertrophy, large uvula) and nasopharyngeal narrowing.
- Measure neck circumference to document any nuchal obesity.
- If severe obstructive sleep apnea suspected, check for signs of pulmonary HTN and cor pulmonale (e.g., right ventricular heave, loud pulmonic component of S_2, jugular venous distention, leg edema).

LAB STUDIES

- Few routine lab studies are of value. TSH determination is indicated if there is evidence of hypothyroidism. Unless patient has very severe disease with signs of cor pulmonale, measuring hematocrit, arterial blood gases, and pulse oximetry is of little value.
- Definitive and most cost-effective study in symptomatic patients with suspected obstructive sleep apnea is formal polysomnographic study, which includes overnight monitoring of EEG, eye movements, muscle activity, chest movements, air flow, and blood oxygen saturation. High sensitivity and specificity minimize false-positives and false-negatives.
- Home monitoring methods for Dx are improving but still lack sensitivity and specificity of polysomnography.

MANAGEMENT

OVERALL APPROACH

- Positive findings on polysomnography, demonstrating >20 apneic periods/hr in symptomatic patient with arterial desaturation during sleep, provide strongest grounds for Rx; risk for complications of obstructive sleep apnea is high in such persons, particularly those with underlying lung disease.
- Minimally symptomatic patients with no concurrent pulmonary disease or evidence of impairment might first try several potentially useful, noninvasive measures (e.g., weight reduction if obese, sleeping on one's side rather than on back) with expectant follow-up. However, empiric Rx based on clinical suspicion without reference to polysomnography is not recommended.
- CPAP improves survival in persons with >20 apneic episodes/hr. Efficacy in those with less severe disease not yet established.

- Rx of underlying hypothyroidism with thyroid hormone replacement is effective in those with documented hypothyroidism as cause of sleep apnea. Other attempts at pharmacologic Rx have been disappointing.

PATIENT EDUCATION

- Advise patients with sleep apnea and their family members of potential hazards, including 6-fold increased risk for traffic accidents.
- Patient ed also essential regarding Rx. For obese patients, instruction about weight reduction (see Overweight and Obesity) is essential. Also important is advice regarding avoiding sedatives and alcohol.

BIBLIOGRAPHY

- For the current annotated bibliography on sleep apnea, see the print edition of *Primary Care Medicine*, 4th edition, Chapter 46, or www.LWWmedicine.com.

Smoking Cessation

MANAGEMENT

OVERALL APPROACH

- Cigarette smoking is the major preventable cause of death in U.S. Strong evidence documents benefit from smoking cessation, even for the elderly and patients with chronic tobacco-related disease.
- PCP needs to be expert in motivating patients to quit and in advising them on best means to accomplish goal.
- Receiving advice from PCP about smoking cessation doubles chance of patient trying to quit. Those who benefit most from assisted method are heavy, more addicted smokers. Their chance of successfully quitting is about half that of smokers who quit on their own.
- Most effective approaches to assisted smoking cessation address nicotine addiction and behavioral cigarette dependency. Short-term cessation rates of 70–80% are common, but people restart. A 1-yr stay-quit rate of 30–35% is usual for effective programs.
- Cornerstone of pharmacologic Rx is relief of withdrawal symptoms by continuing some nicotine exposure at reduced and tapering doses. Transdermal patches, chewing gum, nasal spray, or inhalers can deliver nicotine. Patches and gum are available without prescription. But for those who prefer not to use nicotine replacement Rx, bupropion, an antidepressant, is just as effective.
- Smoking cessation strategies should include these elements:
  - Assessment of smoking habits, including level of nicotine addiction and readiness to quit.
  - Firm statement of advice to quit.
  - Brief motivational interview, eliciting from patients self-motivating expressions of why they might want to quit.
  - Request for commitment to quit.
  - Offer of personalized program that addresses addiction and behavioral needs.
  - Agreed-on plan for follow-up.
- Follow-up is critical to manage nicotine withdrawal, weight gain, and depression that may accompany smoking cessation and to increase patients' success rates. Schedule first follow-up shortly after quit date.

NICOTINE PATCH

- Patients use nicotine patches for 2–3 mos beginning on agreed-on quit date, starting with strongest dose (21 mg/day) for 4–6 wks, then tapering to lower doses (14 mg/day and 7 mg/day) for 2–4 wks each. Small patients (<100 lbs) should start with lower dose. Patients using patches should not smoke and must understand importance of concomitant behavior change.
- Side effects include skin irritation and insomnia. Patients should rotate location of patch. Those bothered by insomnia should use 16-hr patch or remove 24-hr patch at night.

NICOTINE GUM

- Nicotine gum available in 4-mg and 2-mg preparations. Patient chews it beginning on quit date when there is urge to smoke, usually at rate of 12 pieces/day at outset, tapering over 2–3 mos.
- Side effects include sore jaw, mouth irritation or ulcers, nervousness, dizziness, nausea, vomiting, hiccups, intestinal distress, headache, and excess salivation, but these resolve when patient chews the gum properly.
- Patients should avoid drinking acidic beverages before or during gum use; decreased saliva pH blocks nicotine absorption.
- Pregnant or breast-feeding patients and those with recent MI, unstable angina, peripheral vascular disease, or serious arrhythmias should not use nicotine patches or gum.

PHARMACOLOGIC THERAPY

- Role of prescription nicotine nasal sprays and inhalers as alternative to patch and gum is still undefined.
- Patient starts bupropion 1 wk before agreed on quit date with usual dosage of 300 mg/day for 2–3 mos. Patient can use it alone or with nicotine replacement.
- Most common side effects are dry mouth and insomnia. Risk for seizure has decreased with use of slow-release preparation, but alternative Rx is advisable in patients with Hx of seizure or other risk factors.

BEHAVIOR MODIFICATION

- Behavioral methods center on strategies for stimulus control. Patients self-monitor for cues that trigger smoking during course of day, then work to separate themselves from cues by progressive restriction of situations in which smoking is triggered and permitted.
- Various aversive conditioning techniques including rapid smoking have high short-term quit rates, but relapse is common without other techniques.
- Hypnosis and acupuncture are used and often requested. There is more evidence for effectiveness of former than latter.

BIBLIOGRAPHY

- For the current annotated bibliography on smoking cessation, see the print edition of *Primary Care Medicine*, 4th edition, Chapter 54, or www.LWWmedicine.com.

Solitary Pulmonary Nodule

DIFFERENTIAL DIAGNOSIS

- Solitary nodules are found at rate of 1–2/1,000 routine CXRs. They are a concern for doctor and patient because of possibilities of primary lung cancer and solitary metastasis from nonpulmonary cancer. Referral for consideration of bronchoscopy, percutaneous needle biopsy, or thoracotomy depends on determination of likelihood of malignancy based on clinical and radiologic findings.
- Because malignant nodules take 1–18 mos to double, and benign nodules take longer, consider solitary nodule benign if size unchanged for 2 yrs.
- Likelihood of malignant nodule increases with patient age; probability is <2% if patient aged <30 and increases by 10–15% with each decade.
- Calcification patterns helpful. Benign lesions tend to have calcium deposited in central, peripheral, concentric, "popcorn," or homogeneous patterns. Eccentric patterns of calcification more suggestive of malignancies.
- Of all solitary nodules, 60–80% are benign (mostly healed infectious granulomas). Of 20–40% of nodules that are cancerous, >75% are primary lung cancers, and remainder are metastatic lesions. Tumors of breast, colon, and testicles particularly prone to lung metastases.

WORKUP

OVERALL STRATEGY

- Approaches to pulmonary nodules range from early thoracotomy and resection to more conservative management including review of old CXRs and/or close follow-up of lesion, with definitive tissue Dx (by needle biopsy or bronchoscopy) reserved for those with worrisome findings and/or progression.
- Withholding invasive study is legitimate in patients with lesions that have not enlarged in 5 yrs and in young, nonsmoking patients with CXR evidence that suggests benignity (central, laminated, diffuse, or popcorn pattern of calcification; sharp borders). Careful follow-up with serial CXR essential because some malignancies grow slowly.
- Transthoracic needle aspiration is most effective Dx approach short of thoracotomy and resection. Sensitivity for detection of malignancy approaches 95% when nodule is accessible to transthoracic approach. Bronchoscopy with bronchial brushing is far less sensitive.
- Thoracotomy with resection represents most direct and definitive means of Dx (and Rx) but is associated with perioperative mortality risk of 1–10% and considerable morbidity (see Lung Cancer).
- Patients for whom probability of malignancy is neither low enough for conservative follow-up nor high enough for surgery face a dilemma.

Share uncertainty and possible outcomes of alternative approaches with these patients to devise satisfactory plan.

HISTORY

- Age and smoking Hx are most important determinants of cancer risk. Hx of TB exposure or geographic exposure to histoplasmosis or coccidioidomycosis lowers cancer risk by providing alternative etiologic explanation.
- Although symptoms are often absent, inquire into bone pain, headache, weight loss, and other symptoms suggesting malignancy.
- Hx of hemoptysis, even if minimal (see Hemoptysis), and of known previous breast, bowel, or testicular cancer increases likelihood of malignancy.
- Family Hx of hemorrhagic telangiectasia can be valuable clue.

PHYSICAL EXAM

- PE is generally unrevealing, but exclude breast or testicular mass, occult blood in stool, clubbing (see Clubbing), cutaneous or mucosal telangiectasia, or audible bruit over chest wall (suggesting vascular etiology).
- Palpate lymph nodes, particularly in supraclavicular and axillary regions. If enlarged, nodes can be sampled by biopsy, which may eliminate need for thoracotomy or other invasive procedures.

LAB STUDIES

- Assessment of doubling time, ideally by assessing old CXRs, can be especially helpful. Doubling of tumor volume results in 28% increase in nodule diameter. Doubling time >2 yrs or <30 days makes malignancy unlikely.
- Location, size, and shape of nodule on CXR are less valuable distinguishing signs.
- CT is imaging technique of choice for evaluating solitary pulmonary nodule. MRI does not detect calcification well but reveals mediastinum better than does CT, and it is useful for imaging chest wall invasion, aortopulmonic window adenopathy, and superior sulcus tumors.
- PET + ^{18}F-2-fluoro-2-deoxy-D-glucose (FDG) adds useful information for nodules indeterminate on CXR. CT + FDG-PET strategy may be most effective and may be cost-saving among patients for whom cancer probability is 0.12–0.69.
- Implant intermediate-strength TB skin test (see Tuberculosis). If sputum available, stain for acid-fast organisms and culture for TB. In endemic areas, fungal cultures and histoplasmin complement fixation titers may be important.
- Sputum cytology of limited value except in patients too ill for invasive study.

BIBLIOGRAPHY

- For the current annotated bibliography on solitary pulmonary nodule, see the print edition of *Primary Care Medicine*, 4th edition, Chapter 44, or www.LWWmedicine.com.

Tuberculosis

SCREENING AND/OR PREVENTION

- As long as tuberculin skin test and INH remain useful for case finding and prophylaxis, respectively, biologic prophylaxis with BCG for PPD-negative patients is not recommended.
- Perform annual PPD testing in HIV-infected patients. Test other high-risk persons as well, including IV drug abusers, homeless persons, immigrants from countries with high TB incidence, prisoners, residents of long-term care facilities, and persons who are immunosuppressed or have chronic illnesses known to increase risk for active TB.
- Healthy persons with high risk for TB exposure, such as health care professionals, should undergo annual tuberculin testing so long as they remain PPD-negative.
- Consider INH prophylaxis for tuberculin-positive persons based on strength of PPD reaction, presence of risk factors, and age. Positive reactors require 6 mos of daily INH prophylaxis (300 mg/day); those at highest risk (HIV-positive, old TB on CXRs) require 12 mos of daily prophylactic Rx. Take care to ensure compliance to prevent emergence of drug-resistant strains; twice-weekly DOT may be appropriate.
- Rx with rifampin (RIF) and pyrazinamide (PZA) for 2 mos is as effective as Rx with isoniazid (INH) alone for 12 mos in HIV-infected patients, although side effects are more common.
- Exclude active TB before starting INH chemoprophylaxis.
- In deciding to use INH for prophylaxis, weigh risk for drug-induced hepatotoxicity against benefit of preventing active disease. The older the patient, the greater the risk for hepatitis, although benefit usually outweighs risk, especially in populations with high incidence of infection and active disease.
- Prompt Dx and effective, individualized Rx program are essential to preventing spread of disease and emergence of resistant organisms. Of particular importance is early recognition of TB in HIV-infected patients. High index of suspicion and awareness of potentially atypical presentations of TB in these patients (e.g., disseminated disease, meningitis) are essential.

WORKUP

- See Bronchitis and Pneumonia; Chronic Cough.

MANAGEMENT

- Treat patients with active pulmonary or extrapulmonary TB with INH, RIF, and PZA for 2 mos, followed by INH and RIF for 4 mos, for total Rx of 6 mos.
- Because nearly all U.S. centers currently report >4% resistance to 1 of these drugs, and because of now-recognized importance of newly

acquired infection, include ethambutol (or streptomycin) in initial regimen until results of drug susceptibility tests are known; if presence of sensitive organism is confirmed, stop ethambutol Rx.

- The above Rx regimen applies to patients with or without HIV infection. Because relapse rates are higher in HIV-infected patients, however, careful clinical follow-up should be the rule. Many authorities advocate continuing INH and RIF for 6 mos after sputum conversion.

- If INH and RIF cannot be administered simultaneously because of patient intolerance or drug resistance, continue multiple-drug Rx for 18–24 mos. Refer such patients to infectious disease specialist or to local public health authority for optimal management. For patients relapsing after previous course of antituberculous chemotherapy, or for patients in whom you suspect more widespread drug resistance, initial Rx may involve ≥6 drugs and should be coordinated by infectious disease specialist or public health authority.

- Consider DOT initially for all patients with active TB. Twice- and thrice-weekly regimens have established efficacy when given as part of DOT.

- INH, RIF, and ethambutol all appear to be safe for pregnant patients.

- After completing Rx, follow all patients for 1 yr, monitoring for evidence of recurrence. Longer follow-up is appropriate for those with drug-resistant organisms, HIV positivity, or suspected poor compliance.

- Consider hospitalization during initial stages of active pulmonary disease to minimize risk for spread. Chemotherapy for 2 wks usually suffices to render patient noninfectious.

BIBLIOGRAPHY

- For the current annotated bibliography on tuberculosis, see the print edition of *Primary Care Medicine*, 4th edition, Chapters 38 and 49, or www.LWWmedicine.com.

Gastrointestinal Problems

Abdominal Pain

WORKUP

GENERAL STRATEGY

- Match speed and extent of workup to pace of illness and underlying risk of serious pathophysiology.
- Examine patients with acute pain promptly for evidence of obstruction, peritoneal irritation, vascular compromise, and cardiopulmonary disease.
- For those with chronic pain, proceed at more gradual pace, taking time to get to know patient and problem before undertaking extensive testing.

HISTORY

- Obtain complete description of pain, including localization, characterization, area of referral, onset, duration, timing, clinical course, and precipitating and alleviating factors.
- Check for evidence of and risk factors for serious underlying pathology; ask about prior abdominal surgery or bowel obstruction, gallbladder or kidney stones, vomiting, rectal bleeding, melena, diarrhea, marked change in bowel habits, fever, chills, abdominal distention, difficulty urinating, known atherosclerotic disease or risk factors, and cardiac or pulmonary symptoms.
- Note symptoms of pelvic pathology, such as dyspareunia, abnormal vaginal discharge, and irregular menstrual bleeding; inquire into chance of pregnancy.
- Explore psychosocial Hx, noting any ethnic or psychological factors that might color clinical presentation.
- Elicit patient fears, concerns, and expectations.

For Diagnosis of Irritable Bowel Syndrome

- Start with Manning criteria (pain relief with defecation, more frequent stools with onset of pain, looser stools with onset of pain, rectal passage of mucus, and feeling of incomplete evacuation, visible abdominal distention).
- Refine probability estimate using Rome diagnostic criteria:
  - \>3 mos continuous or recurrent symptoms of abdominal pain or discomfort associated with >1 of the following:
    - Relief with defecation,
    - Change in stool frequency, or
    - Change in stool consistency,
  - + ≥2 of the following:
    - Altered stool frequency (>3 bowel movements/day or <3/wk),
    - Altered stool form (lumpy and hard or loose and watery),
    - Altered stool passage (straining, urgency, or incomplete evacuation),
    - Passage of mucus, or
    - Bloating or feeling of abdominal distention.

For Diagnosis of Functional Dyspepsia

- Use Rome criteria; for ulcerlike variant (in which abdominal pain dominates), principal criterion is ≥3 mos of upper abdominal pain with no evidence of organic disease + ≥3 of the following:
  - Very well-localized pain,
  - Pain relieved by food (>25% of time),
  - Pain relieved by antacids or H_2 blockers,
  - Pain that awakens patient from sleep,
  - Periods of remission and relapse (≥2 wks remission).

PHYSICAL EXAM

For All Patients

- Pay particular attention to general appearance; note reluctance to change position (peritonitis) or restlessness (obstruction).
- Check vital signs for postural changes in BP or heart rate, fever, and heart rhythm abnormalities.
- Examine skin for jaundice, other stigmata of chronic liver disease, clubbing or spooning of fingernails, signs of trauma, excoriations, prior surgical scars, and evidence of dehydration, edema, or dermatomal rash.
- Check chest for splinting, pleural friction rub, and signs of consolidation (particularly in lower lobes), and heart for murmurs, chamber enlargement, and signs of CHF (see Congestive Heart Failure).
- Perform detailed but gentle abdominal exam to avoid unnecessary discomfort; note pain with coughing, ascites, altered bowel sounds (increased or absent), hepatic rub, vascular bruit, prominent venous pattern, tenderness, guarding, rebound, hepatosplenomegaly, inguinal hernia, and masses [including dilated aorta (diameter >4 cm), loops of bowel, stool, distended bladder or uterus, and periumbilical adenopathy (pancreatic or ovarian cancer)].
- On pelvic and rectal exams check gently for masses and tenderness and perform fecal occult blood testing.
- Examine for nerve injury; note any dermatomal distribution and hyperesthesia (herpes zoster, nerve root impingement, focal peritoneal irritation).
- Carefully palpate abdominal wall for masses and muscle tenderness and note any exacerbation of pain when muscles are contracted, as on sitting up.

In the Elderly

- Remember that signs of acute peritoneal irritation may be absent in the elderly, especially initially; only manifestation may be unexplained mild fever, tachycardia, reduction in bowel sounds, and vague abdominal discomfort without frank rebound or guarding.
- Consider vascular compromise when you find acute abdominal pain out of proportion to tenderness on PE of person with known atherosclerotic disease.

In Suspected Psychogenic Pain

- Use deep palpation while patient is distracted; lack of tenderness is characteristic.
- Push down slowly, firmly, and deeply with stethoscope, distracting patient by appearing to auscultate; perform only after ruling out more serious pathology by Hx and PE.

LAB STUDIES

Initial Testing in the Office Setting

- Obtain CBC and differential.
- For patients with diarrhea, perform microscopic exam of stool for WBC (see Diarrhea).
- If pregnancy possible, obtain serum hCG β-subunit determination.
- Check plain films of abdomen in patients with moderate to severe tenderness or who are strongly suspected of having bowel obstruction, urinary tract calculi, trauma, ischemia, or gallbladder disease; note any
  - free air under diaphragm (perforation),
  - absent psoas shadow (retroperitoneal bleeding, abscess, or mass), or
  - displaced stomach or bowel (tumor).
- Obtain urinalysis and basic chemistries; note any pyuria, hematuria, bacteriuria, glycosuria, ketonuria, and any disturbances in electrolytes, liver or hepatic function, blood sugar, and amylase.
- Order CXR and ECG in persons with upper abdominal pain, looking for pleuropulmonary disease in lower lobes and acute ischemic changes in inferior myocardium.

Testing in the Emergent Setting

- Immediately hospitalize and urgently test patients with evidence of acute obstruction, peritonitis, bowel ischemia, or worrisome metabolic or cardiopulmonary disease; consider:
  - paracentesis in subset of patients with acute pain who have ascites or abdominal trauma;
  - abdominal CT with meglumine diatrizoate (Gastrografin) oral contrast in patients with suspected diverticulitis, especially if there is clinical concern for abscess formation;
  - CT with IV contrast for suspected dissecting aortic aneurysm;
  - helical CT of appendix (with Gastrografin) for suspected appendicitis;
  - abdominal ultrasonography (U/S) for suspected acute cholecystitis, choledocholithiasis, and aortic aneurysm;
  - renal U/S for suspected urinary tract obstruction or if ureterolithiasis is suspected.

Subsequent Outpatient Testing

- Continue outpatient workup of patients without sufficient evidence of serious acute pathology.
- Provide careful follow-up to any patient sent home with undiagnosed acute abdominal pain, and repeat Hx and PE each time because several serious etiologies (e.g., bowel ischemia, cholecystitis) may initially present with indolent picture, particularly in the elderly.
- Note degree of distress, any elevation in temp or WBC, other lab abnormalities, and ability of patient to eat and drink.
- Proceed with more extensive evaluation in patients with unexplained abdominal pain with recurrent nausea and vomiting, jaundice, fever, weight loss >10% body weight, or blood in stool.
- Test selectively based on specific working hypotheses suggested by clinical findings and initial testing. Avoid "running the bowel" in absence of suggestive clinical evidence because it is wasteful and potentially misleading, and may subject patient to unnecessary risk.

Consider Further Testing in Terms of Location of Pain

Epigastric Pain

- If patient is aged <40 and shows little clinical evidence for malignancy (i.e., no dysphagia, weight loss, melena, hematemesis), consider serologic testing for *H. pylori* and symptomatic Rx for presumed ulcer disease (see Peptic Ulcer Disease), especially if pain parallels acid secretory cycle.
- Failure to respond to 4- to 8-wk course of empiric Rx or development of worrisome symptoms, especially in older patients (who are at increased risk for esophageal and gastric cancers), necessitates direct visualization of upper GI tract by upper GI series or EGD.
- For recurrent bouts of epigastric or right upper quadrant pain, consider abdominal U/S.
- Consider duplex scanning (combination of Doppler with B-mode U/S) for suspected mesenteric insufficiency (postprandial pain in those with systemic vascular disease or its risk factors).

Periumbilical Pain

- Consider small-bowel pathology and upper GI series with small-bowel follow-through.
- If postprandial, use duplex scanning by Doppler U/S for mesenteric ischemia.

Lower Abdominal Pain

- If pain accompanies signs of rectal bleeding (gross or occult), perform colonoscopy or combination of barium enema and sigmoidoscopy to identify source (see Gastrointestinal Bleeding).
- If patient is young (<40) with constipation, obvious hemorrhoidal bleeding, and no risk factors for colorectal cancer (CRC), limit study to sigmoidoscopy to rule out associated rectosigmoid pathology, such as that of inflammatory bowel disease.
- Avoid radiologic or endoscopic evaluation in patients with lower abdominal pain in absence of bleeding, weight loss, or change in bowel habits unless symptoms are particularly severe or chronic; age-appropriate screening for CRC (see Colorectal Cancer) helps provide appropriate reassurance without excessive testing.

Flank and Adnexal Pains

- Consider
  - IV pyelogram for detecting kidney or ureter disease or displacement of ureter by abdominal or retroperitoneal mass.
  - Renal U/S for suspected stone, tumor, or ureteral dilatation.
  - Pelvic U/S when there is adnexal pain with tenderness or mass noted on bimanual exam.

Suspected Pancreatic Cancer

- Screen with U/S; add needle biopsy of any suspected lesion.
- Order abdominal CT if you need further delineation (e.g., U/S indeterminate or suggestive of mass lesion).
- Consider ERCP with biopsy as alternative to abdominal CT.

Suspected Functional Disease

- For suspected IBS, obtain flexible sigmoidoscopy to rule out inflammatory bowel disease and CRC.

- Omit routine ordering of chemistry profiles, blood counts, thyroid indices, urinalyses, and tests for O&P in absence of clinical evidence or risk factors for these conditions.
- For suspected functional dyspepsia, consider empiric trial of Rx for peptic ulcer disease; alternatively, perform serologic testing for *H. pylori* infection; usefulness of upper GI endoscopy in this setting remains controversial; best reserved for onset of symptoms after age 40, especially in persons whose symptoms persist without remission for >8 wks.

Suspected Lead Poisoning and Porphyria

- If acute colicky pain but no signs of obstruction or inflammation, check urine for coproporphyrin (indicative of lead excess).
- Omit serum lead levels because they are unreliable.
- For patients with periodic attacks of cramping pain, constipation, nausea and vomiting, and neuromuscular symptoms in conjunction with altered psychological state, screen for acute intermittent porphyria with Watson-Schwartz test for urinary porphobilinogen.

Undiagnosed Abdominal Pain

- Conduct further anatomic study in patients with strongly positive family Hx of bowel malignancy, significant weight loss, presence of mass, unexplained iron deficiency anemia, or stool test positive for occult blood.
- If you do not uncover cause, plan follow-up for observation and repeat Hx and PE.
- Note clues suggesting possible contributory psychopathology (see Somatization Disorders) in subsequent follow-up. Pay particular attention to Hx of multiple bodily complaints, chronic nonprogressive clinical course that may span many yrs, lack of relation between symptoms and physiologic stimuli, inconsistent or distractible physical findings, and presence of somatic symptoms of depression (e.g., early morning awakening, fatigue, decreased libido, altered appetite).
- In absence of worrisome objective findings, avoid exhaustive testing of patients and concentrate on underlying psychosocial problems.
- Elicit patient's perspective, particularly concerns, beliefs, and expectations, as well as details of daily functioning at work and at home, social supports, and psychological state; note any evidence of psychosocial suffering.
- Inquire into psychosocial issues, such as concurrent stresses, losses, and effect of pain on patient's life and daily activities; avoid suggesting at outset that problem is probably psychogenic.
- Avoid taking adversarial stance or denying reality of patient's pain and suffering. Demonstrate caring response and open-minded attitude.
- Rebuff requests for aggressive testing if detailed Hx, careful PE, and pertinent screening tests have been performed; supplement with plan for careful longitudinal follow-up.
- Continue observation, watching for signs of worrisome disease (see above).
- Avoid extensive invasive testing (e.g., resorting to exploratory laparoscopy/laparotomy and as long as there is no corroborating evidence of serious underlying pathology.
- Give thorough reassurance that specifically addresses patient concerns.

MANAGEMENT

■ For management of a specific condition, see appropriate chapter.

ANALGESICS

■ Avoid in patients with acute abdominal pain of unknown etiology, except in those with terminal cancer [see Cancer (General)].

■ Avoid in patients with undiagnosed chronic pain, especially those who request pain medication (high probability of underlying psychopathology and strong potential for narcotic abuse).

THERAPEUTIC TRIALS

■ For suspected peptic ulcer disease and no evidence of malignancy, begin 4-wk course of PPI Rx (see Peptic Ulcer Disease).

■ For probable IBS, initiate high-fiber program, such as 1 tbsp psyllium/8 oz water bid–tid (see Irritable Bowel Syndrome).

■ Consider trial of antidepressant Rx using agent low in anticholinergic activity (e.g., SSRI; see Depression) in patients with symptoms of major depression as predominant pathology.

BIBLIOGRAPHY

■ For the current annotated bibliography on abdominal pain, see the print edition of *Primary Care Medicine*, 4th edition, Chapter 58, or www.LWWmedicine.com.

Anorectal Complaints

SCREENING AND/OR PREVENTION

PROPER DIETARY HABITS

- Advise increase in intake of dietary fiber; suggest bran, carrots, green vegetables, and fruits with skin.
- Consider use of psyllium preparation.
- For those finding such foods as chili, onions, or alcohol irritating, suggest that they be avoided.

BOWEL HABITS

- Suggest regular time each day to have unhurried bowel movement, with avoidance of straining and lingering too long on toilet.
- Advise avoidance of vigorous wiping after bowel movement.
- Teach patting dry rather than wiping or rubbing after bathing.
- Instruct avoidance of irritant laxatives.
- Suggest using sitz baths at first sign of recurrent symptoms.

DIFFERENTIAL DIAGNOSIS

GENERAL

- Anal discomfort
  - Hemorrhoids
  - Fissure-in-ano (hard bowel movement, cancer, venereal disease)
  - Fistula-in-ano (perirectal abscess, Crohn's disease, carcinoma, radiation, TB, lymphogranuloma venereum)
  - Perirectal abscess (Crohn's disease, immunodeficiency, hematologic disorders)
  - Infected pilonidal cyst
  - Carcinoma of anal epidermis
  - Infections (syphilis, candidiasis, condylomata acuminata)
- Rectal discomfort
  - Proctitis (ulcerative, gonococcal, amebic, herpetic), often accompanied by discharge and bleeding
  - Perirectal abscess
  - Impaction
  - Proctalgia fugax
  - Solitary rectal ulcer
- Pruritus ani
  - Excess moisture (poor hygiene)
  - Pinworms
  - Eczema
  - Scabies
  - Diabetes mellitus
  - Liver failure
  - Irritants (topical agents, alkaline stools)

- Fissure
- Early cancer
- Neurodermatitis
- Infections
- Incontinence
  - Rectal surgery
  - Neurologic disease
  - Perianal disease

ADDITIONAL CONSIDERATIONS IN MALE HOMOSEXUALS

- Proctitis
  - *N. gonorrhoeae*
  - Herpes simplex
  - *Chlamydia* (nonlymphogranuloma strains)
  - Syphilis
  - Condylomata acuminata
  - Trauma
  - Chemical irritants
- Proctocolitis
  - *Campylobacter*
  - *Shigella*
  - *E. histolytica*
  - *Chlamydia* (lymphogranuloma strains)
- Enteritis
  - *G. lamblia*

WORKUP

HISTORY

- Determine whether complaint is predominantly anal (local pain only), anorectal (local anal pain plus rectal discomfort, tenesmus, rectal discharge, constipation), or rectocolonic (rectal discomfort, tenesmus, and rectal discharge + diarrhea, abdominal pain, bloating, nausea).
- Ask patients with anal complaints about masses, nodules, focal tenderness, Hx of hemorrhoids, psoriasis, passage of hard stool, bleeding, discharge, generalized itching, nocturnal pattern, and recent trauma.
- Inquire into use of topical medications (many of which are sensitizing), involvement of other household members or sexual partners, and hygienic practices.
- For patients with anorectal involvement, check for symptoms of inflammatory bowel disease (see Inflammatory Bowel Disease), obtain detailed sexual Hx focusing on number of partners and practice of receptive rectal intercourse, and note any reports of inguinal adenopathy (seen with herpes and lymphogranuloma), sacral root paresthesias, and difficulty with micturition (other telltale symptoms of herpes simplex infection).
- For those with rectocolonic symptoms, consider inflammatory bowel disease and a polymicrobial infection from rectal intercourse; review associated symptoms and risk factors.

PHYSICAL EXAM

- Gently inspect anus and perianal region; note anal skin for erythema, eczema, psoriatic patches, ulcerations, vesicles, fistulas, fissures, condylomata, nodules, hemorrhoids, and inflammatory changes.
- Check for perianal or rectal ulcers in association with proctitis in male homosexuals (indicative of syphilis or herpes simplex). If scaling plaques found, check extensor surfaces of extremities for additional evidence of psoriasis.
- In very anxious patient with multiple excoriations over other parts of body, suspect neurodermatitis as cause of pruritus ani.
- If inflamed anorectal mucosa is encountered, consider gonorrhea and inquire into rectal intercourse.
- Stretch perianal skin to reveal any fissures, which come into view at anal verge, most often in posterior midline but occasionally in anterior midline.
- Note any scarring and induration seen with chronic fissures, in addition to hypertrophied anal papilla at pectinate line; skin tag marks external limit.
- Consider Crohn's disease in those with multiple fissures, recurrent fistulas, or perirectal abscesses.
- Check for painless hard nodule or plaque (carcinoma); if such a lesion is ulcerated, Dx is more obvious and disease more advanced.
- Perform digital rectal exam, being especially gentle in setting of a painful fissure. Check for masses (both fluctuant and firm), discharges, ulcerations, and other mucosal changes and also test stool for occult blood. Do not ascribe anorectal symptoms to hemorrhoids without ruling out cancer.
- Palpate for inguinal adenopathy (herpetic and chlamydial infections).

LAB STUDIES

- Perform anoscopy unless patient has very painful lesion. Inspect for mucosal inflammation, fissure, fistula, mass, plaque, ulcer, and discharge. In male homosexuals engaging in receptive anal intercourse with many sexual partners, obtain samples of mucus for Gram's stain (looking for gonococci) and culture (Thayer-Martin media).
- Consider biopsy of atypical fissures (especially those that do not heal), painless hard anorectal nodules, and mucosal ulcerations to rule out malignancy, inflammatory bowel disease, and chronic infection (syphilis, tuberculosis). Subject any chancrelike lesions to dark field examination for spirochetes and obtain serologic test for syphilis.
- Proceed to sigmoidoscopy if rectal inflammation, fistula, nonhealing fissures, bleeding, or diarrhea are noted.
- In homosexuals with proctocolitis on sigmoidoscopy extending above 15 cm or symptoms of colitis (diarrhea, nausea, abdominal cramping), culture for *Campylobacter*, *Chlamydia* (lymphogranuloma strains), and *Shigella* and have stools examined for O&P (*E. histolytica*). In those with proctitis only (no mucosal disease above 15 cm), limit culturing to gonorrhea, herpes simplex, and chlamydia (nonlymphogranuloma strains). No need to culture for herpes if characteristic clinical features present (severe anorectal pain, multiple perianal ulcers, rectal ulceration, inguinal adenopathy, difficult micturition, impotence, and paresthesias in S-4 and S-5 distributions).
- Take cellophane tape impression of anus of children with nocturnal pruritus ani and examine microscopically for pinworms.

MANAGEMENT

SYMPTOMATIC MEASURES

■ Treat etiologically whenever possible (see specific conditions), but in absence of serious underlying pathology, consider symptomatic measures:

- Application of cold pack for first few hrs after onset of pain.
- Frequent hot sitz baths 3–4 × day following initial application of cold.
- Topical steroid suppository (e.g., hydrocortisone) if inflammation and itching are marked. If symptoms are predominantly external, prescribe 1–2.5% hydrocortisone cream.
- Topical anesthetic if pain acutely severe; if used, choose minimally sensitizing agent (e.g., pramoxine).
- Dietary fiber and stool softener (e.g., 100 mg docusate sodium tid), with continuation of high-fiber diet afterwards.

FOR THROMBOSED HEMORRHOIDS

■ Instruct patient to lie prone with ice applied to thrombosed hemorrhoid.

■ Prescribe PO analgesics; patient may require codeine.

■ Prescribe stool softeners.

■ Conservative Rx should be successful in 3–5 days; otherwise, refer patient for surgical removal of clot, which will relieve pain promptly.

■ For intractable symptoms, refer for consideration of surgical intervention. Specific method depends on surgical expertise available.

BIBLIOGRAPHY

■ For the current annotated bibliography on anorectal complaints, see the print edition of *Primary Care Medicine*, 4th edition, Chapter 66, or www.LWWmedicine.com.

Cirrhosis and Chronic Liver Failure

WORKUP

- See Jaundice; Viral Hepatitis.

MANAGEMENT

GENERAL MEASURES

- Advise maintaining caloric intake of ≥2,000–3,000 kcal/day.
- Prohibit use of alcohol or other hepatotoxic agents.
- Avoid prescribing tranquilizers and sedatives.
- Monitor prothrombin time, serum albumin, and bilirubin to assess severity and progression of hepatocellular dysfunction.
- Have patient record daily weight.
- At each visit, check for occult bleeding, ascites (shifting dullness, fluid wave, bulging flanks), asterixis, and other signs of encephalopathy.
- Order ultrasound exam to confirm suspected ascites and rule out portal vein thrombosis.

MANAGEMENT OF ASCITES

- Perform diagnostic paracentesis in patients with new onset of ascites or clinical deterioration in setting of preexisting ascites.
- Send fluid for cell count and differential, total protein and albumin concentrations, culture, and cytologic exam.
- Instruct patients with ascites to restrict daily sodium intake to ≤2 g and consume ≥50 g protein/day. Consult with dietitian and provide patient and family with specific menus and food lists.
- Restrict fluid intake to 1,500 mL when there is marked hyponatremia (serum sodium concentration <125 mEq/L.
- If salt restriction does not result in diuresis, begin spironolactone, 100 mg/day in divided doses. If natriuresis and diuresis do not occur after 1 wk, increase daily dose of spironolactone by 100 mg q4–5d to maximum of 400 mg/day.
- If spironolactone alone is ineffective in causing diuresis, add furosemide 20–40 mg/day and cautiously increase dosage as necessary.
- Adjust diuretic dose so that no more than 0.5 kg/day of fluid (approximately 1 lb) is lost in patients with ascites alone, and no more than 1 kg/day (2 lb) in those with ascites and peripheral edema.
- Halt diuretics at first sign of intravascular volume depletion.
- Monitor serum potassium, BUN, creatinine, daily weight, and postural signs to avoid inducing intravascular volume depletion, renal failure, hypokalemia, and encephalopathy. Be aware that in some patients serum creatinine may be falsely normal despite worsening renal function.
- Consider daily potassium supplementation (20–40 mEq potassium chloride elixir) in patients receiving furosemide; administer cautiously,

if at all, to patients concurrently taking potassium-sparing diuretic such as spironolactone.

- Consider large-volume paracentesis (5–6 L) with concurrent IV albumin infusion (6–8 g/L fluid removed) for patients with refractory, disabling ascites. Admit patient for procedure.

ENCEPHALOPATHY

- At first sign, restrict dietary protein intake to 20–30 g/day.
- Obtain dietary consultation to construct diet emphasizing plant protein over animal protein. Consider using PO supplement rich in branched-chain amino acids if protein intake is insufficient.
- Monitor mental status and check for asterixis; use 5-point star or signature testing. Monitoring venous ammonia levels is less useful; in drawing blood for ammonia determination, avoid prolonged tourniquet application.
- When protein restriction fails to control encephalopathy, begin PO lactulose, 15–30 mL q4–6h, with subsequent adjustments in dosage to allow 2–3 soft stools/day.
- Add oral neomycin, 1 g bid; or metronidazole, 250 mg tid, if lactulose alone is insufficient. Metronidazole is probably better tolerated for short-term use.
- Consider dietary supplementation with ornithine, aspartate, benzoate, or phenylacetate in patients with mild encephalopathy.

PREVENTION OF VARICEAL BLEEDING AND BLEEDING DUE TO CLOTTING FACTOR DEFICIENCY

- Begin beta blocker (e.g., propranolol, 80 mg/day) for primary prevention in patients at risk for variceal bleeding (marked hepatocellular dysfunction, ascites, encephalopathy, large varices, and presence of dilated venules on varices).
- Consider endoscopic sclerotherapy, endoscopic variceal banding, and shunt procedures (e.g., TIPS) for prevention of recurrent variceal bleeding.
- Monitor PT and platelet count. Administer vitamin K (10 mg/day SQ × 3 days) if there is prolongation of PT due to drug-induced bile salt malabsorption, neomycin, or malnutrition. Platelet transfusions are unwarranted unless there is active bleeding in context of very low platelet count (see Bleeding Problems).

INDICATIONS FOR ADMISSION AND REFERRAL

- Promptly hospitalize patients with GI bleeding, worsening encephalopathy, increasing azotemia, signs of peritoneal irritation, or unexplained fever; intractable ascites may respond to elective admission for large-volume paracentesis.
- Make decisions about management of refractory ascites, encephalopathy, variceal bleeding, and uncommon etiologies of cirrhosis (e.g., primary biliary cirrhosis, Wilson's disease, hemochromatosis), and liver transplantation in consultation with gastroenterologist skilled in treating liver disease.
- Nephrologic consultation may be of considerable help when urine output falls unexplainably (creatinine level may not adequately reflect renal function).

PATIENT EDUCATION

- Emphasize to patient and family that prognosis can often be greatly improved and symptoms lessened by careful adherence to prescribed medical program, particularly dietary discipline and omission of alcohol.
- Many of these patients are chronic alcoholics with low self-esteem. Provide sympathetic support to raise self-esteem and improve chances of compliance (see Alcohol Abuse).
- Depression frequently accompanies later stages of chronic liver disease and is manifested by noncompliance with medical regimen and expressions of wanting to die. Rx is difficult; antidepressants may cause oversedation and are risky. Concern and support can help enormously (see Depression).

BIBLIOGRAPHY

- For the current annotated bibliography on cirrhosis and chronic liver failure, see the print edition of *Primary Care Medicine*, 4th edition, Chapter 71, or www.LWWmedicine.com.

Constipation

SCREENING AND/OR PREVENTION

- During illness, prevent constipation by use of high-fiber diet, bulk agents, and use of commode in preference to bedpan. Correct coincident hypokalemia.
- Avoid prophylactic use of laxatives or stool softeners.
- When severe depression requires antidepressant Rx, choose an agent that is not constipating (see Depression).

DIFFERENTIAL DIAGNOSIS

IMPORTANT CAUSES OF CONSTIPATION

- Impaired motility
  - Inadequate dietary fiber
  - Inactivity
  - Laxative abuse
  - Irritable colon syndrome
  - Diverticulitis
  - Hypothyroidism
  - Hypokalemia
  - Diabetes mellitus
  - Hypercalcemia
  - Pregnancy
  - Scleroderma
  - Drugs (opiates, anticholinergics, tricyclic antidepressants, ganglionic blockers, calcium- and aluminum-containing antacids, sucralfate, disopyramide, calcium channel blockers, antihistamines)
- Neurologic dysfunction
  - Multiple sclerosis
  - Spinal cord injury
  - Neurogangliomatosis
- Psychosocial dysfunction
  - Depression
  - Situational stress
  - Anxiety
  - Somatization
  - Phobias

WORKUP

HISTORY

- Review size, character, and frequency of bowel movements and chronicity of problem.

- Check for symptoms that suggest underlying GI problem, such as abdominal pain, nausea, cramping, vomiting, weight loss, melena, rectal bleeding or pain, and fever.
- Note any anorexia, bloating, belching, flatus, mucus in stool, headache, depression, and anxiety, all suggestive of functional disorders.
- At first visit, take Hx of working, eating, and bowel habits; inquire into dietary fiber intake, physical activity, and use of medications, including nonprescription agents (especially laxatives and antacids).
- Elicit patient's perspective and concerns and psychosocial Hx, with attention to situational stresses, anxieties, and methods of coping.

PHYSICAL EXAM

- Record weight and note overall nutritional status.
- Check skin for pallor and signs of hypothyroidism (see Hypothyroidism); check abdomen for masses, distention, tenderness, and high-pitched or absent bowel sounds.
- Examine rectum for masses, fissures, inflammation, and hard stool in ampulla; check anal sensitivity and reflexes. Note any anal canal patulousness, especially when puborectalis muscle is pulled posteriorly.
- Perform neurologic exam to search for focal deficits and delayed relaxation phase of ankle jerks, suggestive of hypothyroidism. On mental status exam, check for signs of depression (see Depression), anxiety (see Anxiety), and somatization (see Somatization Disorders).
- Note stool color and consistency and test for occult blood.
- Perform anoscopy to identify internal hemorrhoids, fissures, tumors, hyperpigmentation, and other local pathology. Finding melanosis coli on direct visualization of bowel lumen suggests abuse of anthraquinone laxatives such as castor oil or senna.

LAB STUDIES

- Limit radiologic investigation to cases in which evidence from Hx and PE suggests obstruction or other serious pathology.
- For acute onset of constipation in setting of abdominal pain, rule out obstruction and ileus with supine and upright abdominal films + serum potassium and calcium measurements.
- For more chronic or recurrent constipation, check serum glucose and TSH.
- If you suspect subacute or chronic colonic obstruction (especially if Crohn's disease or cancer is possible), proceed to colonoscopy or sigmoidoscopy plus barium enema.
- Follow expectantly for several wks elderly persons presenting with no evidence of obstruction, anemia, or occult blood loss.
  - During this time implement empiric program of increased dietary fiber, exercise, and monitoring with stool guaiac tests.
  - If symptoms resolve and no other risk factors or findings suggestive of colorectal cancer are present, forego further study and schedule return visit for repeated assessment in 4–8 wks.
  - When cause of constipation is obscure, stop all nonessential medications including codeine cough suppressants, OTC calcium-containing antacids, and iron supplements.

MANAGEMENT

GENERAL

■ Consider empiric symptomatic management only after ruling out obstruction and other forms of serious organic pathology.

■ Reassure patient that you have found no evidence of serious underlying illness (including cancer).

■ Educate patient about diet, exercise, and proper laxative use.

■ Reassure patient that daily bowel movement is not essential to good health and that comfortable elimination patterns depend on healthy living and eating habits.

■ Prescribe daily exercise based on patient's physical capacity (see Exercise).

■ Advise adequate fluid intake (1.5–2.0 L/day; 6–8 glasses of water), particularly if prescribing high-fiber diet.

■ Recommend cessation of laxatives, enemas, and nonessential drugs that may suppress colonic motility.

■ Advise establishing convenient, uninterrupted time for defecation each day.

■ Inform patient that it may be wks to mos before better bowel habits ensue.

DIETARY FIBER AND FIBER SUPPLEMENTS

■ Start with fiber before resorting to bulk laxatives.

■ Increase fiber content of diet by adding bran, fruits, green vegetables, and whole-grain cereals and breads.

■ Aim for 15 g fiber/day.

■ Reassure patient that initial bloating is likely to resolve after several wks of continued use.

■ If dietary and exercise efforts fail or patient insists on medication, consider indigestible fiber residue such as Metamucil, Citrucel, or polycarbophil; usual dose: one tsp/8 oz liquid tid).

■ Use with plenty of fluids to prevent obstructing bolus formation.

LAXATIVES

■ Consider laxatives only if other means have failed and serious underlying pathology has been ruled out.

■ For the elderly, consider nonabsorbable saccharide/bulk laxative (e.g., sorbitol, lactulose) that creates osmotic effect; prefer sorbitol (30–60 mL qhs) to lactulose because of cost.

　• Use magnesium-containing laxatives (e.g., milk of magnesia, magnesium citrate) if necessary but with caution because they may induce magnesium and sodium overload in older persons with renal dysfunction.

　• Consider surfactant laxatives such as docusate to soften stool in patients reporting hard stools.

■ Try to avoid regular use of stimulant/irritant laxatives [derivatives of diphenylmethane (bisacodyl), anthraquinone (senna), and cascara] because of potential for bowel refractoriness and worsening constipation.

- Resort to prokinetic agents (e.g., cisapride) with caution because of proarrhythmic effects, especially in the elderly.

ENEMAS

- When fecal impaction is present, prescribe hypertonic enema (e.g., Fleet). Avoid soapsuds enemas because of risk of colitis with their use.
- Instruct patient with impaction who is taking enema to squat over toilet by standing on chair in front of bowl, which provides more favorable position for evacuating rectum. Only rarely does one need to resort to disimpaction.
- For patients with constipation due to IBS, establish trusting, therapeutic patient-doctor relationship; elicit and respond to concerns and perspectives; take time to explain and answer questions; provide a clear rationale for recommendations; counsel patience and realistic expectations; and exhibit sympathetic support.

BIBLIOGRAPHY

- For the current annotated bibliography on constipation, see the print edition of *Primary Care Medicine*, 4th edition, Chapter 65, or www.LWWmedicine.com.

Diarrhea

SCREENING AND/OR PREVENTION

- Traveler's diarrhea
  - Advise care in eating and drinking, using bottled water and avoiding local water supplies, foregoing fresh vegetables washed in local water and even ice cubes.
  - Consider chemoprophylaxis for most common pathogen, enterotoxigenic *E. coli*; prescribe TMP-SMX DS (1 tab/day) or ciprofloxacin (500 mg/day).
  - Consider Pepto-Bismol for prophylaxis and Rx when given in large doses (60 mL qid).

DIFFERENTIAL DIAGNOSIS

- Acute diarrhea
  - Viruses
  - Bacterial toxins
    - Staphylococcus
    - Clostridium
  - Bacteria
    - Salmonella
    - Shigella
    - *E. coli* (including O157:H7)
    - Campylobacter
    - Yersinia
    - *B. cereus*
    - *V. parahaemolyticus*
    - *V. cholerae*
    - Listeria
  - Protozoa
    - *G. lamblia*
    - *E. histolytica*
    - Cryptosporidium
    - Microsporidia
  - Drugs
    - Laxatives
    - Antibiotics
    - Caffeine
    - Alcohol
    - Antacids
  - Functional
    - Anxiety
    - Acute presentations of chronic or recurrent diarrhea
- Chronic or recurrent diarrhea
  - Protozoa
    - *G. lamblia*
    - *E. histolytica*
    - Cryptosporidium

173

- Inflammation
  - Ulcerative colitis
  - Crohn's disease
  - Ischemic colitis
  - Pseudomembranous colitis
  - Collagenous colitis
  - Lymphocytic colitis
- Drugs
  - Laxatives
  - Antibiotics
  - Quinidine
  - Guanethidine; other antihypertensive agents
  - Caffeine
  - Digitalis
- Functional
  - Irritable bowel syndrome
  - Diverticulosis
- Tumors
  - Bowel carcinoma
  - Villous adenoma
  - Islet cell tumors
  - Carcinoid syndrome
  - Medullary carcinoma of thyroid
- Malabsorption
  - Sprue
  - Intestinal lymphoma
  - Bile salt malabsorption
  - Whipple's disease
  - Pancreatic insufficiency
  - Lactase deficiency
  - Other disaccharidase deficiencies
  - Alpha-beta lipoproteinemia
- Postsurgical
  - Postgastrectomy dumping syndrome
  - Enteroenteric fistulas
  - Blind loops
  - Parasympathetic denervation
  - Short-bowel syndrome
  - Bile and diarrhea
- Other
  - Cirrhosis
  - Diabetes mellitus
  - Heavy metal intoxication
  - Other neurogenic diarrheas
  - Hyperthyroidism
  - Addison's disease
  - Pellagra
  - Scleroderma
  - Amyloidosis

WORKUP

OVERALL STRATEGY

■ Before starting workup, confirm that problem is diarrhea and not simply occasional loose stools or frequent defecation of formed stools.

- Diarrhea in AIDS patients
  - Consider Cryptosporidium, *M. avium-intracellulare*, HSV, CMV, *N. gonorrhoeae*, and *C. trachomatis*.
  - Focus evaluation on finding pathogen.
  - Consider bowel biopsy to obtain tissue for viral and mycobacterial culture (see HIV-1 Infection).

HISTORY

Acute and Traveler's Diarrheas

- Determine nature of bowel movements, including frequency, consistency, volume, and presence of gross blood, pus, or mucus (see Tables 64-2 and 64-3 in *Primary Care Medicine*, 4th edition).
- Check for associated symptoms such as fever, rash, abdominal pain, and late onset of neurologic deficits or meningeal symptoms (listeriosis).
- Review travel (international and domestic), personal contacts, and food intake. Ask whether patient has recently eaten custard-filled pastries, undercooked processed meats, foods warmed on steam tables, eggs, poultry, raw seafood, unpasteurized milk and fruit juices, rice, or bean sprouts.
- Check important contacts, including sexual contacts and children who attend day care centers.
- Note onset and associated symptoms.
- Check drug Hx, especially use of laxatives, magnesium-containing antacids, excess alcohol, caffeine-containing beverages, herbal teas, antibiotics, digitalis, quinidine, loop diuretics (furosemide, ethacrynic acid), and antihypertensive agents, and excessive intake of sorbitol-containing "sugar-free" gums and mints.

Chronic or Recurrent Diarrhea

- Assess for etiology (see above) by characterizing diarrhea and eliciting important associated symptoms.
- Consider rectosigmoid pathology if there is frequent passage of small volumes of loose stools associated with left lower quadrant crampy abdominal pain or tenesmus points.
- Suspect small-bowel pathology if there are large volumes of loose stools with periumbilical or right lower quadrant pain or diarrhea occurring shortly after meal or ingestion of certain foods.
- Search for malabsorption, osmotic etiology, dumping syndrome, and fistula if diarrhea follows meals.
- If stools are bloody, investigate for neoplasm, invasive infection, and inflammatory bowel disease.
- Consider IBS and Crohn's disease for alternating diarrhea and constipation.
- Test for giardiasis if there are frothy stools and excessive flatus (signs of fermentation of unabsorbed carbohydrates), especially in conjunction with recent travel.
- Assess for pseudomembranous colitis if there is antibiotic use within past wks to mos.
- Consider postdysentery lactase deficiency and IBS when there is slowly resolving traveler's diarrhea.
- Thoroughly review drug intake (especially antibiotics) and any surreptitious laxative abuse.

- Take note of previous abdominal surgery, particularly procedures that may have produced blind loops and allowed for bacterial overgrowth.

Chronic Diarrhea of Unknown Etiology

- Consider surreptitious laxative abuse (see Eating Disorders), subtle forms of inflammatory bowel disease, and IBS in young women with undiagnosed diarrhea.
- Consider collagenous and lymphocytic forms of colitis in women with chronic watery diarrhea complicated by steatorrhea and malabsorption, especially those who are thought to have sprue but who do not respond to gluten-free diet.

PHYSICAL EXAM

Acute and Traveler's Diarrheas

- Check vital signs for postural hypotension, fever, weight loss.
- Examine for symptoms of sepsis (including truncal macular "rose spot" rash); lymph node enlargement; abdominal tenderness, guarding, or rebound; abnormal bowel sounds; organomegaly; masses; rectal pathology; positive fecal occult blood test; meningeal irritation; and focal neurologic deficits.

Chronic or Recurrent Diarrhea

- Check for fever, dehydration, postural hypotension, cachexia, jaundice, pallor, rash, dermal manifestations of inflammatory bowel disease, abdominal distention, ascites, hepatomegaly, tenderness, rebound, and masses. Note any fecal impaction, perirectal fistula, or patulous anal sphincter; test stool for occult blood.

LAB STUDIES

Acute and Traveler's Diarrheas

Initial Evaluation

- Individualize lab workup.
- Omit immediate testing for patient who feels well except for frequent loose stools.
- For patient with fever, nausea, abdominal cramps, or other systemic symptoms, begin with stool test for WBCs (drop of sample on microscope slide mixed thoroughly with 2 drops methylene blue or Wright's or Gram's stain and topped with cover slip).
- Consider stool Gram's stain for suspected *Campylobacter* infection (gull-wing gram-negative rods).
- Omit stool cultures except if patient appears ill and occult blood or WBCs are present in stool; notify lab if *E. coli* O157:H7 is consideration.
- Consider sigmoidoscopy in patients with severe illness and gross blood or large numbers of WBCs in stool; avoid preparatory enemas and cathartics.

Subsequent Evaluation

- If diarrhea persists >2 wks, check stools for blood and WBCs and send samples for bacterial culture and for O&P.
- If giardiasis is consideration, send ≥3 stool samples and consider therapeutic trial of metronidazole.

- In persons with neurologic deficits or meningeal signs, culture blood and CSF for *Listeria*.
  - If symptoms persist and Dx remains uncertain, proceed to workup for chronic or recurrent diarrhea (see below).

Chronic or Recurrent Diarrhea

- Consider CBC, LFTs, serum electrolytes, amylase, PT, calcium, albumin, and glucose levels, and stool exam for WBCs and RBCs.
- If blood or pus in stool or other evidence of rectosigmoid pathology is present, proceed to sigmoidoscopy (see below).
- For suspected laxative abuse, alkalinize stool: If it contains phenolphthalein (a common ingredient of many OTC laxatives), it will turn pink.
- For suspected fat malabsorption, order qualitative stool fat determination, and if positive, consider 72-hr quantitative stool fat determination.
- In persons suspected of having inflammatory bowel disease, amebiasis, or IBS, perform sigmoidoscopy without cleansing enemas, and note any mucus, mucosal ulceration, plaques, friability, or bleeding.
- If you suspect Crohn's disease or neoplasia, substitute colonoscopy for sigmoidoscopy.
- Reserve barium enema and upper GI series for demonstrating anatomic abnormalities (blind loops, fistulas, and tumors). Complete stool collections for O&P before obtaining barium study.
- Submit up to 3 stool samples for *C. difficile* toxin detection from patients with recent antibiotic exposure or inflammatory exudate on sigmoidoscopy.
- If ulceration of rectosigmoid mucosa is present and epidemiologic data suggest amebic disease, have fresh mucosal smears prepared by sampling periphery of ulcers with glass rod or metal spatula.
- Order stool analysis for O&P for those with travel Hx, anal intercourse, or immunocompromise. Labs require fresh specimens for identification of trophozoites.
- Consider indirect hemagglutination assay for amebiasis when clinical and epidemiologic suspicion persists despite negative exams for O&P.
- Order immunologic ELISA assay of stool to identify *Giardia* antigen if stool exam does not detect organisms; avoid empiric therapeutic trial.
- Consider small-bowel aspiration or even biopsy for Dx of giardiasis or cryptosporidiosis.
- Consider small-bowel biopsy to confirm sprue rather than depending on empiric trial of gluten-free diet.
- Consider therapeutic trial for Dx:
  - Restriction of milk products for suspected lactose intolerance.
  - Course of antibiotic Rx in patients with suspected blind loop syndrome.
  - Use of pancreatic enzymes in patients with suspected pancreatic insufficiency.

Chronic Diarrhea of Unknown Etiology

- Order stool analysis and colonoscopy when Dx is elusive; request measurement of stool volume, osmolality, and electrolyte content to help differentiate IBS, osmotic diarrhea (due to magnesium, bran), maldigestion of food, and malabsorption of osmotically active substances (e.g., carbohydrates).

- Use stool analysis to help identify secretory diarrhea such as surreptitious laxative abuse, villous adenoma, carcinoid syndrome, and pancreatic cholera.
- For suspected collagenous colitis and lymphocytic colitis, proceed to biopsy, especially in women with unexplained watery diarrhea complicated by steatorrhea and malabsorption.
- Consider inpatient evaluation with imposition of 24- to 72-hr fast and IV hydration in patients without Dx. Use fast to differentiate osmotic and secretory causes; perform stool analysis.

MANAGEMENT

ACUTE DIARRHEAS

- Maintain hydration and wait for spontaneous resolution of symptoms.
- Use oral fluids rich in electrolytes and sugar to facilitate water absorption (e.g., 8-oz glass of fruit juice or flat nondiet cola drink, to which is added pinch of table salt + 1/2 tsp honey or 1 tsp table sugar).
- Take fruit juice or cola with equal amount of water containing 1/4 tsp baking soda to replenish losses in stool electrolytes.
- For disabling diarrhea, consider Imodium (2–4 mg q4h, ≤16 mg/day) or diphenoxylate (Lomotil, which contains atropine to discourage abuse, 2.5–5.0 mg q4h, ≤20 mg/day); use cautiously, if at all, in inflammatory bowel disease and certain bacterial diarrheas (e.g., shigellosis); avoid in outbreaks of *E. coli* O157:H7 infection.
- Avoid empiric antibiotic Rx; reserve antibiotics for very ill patients with positive stool cultures or other evidence for specific bacterial etiology.
- For *Salmonella*, consider course of trimethoprim/sulfamethoxazole double strength (TMP-SMX DS) PO bid × 2 wks to limit metastatic infection in vulnerable patients (elderly, vascular prostheses, sickle cell anemia). For bacteremia and typhoid fever, treat with parenteral ampicillin or PO chloramphenicol.
- For *Shigella* complicated by severe dysentery, begin PO amoxicillin (500 mg tid × 3–5 days) or TMP-SMX DS (1 tab bid × 3–5 days) but perform antibiotic sensitivity for resistant strains. Avoid antiperistaltic drugs.
- For *Campylobacter*, consider PO erythromycin (500 mg qid × 7 days).
- For *Yersinia*, treat only toxic patients; use PO chloramphenicol (50 mg/kg/day in 4 divided doses × 7 days) or parenteral Rx.
- For pseudomembranous colitis, treat only sick patients; use metronidazole (250 mg tid × 5–10 days) or PO vancomycin in liquid suspension (125 mg qid × 7–10 days); retreatment is sometimes necessary. Add cholestyramine (1 packet in water tid) to help bind enterotoxin.
- For *E. histolytica*, use metronidazole (750 mg tid × 5–10 days) for trophozoites and diiodohydroxyquin (iodoquinol) (650 mg tid × 21 days) for elimination of cysts.
- For giardiasis, begin metronidazole (250 mg tid × 7–10 days) or quinacrine (100 mg tid × 7 days); retreat as needed.

TRAVELER'S DIARRHEA

- For symptomatic relief of acute diarrhea, ciprofloxacin (500 mg bid × 3 days) or TMP-SMX DS (1 tab bid × 3 days).

- For symptomatic relief in addition to antibiotics, consider diphenoxylate or loperamide, except when *Shigella* or *Salmonella* infection is serious consideration (i.e., fever, rectal bleeding).

CHRONIC DIARRHEA

- Treat etiologically; reserve empiric trials for Dx only.
- For exacerbations of inflammatory bowel disease, begin steroids and sulfasalazine; collagenous and lymphocytic forms appear to benefit from course of bismuth subsalicylate (see Inflammatory Bowel Disease).
- For malabsorption associated with pancreatic insufficiency, use enzyme supplements (see Pancreatitis).
- For steatorrhea caused by sprue, initiate gluten-free diet.
- For lactase deficiency, limit milk products or prescribe exogenous lactase.
- For dumping syndrome, advise small feedings.
- For surreptitious laxative abuse, work toward total cessation of laxative use (see Eating Disorders).
- For IBS, consider loperamide if diarrhea predominates (see Irritable Bowel Syndrome).

CHRONIC DIARRHEA OF UNKNOWN ETIOLOGY

- For patients who remain undiagnosed after extensive workup but who appear otherwise well, trial of IBS Rx is reasonable (see Irritable Bowel Syndrome).
- If patient does not respond after 4 wks of management, obtain gastro-enterologic consultation.
- Avoid nonspecific antidiarrheal agents to treat undiagnosed patients.

BIBLIOGRAPHY

- For the current annotated bibliography on diarrhea, see the print edition of *Primary Care Medicine*, 4th edition, Chapter 64, or www.LWWmedicine.com.

Diverticular Disease

DIFFERENTIAL DIAGNOSIS

- See Abdominal Pain.

WORKUP

DIVERTICULOSIS

- Consider in patient with painless but brisk rectal bleeding.
- Obtain flexible sigmoidoscopy (or barium enema, if cancer is not a concern).

DIVERTICULITIS

- Suspect in older patients with new-onset left lower quadrant abdominal pain.
- Consider atypical presentations in patients who report suprapubic pain or pain localized to right lower quadrant (redundant sigmoid or right-sided diverticulum). Also, in rare instances, there may be nausea, vomiting, and diarrhea or constipation simulating gastroenteritis.
- Check for low-grade fever, focal tenderness with or without guarding, and loss of bowel sounds (indicative of peritoneal irritation).
- Obtain WBC count.
- In situations of diagnostic uncertainty, consider confirmatory testing:
  - Abdominal CT: test of choice for immediate confirmation of acute diverticulitis; has supplanted barium enema; more cost-effective and safer. Diagnostic findings include inflammation of pericolic fat, peridiverticular abscess, thickening of bowel wall >4 mm, and presence of diverticula; use to differentiate cancer from diverticulitis, but sensitivity falls in setting of marked bowel wall thickening.
  - Flexible sigmoidoscopy: when essential to rule out inflammatory bowel disease and cancer. Inability to pass sigmoidoscope beyond rectosigmoid junction strongly suggestive of acute diverticulitis.
- Differentiate diverticulitis from colon cancer. Both produce similar clinical presentations and similar radiologic findings on barium enema. CT at time of initial Dx sometimes can help make distinction. Lower GI endoscopy is more definitive test, allowing for direct visualization and biopsy if tumor is present. Test is usually done after acute symptoms have subsided.

MANAGEMENT

DIVERTICULOSIS

- Increase dietary fiber. Best sources are bran, root vegetables (particularly raw carrots), and fruits with skin.

- For patients who cannot tolerate bran, recommend bulk laxatives such as psyllium hydrophilic mucilloid (Metamucil), but they are relatively expensive.
- Inform patients that bloating or flatulence due to bran intake usually resolves with continued use.
- Advise patients to avoid foods with seeds or indigestible material (e.g., nuts, corn, popcorn, cucumbers, tomatoes, figs, strawberries, and caraway seeds) that may block neck of diverticula.
- Have patients avoid laxatives, enemas, and opiates because they are potent constipating agents.
- Consider anticholinergics in patients with recurrent cramping, but caution about risks of increased constipation and inspissation of fecal material.
- Instruct patients to report fever, tenderness, or bleeding without delay.

DIVERTICULITIS

- For patients with mild diverticulitis (temp <101°F, WBC count <13,000–15,000):
  - Prescribe bed rest and clear liquid diet.
  - Use mild nonopiate analgesics for pain.
  - Monitor temp, pain, and WBC count, and examine abdomen for signs of peritonitis.
  - If patient is febrile, consider broad-spectrum antibiotic [e.g., TMP-SMX DS (1 tab bid); or ciprofloxacin (500 mg bid) + metronidazole (500 mg qid)].
  - Continue antibiotic Rx until patient is afebrile for 3–5 days.
- Arrange for prompt hospitalization if temp >101°F despite antibiotics, pain worsens markedly, peritoneal signs develop, or WBC count continues to rise.

BIBLIOGRAPHY

- For the current annotated bibliography on diverticular disease, see the print edition of *Primary Care Medicine*, 4th edition, Chapter 75, or www.LWWmedicine.com.

Dysphagia

DIFFERENTIAL DIAGNOSIS

- Motor disease
  - Pharyngeal (transfer dysphagia)
    - Pseudobulbar palsy
    - Myasthenia gravis
    - Multiple sclerosis
    - Amyotrophic lateral sclerosis
    - Parkinson's disease
  - Transesophageal
    - Achalasia
    - Scleroderma
    - Diffuse esophageal spasm
  - Distal
    - Nutcracker esophagus
    - Hypertensive lower esophageal sphincter
- Obstructing lesions
  - Upper esophageal
    - Tumor
    - Zenker's webs (Plummer-Vinson syndrome)
    - Goiter
    - Enlarged lymph nodes
    - Cervical spine osteophytes
  - Lower esophageal
    - Carcinoma
    - Stricture (chronic reflux, corrosive agents, intubation)
    - Webs and rings
  - Foreign bodies
  - Food impaction
  - Mediastinal tumors
  - Aortic aneurysm
  - Odynophagia
  - Opportunistic esophageal infection (CMV, herpesvirus, *Candida*)
  - Tablet-induced irritation
  - Severe reflux esophagitis

WORKUP

GENERAL STRATEGY

- Differentiate by Hx and PE oropharyngeal from esophageal dysphagia and mechanical esophageal dysphagia from neuromuscular forms.

HISTORY

- Differentiate obstructing lesion from motor dysfunction by taking particular note of duration and progression of symptoms, their relation to ingestion of solids and liquids, effect of cold on swallowing, and response to swallowing a bolus.

- Check pace of illness: very acute dysphagia (suggests infection, irritation, or food impaction); steady quick progression (tumor); slow progression (motor disorder).
- Note weight loss (obstruction).
- Review location of discomfort and hiccups to help localize region of difficulty.
- Note intermittent dysphagia with solid food only, suggestive of lower esophageal (Schatzki's) ring.
- Inquire into pain associated with dysphagia (indicative of spasm, achalasia).
- Check for pain on swallowing saliva alone (mucosal inflammation).
- Note any chronic heartburn in conjunction with difficulty swallowing solids (stricture), or dysphagia after activity accompanied by diplopia or dysphonia (myasthenia).
- Inquire into dysphagia occurring with reflux, skin changes, and cold extremities (scleroderma).
- Note dysphagia accompanied by tremor or difficulty initiating movement (Parkinson's disease).
- Check for use of inhaled steroid aerosols or broad-spectrum antibiotics, and concurrent HIV infection.

PHYSICAL EXAM

- Check skin for pallor, sclerodactyly, telangiectasia, calcinosis, hyperkeratotic palms and soles (esophageal carcinoma).
- Examine mouth for inflammatory lesions, ill-fitting dentures, and pharyngeal masses; in HIV-positive patients, note any oral candidiasis.
- Palpate lymph nodes and thyroid for enlargement.
- Check abdomen for masses, tenderness, and organomegaly; and check stool for occult blood.
- Test for motor dysfunction, tremor, rigidity, and fatigability in addition to checking for cranial nerve deficits, abnormal Babinski's response, and abnormal gag reflex.

LAB STUDIES

- Consider barium swallow if you suspect structural impediment or motor dysfunction.
- To trace movement of solid food, perform all barium studies with patient supine, and dip piece of bread into barium.
- Obtain video studies of oropharyngeal phase of swallowing both to evaluate suspected oropharyngeal dysphagia and to determine aspiration risk.
- Proceed to referral for endoscopy and biopsy when needing to distinguish between cancer and postinflammatory scarring with stenosis, especially when Hx suggests malignancy (e.g., rapid progression, marked weight loss); consider stretching sphincter at same time; omit endoscopy if barium study normal.
- In setting of odynophagia, obtain endoscopic exam for plaques, vesicles, and pseudomembranes; obtain brushings and biopsy specimens as

needed to detect fungi, giant cells, and intranuclear inclusion bodies. All patients with new-onset odynophagia require endoscopic evaluation.

- Consider manometry if strong clinical suspicion of motor dysfunction or failure of barium swallow to reveal probable etiology.
- Consider provocative testing for assessment of atypical chest pain, using either acid perfusion (Bernstein) test or edrophonium (Tensilon) infusion.
- In cases of atypical chest pain that defies explanation, consider 24-hr continuous ambulatory monitoring of intraesophageal pH and pressures.

MANAGEMENT

SYMPTOMATIC RELIEF

Motility Disorders

- For mild motor disease, advise eating slowly, drinking in small quantities, and avoiding cold foods.
- In patients with mild to moderate motor dysfunction, consider trial of sublingual nitrates or calcium channel blockers before meals.
- Provide thorough explanation and consider trial of nitrates and/or calcium channel blockers in patients with atypical chest pain due to esophageal motor dysfunction.
- Begin antireflux Rx (see Heartburn and Reflux) when workup suggests acid reflux as trigger of symptoms.
- Consider antidepressant with little anticholinergic activity if you suspect psychiatric precipitant of esophageal motor dysfunction. Likewise, consider trial of relaxation techniques and other behavioral methods. Provide thorough reassurance that there is no serious underlying esophageal pathology.
- For patients with severe achalasia unresponsive to diet and drug manipulations, refer for consideration of esophageal dilation or myotomy.

Inflammatory Conditions

- In HIV-infected patients initiate appropriate antifungal or antiviral program (see HIV-1 Infection).
- For severe erosive esophagitis, begin proton pump inhibition (see Heartburn and Reflux).

Obstructing Lesions

- Recommend liquids or soft solids sufficient to provide adequate caloric intake with minimum discomfort.
- Refer for consideration of dilation or surgery.
- For those with lower esophageal ring, restore adequate iron intake.
- For carcinoma of upper or middle third of esophagus, refer for consideration of palliative radiation Rx.
- For Zenker's diverticulum or large goiter, consider surgical correction.

INDICATIONS FOR REFERRAL AND ADMISSION

- Refer for consideration of nonoral nutrition patients with oropharyngeal dysphagia who aspirate >10% of barium test bolus and show barium residue in oropharynx.

■ In those with neuromuscular disease severe enough to cause oropharyngeal dysphagia, obtain neurologic consultation.

■ Refer to gastroenterologist or surgeon for consideration of endoscopic biopsy patients with obstructing lesion of unclear etiology.

■ Regardless of referral, monitor nutritional status in all patients.

BIBLIOGRAPHY

■ For the current annotated bibliography on dysphagia, see the print edition of *Primary Care Medicine*, 4th edition, Chapter 60, or www.LWWmedicine.com.

External Hernia

DIFFERENTIAL DIAGNOSIS

- Entrapped femoral hernia
  - Inguinal hernia
  - Femoral lymphadenopathy
  - Saphenous varix
  - Psoas abscess
  - Hydrocele
- Groin pain or swelling
  - Encarcerated hernia
  - Muscle strain
  - Hip arthritis
  - Inguinal adenopathy
  - Undescended testicle

WORKUP

HISTORY

- Question patient about groin pain, swelling, ability to reduce hernia, circumstances of onset, and aggravating and alleviating factors, such as exacerbation on standing, straining, or coughing.

PHYSICAL EXAM

- On inspection, examine in supine and standing positions and use Valsalva's maneuver to increase intra-abdominal pressure.
- To detect ventral hernias visually, have supine patient lift head from exam table and bear down to tense abdominal wall.
- Palpate with patient standing; in male patient, insert index finger into inguinal canal by following spermatic cord.
- Distinguish direct from indirect hernias; indirect hernia projects more inferiorly, and protrusion into scrotum is almost always a sign.
- To detect femoral hernia, palpate fossa ovalis, inferior to inguinal canal.
- If you detect groin hernia, gently attempt reduction of hernia while patient relaxes abdominal muscles.
- If hernia is irreducible, look for signs of incarceration and strangulation tenderness, discoloration, edema, fever, and signs of small-bowel obstruction.
- Check for inguinal lymphadenopathy and other masses that do not change with position or Valsalva's maneuver.
- If groin pain is present but no mass evident, check for pain reproduced by internal or external rotation of the hip, suggesting hip pathology as source of pain.
- Although it has been suggested that hernia patients routinely undergo screening for colorectal cancer, decide this based on overall risk (see Colorectal Cancer).

- Note any symptoms or signs of prostatism, liver enlargement, or ascites, which sometimes accompany hernia formation.

MANAGEMENT

INGUINAL HERNIA

- Base need for surgery on PE findings.
- For patients with asymptomatic, easily reducible inguinal hernia, manage expectantly; consider surgery if symptomatic patient is young or if pain ensues or signs of incarceration develop.
- For patients with reducible inguinal hernia, refer for elective repair; reduction using truss may be unsatisfactory, even in patients with relative medical contraindications to surgery.
- If hernia is of recent onset and signs of inflammation or bowel obstruction are absent, attempt gentle reduction (taxis); best accomplished with patient supine and hips and knees flexed.
- If gentle pressure over hernia sac does not reduce mass, refer for surgical consultation.
- Refer patients with evidence of strangulated groin hernias for immediate operation regardless of medical contraindications.

FEMORAL HERNIA

- Refer patients with reducible femoral hernia for prompt elective repair.
- If there may be incarcerated femoral hernia, proceed immediately with surgical exploration.

UMBILICAL HERNIA

- For umbilical hernia presenting as small, asymptomatic fascial defect without protrusion, follow expectantly.
- If PE reveals herniation, refer for repair because risk for incarceration and strangulation is high.
- Manage incarcerated umbilical hernias as if they were strangulated.
- Avoid elective umbilical herniorrhaphy in patients with ascites; instead, try to reduce ascites (see Cirrhosis and Chronic Liver Failure).

INCISIONAL HERNIA

- For small-neck incisional hernias or tender incarceration, proceed to urgent repair; same for patients who have trophic changes or ulceration in skin overlying incisional hernias.
- For large incarcerated abdominal incisional hernia in very obese patient, attempt weight reduction before repair.
- If intestinal obstruction is possible or viability of sac contents doubtful, obtain advice of surgeon.

TREATMENT OF CONTRIBUTING FACTORS

- Attend to symptomatic prostatism that leads to straining (see Benign Prostatic Hyperplasia).
- Address causes of chronic cough (see Chronic Cough).

CONVENTIONAL VS LAPAROSCOPIC HERNIA REPAIR

■ If requisite surgical skill is available and patient is capable of undergoing general anesthesia, offer laparoscopic repair.

BIBLIOGRAPHY

■ For the current annotated bibliography on external hernia, see the print edition of *Primary Care Medicine*, 4th edition, Chapter 67, or www.LWWmedicine.com.

Gallstones

DIFFERENTIAL DIAGNOSIS

- See Abdominal Pain; Jaundice.

WORKUP

- See Abdominal Pain; Jaundice.

MANAGEMENT

WATCHFUL WAITING VS TREATING

- Follow patients with asymptomatic cholelithiasis expectantly, because risk of developing symptomatic disease or complication is only 1%/yr.
- Patients with single episode of biliary colic are reasonable candidates for expectant management, as long as they are free of recurrent pain.
- Advise patients with documented gallstones and recurrent biliary colic or Hx of gallstone disease complication (cholecystitis, pancreatitis) to undergo elective cholecystectomy, provided they can tolerate general anesthesia and surgery.
- Dyspeptic symptoms are not grounds for medical or surgical Rx because their relation to gallstone disease is tenuous at best. Dyspeptic symptoms likely to respond better to other measures (see Nonulcer Dyspepsia).

SURGICAL THERAPY

- Consider laparoscopic cholecystectomy surgical procedure of choice for patients with recurrent biliary colic who can tolerate general anesthesia; procedure reduces perioperative morbidity and shortens recovery period when performed by skilled surgeon.

BILE ACID THERAPY

- Consider trial of bile acid Rx with ursodiol (10–15 mg/kg/day) for symptomatic patients who are not good surgical candidates but do have functioning gallbladder and radiolucent (i.e., cholesterol) gallstones.
- Continue bile acid Rx for ≥12 mos and often for 24 mos. Best results in those with <3 stones <2-cm diameter. Presence of calcification rules out bile acid Rx.
- Monitor effects of Rx with gallbladder ultrasound q6mos. Risk of recurrence high after bile acid Rx stops.

LITHOTRIPSY

- Consider referral for consideration of lithotripsy if symptomatic patient with calcium-containing stones is not surgical candidate. Best results in those with <4 stones <3-cm diameter.
- Refer to center with expertise in procedure.

DIETARY AND OTHER PREVENTIVE MEASURES

- Stop or decrease dosages of estrogen preparations, clofibrate, and other drugs that may trigger stone formation in persons with gallstones or high risk of developing them.
- Although restricting fat and cholesterol is of little or no benefit in altering clinical course of established gallstone disease, do advise restricting fat and caloric intake because obesity and caloric excess are major risk factors for development of new stones.
- Advise gradual weight reduction through modest caloric restriction, but caution against fasting and starvation diets, because they make bile more lithogenic.
- Counsel regular exercise and advise that modest alcohol consumption (<1 oz/day) is not harmful.

BIBLIOGRAPHY

- For the current annotated bibliography on gallstones, see the print edition of *Primary Care Medicine*, 4th edition, Chapter 69, or www.LWWmedicine.com.

Gastrointestinal Bleeding

DIFFERENTIAL DIAGNOSIS

- Hematemesis
  - Esophageal varices
  - Esophagitis
  - Esophageal ulceration
  - Mallory-Weiss tear
  - Esophageal cancer
  - Gastritis or duodenitis
  - Gastric or duodenal ulcer
  - Gastric neoplasm (carcinoma, lymphoma, or rarely leiomyoma/sarcoma)
  - Telangiectasia
  - Angiodysplasia, especially in patients with renal failure
- Melena
  - All causes of hematemesis
  - Meckel's diverticulum
  - Crohn's disease
  - Small-bowel neoplasms (rare)
- Hematochezia
  - Hemorrhoid
  - Anal fissure
  - Colonic polyp
  - Colorectal carcinoma
  - Angiodysplasia
  - Diverticular disease
  - Inflammatory bowel disease
  - Any upper GI or small-bowel lesion if bleeding is brisk

WORKUP

OVERALL STRATEGY

- Rule out serious acute blood loss; ask about postural light-headedness and check for postural hypotension.
- If degree of blood loss poses no immediate hazard, proceed with office evaluation.

HISTORY

- Clarify nature of bleeding (melena, hematemesis, or hematochezia).
- Review for intake of substances that may turn stool black (Pepto-Bismol, iron, charcoal, or spinach) or red (beets).
- Consider factors that can produce false-positive fecal occult blood test (e.g., use of cough syrup containing glycerol guaiacolate, recent meal of rare red meat).
- If patient reports hematemesis, review Hx for bleeding diathesis, cirrhosis, chronic liver disease, alcoholism, aspirin use, acute alcohol excess, NSAID use, Hx of peptic ulcer disease, and epigastric pain.

- With frank rectal bleeding, review Hx for diarrhea, urgency, tenesmus, or lower abdominal cramping suggesting inflammatory bowel disease; also check for Hx of diverticulosis, cancer, polyps, and other rectosigmoid pathology; note any weight loss and change in bowel habits; even if Hx of hemorrhoids, continue to search for other etiologies.

PHYSICAL EXAM

- Repeat determination of postural signs.
- Inspect skin for pallor, ecchymoses, petechiae, telangiectasias, and stigmata of chronic liver disease (e.g., jaundice, palmar erythema, spider angiomata).
- Check nose and pharynx for bleeding sources; lymph nodes for enlargement (especially Virchow's node); abdomen for organomegaly, ascites, and masses; anorectal area for lesions; and stool for color and occult blood (see Colorectal Cancer).
- Perform anoscopy on patients who complain of anal symptoms.
- Consider passing nasogastric tube if significant acute blood loss of unclear origin. Neutralize guaiac test of aspirate with drops of sodium hydroxide to assure adequate test sensitivity.

LAB STUDIES

- Obtain hemoglobin concentration, CBC, and RBC indices.
- Check platelet count, PT, and PTT.
- Check liver and renal function.
- For hematochezia in person aged >50, search for tumor, even in presence of hemorrhoids, by ordering colonoscopy. Consider air-contrast barium enema plus sigmoidoscopy if colonoscopy unavailable.
- For suspected acute brisk upper GI bleeding, obtain prompt upper GI endoscopy. Also consider endoscopy for patients at high risk for recurrent bleeding (evidence of chronic liver disease or initial bleed that requires transfusion) and those with persistent bleeding despite medical Rx.
- Reserve upper GI barium study as supplementary procedure for patients with inactive bleeding, unexplained chronic blood loss, or suspected small-bowel disease.
- Consider empiric Rx for *H. pylori*– or NSAID-induced peptic ulcer (see Peptic Ulcer Disease) for patients with small bleeds who are hemodynamically stable and do not have liver disease or significant risk for gastric cancer.
- Patients at high risk for recurrent bleeding (e.g., chronic liver disease, transfusion requirement) and those with persistent bleeding should undergo upper GI endoscopy.
- For melena, determine whether source is more likely upper or lower GI tract and proceed accordingly.
- For occult bleeding in absence of suggestive symptoms or risk factors, begin with colonoscopy to focus on detecting asymptomatic neoplasms at curable stage. If no identifiable cause of occult bleeding within colon, consider evaluation of upper GI tract and small bowel, although yield for detection of cancer is likely low.

MANAGEMENT

- Consider prophylactic measures for patients at high risk for upper GI bleeding (such as those with varices or Hx of upper GI bleeding, especially if exposed to anticoagulants or high doses of NSAIDs).
- In patients with known varices, begin propranolol (e.g., 40 mg bid) to reduce risk of first bleed (see Cirrhosis and Chronic Liver Failure).
- In selected patients with Hx of bleeding from ulcer or gastritis, begin H_2 blocker or omeprazole (see Peptic Ulcer Disease).
- Treat modest falls in hematocrit with PO iron (300 mg ferrous sulfate tid) to treat resulting iron deficiency (see Anemia).
- For patients with presumed anal bleeding, recommend fiber supplement and stool softeners to decrease mechanical trauma (see Constipation).
- Admit emergently for recent or ongoing brisk bleeding, especially if it is accompanied by orthostatic hypotension or other symptoms or signs of hemodynamic compromise.
- Hospitalize those with profound anemia, even in absence of evidence for dramatic blood loss, especially if there is underlying cardiopulmonary disease.
- Refer to gastroenterologist patients who may be candidates for endoscopy, and those whose bleeding source remains elusive after initial evaluation.

BIBLIOGRAPHY

- For the current annotated bibliography on gastrointestinal bleeding, see the print edition of *Primary Care Medicine*, 4th edition, Chapter 63, or www.LWWmedicine.com.

Heartburn and Reflux

DIFFERENTIAL DIAGNOSIS

- Esophageal spasm
- Myocardial ischemia
- Peptic ulcer disease
- Esophageal cancer
- Esophageal infection (viral, fungal)
- Reflux secondary to underlying disease (DM, scleroderma, peptic ulcer, cancer)

WORKUP

HISTORY

- Check for characteristic Hx of retrosternal burning sensation radiating upward associated with large meals and supine posture that is virtually diagnostic of reflux disease.
- Identify aggravating factors, such as intake of fatty foods, concentrated sweets, alcohol, peppermint, coffee, tea, anticholinergics, calcium channel blockers, and theophylline compounds.
- Note any gastroesophageal surgery or use of drugs capable of causing esophageal injury (NSAIDs, quinidine, wax matrix potassium chloride tablets, tetracycline).
- Inquire into antacid response.
- Check for concurrent Raynaud's phenomenon, raising possibility of scleroderma.
- Consider achalasia, malignancy, esophagitis, and stricture if dysphagia is part of clinical presentation (see Dysphagia).

PHYSICAL EXAM

- Examine hands for sclerodactyly, calcinosis, and telangiectasia.
- Check epigastrium for mass lesion; check stool for occult blood.

LAB STUDIES

- Establish Dx of reflux disease by careful Hx; use lab testing only in atypical or severe cases.
- When Hx reveals story indicating classic uncomplicated reflux with no clinical evidence of underlying disease, proceed directly to management.
- When Hx is less straightforward (e.g., atypical chest pain), consider 24-hr esophageal pH monitoring to determine if symptoms correlate with acid reflux (see Dysphagia).
- Obtain barium swallow and/or esophagoscopy if dysphagia, painful swallowing, significant weight loss, or occult blood loss is present; for suspected esophageal mucosa injury, order endoscopy with biopsy.
- Reserve Bernstein acid perfusion test for determining whether atypical chest pain is consequence of acid reflux (see Dysphagia).

MANAGEMENT

- Consider empirical Rx of otherwise healthy patients who give classic Hx of uncomplicated reflux.
- Treat in stepwise fashion, beginning with simple nonpharmacologic measures, then adding pharmacologic intervention as needed (see below).
- If patient does not respond, if heartburn is complicated by dysphagia, weight loss, or anemia, or if stool tests positive for occult bleeding, then proceed to endoscopic evaluation, especially in older patients at risk for malignancy.

NONPHARMACOLOGIC MEASURES

- Begin dietary intervention, lifestyle modification, and antacids:
  - Dietary manipulations: avoid high-fat, high-carbohydrate foods (chocolate can be particularly problematic); avoid cigarettes, alcohol, and coffee.
  - Reduce weight if obese.
  - Avoid large evening meals near bedtime or before exercise.
  - Elevate head of bed with 6-in. blocks under bedposts (pillows are inadequate).
  - Avoid medications that decrease sphincter tone (including theophylline compounds, calcium channel blockers, meperidine, and anticholinergics), and those that may injure esophageal mucosa (tetracycline, quinidine, wax matrix potassium chloride tablets, NSAIDs, bisphosphonates).
  - Suggest liquid antacids pc and qhs.
- When above measures are insufficient, implement initial pharmacologic measures.

PHARMACOLOGIC MEASURES

Suppression of Gastric Acid Production

- Prescribe H_2 blocker in place of or in combination with antacid; advise taking separately from antacids.
- For best results, consider full-dose regimen bid (e.g., 800 mg cimetidine, 150 mg ranitidine, or 20 mg famotidine). For milder reflux, use once-daily dose at time of maximal symptoms, supplemented when necessary by antacids for prompt relief of breakthrough heartburn.
- Begin PPI (e.g., omeprazole, 20 mg/day) for symptoms refractory to full implementation of nonpharmacologic measures and H_2 blocker Rx (see above) and for those with erosive esophagitis (see below).
- Double PPI dose if symptoms not fully controlled.
- Consider long-term maintenance Rx if patient relapses on tapering, especially in persons with erosive esophagitis (see below).

Prokinetic Therapy

- Consider when symptoms persist despite above measures, choosing either metoclopramide (10–15 mg qid) or cisapride (10–20 mg qid).
- Use with caution due to CNS side effects in metoclopramide and proarrhythmic effects (QT prolongation) in cisapride; obtain ECG for arrhythmias and prolongation of QT interval before and during cisapride Rx.

ANTIREFLUX SURGERY

- Refer patients who experience disablingly refractory symptoms or complications such as stricture, bleeding, Barrett's esophagus, or pulmonary aspiration.
- Check for preserved function of esophageal body and normal gastric emptying before subjecting patient to surgery.
- Consider reoperation if reflux recurs.

EROSIVE ESOPHAGITIS

- Treat persons with endoscopically documented erosive esophagitis with long-term maintenance PPI but only after patient experiences symptomatic recurrence and only if recurrence takes place in context of full implementation of dietary and other nonpharmacologic measures.
- Implement PPI maintenance Rx before symptomatic recurrence only in those with severe erosion (grade 4) and those in whom symptoms reduce quality of life (>25%).
- Check for and eradicate *H. pylori* infection (see Peptic Ulcer Disease), a risk factor for gastric cancer in setting of atrophic gastritis, which may result from chronic PPI Rx.
- If prolonged PPI use is concern, consider maintenance program of long-term H_2 blocker Rx (e.g., ranitidine, 150 mg qhs or bid).
- For refractory erosive disease, consider antireflux surgery.

BARRETT'S ESOPHAGUS

- Screen persons who have had symptomatic GERD for ≥5 years and are sufficiently fit and willing to undergo surgery should severe dysplasia or early cancer be found.
- Obtain endoscopy and include biopsy even if mucosal changes are not visible.
- For those with changes of Barrett's esophagus without dysplastic transformation, continue surveillance endoscopy q3yrs thereafter.
- For those with low-grade dysplasia, screen more frequently (e.g., q6mos).
- For finding of high-grade dysplasia, refer for surgical consideration.
- Treat medically as for erosive disease (e.g., long-term PPI Rx; see above).
- Consider variety of ablative approaches as alternatives to surgery as new efficacy data become available.

CHRONIC COUGH DUE TO REFLUX

- Consider trial of antireflux Rx when patient with chronic pulmonary complaints reports symptoms of reflux.
- Continue for several wks to allow airway healing before deciding on efficacy.
- Avoid use of theophylline for pulmonary complaints because it can aggravate problem by reducing lower esophageal sphincter pressure (see Asthma).

PATIENT EDUCATION AND INDICATIONS FOR REFERRAL

- Stress importance of compliance with all elements of program because no single measure is likely to suffice.

- Point out lack of direct connection between hiatus hernia and reflux and the likelihood that surgery will be unnecessary.
- Refer when considering endoscopy (chronic symptomatic disease of duration ≥5 yrs, dysphagia, odynophagia, unexplained weight loss, or iron deficiency anemia).
- Consider surgical referral for persons who remain symptomatic despite max medical Rx.

BIBLIOGRAPHY

- For the current annotated bibliography on heartburn and reflux, see the print edition of *Primary Care Medicine*, 4th edition, Chapter 61, or www.LWWmedicine.com.

Inflammatory Bowel Disease

DIFFERENTIAL DIAGNOSIS

- See Abdominal Pain; Diarrhea.

WORKUP

- See Abdominal Pain; Diarrhea.

MANAGEMENT

ULCERATIVE COLITIS

General Measures

- Periodically document activity of disease with endoscopic evaluation.
- Reduce dietary fiber during exacerbations.
- Advise adequate rest and sleep.
- Prescribe folic acid supplement (1 mg/day) when leafy vegetables are restricted or sulfasalazine is being used.
- Add iron supplement (e.g., ferrous sulfate, 300 mg PO tid) when there is considerable rectal bleeding and documented iron deficiency anemia.
- Schedule visits frequently in early phases of illness to provide psychological support and close monitoring. Phone checks help.
- Prescribe short course of opiate Rx (e.g., loperamide, 2–4 mg; or codeine, 15 mg ac and qhs) for temporary symptomatic control of troublesome diarrhea in patients with mild to moderate disease; avoid prolonged use and use in patients with severe disease (high risk of toxic dilatation).
- If mild diarrhea persists during remissions, initiate trial of psyllium hydrophilic colloid (1 tsp/8 oz water qd or bid); if unsuccessful, try restricting milk products.
- Refer for consideration of periodic colonoscopy and biopsy those patients who have pancolitis lasting >8 yrs.

Mild to Moderate Disease

- Begin sulfasalazine, 500 mg qid, taken with meals and qhs.
- Increase dosage as tolerated over several days to 1 g qid. Continue dosage for 2–4 wks until symptoms abate, then decrease to smallest dosage that controls symptoms (usually 2 g/day, but up to 4 g/day).
- Substitute a nonsulfa 5-ASA (e.g., mesalamine, 1 g qid) in sulfa-allergic patients and those who cannot tolerate or experience suboptimal response from sulfasalazine.
- If sulfasalazine or another 5-ASA fails to achieve control within several wks, begin PO prednisone, 40 mg/day. Initially give in divided doses for patients with round-the-clock symptoms, but change to a qam program as soon as possible to limit adrenal suppression. Continue dosage 7–10 days.
- If control is achieved, begin tapering prednisone by 5–10 mg q2wks to lowest dosage necessary to suppress disease activity.

- To minimize adverse effects of chronic steroid Rx, try qod program (using same total weekly dose that maintains control) (see Glucocorticoid Therapy).
- Once you taper steroids and disease activity ceases, decrease sulfasalazine to maintenance dose of 2 g/day and continue for at least 1 yr to maintain remission. If mesalamine is used, prescribe 1–2 g/day for maintenance.

Moderate to Severe Disease

- Start with prednisone, 60 mg/day in divided doses; and sulfasalazine, 4 g/day.
- Once symptoms are controlled, give entire prednisone dose in the morning and begin tapering empirically by 5 mg/wk. Continue sulfasalazine, 1 g qid, indefinitely.
- If nausea or abdominal pain causes inadequate food intake, consider supplementing diet with nutritionally balanced low-residue liquid dietary preparation (e.g., Magnacal, Ensure, Sustacal, Isocal).
- Monitor carefully for marked blood loss, volume depletion, severe abdominal pain, distention, and peritoneal signs; these are indications for prompt hospital admission, parenteral Rx, and urgent surgical consultation.
- Refer for consideration of steroid-sparing immunosuppressive Rx patients requiring persistently high doses of steroids.
- Refer for consideration of elective surgery patients refractory to maximal medical Rx, those requiring daily steroids for prolonged periods (>6 mos), and those found on cancer screening to have stricture or dysplasia.

Ulcerative Proctocolitis

- If disease is limited to rectosigmoid, begin Rx with PO sulfasalazine (as above) or topical agent. Enemas of hydrocortisone or 5-ASA are effective topically.
- If choosing topical hydrocortisone, base selection of preparation on patient preference and empirical results. Choices include 100-mg retention enema qhs, 25-mg suppository inserted qd–bid, and 90-mg foam preparation administered qd–tid.
- Consider using 5-ASA enemas (2–4 g/day for acute symptoms; 1 g/day for maintenance) if concerned about steroid absorption and systemic side effects. Continue Rx until symptoms clear.
- Continue sulfasalazine or one of its substitutes for prophylaxis.

CROHN'S DISEASE

General Measures

- Document extent of disease by barium studies or colonoscopy. Postpone barium enema and colonoscopy until disease activity subsides.
- Limit dietary fiber content in patients with cramps and diarrhea.
- Decrease fat intake to <80 mg/day when there is steatorrhea.
- Try restricting milk products in patients with diarrhea; if diarrhea promptly improves, continue lactose-restricted diet.
- Supplement diet with multivitamin containing 5× normal RDA + iron, calcium, magnesium, and zinc.
- Consider short-course opiate Rx (e.g., loperamide, 2–4 g; or codeine, 15 mg with meals and qhs) for symptomatic relief of diarrhea; use caution; Rx may aggravate obstruction, and prolonged use can lead to narcotic dependence.

- Advise partial bowel rest and use of elemental low-residue dietary preparations for severe cramps and diarrhea.
- Admit for surgical consultation patients with refractory disease, severe bleeding, toxicity, abdominal pain, abscess formation, or evidence of obstruction.

Colonic Disease

- Begin sulfasalazine (500 mg qid) and quickly increase dosage to 1 g qid over several days; continue for 4–8 wks. Use olsalazine (500 mg bid) or mesalamine (up to 4.8 g/day) for sulfa-intolerant patients or patients unresponsive to sulfasalazine.
- If there is response to sulfasalazine, continue 4–6 mos, then stop if symptoms cease.
- For maintenance, prescribe mesalamine at lowest dose that sustains remission (usually 2.4–3.6 g/day). Sulfasalazine and olsalazine do not prevent recurrences.
- If no initial response to 5-ASAs, switch to metronidazole, 10–20 mg/kg/day (e.g., 250–500 mg tid) and continue for 4-wk trial. If response is satisfactory, continue 4–6 mos, then stop if symptoms cease.
- If inadequate response to metronidazole, switch to prednisone 60 mg/day; patient may initially require qid dosages for round-the-clock control.
- As disease activity subsides, give entire dosage in the morning and begin tapering to lowest dosage that controls symptoms (often as little as 5 mg/day). Continue dosage until all evidence of disease activity ceases (then for at least 1 yr); a qod schedule may suffice.
- For refractory disease or patients requiring chronic steroid Rx, refer for consideration of immunosuppressive Rx with 6-MP or azathioprine (50 mg/day), or one of newer antiinflammatories/immunomodulators (e.g., methotrexate, infliximab).

Perianal Disease

- Prescribe metronidazole (750–2,000 mg/day) for refractory perianal disease; prolonged course of Rx may be necessary.

Ileal Disease

- Begin with 4- to 6-wk trial of olsalazine (500 mg bid) or mesalamine (up to 4.8 g/day). Effectiveness of sulfasalazine is not well established.
- If no response or if severe ileal symptoms, prescribe prednisone (60 mg/day) and use as for colonic involvement (see above).
- Consider use of 6-MP or azathioprine (50 mg/day) for patients with fistulas, refractory symptoms, or persistent requirements for very high steroid dosages. A 6-month trial is often necessary. Continue Rx for 12 mos, then attempt cessation, although long-term Rx is sometimes necessary and successful in maintaining remission.
- Because immunosuppressive Rx can cause marrow suppression and carcinogenesis, obtain gastroenterologic consultation if considering such Rx.

BIBLIOGRAPHY

- For the current annotated bibliography on inflammatory bowel disease, see the print edition of *Primary Care Medicine*, 4th edition, Chapter 73, or www.LWWmedicine.com.

Irritable Bowel Syndrome

DIFFERENTIAL DIAGNOSIS

- See Abdominal Pain; Constipation.

WORKUP

- Take patient's bowel complaints seriously; do not minimize their importance or deny their reality.
- Minimize patient requests for costly testing by conducting detailed Hx and careful PE that specifically elicit and address patient concerns, and check specifically for malignancy and inflammatory bowel disease (see Abdominal Pain; Constipation; Diarrhea; Gastrointestinal Bleeding).
- Thoroughly review key findings and their significance with patient, using clinical presentation to determine need for further diagnostic testing.
- When there are no risk factors or clinical findings suggestive of malignancy or inflammatory bowel disease, fecal occult blood testing is negative, and CBC is normal, consider halting workup and proceeding to Rx.
- When there are risk factors for serious underlying illness (e.g., positive family Hx of colorectal cancer, age >50) or suggestive symptoms (weight loss, new-onset constipation, hematochezia), proceed to colonoscopy.
- If problem is predominantly constipation in absence of evidence for serious organic disease, consider diagnostic trial of increased dietary fiber, stool softeners (dioctyl sodium sulfosuccinate), or osmotic laxative (psyllium); check serum potassium in patients taking diuretics to rule out hypokalemia, which may exacerbate constipation.
- Rule out partial obstruction if constipation is accompanied by severe abdominal pain and marked distention; obtain plain film of abdomen during symptoms.
- When diarrhea predominates, consider workup for common etiologies of chronic diarrhea (see Diarrhea).
- Take time to identify psychological difficulties or social stresses by taking detailed psychosocial Hx; note frustrations, losses, concerns, fears, expectations, and responses to life stresses.
- Assess specifically for underlying anxiety (see Anxiety), depression (see Depression), and somatization (see Somatization Disorders).

MANAGEMENT

GENERAL MEASURES

- After conducting thorough workup that includes detailed investigation of all possible etiologies (both organic and psychological), provide thorough explanation of Dx and directly address patient's concerns and fears.

- Establish supportive relationship and begin supportive psychotherapy for patients with underlying situational or psychosocial stresses.
- Help redirect patient's attention away from bowel symptoms and endless searches for cure and toward better coping with daily stresses; focus on accomplishments rather than symptoms, and on taking control through exercise, good eating habits, and behavioral changes rather than on repeated recitation of symptoms.
- See patient at regular intervals and be available for help at times of increased stress.
- Stop or minimize nonessential medicines that may affect bowel function, especially irritant laxatives.

CONCURRENT DEPRESSION, ANXIETY, OR SOMATIZATION DISORDERS

- Treat specifically and etiologically any concurrent depression (see Depression), anxiety (see Anxiety), or somatization disorder (see Somatization Disorders).
- When treating IBS patient with concurrent depression, consider patient's bowel symptomatology when choosing antidepressant agent [e.g., tricyclic for patient with frequent loose stools; SSRI if constipation is predominant problem (see Depression)].
- For chronic anxiety, consider anxiolytic antidepressants [e.g., amitriptyline, trazodone, and doxepin, as well as nonaddicting anxiolytics (e.g., buspirone)]. Avoid use of sedatives, tranquilizers, and combination preparations containing benzodiazepines or barbiturates (risks of habituation and withdrawal usually outweigh benefit).
- For motivated patients with well-identified psychosocial stressors, consider referral for combination of behavioral techniques and psychotherapy.

FOR IRRITABLE BOWEL SYNDROME WITH CONSTIPATION PREDOMINATING

- Increase dietary fiber and recommend regular exercise.
- Add bulking agent such as psyllium (Metamucil, 1 rounded tsp/8 oz water tid, prn).
- Try stool softener (e.g., dioctyl sodium sulfosuccinate) if hard stool is problematic.

FOR IRRITABLE BOWEL SYNDROME WITH DIARRHEA PREDOMINATING

- Limit intake of potentially contributing substances such as caffeine, sorbitol-containing candies and chewing gums, and alcohol.
- Give short trial (1–2 wks) of restricting dairy products (except for yogurt with live cultures).
- Consider need for short-term symptomatic relief and if necessary prescribe short course of loperamide (1 tab bid × 2–5 days prn); avoid opiates because of addiction potential in this chronic condition.
- For refractory diarrhea, consider diagnostic trial of cholestyramine (4 g tid–qid).

- If cholestyramine does not suffice, consider trial of anticholinergic Rx [e.g., dicyclomine, 20 mg qid; or anticholinergic tricyclic antidepressant (e.g., amitriptyline, 50 mg qhs)], but only if patient finds abdominal pain and distention intolerable and condition is refractory after other measures; avoid these if constipation is bothersome.
- At this time there is insufficient evidence to recommend trial of Chinese herbal medicine.

BIBLIOGRAPHY

- For the current annotated bibliography on irritable bowel syndrome, see the print edition of *Primary Care Medicine*, 4th edition, Chapter 74, or www.LWWmedicine.com.

Jaundice

DIFFERENTIAL DIAGNOSIS

- Unconjugated hyperbilirubinemias (urine negative for bilirubin)
  - Increased bilirubin production
  - Decreased hepatic uptake of bilirubin
  - Decreased conjugation
- Conjugated hyperbilirubinemias (urine positive for bilirubin)
  - Hepatocellular disease
  - Intrahepatic cholestasis
  - Extrahepatic obstruction

WORKUP

HISTORY

- Check for abdominal pain (indicative of acute biliary tract obstruction), Hx of alcoholism, exposure to hepatitis, and flulike onset (all suggestive of hepatocellular etiology).
- Note other hepatocellular disease risk factors (e.g., blood transfusion, travel to area endemic for hepatitis, consumption of raw shellfish, IV drug abuse, high-risk sexual practices, use of potentially hepatotoxic drugs).
- Inquire into risk factors for obstruction, such as gallstones, previous biliary tract surgery, and high fever.
- Review risk factors for intrahepatic cholestasis, such as use of estrogen, phenothiazines, and other drugs that can cause cholestasis.
- Review family Hx for episodic jaundice in setting of intercurrent illness (Gilbert's disease).

PHYSICAL EXAM

- Note findings of hepatocellular failure (e.g., spider angiomata, gynecomastia, and palmar erythema), small liver, splenomegaly, prominent abdominal venous pattern, asterixis, and peripheral edema; also signs of early or mild hepatocellular disease (mild to moderate hepatic enlargement and mild tenderness to punch).
- Check for signs of extrahepatic obstruction, including palpable gallbladder (Courvoisier's sign) and marked hepatic enlargement (≥6 cm below inferior costal margin); guarding, rebound tenderness, and fever suggest acute obstruction.

LAB STUDIES

- Check urine for bilirubin and obtain direct and indirect serum bilirubin levels.
- If evidence of unconjugated hyperbilirubinemia, initiate search for hemolysis (see Anemia), ineffective erythropoiesis, hereditary causes of jaundice, and concurrent systemic illness.

- If conjugated hyperbilirubinemia, obtain serum SGOT, SGPT, alkaline phosphatase, PT, and serum albumin and check for patterns suggestive of each mechanism [e.g., marked rises in alkaline phosphatase (>4–5x) and modest elevations in transaminases (2–3x) = cholestasis or extrahepatic obstruction].
- Consider response to IM or SQ administration of vitamin K to help differentiate hepatocellular disease from cholestatic and obstructive conditions.
- If marked elevation in alkaline phosphatase, differentiate extrahepatic obstruction from intrahepatic cholestasis by ultrasonography (U/S).
- If initial U/S study is technically unsuccessful, repeat or proceed to CT, especially if surgery is consideration.
- If you strongly suspect common duct obstruction (even if U/S or CT is nondiagnostic), or if additional anatomic detail is required for planning Rx, consider percutaneous transhepatic cholangiography or endoscopic retrograde cholangiopancreatography, and magnetic resonance cholangiopancreatography; select in consultation with surgeon, radiologist, or gastroenterologist experienced in evaluating obstructive jaundice.
- Consider liver biopsy in cases of persistent severe hepatocellular injury of unknown etiology, but only after ruling out obstruction and only if result will affect management.
- Avoid hepatobiliary scintigraphy, which although useful in suspected acute cholecystitis and cystic duct obstruction (see Gallstones), has no value in evaluation of jaundice.

MANAGEMENT

SYMPTOMATIC RELIEF

- Consider trial of cholestyramine for severe pruritus (9-g packet of powder in orange juice or applesauce tid).
- Avoid vitamin deficiency by supplementing with fat-soluble vitamins (A, D, and K).

BIBLIOGRAPHY

- For the current annotated bibliography on jaundice, see the print edition of *Primary Care Medicine*, 4th edition, Chapter 62, or www.LWWmedicine.com.

DIFFERENTIAL DIAGNOSIS

SOME IMPORTANT CAUSES OF NAUSEA AND VOMITING

- Nausea/vomiting as predominant or initial symptom
  - Acute
    - Digitalis toxicity
    - Ketoacidosis
    - Opiate use
    - Cancer chemotherapy
    - Early pregnancy
    - Inferior myocardial ischemia
    - Drug withdrawal
    - Binge drinking
    - Hepatitis
  - Recurrent or chronic
    - Psychogenic vomiting
    - Metabolic disturbances (uremia, adrenal insufficiency)
    - Gastric retention (gastroparesis, outlet obstruction)
    - Bile reflux after gastric surgery
    - Pregnancy
- Nausea/vomiting associated with abdominal pain (abdominal pain sometimes absent)
  - Viral gastroenteritis
  - Acute gastritis
  - Food poisoning
  - Peptic ulcer disease
  - Acute pancreatitis
  - Small-bowel obstruction and pseudo-obstruction
  - Acute appendicitis
  - Acute cholecystitis
  - Acute cholangitis
  - Acute pyelonephritis
  - Inferior MI
- Nausea/vomiting associated with neurologic symptoms
  - Increased intracranial pressure
  - Midline cerebellar hemorrhage
  - Vestibular disturbances
  - Migraine headaches
  - Autonomic dysfunction

WORKUP

HISTORY

- Focus on timing of symptoms, their relation to meals, characteristics of vomitus, and associated complaints.

- Check for early morning onset (metabolic disturbances, alcoholic binge, early pregnancy); precipitation by meals (psychogenic, pyloric channel ulcer, gastritis); onset several hrs after eating (obstruction, gastric atony); emesis of food ingested >12 hrs earlier (gastric stasis); vomiting of large volumes (>1,500 mL/day).
- Inquire about blood or "coffee ground" material, bilious vomitus (pyloric channel open), pure gastric juice (peptic ulcer disease, Zollinger-Ellison syndrome), lack of acid (atrophic gastritis, gastric cancer), feculent material (distal small-bowel obstruction and blind-loop syndrome).
- Check Hx for abdominal pain, fever, jaundice, weight loss, abdominal surgery, external hernias, family Hx of emesis, symptoms of DM, prior renal disease, ischemic heart disease, drug use (e.g., digitalis, narcotics), visual disturbances, headache, ataxia, vertigo, and last menstrual period.
- Ask about concurrent emotional and social stresses; if you suspect bulimia, gently inquire into self-image, binge eating, and self-induced emesis (see Eating Disorders).
- Note any acute hepatitis risk factors (sick contacts; IV drug abuse; exposure to raw shellfish, pastries, poultry; travel to area with poor sanitation or cholera).

PHYSICAL EXAM

- Check for postural hypotension, elevated BP, irregularities of rate and rhythm, Kussmaul's respiration, pallor, hyperpigmentation, jaundice, papilledema, retinopathy, nystagmus, stiff neck, abdominal distention, visible peristalsis, abnormal bowel sounds, succussion splash, peritoneal signs, focal tenderness, organomegaly, masses, flank tenderness, muscle weakness, ataxia of gait, and asterixis.
- If Hx of vertigo with nausea, perform Bárány's maneuver (see Dizziness).
- In patients with suspected bowel motility disorder, check for signs of autonomic insufficiency (postural hypotension without increase in heart rate, lack of sweat, blunted pulse and BP responses to Valsalva's maneuver).

LAB STUDIES

- Test by suspected etiology rather than by routine ordering of "nausea and vomiting studies."

Acute Emesis with Abdominal Pain

- Check plain and upright abdominal films to rule out acute surgical cause such as bowel obstruction, peritonitis, or blockage of hollow viscus (see Abdominal Pain).
- If pancreatitis suspected, obtain serum amylase.
- For suspected acute cholecystitis or choledocholithiasis, order liver function studies (e.g., alkaline phosphatase, AST) and promptly proceed to abdominal ultrasonography.

Acute Nausea and Vomiting without Abdominal Pain

- Check for associated gait ataxia and nuchal rigidity (midline cerebellar hemorrhage); if present proceed immediately to emergency CT of posterior fossa (see Headache).
- If patient has type I DM, consider ketoacidosis and obtain urine and serum ketones and blood glucose determinations (see Diabetes Mellitus).

- In patient with risk factors for CAD, perform ECG (see Chest Pain).
- Consider hepatitis and obtain transaminase (aminotransferase) determination.
- If patient is taking medication that may cause nausea and vomiting, order serum drug level. If patient takes digitalis, halt intake of drug, and check ECG and levels of drug and potassium.

Recurrent Vomiting

- Consider psychogenic cause, but first rule out pregnancy, metabolic derangements, and chronic gastroesophageal disease.
- If early morning vomiting, obtain urinalysis and determinations of serum BUN, creatinine, electrolytes, glucose, and, in women of childbearing age, hCG β-subunit.
- For patients with postprandial symptoms, order upper GI series if concerned about gastric outlet obstruction or retention, and consider endoscopy if mucosal injury is possible.
- For suspected psychogenic vomiting, individualize testing; some patients may insist on further testing; others are comforted knowing that extensive studies are unnecessary.

MANAGEMENT

THERAPEUTIC TRIALS

- If you suspect gastroesophageal motility disorder, consider short course of prokinetic agent such as metoclopramide or cisapride (e.g., 10 mg, 30 mins ac) supplemented by a proton pump inhibitor (e.g., 20 mg/day omeprazole).
- Patients with suspected underlying affective disorder sometimes respond to 4- to 8-wk trial of antidepressant; select agent with minimal anticholinergic activity (e.g., trazodone, desipramine, or fluoxetine).

SYMPTOMATIC RELIEF

- Whenever possible, treat etiologically.
- Consider symptomatic measures only when you have identified cause but Rx of underlying condition does not adequately control symptoms; do not use symptomatic Rx in lieu of Dx.

Phenothiazines

- For initial symptomatic Rx of vomiting caused by drugs, metabolic disorders, and gastroenteritis; use with caution in emesis due to hepatitis and cholestasis because drug is hepatically metabolized.
- Consider prochlorperazine (Compazine, 5–10 mg q6h prn, or rectally 25 mg tid prn) or promethazine (Phenergan, 12.5–25 mg q6–8h, or rectally 25 mg tid prn).

Other Centrally Acting Agents

- For emesis due to motion sickness or vestibular disease, consider trimethobenzamide (Tigan, 250 mg tid prn, or rectal suppositories tid prn).

Antihistamines

- Consider meclizine (Antivert, 12.5–25 mg tid prn) for symptomatic relief of emesis due to vestibular disturbances.

- For more rapid onset of action, consider dimenhydrinate (Dramamine) just before or with onset of symptoms; for more prolonged effect, consider transdermal scopolamine (single transdermal patch applied behind ear several hrs before travel and left on for ≤3 days).
- Avoid use before driving or using machinery.

Prokinetic Agents

- For patients with emesis resulting from gastroparesis.
- Consider metoclopramide (10 mg pc and qhs) or cisapride (10 mg pc and qhs); cisapride causes fewer CNS effects but can prolong QT interval.

Antiemetics for Cancer Chemotherapy

- See Cancer (General).

Drugs for Morning Sickness

- Recommend small morning feedings and try to avoid or minimize antiemetic use.
- For more prolonged, severe forms (hyperemesis gravidarum), first consider supportive psychotherapy and trial of hypnosis, but drug Rx is sometimes necessary.
- Consider trial of vitamin B_6 (25 mg/day).
- Alternatively, try short course of metoclopramide (see above). Approval for Bendectin has been withdrawn because of concern for teratogenic effects.

PSYCHOGENIC VOMITING

- Focus attention on underlying conflicts and stresses troubling patient.
- Avoid antiemetics.

INDICATIONS FOR REFERRAL AND ADMISSION

- Refer patient with suspected refractory motility disorder for consideration of specialized motility studies.
- Patients suspected of psychogenic vomiting require psychiatric consultation because they may be seriously disturbed and potentially suicidal. Referral to mental health professional skilled and experienced in Rx of patients with eating disorders is optimal for those suffering from bulimia (see Eating Disorders).
- Hospitalize for parenteral fluid and electrolyte replacement and additional workup if postural hypotension is present, especially if patient is elderly.
- Treat similarly if evidence of bowel obstruction, increased ICP, or any other GI, neurologic, or metabolic emergency.
- Consider hospitalizing for observation patients who remain undiagnosed after extensive evaluation and are unresponsive to therapeutic trials.

BIBLIOGRAPHY

- For the current annotated bibliography on nausea and vomiting, see the print edition of *Primary Care Medicine*, 4th edition, Chapter 59, or www.LWWmedicine.com.

Nonulcer Dyspepsia

DIFFERENTIAL DIAGNOSIS

- See Abdominal Pain.

WORKUP

- As with any disorder that can mimic more worrisome illness, take patient's concerns seriously and address them directly.
- Check for evidence of serious underlying pathology by reviewing upper GI cancer risk factors (e.g., age >50, unexplained weight loss, persistent nausea and vomiting, decades of severe heartburn, dysphagia, odynophagia, jaundice, iron deficiency anemia, or positive guaiac stool test).
- Order prompt upper GI endoscopy if any of these features are present.
- For patients with paroxysmal attacks of steady epigastric or right upper quadrant pain lasting several hrs and radiating into back, with or without nausea and vomiting, proceed to abdominal ultrasound (U/S) and check LFTs for biliary tract disease (see Abdominal Pain).
- For those with upper abdominal pain radiating into back, especially if alcohol related, check serum amylase and abdominal U/S for possible pancreatitis (see Abdominal Pain; Pancreatitis).
- For those with altered bowel habits and upper abdominal pain, consider colonoscopy or barium enema to rule out transverse colon pathology (e.g., colitis, bowel cancer) if there is additional supporting data (see Abdominal Pain).
- For those with low risk for serious underlying pathology and without Hx of NSAID use, skip above studies and proceed to serologic study for *H. pylori* antibodies (see Peptic Ulcer Disease).
- If there is NSAID use, evaluate and treat for peptic ulcer disease (see Peptic Ulcer Disease).
- Revisit need for endoscopy in low-risk patients if they do not respond to trial of empiric Rx or later develop manifestations suggestive of more serious disease.
- For patients with persistent heartburn, perform assessment appropriate for GERD (see Heartburn and Reflux).

MANAGEMENT

- Consider GI consultation for low-risk but overly concerned patient, but minimize need for such referrals with thorough patient ed and support.
- Select from available Rx options based on best estimate of underlying pathophysiology. Options include eradication of *H. pylori* infection, chronic acid suppression, prokinetic Rx, dietary manipulations, and psychotherapy.
- For those with *H. pylori*, consider eradication of *H. pylori* infection (see Peptic Ulcer Disease).

- In suspected acid-peptic mechanism, consider trial of acid suppression Rx (see Peptic Ulcer Disease); give 4- to 8-wk trial; if symptoms persist, consider additional workup (e.g., upper GI endoscopy) to rule out more serious underlying pathology (see Abdominal Pain; Peptic Ulcer Disease).
- Consider trial of prokinetic Rx with metoclopramide or cisapride; exert caution in long-term use because of risks of tardive dyskinesia and cardiac dysrhythmias, respectively (see Heartburn and Reflux).
- Eliminate only foods and beverages that are clear-cut precipitants identified by careful dietary Hx; avoid recommending special or overly restricted diets.
- In otherwise refractory cases with clear-cut association between dyspepsia and psychosocial factors, address latter thoroughly and specifically (see Anxiety; Depression; Somatization Disorders).
- Refer to gastroenterologist when endoscopy is appropriate (see above).

BIBLIOGRAPHY

- For the current annotated bibliography on nonulcer dyspepsia, see the print edition of *Primary Care Medicine*, 4th edition, Chapter 74, or www.LWWmedicine.com.

Pancreatitis

WORKUP

- See Abdominal Pain.

MANAGEMENT

OUTPATIENT/RECOVERY PHASE OF ACUTE PANCREATITIS

- Begin feedings with carbohydrate-rich, low-fat, low-protein foods. Gradually increase amount of protein in diet as tolerated, followed by slow resumption of fat intake.
- Check for and treat any underlying alcohol abuse (see Alcohol Abuse), hypertriglyceridemia (see Hypercholesterolemia), or hypercalcemia (see Hypercalcemia).
- Eliminate, if possible, use of drugs associated with pancreatitis (azathioprine, estrogens, thiazides, corticosteroids).
- In HIV-infected patients, check for and treat toxoplasmosis or CMV infection and eliminate, if possible, such potentially inciting medications as didanosine, pentamidine, sulfonamides, and corticosteroids.
- Obtain ultrasound (U/S) exam of gallbladder and biliary tract; refer patient for surgical consideration if stones are found. There is no benefit to early endoscopic retrograde cholangiopancreatography and stone removal in persons with biliary pancreatitis who are not jaundiced.

CHRONIC PANCREATITIS

- Check for and treat inciting causes, such as alcoholism, biliary tract disease, hypercalcemia, or hyperlipidemia (see above).
- Readmit patient if severe recurrent acute pancreatitis develops.
  - Temporarily limit fat intake during flare-ups.
  - Begin with mild analgesics for pain control, such as aspirin or acetaminophen, 600 mg q4h.
- Pain unrelieved by mild analgesia is indication for narcotic analgesics, such as methadone, 5 or 10 mg q6–8h.
- Evaluate further to rule out carcinoma, pseudocyst, and biliary tract disease. Begin with U/S and proceed to CT if U/S is technically unsatisfactory.
- Refer patient for surgery if you find treatable lesion.
- Aggressive surgical procedures other than sphincteroplasty aimed at relieving ductal obstruction do not reliably relieve pain.
- Consider trial of tricyclic antidepressant Rx (see Depression) for patients with refractory pain. Psychiatric or pain management consultation may also help.

PANCREATIC INSUFFICIENCY

- Give PO pancreatic extract with each feeding in doses of 0.5–2.5 g (2–8 tabs) with full meals and 0.5 g with snacks. Lack of effect may require addition of antacid (e.g., 60 mL Mylanta with each meal) or H_2-receptor antagonist (e.g., ranitidine, 150 mg bid) to neutralize gastric acid and prevent enzymes from becoming inactivated.

- Provide high-calorie, carbohydrate- and protein-rich diet.
- Supplement diet with medium-chain triglyceride preparation. Restrict fat in symptomatic steatorrhea.
- Monitor glucose tolerance and treat any clinical DM; insulin is required, but use cautiously because these patients often exhibit brittle diabetic control.

BIBLIOGRAPHY

- For the current annotated bibliography on pancreatitis, see the print edition of *Primary Care Medicine*, 4th edition, Chapter 72, or www.LWWmedicine.com.

Peptic Ulcer Disease

WORKUP

- Check for use of NSAIDs (including nonprescription use), aspirin, alcohol, tobacco, and systemic corticosteroids.
- Review Hx for prior peptic ulcer disease or symptoms suggesting it.
- Check for symptoms of malignancy and complicated peptic ulcer disease (weight loss, GI bleeding, persistent nausea and vomiting).
- Check weight.
- Perform stool guaiac exam.
- Test for *H. pylori* infection if there is no obvious inciting factor such as aspirin or NSAID use.
- For initial noninvasive testing, obtain quantitative *H. pylori* serology, using reference lab for the determination.
- Alternatively and to test for eradication of infection, perform ^{14}C or ^{13}C breath test.
- If endoscopy is required, have rapid urease test (e.g., CLO test) performed at same time.
- Order upper GI endoscopy or barium study before initiating Rx if clinical findings suggest malignancy or complicated disease.

MANAGEMENT

NONPHARMACOLOGIC MEASURES

- Avoid, or at least limit to extent medically possible, use of agents potentially injurious to mucosa, including aspirin, excess alcohol, NSAIDs, and perhaps long-term, high-dose glucocorticosteroids.
- Insist on total smoking cessation (see Smoking Cessation).
- Suggest decreased intake of coffee (including decaffeinated) and other caffeine-containing beverages; complete cessation is unnecessary.
- Do not restrict any foods or insist on bland or milk-laden diet. Frequent small feedings are unnecessary, and bedtime snack may actually stimulate nocturnal acid secretion. Patient should avoid only foods that cause discomfort.
- Attend to stress-related issues, but avoid recommending major job or geographic change.

INITIAL PHARMACOLOGIC MEASURES

For All Patients

- Begin acid suppression program to assist ulcer healing, especially those who are *H. pylori* negative. Prescribe proton pump inhibitor (PPI) (e.g., esomeprazole, 40 mg/day; or lansoprazole, 30 mg/day), H_2-receptor antagonist (e.g., cimetidine, 400 mg tid), or high-potency magnesium hydroxide/aluminum hydroxide liquid antacid (30 cc pc and qhs). Base selection on affordability, severity of disease, capacity for compliance, and potential for interaction with other medications.

If NSAID-Induced Ulcer

- Start program of PPI Rx (e.g., esomeprazole, 20 mg/day) or misoprostol (200 mg with each meal and qhs); continue for 4–8 wks, depending on severity at time of presentation. There is no need to test for or treat *H. pylori* infection because its eradication does not improve outcome in NSAID-induced disease.

- For patients with prior Hx of NSAID-induced peptic ulceration or of upper GI bleeding who absolutely require continuous NSAID Rx for maintenance of function, initiate prophylaxis with PPI (e.g., omeprazole 20 mg/day).

- Consider misoprostol (200 mg with breakfast and supper) as slightly less effective alternative for secondary prevention of NSAID-induced disease but as reasonable (although not very cost-effective) first choice for primary prevention.

- Thoroughly instruct patient on how to carry out therapeutic program and review common misconceptions to maximize compliance.

If *H. pylori* Positive

- Begin multidrug antibiotic program.

- When cost is major consideration but compliance is not, prescribe metronidazole (250 mg qid), + tetracycline (500 mg qid) or amoxicillin (500 mg qid) if patient cannot tolerate tetracycline, + bismuth subsalicylate (two tablets, 525 mg, qid). Continue for 2 wks or limit to 1 wk by adding concurrent course of daily PPI Rx (e.g., omeprazole, 20 mg/day; or lansoprazole, 30 mg/day).

- When side effects and compliance with qid regimen are major concerns but cost is not, consider 2-wk, bid program of clarithromycin (500 mg bid), + PPI (e.g., omeprazole, 20 mg bid), + metronidazole (500 mg bid) or amoxicillin (500 mg bid).

- Acid suppression Rx not required for ulcer healing in patients with *H. pylori* infection, but it speeds healing and attainment of symptomatic relief.

REFRACTORY OR RECURRENT DISEASE

- Check for failure to eradicate *H. pylori* infection, preferably by breath test (if available); alternatively, repeat quantitative serology and compare pretreatment titers with current titers (seroconversion from positive to negative is highly specific but not sensitive).

- If *H. pylori* infection persists, retreat with new antibiotic regimen rather than repeating original program.

- Reemphasize importance of compliance, smoking cessation, and avoidance of NSAIDs.

- Institute high-dose PPI Rx (e.g., esomeprazole, 40 mg/day), but limit its duration if possible; if not possible, check for and eradicate any concurrent *H. pylori* infection to avoid development of atrophic gastritis.

- Institute long-term PPI Rx for Zollinger-Ellison syndrome Rx.

- For persistent or recurrent disease unresponsive to Rx, refer for endoscopic exam and biopsy to rule out malignancy and complicated disease, especially if endoscopy was not performed initially.

- Refer patient with refractory multiple ulcers, frequent recurrences, or associated secretory diarrhea for consideration of Zollinger-Ellison syndrome when symptoms are accompanied by marked hypergastrinemia in context of acid hypersecretion.

- Admit patients with evidence of bleeding, gastric outlet obstruction, or perforation and obtain surgical consultation.

BIBLIOGRAPHY

- For the current annotated bibliography on peptic ulcer disease, see the print edition of *Primary Care Medicine*, 4th edition, Chapter 68, or www.LWWmedicine.com.

Serum Transaminase (Aminotransferase) Elevation

DIFFERENTIAL DIAGNOSIS

- Hepatitis C
- Hepatitis B
- Autoimmune disease (including primary biliary cirrhosis)
- Hereditary hemochromatosis
- Alcohol abuse
- Nonalcoholic steatohepatitis
- Wilson's disease

WORKUP

- Repeat determination in 4 wks with patient refraining from alcohol and all noncritical drugs with potential to cause hepatocellular injury.
- Proceed with workup only after confirming elevation.

HISTORY

- Inquire into viral hepatitis risk factors, alcohol abuse, and symptoms of autoimmune disease (see Polyarticular Complaints).
- Note any symptoms, risk factors, or complications of hemochromatosis (fatigue, arthritis, DM, poor libido, family Hx, cirrhosis, heart failure, arthritis) not explained by other causes.
- Note risk factors for nonalcoholic steatosis, such as obesity, hyperlipidemia, and DM.
- Check medications for potentially toxic drugs.
- Review symptoms pertinent to estimating severity of hepatocellular injury (fatigue, easy bruising, jaundice).

PHYSICAL EXAM

- Check for signs of hemochromatosis (hyperpigmentation, arthritis, liver enlargement) and hepatocellular injury (jaundice, ecchymoses, spider angiomata).

LAB STUDIES

- Check alkaline phosphatase, serum albumin and PT as well as SGOT and SGPT.
- If you suspect alcohol abuse, check SGPT to SGOT ratio (2:1 characteristic of alcoholic liver injury).
- Check hepatitis serology (e.g., antibodies to HBV and HCV, and HBsAg).
- Consider ANA and antimitochondrial antibody determinations if Hx suggests autoimmune disease.

- Obtain ultrasonography to check for fatty liver and extrahepatic cholestasis.
- If patient has family Hx of idiopathic cirrhosis or other features suggestive of hemochromatosis, check serum iron, transferrin (TIBC), and ferritin.
- If young patient presents with concurrent neuropsychiatric disease, consider serum ceruloplasmin determination.
- Consider liver biopsy if result will change management.
- Given high frequency of occult steatosis, consider alternative approach to biopsy in obese or diabetic person, recommending exercise, diet, and weight loss followed by repetition of LFTs.

BIBLIOGRAPHY

- For the current annotated bibliography on serum transaminase (aminotransferase) elevation, see the print edition of *Primary Care Medicine*, 4th edition, Chapter 62 appendix, or www.LWWmedicine.com.

SCREENING AND/OR PREVENTION

HEPATITIS A PRECAUTIONS (CONTINUE UNTIL 1 WK AFTER ONSET OF JAUNDICE)

- Advise patient to wash hands thoroughly after toilet use and refrain from intimate contact and handling and serving food to others. Patient need not be confined to home.
- Advise others to avoid contact with patient's fecal material and to wash hands thoroughly if contact is made.

HEPATITIS A PROPHYLAXIS

- For preexposure prophylaxis, administer 2 IM injections of hepatitis A vaccine at least 6 mos apart (dose recommendations vary between 2 vaccine manufacturers).
- For imminent travel to endemic areas, when time is too short to achieve vaccine-induced immunization, administer immune globulin (IG) at dose of 0.02 mL/kg (average adult dose, 2 mL IM) along with first dose of vaccine.
- For postexposure prophylaxis, administer IG to household contacts within 2 wks of exposure at dose of 0.02 mL/kg (average adult dose, 2 mL IM).

HEPATITIS B PRECAUTIONS (CONTINUE UNTIL HBsAG CLEARS SERUM)

- Screen all blood donors for HBsAg.
- Use volunteer blood rather than blood from commercial donors.
- Use disposable syringes and needles.
- Have patient use separate razor, toothbrush, and other personal items.
- Handle carefully any materials containing HBsAg, particularly blood samples and other body fluids; use of gloves required. Following universal precautions when handling clinical materials makes additional precautions unnecessary.
- Recommend avoidance of intimate contact, but confinement to home is unnecessary.
- Wash hands thoroughly after direct contact with patient or with patient's blood or body fluids.

HEPATITIS B PROPHYLAXIS

Preexposure

- Identify high-risk persons: health workers exposed to blood, residents and staff of custodial institutions, household and sexual contacts of chronic HBsAg carriers, promiscuous male homosexuals and promiscuous heterosexuals, patients with hereditary hemoglobinopathies and clotting disorders who require long-term Rx with blood products, and hemodialysis patients.

- For high-risk groups, administer hepatitis B vaccine (1mL IM at 0, 1, and 6 mos; doses for specific age groups may vary according to manufacturer).

Postexposure

- Administer HBIG [0.06 mL/kg body weight (approximately 5 mL)] to those who sustain accidental percutaneous or transmucosal exposure to HBsAg-positive blood or body secretions or needles and instruments contaminated with HBsAg-positive material.

- Administer as soon after exposure as possible. Although globulin injections are recommended up to 7 days after inoculation, their efficacy is nil beyond 2 days.

- Follow passive HBIG immunoprophylaxis by complete 3-injection course of hepatitis B vaccine; start vaccine at same time as HBIG or within first few days to 1 wk after exposure.

- Administer HBIG at dose cited above to sexual contacts of patients with acute hepatitis B as soon after exposure as is practical. Because recognition of hepatitis in sexual contacts is often delayed, be aware that early prophylaxis is usually impossible. Current recommendations call for prophylaxis within 14 days of exposure. After HBIG, give complete 3-injection course of hepatitis B vaccine to all sexual contacts of patients with acute hepatitis B.

- Administer 0.5 mL of HBIG IM to newborns of HBsAg-positive mothers immediately after birth, preferably in delivery room. Follow this Rx by complete 3-injection course of hepatitis B vaccine, 0.5 mL per dose, preferably starting within 7 days of birth (dose may vary according to manufacturer).

- No prophylaxis necessary for casual contacts or nonintimate household contacts.

- Universal vaccination of all children, in conjunction with routine vaccinations of childhood, is recommended. For children without hepatitis B vaccination, vaccinate during adolescence.

HEPATITIS D PROPHYLAXIS

- For those already infected with hepatitis B, prevent hepatitis D by limiting percutaneous and intimate contact with persons known to harbor HDV infection.

- In those susceptible to hepatitis B, vaccinate against hepatitis B to prevent hepatitis D.

HEPATITIS C PRECAUTIONS AND PROPHYLAXIS

- Institute same precautions as for hepatitis B (i.e., limit exposure to blood and body fluids of infected patients).

- Limit transfusion-associated hepatitis C by relying exclusively on volunteer rather than commercial blood donations and screening donors for anti-HCV.

- Do not administer IG to those who sustain needlestick injury, have sexual contact, or are born to infected mothers (not shown effective in preventing hepatitis C; effective hepatitis C vaccine is yet to be developed).

HEPATITIS E PROPHYLAXIS

- To prevent exposure, use same approaches as for hepatitis A (see above).

- Neither IG nor vaccine is available for prevention of hepatitis E.

MANAGEMENT

ACUTE VIRAL HEPATITIS

- Maintain adequate caloric intake and balanced diet. Small feedings are tolerated best, especially in the morning. No foods need be restricted.
- Ensure adequate rest, but activity need not be unduly restricted if patient feels capable.
- Omit potentially hepatotoxic agents, especially alcohol.
- Treat severe pruritus with cholestyramine.
- Treat severe nausea and vomiting with nonphenothiazine antiemetic, such as trimethobenzamide (Tigan) suppositories.
- Admit to hospital if signs of hepatocellular failure develop (e.g., marked prolongation of PT, ecchymoses, encephalopathy). Also consider admission for maintaining adequate caloric and fluid intake when symptoms are severe or for managing complicated underlying diseases.
- Refer patients with fulminant hepatitis for consideration of liver transplantation. In cases of hepatitis B, consider trial of lamivudine, but it should not interfere with transplantation evaluation.
- For patients with acute hepatitis C, initiate IFN-α + ribavirin Rx as soon as possible.
- Check aminotransferase, PT, bilirubin, albumin/globulin, and HBsAg at onset and 12 wks; monitor aminotransferase at 1- to 4-wk intervals during acute illness.
- Retest q4wks any patient with evidence of persistent symptoms or lab abnormalities.
- Refer for liver biopsy those with combination of failure to resolve infection and inflammation by 6–12 mos and persistence of disabling symptoms.

DRUG-INDUCED HEPATITIS

- Stop drugs that might be responsible and institute supportive measures.
- Avoid rechallenging patient with same agent.

NONVIRAL CHRONIC HEPATITIS

- Follow patients with mild chronic hepatitis at regular intervals and rebiopsy if signs of marked worsening.
- For patients with severe chronic hepatitis (multilobular or bridging necrosis on biopsy, disabling symptoms, and marked aminotransferase and globulin elevations), begin high-dose prednisone (60 mg/day) or combination prednisone (30 mg/day) plus azathioprine (50 mg/day). Combination Rx preferred for the elderly, diabetics, and others who cannot tolerate long-term high-dose steroids. Because of impact of azathioprine on fertility, avoid using drug if possible in young adults.
- Taper prednisone in 5- to 10-mg increments over course of 1 mo until you establish maintenance dose of 10 mg/day (with 50 mg/day azathioprine) or 20 mg/day.
- Monitor aminotransferase, bilirubin, and globulins at 2 wks, then q1–3mos. If patient is taking azathioprine, obtain platelet and WBC counts at wks 1 and 2, then once/mo.

- Continue maintenance Rx for at least 24–36 mos, then consider attempting Rx discontinuation with 6-wk period tapering medication.
- Obtain consultation if no clinical improvement within 2–8 mos of initiating Rx; high-dose treatment may be indicated.
- Treat relapses as new cases.

CHRONIC VIRAL HEPATITIS

- Avoid immunosuppressive Rx in patients with chronic viral hepatitis.

Hepatitis B

- Refer for consideration of IFN-α Rx patients with compensated chronic hepatitis B who demonstrate sustained presence of HBV DNA and HBeAg.
- If deemed appropriate by consultant, begin 6-wk course of IFN-α (5 million U/day of SQ or 10 million U qod).
- For chronic "replicative" hepatitis B, consider lamivudine Rx. Treatment consists of 100 mg/day PO for 12 mos. Stop Rx in patients who lose HBeAg; in those who retain HBeAg, continue lamivudine.

Hepatitis C

- Treat patients with compensated chronic hepatitis C with sustained aminotransferase elevations and detectable HCV RNA with IFN-α (3 million U SQ 3 × wk) plus oral ribavirin, 1,000 mg/day (for those weighing <75 kg), or 1,200 mg/day (for those weighing ≥75 kg) for 1 yr.
- In patients with genotypes other than 1 and with low viral load (<2 million viral copies), consider 6-mo Rx course, which may suffice.
- For nonresponding patients and those who relapse whenever Rx stops, refer for determination of need for long-term maintenance IFN Rx.

Hepatitis D

- Consider IFN-α for patients with hepatitis D. Long-term high-dose Rx (as much as 9 million U 3 × wk for 1 yr) is required. Some patients may benefit from indefinite maintenance Rx.

Monitoring Treatment

- Monitor patients receiving IFN by checking WBC, granulocyte, and platelet counts at wks 1, 2, and 4, then once/mo.
- Check aminotransferase levels monthly and thyroid-stimulating hormone every q1–3mos.
- In patients with hepatitis B treated with IFN or lamivudine, monitor HBV DNA q1–3mos and measure HBeAg periodically.
- In patients being treated for hepatitis C, monitor HCV RNA at approximate 3-mo intervals. Those receiving ribavirin need close monitoring of hematocrit/hemoglobin.

INDICATIONS FOR ADMISSION AND REFERRAL

- Admit patient to hospital if evidence of worsening hepatocellular function.
- Consider liver transplantation for patients with hepatic decompensation.

BIBLIOGRAPHY

- For the current annotated bibliography on viral hepatitis, see the print edition of *Primary Care Medicine*, 4th edition, Chapters 57 and 70, or www.LWWmedicine.com.

Hematologic Problems

Anticoagulant Therapy

MANAGEMENT

WARFARIN

Indications and Use

- Warfarin Rx is preferred means of oral anticoagulation. Recommended intensity of anticoagulation for most indications is a PT INR of 2–3.
- Use target INR of 2.5–3.5 in patients with metallic prosthetic heart valves; in highest-risk patients, add aspirin to warfarin Rx.
- Prescribe warfarin for stroke prophylaxis in most cases of AF; substitute aspirin only in those at low risk for stroke and in those in whom warfarin Rx is contraindicated.
- Treat patients with known cause for DVT or pulmonary embolism with warfarin for 3–6 mos.
- Treat patients with idiopathic DVT or idiopathic pulmonary embolism for more prolonged period (i.e., ≥6 mos).
- Continue warfarin indefinitely for patients with recurrent DVT, recurrent pulmonary embolism, ongoing hypercoagulable state, or known homozygosity for activated protein C resistance.
- Perform rapid reversal of oral anticoagulation Rx for severe bleeding, INR >20, or need for urgent surgery. Administration of FFP achieves reversal within hrs. Vitamin K accomplishes same in 6–48 hrs, depending on dose and route of administration.
- Individualize decision to discontinue anticoagulant Rx in context of nonemergent bleeding or elective surgery. Balance risk for embolization against risk for hemorrhage.
- Reverse oral anticoagulation for elective surgery simply by withholding warfarin for 4 days or until INR <1.5, level at which risk for hemorrhage becomes minimal in most surgeries.
- For high-risk patients, consider perioperative heparinization to maintain full anticoagulation for longest period of time possible pre- and postoperatively.
- Anticoagulant Rx mandates frequent monitoring, lifestyle changes, and commitment by patient and health care team to optimize safety and efficacy.

Contraindications to Warfarin Therapy

- Absolute contraindications
  - Previous CNS bleeding
  - Recent neurosurgery
  - Active frank bleeding
  - Early pregnancy and delivery
- Relative contraindications
  - Active peptic ulcer disease
  - Chronic alcoholism
  - Bleeding diathesis
  - Severe HTN

Common Drugs That Interact with Oral Coagulants
- Metronidazole
- TMP-SMX
- Cimetidine
- Omeprazole
- Sulfinpyrazone
- Disulfiram
- Anabolic steroids
- Second- and third-generation cephalosporins
- L-Thyroxine
- Erythromycin
- ? Tamoxifen
- ? Phenytoin
- ? Isoniazid
- ? Ketoconazole
- ? Piroxicam
- Barbiturates
- Carbamazepine
- Rifampin
- Cholestyramine
- Estrogens
- Penicillins

ASPIRIN AND OTHER PLATELET INHIBITORS
- Consider use of aspirin in all persons at risk for atherothrombosis; reduces risk for vascular events, including MI, stroke, and TIA.
- Prescribe aspirin combined with clopidogrel or ticlopidine for ≥14 days after coronary stent implantation.

BIBLIOGRAPHY

- For the current annotated bibliography on anticoagulant therapy, see the print edition of *Primary Care Medicine*, 4th edition, Chapter 83, or www.LWWmedicine.com.

Anemia

SCREENING AND/OR PREVENTION

CANDIDATES FOR SCREENING

- Do not perform routine screening for anemia in nonpregnant, asymptomatic patients. Although determination of hemoglobin concentration or hematocrit is important to evaluating a variety of complaints (e.g., fatigue, weight loss, abdominal pain, GI bleeding) and may provide clues in asymptomatic patients to presence of treatable disease (e.g., GI malignancy), these determinations are less sensitive and less specific than well-recognized screening methods identified for such conditions (e.g., stool guaiac testing, sigmoidoscopy, colonoscopy).
- Obtain screening hematocrit or hemoglobin concentration at time of first prenatal visit in pregnant women, because iron deficiency anemia is common in this setting and associated with poorer pregnancy outcomes.
- Do not screen for anemia in menstruating nonpregnant women because there is no clear relationship between mild to moderate degrees of anemia and symptoms and no clearly measurable benefits from treating iron deficiency anemia.

PREVENTION

Iron Deficiency

- Advise adequate iron intake to prevent iron deficiency in those with increased needs (e.g., pregnant women and young children).
- Recommend iron-rich foods to avoid need for iron supplements (e.g., liver, oysters, moderately to heavily iron-enriched cereals, lean beef, veal, and beans). Green vegetables are rich in iron, but iron absorption is poor because of binding to plant phytates and phosphates.
- When diet alone seems inadequate and needs are very high (e.g., pregnancy), prescribe 150–300 mg/day ferrous sulfate.
- Counsel against iron supplement use in most other instances; supplementation is unnecessary, expensive, and associated with increased risks for malignancy and atherosclerotic disease.

B_{12} Deficiency

- Prevent vitamin B_{12} deficiency in the elderly by recommending frequent feedings and total intake of ≥25 μg/day cyanocobalamin PO.

DIFFERENTIAL DIAGNOSIS

MICROCYTIC ANEMIA (MCV <82)

- Iron deficiency
- Anemia of chronic disease
- Thalassemia trait
- Sideroblastic anemia

MACROCYTIC ANEMIA (MCV >95)

- Vitamin B_{12} deficiency
- Folate deficiency
- Aplastic anemia
- Acute hemolysis or hemorrhage with brisk reticulocytosis
- Chronic liver disease
- Myelodysplastic syndromes
- Severe hypothyroidism

NORMOCYTIC ANEMIA (MCV 82–95)

- Hemolysis
  - Drug induced
  - Autoimmune (idiopathic, collagen disease, lymphoma)
  - Cold agglutinin–induced (viral infection, lymphoma)
  - Hemoglobinopathy (sickle cell disease, G-6-PD deficiency)
  - Hereditary spherocytosis
  - Microangiopathy (heart valve, jogging, vasculitis, dissented intravascular coagulation)
- Chronic disease, including HIV infection
- Renal failure
- Hypothyroidism
- Myelofibrosis
- Early stage of iron deficiency
- Sideroblastic anemia
- Mixed anemia (e.g., iron and vitamin B_{12} deficiencies)

WORKUP

GENERAL STRATEGY

- Classify anemia and conduct workup based on peripheral smear appearance and MCV:
  - Microcytic if MCV <82 fL and RBCs are small
  - Macrocytic if MCV >95 fL and RBCs are large
  - Normocytic if MCV is 82–95 fL and RBCs are normal size.

LAB STUDIES

Microcytic Anemia

- Test first for iron deficiency by obtaining serum ferritin (test of choice for iron deficiency). No need to order serum iron or TIBC for Dx of iron deficiency unless there is concurrent inflammation (ferritin is an acute-phase reactant and its level may be elevated in the setting of inflammatory disease).
- If iron deficiency identified, but cause is not evident, begin search of GI tract for source of occult blood loss (see Gastrointestinal Bleeding).
- If iron deficiency ruled out, assess for thalassemia. Check for Mediterranean extraction and family Hx of anemia or thalassemia. Examine peripheral smear and RBC indices for characteristic manifestations (e.g., target cells, teardrops, increased RBC count, reduced MCHC), and consider testing for hemoglobin A_2 level.

- If iron deficiency and thalassemia have been ruled out, review ferritin level and obtain transferrin saturation (iron/TIBC) to help differentiate anemia of chronic disease (ferritin normal, transferrin saturation low to normal) from sideroblastic anemia (ferritin high, transferrin saturation high).
- If sideroblastic anemia suspected, obtain hematologic consultation for consideration of bone marrow aspirate to check for ringed sideroblasts.

Macrocytic Anemia

- Examine peripheral smear for hypersegmented polymorphonuclear leukocytes and oval macrocytes. If present, obtain serum vitamin B_{12} and folate levels.
- If serum vitamin levels are not diagnostic, obtain serum homocysteine and methylmalonate levels to enhance diagnostic sensitivity, or perform diagnostic trial with small dose of vitamin B_{12} or folate, monitoring reticulocyte count.
- If you detect vitamin B_{12} deficiency, consider Schilling test to differentiate lack of intrinsic factor from malabsorption.
- If macrocytic anemia is nonmegaloblastic, obtain reticulocyte count and examine peripheral smear to determine if marrow activity is increased, normal, or decreased.
- If reticulocyte count is high in absence of hemorrhage, check for hemolysis (haptoglobin, bilirubin, LDH); if normal or slightly reduced, consider hepatic and thyroid dysfunction; if markedly reduced, review peripheral smear for teardrops and ringed sideroblasts, and consider bone marrow biopsy.

Normocytic Anemia

- Determine whether reticulocyte count is elevated, inappropriately normal, or low.
- If count is elevated, evaluate for evidence of recent hemorrhage; if none, confirm hemolysis with haptoglobin, bilirubin, and lactate dehydrogenase determinations.
- If hemolysis confirmed, check for drug-induced cause (direct Coombs' test), autoimmune mechanism (IgG or cold agglutinins), or hemoglobinopathy (sickle cell disease, G-6-PD deficiency).
- If reticulocyte count is not elevated, search for underlying hepatocellular, endocrine, and renal causes and for early iron deficiency anemia and anemia of chronic disease (see above).
- If reticulocyte count is nil, if peripheral blood count and smear show pancytopenia, teardrop forms, and fragmented cells, and if halting all potentially offending medications does not promptly restore marrow function, obtain hematology consultation for bone marrow biopsy.

MANAGEMENT

IRON DEFICIENCY ANEMIA

- Never treat empirically until underlying etiology identified. Correcting iron deficiency without attending to underlying cause can mask important clues to treatable disease and compromise timely Rx.
- Begin replacement Rx when
  - symptomatic
  - underlying cardiac or pulmonary disease

- anemia moderately severe (hemoglobin level 8–9 g/dL)
- pregnant
- subtotal gastrectomy and gastrojejunostomy
- continued heavy blood loss anticipated
- recovering from megaloblastic anemia

■ For maximum cost-effectiveness, prescribe generic ferrous sulfate tablets.

■ Maximize compliance by starting with small dose of ferrous sulfate (e.g., 300 mg/day) and building to 900 mg/day to minimize GI upset.

■ Minimize upper GI side effects by taking iron with meals and using lowest effective dose; reducing frequency of dosing is less effective than reducing dose itself.

■ Avoid use of slow-release and enteric-coated preparations because they dissolve slowly and can bypass proximal small bowel (in which most absorption takes place).

■ Limit use of parenteral iron to patients who have had adequate trial of PO iron and have shown genuine intolerance to all available preparations (e.g., patients with inflammatory bowel disease).

■ If parenteral iron required, administer using IV route, first by very small test dose and then by slow drip; draw up syringe with epinephrine at same time and keep it on hand.

■ Avoid IM administration of iron (sarcomas at injection sites).

■ Consider effect of iron on absorption of other drugs when taken simultaneously (e.g., levodopa, methyldopa, tetracycline, and fluoroquinolone antibiotics). Delay iron intake for several hrs after intake of these other medications.

■ Take iron with orange juice (rich in ascorbic acid) or use ascorbic acid–containing preparation when gastric acid suppression is necessary.

■ Watch for reticulocytosis at 10 days into Rx followed by daily rise in hemoglobin concentration of 0.1–0.2 g/dL.

■ Continue Rx at maximum tolerated doses for several wks until hemoglobin level is normal; fully replenishing iron stores may take several mos: educate patient to maximize compliance.

■ If speed of replacement is an issue, consider blood transfusion rather than iron Rx (response to parenteral iron Rx is no more rapid with PO preparations).

FOLATE DEFICIENCY

■ Treat with pharmacologic doses of folic acid (1–2 mg/day PO). Continue for 4–5 wks.

■ When underlying cause persists (e.g., malabsorption, malignancy, psoriasis, hemodialysis), continue Rx indefinitely.

■ Prescribe folinic acid for patients taking methotrexate.

■ Avoid nonspecific folic acid monotherapy to treat megaloblastic anemia.

■ If alcoholism is basis of folate deficiency, address drinking problem (see Alcohol Abuse).

■ Provide dietary counseling and perhaps referral to nutritionist.

■ Avoid large empiric doses of PO folate monotherapy (e.g., 5 mg) for megaloblastic anemia because of risk of partial and nonspecific correction of anemia while masking underlying vitamin B_{12} deficiency.

VITAMIN B$_{12}$ DEFICIENCY

- For patients with vitamin B$_{12}$ deficiency caused by bacterial over-growth or terminal ileum disease, treat underlying bowel problem [e.g., oral tetracycline or amoxicillin for bacterial overgrowth; steroids and sulfa drugs for inflammatory bowel disease (see Inflammatory Bowel Disease)].
- Promptly recognize and treat vitamin B$_{12}$ deficiency to minimize risk of permanent neurologic damage (see Anemia; Dementia; Focal Neuro-logic Complaints).
- Prescribe parenteral Rx (except in rare patient with poor intake) because most vitamin B$_{12}$ deficiency is secondary to impaired absorption.
- In some cases, use of large oral doses (>100 µg/day) may result in sufficient absorption of vitamin B$_{12}$.
- Consider use of parenteral cyanocobalamin or hydroxocobalamin (bet-ter bound to serum proteins and less rapidly excreted, requiring less frequent administration).
- Choose from host of initial replacement regimens; all are adequate.
- For pernicious anemia, begin with 100–1,000 µg/day IM cyanocobal-amin or hydroxocobalamin for 1–2 wks, repeated 2 × wk for 1 mo, then monthly for remainder of patient's life.
- Alternatively, consider follow-up injection q3–4mos, which suffices for many patients; if neurologic symptoms are present, administer twice/mo follow-up dose for 6 mos.
- More important than interval of Rx is its indefinite continuation; ensure long-term administration; have visiting nurse or family member give injection.
- Avoid empiric use of parenteral vitamin B$_{12}$ as nonspecific Rx for fatigue.
- During Rx, monitor serum potassium and replace if low (see Conges-tive Heart Failure) because serious hypokalemia can develop in patients who have had severe B$_{12}$ depletion.

ERYTHROPOIETIN DEFICIENCY STATES

- Consider erythropoietin in dialysis patients with regular transfusion requirements (IV injections of recombinant erythropoietin, 150 U/kg, 3 × wk). Concurrent iron supplementation is often necessary.
- Also consider in situations associated with severe anemia and reduced serum erythropoietin levels (e.g., HIV infection, malignancy, cancer chemotherapy).

PREOPERATIVE ANEMIA

- Consider allogeneic transfusion for patients undergoing elective sur-gery if there is anemia before surgery and expected operative blood loss.
- Alternatively, consider preoperative erythropoietin Rx (erythropoietin, 300–600 U/kg SQ, 2–4 × wk) if you want to limit allogeneic transfusion requirements and facilitate donation of autologous blood. Best candi-dates have preoperative hematocrit of 33–39% and expected blood loss of 1–3 L.

SICKLE CELL ANEMIA

- See Sickle Cell Disease.

BIBLIOGRAPHY

■ For the current annotated bibliography on anemia, see the print edition of *Primary Care Medicine*, 4th edition, Chapters 77, 79, and 82, or www.LWWmedicine.com.

Bleeding Problems

SCREENING AND/OR PREVENTION

- Always perform preoperative screening for a bleeding disorder.
- Screen by Hx for bleeding diathesis, especially for abnormal bleeding during previous surgery.
- Review current medications, especially NSAIDs, salicylates, and drugs that precipitate thrombocytopenia.
- Obtain platelet count, PT, and PTT, although their value in absence of condition known to compromise hemostasis remains unproved.

DIFFERENTIAL DIAGNOSIS

QUALITATIVE PLATELET DISORDERS

- Defective adhesion
  - von Willebrand's disease
  - High doses of semisynthetic penicillins and cephalosporins
- Defective aggregation
  - Glanzmann's thrombasthenia
  - High doses of semisynthetic penicillins and cephalosporins
- Defective activation
  - NSAIDs
  - Dipyridamole
  - Cardiopulmonary bypass
- Defective acceleration
  - Factor V deficiency

QUANTITATIVE PLATELET DISORDERS

- Thrombocytosis
  - Myeloproliferative disease
  - Reactive (rarely pathologic)
- Thrombocytopenia
  - Decreased production
    - Thiazides
    - Alcohol
    - Viral infection
    - Marrow failure
    - Megaloblastic anemia
    - Myelophthisic process
  - Increased destruction
    - Drugs (quinidine, methyldopa, sulfa, phenytoin, barbiturates)
    - Lupus
    - Infection
    - Idiopathic thrombocytopenic purpura
    - Chronic lymphocytic leukemia
  - Increased sequestration
    - Hypersplenism

INTRINSIC PATHWAY DEFECTS

- Factor VIII deficiency
  - Hemophilia A
- Factor IX deficiency
  - Hemophilia B
- Factor XI deficiency
  - Ashkenazi Jews

EXTRINSIC PATHWAY DEFECTS

- Vitamin K–dependent factor deficiency
  - Poor diet
  - Cholestasis
  - Hepatocellular failure
  - Drugs (coumarin, broad-spectrum antibiotics)

VASCULAR DEFECTS

- Connective tissue fragility
  - Age
  - Cushing's syndrome
  - Scurvy
  - Purpura simplex
- Hereditary defect
  - Marfan syndrome
  - Osler-Weber-Rendu disease
- Drug-induced (procaine, penicillin, sulfa, thiazides, quinine, iodides, coumarin)
- Paraproteinemia
  - Myeloma
  - Macroglobulinemia
  - Cryoglobulinemia
- Connective tissue disease
  - Lupus
  - RA
  - Sjögren's syndrome

MULTIPLE DEFECTS

- Uremia
- Chronic hepatocellular failure
- Disseminated intravascular coagulation
- HIV infection

WORKUP

OVERALL STRATEGY

- Ascertain likelihood of underlying hemostasis defect by checking for bleeding from multiple sites, easy bruising, spontaneous bleeding, ecchymoses diameter >6 cm, or prolonged bleeding after surgical or dental procedure.

- Before starting detailed office evaluation, check that no serious hemorrhage or major volume depletion is present by inquiring into dyspnea, light-headedness, marked postural fatigue, and large volume of visible blood loss; also examine postural signs, skin color, and skin temp.
- Ascertain which segment(s) of hemostatic system are at fault (see Table 81-2 in *Primary Care Medicine*, 4th edition).

HISTORY

- Obtain detailed Hx of bleeding problem, including onset, precipitants, location, clinical course, and medical Hx, associated family Hx, and drug Hx.
- In reviewing drug Hx, note medications capable of interfering with platelet function (aspirin, NSAIDs, semisynthetic penicillins, cephalosporins, dipyridamole), platelet number (thiazides, alcohol, quinidine, methyldopa, sulfa, phenytoin, barbiturates), or coagulation factor synthesis (warfarin).
- Inquire into past surgery, childbirth, menstruation, nosebleed (both nostrils), dental extraction, trauma, laceration, and injection. Note any Hx of transfusion requirement after minor trauma or surgery when such transfusion would not ordinarily be necessary.
- In patient with suspected hereditary cause, note gender of those involved to check for sex-linked defects, especially those involving clotting factors.
- Check for recent or concurrent illness that might affect hemostasis, including chronic liver disease, uremia, viral infection, connective tissue disease, myeloproliferative states, and paraproteinemias.

PHYSICAL EXAM

- Observe general appearance for cushingoid habitus and marfanoid appearance.
- Examine skin for size, number, and location of any purpuric lesions, noting whether they are petechial (<3 mm) or ecchymotic (>3 mm), and if ecchymotic, >6 cm.
- If petechial, note whether lesions are palpable, tender, or pruritic, and surrounded by erythematous flush (vasculitic).
- Distinguish petechiae from nonpurpuric erythematous skin lesions by failure to blanch when compressed with glass slide. Do not dismiss all blanching lesions; telangiectases blanch and are clues to Osler-Weber-Rendu syndrome.
- Check skin for signs of chronic liver disease (spider angiomas, jaundice).
- Examine mucous membranes for bleeding, lymph nodes for enlargement, abdomen for hepatosplenomegaly, and joints and muscles for hematomas and hemarthroses.
- Conduct rectal and pelvic exams to check for bleeding.
- Examine patients with thrombocytopenia for splenomegaly: with patient in right lateral decubitus position, palpate spleen and percuss Traube's space (area of resonance over stomach) for dullness.

LAB STUDIES

- Use to classify further cause of bleeding.
- Assess primary hemostasis by platelet count and bleeding time, extrinsic clotting system by PT, and intrinsic clotting system by PTT.

Finding platelets on exam of peripheral smear is evidence of adequate quantity.

- To test for suspected qualitative platelet defect (normal platelet count, normal PT and PTT), perform bleeding time using Ivy's method (template to ensure 1-cm long and 1-mm deep incision while obstructing venous return with blood pressure cuff inflated to 40 mm Hg; apply blotting paper to edge of incision; normal result is cessation of blotter-detected oozing by 9 mins).

- If bleeding time is prolonged in absence of extrahematologic cause, and PT and PTT are normal, follow with in vitro testing of platelet function, including aggregation testing and hematologic consultation.

- If bleeding time and PTT are prolonged, obtain hematologic consultation to perform ristocetin-induced agglutination of platelets for suspected von Willebrand's disease (platelets fail to agglutinate, but aggregation is normal).

- If clotting factor inhibitor is suspected, order mixing equal volumes of patient and normal donor plasma to see if prolongation in PT or PTT is corrected. If corrected, proceed with hematologic consultation to determine missing clotting factor. If not corrected, proceed with identification of inhibitor.

For Thrombocytopenia

- Rule out pseudothrombocytopenia by examining peripheral smear for clumping.

- Check peripheral blood smear for pancytopenia (marrow failure) and large immature platelets (increased destruction).

- Check for sequestration by examining for enlarged spleen.

- If uncertainty persists, consider bone marrow exam.

- For suspected increased destruction, withdraw potentially offending drugs (e.g., quinidine, gold, TMP-SMX) and check HIV antibodies (see HIV-1 Infection), ANA, and heterophile when there is supporting clinical evidence.

- In absence of such common precipitants and presence of otherwise normal CBC (mild lymphocytosis included), consider idiopathic thrombocytopenic purpura and testing whole blood for platelet-bound IgG autoantibodies.

- To check for platelet consumption, examine peripheral smear for RBC schistocytes (microangiopathy) as occurs with thrombotic thrombocytopenic purpura and disseminated intravascular coagulation (PTT is normal in former and abnormal in latter).

MANAGEMENT

VASCULAR DEFECTS

- Reassure patients with purpura simplex and senile purpura and advise against need for large doses of vitamins C and K; suggest withholding nonprescription use of NSAIDs if easy bruising disturbs patient but not if medically indicated.

- Advise patients with recurrent bleeding from serious vascular disease (e.g., hereditary hemorrhagic telangiectasia) to avoid agents that might compromise hemostasis and to use compression for bleeding episodes; prescribe iron replacement (see Anemia) if patient has had recurrent bleeding.

PLATELET DISORDERS

- Counsel avoidance of NSAIDs if patient has Hx of bleeding; if not, continue NSAID use if necessary but stop before surgery.
- Postpone surgery, dental extraction, and contact sports in patients with platelet counts <50,000 until problem is corrected; recommend use of stool softeners and soft toothbrush.
- Hospitalize those with counts <20,000; halt all but most essential medications and exposures (solvents, insecticides, alcohol), and prohibit NSAIDs and salicylates.
- Treat etiologically and with hematologic consultation.
- For thrombocytopenia associated with HIV infection, begin antiretroviral Rx (see HIV-1 Infection).
- For idiopathic thrombocytopenic purpura, start high-dose steroid Rx (e.g., prednisone, 1 mg/kg/day), especially if patient is symptomatic; taper after 1–2 wks if platelet count normalizes; if it does not, consider splenectomy.

CLOTTING FACTOR PROBLEMS

- For patients on warfarin who exhibit mild bleeding from excessive anticoagulation, recommend halting Rx until PT drifts back into therapeutic range (see Anticoagulant Therapy); avoid large doses of vitamin K, but give small doses if clinically indicated. Infuse FFP if urgent reversal of anticoagulation is necessary.
- Consider oral vitamin K supplements (2.5–10.0 mg/day) or parenteral doses (10–25 mg IM) for patients with poor vitamin K intake or malabsorption; attend to underlying cause of malabsorption (see Diarrhea).

HEMOPHILIA

- Specify permissible physical activity and teach proper first aid.
- If degree of bleeding has been only mild to moderate, encourage participation in noncontact sports and other low-risk activities.
- Teach family about first aid for acute hemarthrosis (immobilization, ice packs, splinting, and elastic bandages).
- Do not attempt to aspirate hemarthrosis because of high risk for causing further bleeding and introducing infection.
- Prohibit aspirin and NSAID use; use acetaminophen and codeine for short periods prn.
- Refer promptly for administration of factor VIII concentrate for acute bleeding and before surgery and dental work.
- To treat patients with mild to moderate hemophilia or von Willebrand's disease, consider desmopressin in place of factor VIII.
- Provide genetic counseling; consider DNA testing to identify women who are hemophilia gene carriers.

INDICATIONS FOR ADMISSION AND REFERRAL

- If severity of condition is obviously marked or unclear, promptly admit.
- Admit emergently for evidence of volume depletion, ischemia, gross bleeding, bleeding from multiple sites, or mental status change.

- Consider admission for dangerously low platelet count (<20,000), absence of platelets on smear, or markedly prolonged bleeding time.
- Admit hemophiliacs with acute bleeding for emergency transfusion of factor VIII.
- Refer for hematologic consultation to aid test selection when patient with clinical bleeding is suspected of having qualitative platelet disorder, as well as for patients with unexplained, clinically significant clotting factor deficiencies, severe thrombocytopenia, or suspected hemophilia or von Willebrand's disease.

BIBLIOGRAPHY

- For the current annotated bibliography on bleeding problems, see the print edition of *Primary Care Medicine*, 4th edition, Chapter 81, or www.LWWmedicine.com.

Erythrocytosis

DIFFERENTIAL DIAGNOSIS

- Polycythemia vera
- Secondary polycythemia
  - Physiologic (systemic hypoxia)
    - High altitude
    - Right-to-left shunt
    - Heavy smoking
    - Severe pulmonary disease
    - Abnormal hemoglobin with high oxygen affinity
  - Pathologic (no systemic hypoxia)
    - Renal cell carcinoma
    - Uterine myoma
    - Cerebellar hemangioma
    - Hepatoma
    - Hydronephrosis
    - Cystic kidney disease
    - Renal artery stenosis
- Relative polycythemia
  - Marked volume depletion
    - Protracted vomiting
    - Persistent diarrhea
    - Excessive diuretic use
    - Diuretic phase of renal failure
  - High to normal erythrocyte mass, low to normal volume: hypertensive, obese, middle-aged, male smoker

WORKUP

HISTORY

- Check for risk factors for volume depletion (e.g., diuretic use, vomiting, diarrhea) and for precipitants of chronic hypoxemia (e.g., residence at high altitude, known cyanotic heart disease, smoking >2 packs/day, chronic lung disease).
- Inquire into familial occurrence of polycythemia (abnormal hemoglobin) and Hx of renal disease.
- Note important clues for polycythemia vera [e.g., easy bruising, bleeding, and thrombosis (especially in unusual sites such as retina, hepatic or portal vein, mesenteric vasculature)].
- Review for symptoms of hyperviscosity (e.g., lassitude, headache, sweating).
- Ask about pruritus worsened by bathing (classic symptom of polycythemia vera).

PHYSICAL EXAM

- Check postural signs for volume depletion.
- Examine for plethora, cyanosis, clubbing, and ecchymoses, signs of chronic lung disease (see Chronic Dyspnea), structural heart disease with right-to-left shunt (see Asymptomatic Systolic Murmur), hepatic enlargement, splenomegaly, and abdominal and pelvic masses.

LAB STUDIES

- Begin with CBC, platelet count, and peripheral blood smear exam.
- Limit specific testing for polycythemia vera to patients with ≥1–2 characteristic features in addition to elevated hematocrit (e.g., generalized pruritus after bathing, splenomegaly, persistent leukocytosis, persistent thrombocytosis, or atypical thrombosis).
- In patients with increased probability of polycythemia vera, check erythropoietin level and consider hematologic consultation for consideration of in vitro growth of erythroid stem cell colonies.
- If stem cell testing is unavailable, measure total RBC volume, arterial oxygen saturation, leukocyte alkaline phosphatase, serum B_{12}, and unbound B_{12}-binding capacity in addition to CBC and peripheral smear.
- For suspected reactive erythrocytosis, measure arterial blood gas or arterial oxygen saturation.
- For patients with strong family Hx of polycythemia, obtain hemoglobin electrophoresis.
- Obtain cardiac ultrasonography (U/S) with Doppler (and bubble study if available) for suspected structural heart disease with right-to-left shunt.
- For suspected renal lesions and tumors, especially renal cell carcinoma, obtain renal U/S or IV pyelography with nephrotomograms. If positive, follow with contrast-enhanced abdominal CT.
- Consider abdominal and pelvic U/S to screen for hepatoma and uterine myoma.
- For relative erythrocytosis, check BUN to creatinine ratio.
- Consider RBC mass determination only when it is impossible clinically to differentiate relative from absolute erythrocytosis.

MANAGEMENT

SYMPTOMATIC THERAPY

- When possible, direct Rx at underlying cause (e.g., correction of right-to-left shunt, removal of erythropoietin-secreting tumor).
- Order smoking cessation (see Smoking Cessation).
- For selected patients with severe COPD, consider long-term oxygen Rx (see Chronic Obstructive Pulmonary Disease).
- Consider phlebotomy in patients with polycythemia vera and pathologic secondary erythrocytosis if erythrocytosis becomes excessive (hematocrit >60%) and threatens oxygen delivery. Reduce hematocrit to <55%.
- Remove up to 500 mL blood as often as q2–3d to achieve hematocrit <55%. In frail and elderly, limit removal to ≤250 mL 1–2 × wk.
- Do not correct resulting iron deficiency in pathologic secondary erythrocytosis, except to mild degree in cardiopulmonary disease.

- Perform preoperative phlebotomy and administer volume expander in severely erythrocytic patients to prevent compromised hemostasis.

POLYCYTHEMIA VERA

- Initiate phlebotomy, aiming for immediate reduction of hematocrit to 50%, but continue regularly until hematocrit reaches mid-40s in men and low 40s in women; follow with maintenance schedule based on monthly monitoring of hematocrit.
- Treat bothersome pruritus with combination histamine blockers (e.g., fexofenadine, 60 mg qam; chlorpheniramine, 4 mg qhs, + cimetidine, 400 mg tid).
- To counter secondary hyperuricemia, prescribe allopurinol (300 mg/day) when uric acid level >9 mg/dL.
- Refer for consideration of myelosuppressive Rx when phlebotomy is inadequate, thrombocytosis develops, or extramedullary hematopoiesis ensues. Hydroxyurea is preferred. Consider phosphorus 32 for patients who do not respond to hydroxyurea Rx.
- Consider PO anticoagulation if thrombosis ensues but monitor closely due to increased risk of bleeding.
- For painful splenic infarction or congestive splenomegaly, refer to surgery for consideration of splenectomy.

BIBLIOGRAPHY

- For the current annotated bibliography on erythrocytosis, see the print edition of *Primary Care Medicine*, 4th edition, Chapter 80, or www.LWWmedicine.com.

Sickle Cell Disease

SCREENING AND/OR PREVENTION

- Offer screening for sickle trait to African-American adults in reproductive age groups. Explain full implications of test results before screening.
- Screen newborn infants to permit appropriate prophylaxis and immunization, because sickle cell disease is serious health hazard that usually presents during early childhood.
- Screen high-risk pregnant women at first prenatal visit and advise paternal testing as well.
- Screen adults for presence of sickle trait principally for genetic counseling. Otherwise routine screening for sickle trait is not recommended, except perhaps for unconditioned persons who may have to exert extreme physical effort at high altitude; however, absolute risk is extremely low and nil in trained persons.
- Avoid indiscriminate screening and inadequate counseling; may be harmful and unlikely to benefit those who will not revise marriage and parenthood decisions based on test results.

WORKUP

- Order test of sickling (using 2% metabisulfite solution or 1 of the more expensive commercial methods). Tests are positive in presence of hemoglobin S but do not distinguish between homozygotes, heterozygotes, and double heterozygotes (hemoglobin S combined with thalassemia or hemoglobin C).
- Follow positive sickling test with hemoglobin electrophoresis; not substitute for sickling test because some nonsickling hemoglobin variants travel in same electrophoretic band as hemoglobin S (e.g., hemoglobin Lepore).
- Examine peripheral blood smear and check reticulocyte count to obtain supportive data.

MANAGEMENT

- Institute Rx in patients with painful crises.
- Consider low-dose clotrimazole Rx to decrease concentration of hemoglobin S by increasing intracellular water.
- Consider hydroxyurea to increase hemoglobin F.

BIBLIOGRAPHY

- For the current annotated bibliography on sickle cell disease, see the print edition of *Primary Care Medicine*, 4th edition, Chapters 78 and 82, or www.LWWmedicine.com.

Oncologic Problems

Bladder Cancer

SCREENING AND/OR PREVENTION

- Lower urinary tract cancer is associated with significant morbidity and mortality.
- Risks of occupational exposure to dyestuffs, rubber, leather and leather products, paint, and organic chemicals have been well defined. Smoking is also associated with significant risk increase.
- High levels of fluid intake may reduce risk for bladder cancer.
- Urinary cytology is imperfect but useful screening test for high-risk groups.
- There is no evidence that screening significantly advances time of Dx in individual cases or that early Rx influences outcome. Nevertheless, because of relatively high specificity and lack of morbidity associated with cytologic screening, identification of patients at high risk because of occupational exposure, with subsequent yearly cytologic screening, may be indicated in occupational health settings.
- Screening of asymptomatic smokers without risk of occupational exposure is not recommended.

WORKUP

- Cystoscopy and biopsy of multiple sites are required for Dx of bladder cancer. Urine cytology is too insensitive to obviate need for invasive study.
- Staging is performed by cystoscopy with biopsy and bimanual rectal-abdominal exam under anesthesia to determine depth of tumor penetration and infiltration into bladder wall.

MANAGEMENT

- Noninvasive stages of disease are often curable with local measures. Excision at time of cystoscopy in conjunction with fulguration represents most effective Rx for early disease. In setting of multiple tumors, cytotoxic agent can be instilled. Thiotepa has been widely used.
- BCG has emerged as superior Rx for carcinoma *in situ* in patients with superficial transitional cell disease.
- Infiltrative disease carries poor prognosis because of substantial likelihood of lymph node metastases. Options include partial bladder resection, cystectomy with urinary diversion via ileal loop, radical radiation, and combination Rx.
- Although partial cystectomy has attraction of preserving some bladder, few patients are suitable candidates. Combination Rx with preoperative irradiation + cystectomy is often used.
- Those with deeply invasive disease are not candidates for surgery. External beam megavoltage irradiation provides reasonable chance

(50%) for local control and small chance (≤25%) for cure. Rate of bowel and bladder complications is 10–15%.

- In patients with distant metastases, cisplatin with cyclophosphamide and doxorubicin has achieved substantial, but not lasting, regression.
- Monitoring patients treated for early disease is essential. Conduct surveillance cystoscopy and washings q3mos during first yr and then at less-frequent intervals.

BIBLIOGRAPHY

- For the current annotated bibliography on bladder cancer, see the print edition of *Primary Care Medicine*, 4th edition, Chapters 128 and 143, or www.LWWmedicine.com.

Breast Cancer

DIFFERENTIAL DIAGNOSIS

- See Breast Masses and Nipple Discharge.

WORKUP

- See Breast Masses and Nipple Discharge.

SCREENING AND/OR PREVENTION

- Breast cancer is common. Although risk factors allow identification of subgroups at particularly high risk, women without risk factors are also at substantial risk and should be educated about breast cancer and benefits and harms of screening.
- Conduct testing and counseling related to breast cancer susceptibility genes and family Hx with utmost care. Before referring for testing, discuss implications of inherited breast cancer, including limitations of available prevention strategies.
- Mammographic screening among women aged 50–74 reduces breast cancer mortality 25–30%; perform regular mammograms in this age group q1–2yrs.
- Among women aged <50, modest benefit (approximately 10% mortality reduction) seems likely based on trial results, but mammography has not been proved beneficial. Furthermore, younger women face higher likelihood of mammographic detection of DCIS and subsequent difficult therapeutic decisions leading to potentially unnecessary surgery. Engage women in this age group in dialogue about their wishes regarding mammography. Include quantitative estimates of benefits and harms of screening. When regular mammography is performed for women aged <50, shorter screening interval (e.g., yearly) may be more appropriate.
- PE of breast can detect cancers not detected by mammogram. It should not be neglected, especially in younger women.
- Effectiveness of recommendations for breast self-exam depend on breast size, shape, and density as well as patient motivation.

MANAGEMENT

GENERAL APPROACH

- Appropriate Rx choice for each woman is highly dependent on personal preferences and attitudes toward benefits and harms. PCP is critically important source of support, empathy, and information.
- DCIS accounts for 12% of all cancers and 30% of those detected by mammography. Women should understand difference in natural Hx

between noninvasive and invasive cancer, including fact that as many as one-half of DCIS cases do not progress to invasive disease.

- Although oncologists are likely to manage Rx of advanced local and metastatic disease, PCP should continue to play key supportive role, especially as patient confronts decisions that involve trade-offs between quality and length of life.
- Offer information about prognosis, including explicit estimates of recurrence rates based on tumor size and number of positive nodes. Women vary in how much they want to know; elicit and honor their preferences for prognostic information.
- Monitoring after primary Rx should include annual mammograms. Other tests, including bone scans, in asymptomatic women have not been proved beneficial and are not recommended. Be attentive to signs of depression.

PRIMARY THERAPY

- Women with early stage breast cancer must understand that multiple trials have demonstrated same survival with mastectomy or breast-conserving surgery (lumpectomy or quadrantectomy) + radiation. Some relative contraindications to breast-conserving surgery include tumors that are large relative to breast size, cancer that is near or involves nipple, and tumors with extensive intraductal components within or adjacent to primary tumor. Neoadjuvant chemotherapy can reduce tumor size and make breast-conserving surgery possible for some women whose tumors would otherwise be too large.
- Mastectomy is choice of some women who do not want to live with anxiety of ipsilateral recurrence. Others prefer mastectomy because it does not usually involve subsequent radiation and lets them complete primary Rx more quickly, although some recent studies suggest that women at high risk of recurrence (tumor >4 cm or presence of >4 positive nodes) benefit from radiation Rx after mastectomy. After mastectomy, some women opt for breast reconstruction, whereas others feel no need for cosmetic surgery.

ADJUVANT THERAPY

- Adjuvant Rx, chemotherapy or hormonal Rx, is administered to decrease likelihood of or delay cancer recurrence and death. Adjuvant chemotherapy reduces recurrence risk by as much as 35% in some women but confers considerable morbidity. Tamoxifen is effective regardless of age or menopausal status in women who are estrogen receptor or progesterone receptor positive, reducing recurrence risk by as much as 50% when taken for 5 yrs. In these women, effects of chemotherapy and tamoxifen are greater than either intervention used alone.
- It is essential that women understand benefits of adjuvant Rx in terms of relative and absolute risk reduction. Specifically, women with low baseline risk must understand that their absolute risk benefit may be too small to justify morbidity of adjuvant Rx, especially adjuvant chemotherapy.
- Consider biphosphonate Rx to reduce risks of bony metastases, bone pain, and hypercalcemia.
- Hormonal Rx can be very effective in receptor-positive women with advanced breast cancer, although you may not see effect on tumor size for 1–2 mos.

- Chemotherapy is effective in some women who are receptor negative and after failure of hormonal Rx.
- Breast cancers, including bony metastases, are sensitive to radiation Rx.
- Autologous bone marrow transplantation with high-dose chemotherapy has not been shown to produce survival benefit. Do not advise outside of clinical trials.

BIBLIOGRAPHY

- For the current annotated bibliography on breast cancer, see the print edition of *Primary Care Medicine*, 4th edition, Chapters 106 and 122, or www.LWWmedicine.com.

Cancer (General)

WORKUP

STAGING PRINCIPLES

- Stage clinically (by means of Hx, PE, imaging procedures, and serum markers) and pathologically (by direct sampling of tissue); these are complementary.
- If anatomic extent of disease remains unclear after detailed Hx and PE, proceed to imaging studies.
- Choose among CT, MRI, ultrasonography (U/S), and radionuclide scanning (particularly bone scan).

STAGING PROCEDURES

Computed Tomography and Magnetic Resonance Imaging

- Provide improved detection of tumor and better quantification of tumor burden.
- CT is less expensive and more readily available.
- Chest CT particularly useful for staging lung cancer, sarcomas, and testicular cancers.
- Abdominal CT enhances evaluation of retroperitoneal lymph nodes, pancreas, liver, adrenal gland, and kidney.
- Pelvic CT less useful for early ovarian and prostate cancers; lacks sensitivity in detecting early disease and early spread to pelvic nodes.
- Head CT enhanced by iodinated contrast can eliminate need for invasive and radionuclide staging studies of CNS.
- MRI provides enhanced resolution in some areas, particularly CNS (posterior fossa and spinal cord).
- MRI may prove useful for staging pelvic malignancies, but too early to recommend routine use.

Radionuclide Scanning

- Best test for metastases to bone; highly sensitive; specificity sometimes lacking, necessitating confirmatory study.
- Integral part of initial evaluation of cancers with high propensity for bone metastasis (prostate, breast, small cell cancers).
- Liver scans usually add little; routine liver scanning for metastases unwarranted in primary breast or colon cancer.
- Gallium scanning occasionally helpful in staging melanoma and lymphoma.

Ultrasonography

- Useful for assessing prostate, ovaries, testes, liver, pancreas, kidneys, and thyroid.
- Excellent for distinguishing solid from cystic masses; important in evaluation of pelvic, testicular, renal, and thyroid masses; helps guide needle biopsy.

- Resolution for transabdominal studies wanes for lesions <1 cm in diameter; about 20% inadequate due to overlying bowel gas.
- Transrectal U/S comparable to MRI for staging early prostate disease, but at much lower cost.

Standard Radiographs

- Metastatic series has high false-negative rate; not used.
- Contrast studies (IV pyelography, venography, and angiography) infrequently applied to staging, although helpful in planning surgery.
- Conventional CXR supplanted by chest CT (see above).

Lymphangiography

- Replaced by abdominal CT in lymphoma, but still used selectively for staging in Hodgkin's disease (see Hodgkin's Disease; Non-Hodgkin's Lymphoma).

Serum Chemistries and Markers

- Alkaline phosphatase (liver fraction) elevation useful for detecting early hepatic infiltration and often precedes radiologically detectable lesion.

Prostate-Specific Antigen

- Elevation >10 suggests large tumor burden and likelihood of extracapsular spread.

Surgical and Other Invasive Procedures

- Indicated when results alter therapeutic decision making [e.g., laparotomy in ovarian cancer, splenectomy in Hodgkin's disease (see Hodgkin's Disease; Non-Hodgkin's Lymphoma)].
- Mediastinoscopy for operability in lung cancer; more invasive Chamberlain procedure sometimes necessary.
- Bone marrow biopsy in cancers that frequently metastasize to bone marrow (e.g., lymphoma, small cell carcinoma, prostate cancer).
- Lymphadenectomy for primary lesion during surgery does not extend survival, but useful as prognostic and therapeutic determinant in prostate and breast cancers.
- Sentinel node biopsy using radionuclide markers for node identification applied in malignant melanoma and breast cancer as alternative to standard node dissections. This approach involves performing intraoperative lymph node mapping to allow selective lymphadenectomy.
- Lymph node evaluation of distant disease is recognized staging procedure in some tumors (e.g., scalene or retroperitoneal node biopsy in testicular cancer).

MANAGEMENT

TREATMENT MODALITIES

Localized Disease

- Surgery dominant in management of localized cancer.
- Shift toward minimizing surgical procedures, particularly when prognosis is determined by distant metastases so that morbidity is reduced without compromising survival.

- Adjuvant methods (e.g., radiation, cytotoxic agents) being used to limit extent of surgery/improve outcomes.
- Radiation Rx may be curative alone in some localized cancers (e.g., Hodgkin's disease) and in conjunction with surgery (e.g., breast, rectal cancer).
- Combining radiation Rx with surgery or chemotherapy may promote palliation and chances for long-term survival.

Regional Disease

- Adjuvant Rx (chemotherapy and/or radiation) added to surgical procedures in instances in which it improves control and survival (e.g., testicular cancer, osteogenic sarcoma, Hodgkin's disease).
- Not used in patients with generally unresponsive tumors (e.g., regionally advanced lung, renal cell, or pancreatic cancers).
- Radiation promotes local control of presumed residual microscopic tumor.
- Chemotherapy addresses possibility of occult distant disease, treating micrometastases when they are rapidly proliferating and likely to be drug sensitive.

Metastatic Disease

- Rx is largely palliative and involves systemic Rx, mostly chemotherapy.
- Decision to use chemotherapy should involve analysis of host tolerance in addition to potential tumor responsiveness.
- Consider experimental drug Rx when
  - no response to known effective drugs;
  - strong patient desire or insistence on new form of Rx;
  - readily measurable objective disease parameter available.
- Biologic response modifiers (e.g., IL, IFN) may contribute to survival. Designed to promote generalized response that can affect tumors at any site. Offer considerable promise as adjunct to cytotoxic chemotherapy.

Alternative or Complementary Approaches

- To date, few data from randomized, controlled trials are available on which to base their use.
- Most claims of efficacy are based on anecdotal reports at best.
- Triggers of use include depression, fear of recurrence of cancer, and psychosocial distress.
- Elicit and effectively address such fear and distress.
- Valuing informed medical opinions, patients hope their physicians are knowledgeable about safety and efficacy of such practices.
- Follow scientific literature closely and provide patients with best available information when they desire it. In this manner, maximize patient safety and satisfaction and avoid unnecessary expense.

Preterminal and Palliative Care

Preterminal Care
- Terminal cancer designates that death will ensue within 4-wk period.
- Term not particularly useful; imposes tremendous stress on patient and family that often results in withdrawal; many live much longer than 4 wks.

- Thoroughly explore sources of physical and social suffering along with patient's awareness of Dx and prognosis and preferences for end-of-life care.
- Perform differential Dx of uncomfortable symptoms and treat underlying causes to fullest extent consistent with goal of patient comfort (physical and psychological) and dignity (see below).
- Regular visits at home or office very useful psychologically.
- No need to reinforce inevitability of death to patient, but family must be apprised precisely during this period to allow them to pass through grieving process successfully.
- Inform patients with chronic life-threatening illnesses and their families that attentive comfort care can be provided, if desired, in lieu of aggressive, life-sustaining Rx.
- Initiate hospice care.
- Omit hospitalization with curative attempts, lab studies, and life-sustaining Rx.
- Concentrate on psychological and symptomatic support; priorities include pain relief and psychological support of patient and family.
- Consider psychotropic agents, pain control measures, and nutrition support:
  - If patient is depressed, ask about suicidal thoughts and offer SSRI antidepressant Rx (e.g., sertraline, 25–50 mg qam; see Depression) for somatic symptoms of depression (marked fatigue, early morning awakening) and for pain control. Avoid tricyclic antidepressants (overdose risk).
  - For acute situational stress, consider short course of benzodiazepines (e.g., 2 mg diazepam qhs) to help with coping and resultant difficulty falling asleep (see Anxiety).
  - Intensify pain control and other palliative measures (see below).
  - Address artificial nutrition and hydration in manner similar to any other therapeutic intervention, focusing on ratio of benefit to burden and patient's or surrogate's wishes.
- Anticipate sources of terminal distress and make Rx plans in advance.

Palliative Care

- Continuously weigh benefits and burdens of all diagnostic and therapeutic measures and consider recommending omission of the more burdensome measures. No medical, ethical, or legal distinction is made between withdrawing and withholding Rx that is more burdensome than beneficial or not desired by patient.
- Consider Rx that relieves serious refractory symptoms in terminally ill patients, even at risk of unintended but foreseeable side effects, including hastening death.
- Consider referral for inpatient or outpatient hospice services when problematic symptoms and/or psychosocial problems.
- Consider referral of dying patient to hospital when symptoms are refractory and difficult to control at home.
- Care of specific symptoms
  - Dyspnea: treat with PO, sublingual, or rectal morphine; if severe, administer IV or SQ.
  - Excessive respiratory secretions: treat with anticholinergics such as scopolamine or glycopyrrolate.

- Xerostomia: prescribe a saliva substitute around the clock, particularly in dehydrated patients.

Approach to Care of Cancer Survivors

- Provide supportive Rx; counsel patient and family about challenges and potential difficulties they may experience as patient returns to daily life.
- Conduct counseling in honest, open, and supportive manner that characterized discussions in earlier phases of illness.
- Arrange regularly scheduled office visits to check symptoms, physical findings, and progress in returning to normal life; continue supportive visits for mos to yrs.
- In particular, understand and address psychological, psychosocial, and physical consequences, including
  - heightened sense of vulnerability and fear of death, and decreased feeling of control and mastery over life;
  - anxiety about recurrence, hypochondriasis, or avoidance of follow-up health care;
  - rekindled feelings of fear and vulnerability with contact with patients having active disease;
  - marked anxiety over loss of close contact with health care team that characterized active phase of their illness;
  - feelings of anger over perceived shortcomings in Dx and care;
  - depression over consequences of cancer care; may present as fatigue or other physical complaints; preoccupation with bodily sensations; symptoms mistaken for more serious disease;
  - difficulty returning to responsibilities of normal life;
  - awkward relations with family members and colleagues;
  - concern over return to sexual activity; sexual dysfunction;
  - interpersonal isolation, especially among those who are single and reluctant to share information about cancerous past with potential mate; adverse consequences greatest in patients lacking close, supportive relationships;
  - difficulty obtaining affordable health insurance;
  - work difficulties from real or imagined fears of losing job;
  - prolonged absence and perceived inability to perform, compromising previous position and leading to long-term job insecurity.

CHEMOTHERAPY

Types of Chemotherapy Regimens and Their Indications

Neoadjuvant (Preoperative) Chemotherapy

- For preoperative Rx of locally invasive tumors that are moderately sensitive and responsive to drugs (e.g., stage III non-SCLC and stage III breast cancer; see Breast Cancer; Lung Cancer).
- Goals: decrease tumor bulk, make possible more conservative surgical approach, and reduce risk for systemic disease via micrometastasis.
- Early consultation with medical oncologist indicated.

Postoperative Adjuvant Therapy

- Standard form of Rx for stage I and II breast cancer (see Breast Cancer) and Dukes' stage C colorectal cancer (CRC) (see Colorectal Cancer).
- Rationale: reduce frequency of distant micrometastases and local recurrences.

- Applied just after surgery for best results.

Chemotherapy of Advanced Disease

- Evolving from strictly palliative to curative in selected instances (e.g., lymphoma, testicular cancer; see Bladder Cancer; Hodgkin's Disease; Non-Hodgkin's Lymphoma, Prostate Cancer; Renal Cell Carcinoma; Testicular Cancer).
- Rationale: reduce morbidity and prolong survival without placing too heavy a burden on patient.
- Use of chemotherapy in advanced disease is often philosophical and psychological, based on feelings of patient, family, and physician. Worth considering when chemotherapy has potential to prolong life and improve its quality with acceptable morbidity; obtain patient consent and oncologic consultation.
- Primary indications for chemotherapy in advanced disease
  - Probability of tumor responsiveness to chemotherapy of >30% for partial response and >5% for complete response.
  - Progressive tumor growth during period of observation (e.g., pulmonary nodules doubling in <30 days).
  - Symptomatic metastatic disease (e.g., pleural effusion).
- Program stopped or changed if no clinically meaningful response.

Basic Chemotherapy Strategies

Combination Chemotherapy

- Agents with synergistic modes of action.
- Ideally, side effects nonadditive.
- Meaningful response expected within 2 courses of Rx.

Dose Intensification

- Using highest possible doses.
- Treating drug side effects by means other than dose reduction.
- Complementing chemotherapy with marrow-supportive efforts (e.g., BMT, hematopoietic growth factors).

Bone Marrow Transplantation

- Established for lymphomas, myelomas, and leukemias.
- Allogeneic BMT with HLA-matched donor marrow cells for leukemias.
- Autologous BMT with peripheral stem cells for some solid tumors.
- Risks: life-threatening infection, acute graft-versus-host reactions, lymphomas, and hematopoietic disorders (first several years), and solid tumors (later, especially in patients also receiving radiation).
- Long-term follow-up critical.

Growth Factors

- G-CSF, GM-CSF, and IL-11.
- Lessen risk for infection.
- Cost-effective when used prophylactically in situations in which febrile neutropenia is highly likely; not used routinely to treat neutropenia.
- Recombinant IL-11 approved for severe thrombocytopenia.
- Use of erythropoietin and thrombopoietin is being studied.

Follow-Up

- Essential to determining if continuation of chemotherapy justified.
- Usually conducted within 2 mos of initiation.

Types of Chemotherapeutic Agents

- See also Table 88-1 in *Primary Care Medicine*, 4th edition.
- Cytotoxic agents
  - Plant derivatives
    - Paclitaxel
    - Vincristine
    - Vinblastine
    - VP-16
  - Antibiotics
    - Bleomycin
    - Dactinomycin
    - Daunorubicin
    - Doxorubicin
    - Mitomycin C
  - Antimetabolites
    - Cytarabine (cytosine arabinoside)
    - Fludarabine
    - 5-FU
    - 5-FU with leucovorin
    - Hydroxyurea
    - Methotrexate
    - Methotrexate (high-dose with leucovorin)
    - 6-MP
  - Alkylating agents
    - BCNU
    - Busulfan
    - CCNU
    - Chlorambucil
    - Cisplatinum
    - Carboplatin
    - Cyclophosphamide
    - Ifosfamide and mesna
    - Melphalan
    - Streptozocin
  - Miscellaneous
    - Dacarbazine
    - Mitoxantrone
    - Procarbazine

Mechanisms of Action

- Alkylating agents
  - Broad spectrum of antitumor activity, chemically interacting directly with DNA.
  - Secondary malignancy a concern.
- Antimetabolites
  - Interfere with DNA synthesis by blocking metabolic precursors and cofactors; greatest effect is on rapidly growing cells.
- Topoisomerase inhibitors:
  - Impair action of reversible nucleases (topoisomerases) needed for DNA replication.
  - Spectrum of activity of doxorubicin comparable to that of alkylating drugs, providing synergistic antitumor effect when used with them.

- Mitotic spindle inhibitors
  - Inhibit mitosis; paclitaxel interferes with microtubular function.
- Miscellaneous or mixed-mechanism agents
  - Nitrosoureas cross blood-brain barrier.
  - Cisplatin very effective in Rx of testicular and ovarian cancers.

Adverse Effects

- Benefits of Rx continue to outweigh risks (see Table 88-2 in *Primary Care Medicine*, 4th edition), but lack of selectivity for tumor cell, leads to impairment of normal cells, especially populations with rapid turnover (e.g., bone marrow, GI mucosa, hair follicles).
- Acute marrow suppression
  - Typically, 7–10 days after administration; may last about 1 wk.
  - Dose-related leukopenia, leading to overwhelming sepsis; thrombocytopenia, resulting in hemorrhage; prevented or lessened by dose adjustment.
  - Pattern of suppression a function of drug type, dose, and schedule of administration (see Table 88-3 in *Primary Care Medicine*, 4th edition).
  - Standard approaches include adjustments in dose and timing of chemotherapy.
  - Dose adjustments based on nadir levels observed.
  - Follow-up CBCs on anticipated nadir days.
  - For patients with leukopenia, observation period intensified.
  - Prophylactic PO antibiotics considered (e.g., levofloxacin, 500 mg/day) when absolute neutrophil count <1,000/mm^3.
  - Prophylactic use of growth factors also considered.
- Alopecia
  - Usually partial, but can be total; beginning approximately 2 wks after initiation of Rx and becoming complete by 4–6 wks.
  - Hair loss always transient and often some hair grows during Rx.
  - Total restitution not until chemotherapy stops.
- Secondary malignancy
  - Acute leukemia, especially in younger patients undergoing curative-intent Rx for leukemia or lymphoma; especially when alkylating agents have been used.
- Nausea, vomiting, mucosal injury (stomatitis), and diarrhea
  - Especially with cisplatin, dacarbazine, doxorubicin, nitrogen mustard, and high doses of cyclophosphamide.

Administration

- Requires proper venous access to prevent extravasation.
- Large-diameter veins needed (antecubital fossa or higher) to minimize risk of sclerosis and endothelial damage from repeated use of irritating IV chemotherapy.
- For extravasation when using irritant IV agents (e.g., doxorubicin, vincristine, vinblastine, dacarbazine, BCNU, nitrogen mustard), infusion should be stopped immediately and ice applied.
- Any accumulation of drug removed by aspiration.
- Site monitored closely for inflammation and necrosis over 3–10 days.
- Corticosteroids considered, but definitive evidence of efficacy not demonstrated.

New Cytotoxic Therapies: Biologic Agents

Interleukins
- Naturally occurring cytokines produced by activated T cells.
- Immunostimulatory and antineoplastic effects.
- Adverse effects caused by release of tumor necrosis factor and IL-1; include fever, chills, lethargy, diarrhea, thrombocytopenia, liver dysfunction, myocarditis, and vascular leakage.
- Adverse effects dose-related and rapidly reversible.

Interferons
- Proteins with antiproliferative and immunomodulatory properties.
- Demonstrated antitumor effects, especially in chronic myelogenous leukemia, hairy cell leukemia, and, to lesser extent, Kaposi's sarcoma, and as adjuvant Rx in melanoma, renal cell carcinoma, and multiple myeloma.
- Produces better outcomes in combination with chemotherapeutic agents.
- Side effects dose-dependent; flulike syndrome during first wks of Rx.
- Also anorexia, depression, anxiety, emotional lability, hair loss, tinnitus, reversible hearing loss, thyroid dysfunction, increased susceptibility to bacterial infection and cardiotoxicity.

Monoclonal antibodies
- Still experimental for cancer.
- Possible means of enhancing specificity of chemotherapeutic agents.

Evaluating Response to Therapy

- Use objective tumor measurements whenever possible (see Table 88-4 in *Primary Care Medicine*, 4th edition). Include consideration of tumor markers (see above).
- Measurement can be made from time of Dx, metastasis, or initiation of Rx.
- Median response compared with randomized control or historical control not receiving Rx or receiving alternative Rx.
- Survival as measure of response may be supplemented by measurement of time from Dx to point of recurrence (disease-free survival).

Objective Measures of Response
- Partial response: 50% reduction in product of max perpendicular diameters of most easily measurable lesion without increase in other lesions and for minimum 4 wks.
- Complete response: 100% reduction in all evidence of tumor for minimum 4 wks without appearance of new lesions.
- Stable disease: <25% decrease in measurable disease without development of other lesions.
- No response/progressive disease: >25% increase in size of lesion or development of new lesions.
- Improvement: 25–50% reduction in product of max perpendicular diameters lasting at least 4 wks.

Patient Education

- Establish strong patient-doctor relationship to enhance ability to tolerate chemotherapy.
- Fully educate patient and family about Dx, prognosis, and the rationale and side effects of planned Rx.
- Specifically address concerns about side effects, such as alopecia, sterility, GI upset.
- Review probability of response.
- Ensure comprehensive educational effort appropriate for patient's level of understanding.
- Encourage patient participation in decision making and encourage sense of partnership, which can help sustain patient through this often difficult time.
- Advise asymptotic patient with platelet count of 20,000–50,000 to refrain from contact sports and other avoidable forms of trauma.

Indications for Admission and Referral

- Admit urgently for onset of febrile neutropenia (absolute neutrophil counts = 1,000/mm^3) or significant bleeding in setting of thrombocytopenia.
- Consider admission for platelet transfusion for asymptomatic patient with severe thrombocytopenia (platelet count = 20,000/mm^3).
- Be sure that each patient's Rx program is designed and conducted in conjunction with oncologist. If necessary expertise is not locally available, refer patient to regional center for design and implementation.
- Consider computer-based chemotherapy protocol advisory systems for expert input when it may not otherwise be obtainable.

RADIATION

Modes of Delivery

- External sources (external beam or teletherapy).
- Brachytherapy (encapsulated sources placed directly into body at tumor sites).
- Systemic delivery (via radionuclides).

Specific Applications

As Sole Curative Therapy

- For treating local or regional disease by "sterilizing" primary tumor and likely areas of local and regional spread.
- For preserving function and appearance with comparable survival (as in localized breast cancer, localized prostate cancer, or early head and neck cancers). For example,
  - Hodgkin's disease: stage IA-IIA; 90% 10-yr survival.
  - Lymphoma (indolent): stage I-II; 50% 10-yr survival (see Hodgkin's Disease; Non-Hodgkin's Lymphoma).
  - Cervical cancer: stage IB-IIA; 85% 5-yr disease-free survival.
  - Testicular cancer: early stage seminoma cure rate 95%.
  - Head and neck cancer: early stage disease (T1, T2) with results comparable to those of surgery with less functional and cosmetic loss.
  - Prostate cancer: external beam or brachytherapy excellent alternatives to surgery for organ-confined disease; external beam and hormonal Rx for locally advanced disease.

As Combined Modality with Surgery

■ Preceding surgery: reduces tumor bulk and destroys microscopic disease, thereby facilitating surgical removal and local control; allows lower doses of radiation and less radical surgery.

■ After surgery: destroys microscopic disease and allows immediate surgery; provides definitive pathologic review, avoids radiation effects on wound healing.

■ Intraoperatively: allows moving normal abdominal organs out of the field and preferentially targeting diseased tissue more precisely.

■ Examples
  • Uterine cancer: with surgery, good results for stages I, II, and III; 60–90% 5-yr survival.
  • Head and neck cancer: with surgery and/or chemotherapy in locally advanced cases.
  • Soft-tissue sarcomas: with surgery, often spares function or limb.
  • Breast cancer: with surgery and chemotherapy/hormonal Rx, breast preservation with survival equivalent to that of mastectomy possible for tumors <5 cm.

As Combined Modality with Chemotherapy

■ Rationale: radiation treats local disease, chemotherapy increases efficacy of radiation against primary tumor, targets occult systemic metastases, treats areas not readily accessible to chemotherapy (e.g., brain in SCLC).

■ Toxicities (can be additive): marrow suppression, hemorrhagic cystitis, mucositis of oral cavity, radiation enteritis, acute esophagitis, increased risk of leukemia.

■ Examples
  • Esophageal cancer: cures 25% of patients with localized disease.
  • Lung cancer: cures 15% of patients with locally advanced non-SCLC and 20–25% of patients with limited SCLC.
  • Bladder cancer: organ-sparing option with similar Rx outcome as cystectomy.
  • Rectal cancer: when added to surgery, improves outcome in patients with node-positive or transmural tumors.
  • Anal cancer: replaced surgery as primary Rx, curing 75% of patients.
  • Advanced-stage Hodgkin's disease: potentially curative.
  • Locally advanced cancers of head and neck, lung, esophagus, rectum, anus, and cervix: improves outcomes.

As Palliative Therapy

■ Bony metastases: for pain not controlled by analgesics, chemotherapy, or hormonal Rx.

■ Brain metastases: stereotactic radiosurgery, alternative to craniotomy for patients with 1–2 lesions.

■ Spinal cord compression: patients with myeloma, lymphoma, and small cell cancers respond especially well; treated emergently with steroids especially when single focal obstructing lesion.

■ For localized symptomatic tumor not sensitive to other modalities (e.g., painful bony breast and prostate metastases).

■ Relatively short course required (2 wks).

■ For urgent Rx of certain oncologic emergencies (e.g., spinal cord compression; superior vena cava syndrome).

Adverse Effects

- Tolerance decreases as dose increases.
- Acute radiation toxicity: ≤90 days after start of radiotherapy, usually resolves with supportive care.
- Late toxicity: more serious and clinically significant; may involve irreversible injury to normal tissue.

Major Adverse Effects of Radiotherapy and Dose Limits (cGy, ≤5% Toxicity)

- Bone marrow suppression, >250 cGy; most radiosensitive tissue; usually transient and reversible, unless large marrow volumes irradiated.
- Pneumonitis, >2,000 cGy; usually within 6–12 wks; dyspnea, cough, low-grade fever, hypoxemia, "ground glass" appearance on CXR, straight lines on CT that match field; restrictive physiology, chronic hypoxemia follows if fibrosis occurs. For acute pneumonitis: high-dose steroids (prednisone, 1 mg/kg, initially with taper) + oxygen. Once fibrosis occurs, no Rx available.
- Nephrosclerosis, 2,000
- Hepatitis, 3,000
- Pericarditis, 4,500
- Myelitis, 4,500
- Small intestine ulceration, fibrosis, 4,500
- Skin dermatitis, sclerosis, 5,500
- Brain necrosis, 6,000

Modified from Chabner BA. Principles of cancer therapy. In: Wyngaarden JB, Smith LH, eds. Cecil's textbook of medicine, 16th ed. Philadelphia: Saunders, 1982:1034, with permission.

Other Adverse Effects

- Secondary malignancy: risk usually small (0.2% at 10 yrs).
- Nausea/vomiting: with abdominal irradiation, 1–2 hrs after Rx; helped by prior administration of prochlorperazine, ondansetron, or granisetron, and small, frequent feedings. May require reducing or temporarily stopping Rx.
- Mouth dryness, difficulty with mastication and swallowing: pilocarpine (Salagen) begun at start of radiotherapy; managed by use of pureed meals or liquid dietary supplements.
- Diarrhea: helped by diphenoxylate (Lomotil) or loperamide.
- Skin sensitivity: helped by avoiding heat and excessive sun exposure.

Patient Education and Coordination of Care

- Provide emotional support and patient ed.
- Address fears compounded by awesome machinery and concerns about exposure.
- Directly discuss expected side effects and their control.
- Use printed information, when available.
- Review risks for sterility with patients of reproductive age and chances of second malignancy.
- Provide in conjunction with radiation Rx specialist data on risk-benefit issues to help patient make informed choice.
- Reassure that Rx can be adjusted to one's tolerance.

- Ensure that program is well suited to patient's needs, well explained, and monitored.
- Designate one team member as "go-to" person during this Rx phase (usually radiation therapist), but continue to provide support and advice.

MONITORING CANCER THERAPY

General Strategy

- Monitoring appropriate for asymptomatic patients who have undergone curative Rx; need to check for residual disease and new primary.
- Adds little to care of patients with incurable disease except to objectively document tumor response to palliative Rx.
- Helps to monitor response when undertaking palliation.
- Order only those monitoring activities that affect decision making and improve outcomes.
- Frequency and duration of monitoring depend on rate of disease recurrence, tumor type, response to Rx, stage of disease, and pattern of metastasis.

Methods

- Hx and PE supplemented by several simple lab studies are most cost-effective of monitoring measures; test sensitivity and specificity are important considerations.
- Tumor markers
  - Useful when obtained at baseline and posttreatment; levels repeated and compared at regular intervals.
  - Carcinoembryonic antigen present in normal and malignant tissue; serum levels >2.5 ng/mL suggest tumor; useful for early detection of recurrence, especially for colon, rectum, breast, and lung cancers. Best currently available noninvasive means for identifying recurrent CRC after surgery
  - Alpha fetoprotein (AFP) useful in monitoring hepatomas, testicular carcinomas, and extragonadal germ cell tumors.
  - hCG β-subunit useful for germ cell tumors of testes and ovaries; provides information similar to that obtained from AFP.
  - PSA is unique to prostate tissue but found in normal and malignant cells. Levels increase with tumor burden and rise briefly after needle biopsy or with prostatitis but not after digital rectal exam. Concentration >10 ng/mL strongly suggestive of cancer that might have extended beyond prostate capsule. False-negatives with use of finasteride.
  - CA 125 produced by 80% of epithelial ovarian cancers; detected by monoclonal antibody methods. Levels correlate with clinical course; specificity is high for use in monitoring ovarian cancer.
  - CA 19-9 being applied experimentally in monitoring breast and pancreatic cancers.

Local or Regional Disease

- Most tumors, if they recur, do so at max rate during first 2 yrs after surgery for cure.
- Melanoma, breast, and renal cell carcinomas notorious for late recurrence (>10 yrs).

- Hx and PE are supplemented by more detailed study at routine intervals or as clinically indicated.
- Emphasis more on finding new primary tumors (greater impact on outcome) than on detecting asymptomatic metastases (e.g., endoscopy for CRC, mammography for breast cancer).
- In absence of symptoms or signs of recurrence, monitor at 3-mo intervals for first yr and at 4-mo intervals for second yr.
- Thereafter, follow up q6mos for minimum 5 yrs.

Metastatic Disease

- Used to assess response to systemic Rx; failure to respond and detection of new disease is indication for cessation of current Rx program.
- Requires identifying best objective site of disease to be followed; additional monitoring and staging procedures inappropriate if they do not alter Rx.
- For hormonal breast cancer Rx, check at 3 mos.
- For cytotoxic chemotherapy, check after 2 courses of Rx (4–6 wks), especially for exquisitely responsive tumors (e.g., breast, testicular, ovarian, and oat cell carcinomas).

COMPLICATIONS OF CANCER TREATMENT

Gastrointestinal Complications

Nausea and Vomiting

- Consider prophylactic program; prevention is best approach and also eliminates behaviorally triggered emesis.
- Recommend normal food intake before chemotherapy.
- Prospectively assess need for prophylaxis based on patient's cancer Rx regimen.

EMETIC POTENTIAL

- Low: bleomycin, chlorambucil, VP-16, 5-FU, methotrexate, mitomycin C, vinblastine, vincristine.
- Moderate: carmustine, cytarabine, daunorubicin, doxorubicin, lomustine, procarbazine.
- High: cisplatin, cyclophosphamide, dacarbazine, dactinomycin, mechlorethamine.
- Consider combination program using drugs with synergistic mechanisms (e.g., a serotonin receptor blocker, a corticosteroid, and a benzodiazepine); mix of IV and PO routes can be used; obtain oncologic consultation in program design.

AVAILABLE AGENTS

- Serotonin S_3 receptor blocker (e.g., ondansetron, granisetron, dolasetron): blocks peripheral and central serotonin S_3 receptors; useful for prevention of acute and delayed emesis; effective alone but more so when combined with steroids. Administer IV or PO; ondansetron least expensive of PO preparations; dolasetron least expensive IV agent.
- Glucocorticosteroids: mechanism unknown; ? role of antiinflammatory action; effective for prevention of delayed nausea and vomiting; provides enhanced control when used with serotonin S_3 receptor blockers.
- Benzodiazepines: increases central inhibitory transmission; enhances antiemetic effects of other agents; causes desirable degree of mild

amnesia; useful for psychogenic vomiting in conjunction with behavioral desensitization; short-acting preparation (lorazepam) useful; best as part of combination program.

- Metoclopramide: blocks dopaminergic and serotonergic receptors; helps prevent delayed emesis; promotes gastric emptying and gastroesophageal sphincter closure; less effective than serotonin receptor blockers. Mostly used in combination with other agents.
- Phenothiazines: blocks central dopamine receptors; well established, but less effective if used alone; when combined with other antiemetic agents, useful for prophylaxis; extrapyramidal symptoms (with prochlorperazine doses >50 mg/day).
- Cannabinoids and marijuana: little better than phenothiazines; some antinausea and appetite-stimulant effects with use of purified tetrahydrocannabinol; no evidence that patient must smoke crude marijuana to achieve effects.
- Substance P–blockade (neurokinin-1 receptor antagonists): promising for delayed emesis, but still investigational.

RECOMMENDED PROGRAM

- Select a neurotransmitter blocking agent:
  - ondansetron, or
  - metoclopramide, or
  - phenothiazine.
- Add benzodiazepine or antihistamine:
  - lorazepam or
  - diphenhydramine.
- Add corticosteroid:
  - dexamethasone, or
  - methylprednisolone.

Refractory Emesis

- Rule out bowel obstruction and severe ileus, which require decompression using nasogastric suctioning.
- Check for hypercalcemia and hypokalemia.
- Monitor and correct electrolyte imbalances.

Anorexia and Weight Loss

- Achieve control of underlying malignancy.
- In interim, put the following to immediate use:
  - Small, frequent feedings (about 6/day) of high-calorie, high-protein foods.
  - Liquid dietary supplements, if tolerated.
  - Salty foods, cool, clear beverages, and desserts such as gelatin and popsicles.
  - Toast and crackers.
- Suggest meals served in relaxed family or group setting, attractively prepared and readily available.
- If taste wanes or becomes altered and makes food less palatable, try the following:
  - Substitute dairy products for meat.
  - Try acidic foods, extra seasoning, and spicy foods.
- Avoid overly sweet and greasy, fatty foods when nausea is prominent.

■ Consider use of appetite stimulant [e.g., tricyclic antidepressants (amitriptyline) or anabolic steroids (megasterol)].

Stomatitis

■ Recommend avoidance of smoking, alcohol, and very hot, cold, spicy, or salty foods.

■ Consider mixture of Benadryl elixir and Kaopectate used as mouthwash and chlorhexidine gluconate as antimicrobial oral rinse to prevent infection.

■ Consider viscous lidocaine (Xylocaine) preparation, but usefulness limited by distortion of taste (paste) and transience of benefit (mouthwash).

■ Recommend chewing gum or sucking on hard candy, use of gravies, and avoidance of dry foods when radiation Rx results in xerostomia and mucositis; consider artificial saliva in refractory situations.

Malnutrition

■ Recognize early (10% weight loss, serum albumin <3.5 g/dL, total lymphocyte count <1,500/mm^3, low serum creatinine for size).

■ Recommend pureed meals or nutritionally complete liquid preparation (lactose-free if lactose intolerant) if chewing and swallowing become problematic.

■ Consider temporary enteral hyperalimentation for difficult phases of cancer Rx in carefully selected patients (likely to benefit meaningfully) who have partially obstructed or injured upper alimentary tract, but intact lower GI tract.

■ Use long (43-in.), flexible silicon nasal feeding tube to administer supplement into distal duodenum or proximal jejunum, avoiding aspiration and reflux.

■ Start enteral hyperalimentation formulation at half strength and increase over several days as tolerated: goal: 2,000–3,000 calories/day.

■ Reserve total parenteral nutrition for short-term use in persons whose oral or enteral intake is likely to be inadequate for >10–14 days and who are likely to obtain an extended benefit (e.g., preoperatively in severely malnourished patients). Coordinate with hyperalimentation consultant.

■ Monitor glucose, calcium, phosphate, magnesium, BUN, and creatinine levels.

Diarrhea

■ When self-limited (radiation- or chemotherapy-induced enteritis), explain to patient and follow expectantly.

■ If persistent (>1–2 wks) or troublesome, begin low doses of diphenoxylate (Lomotil) or nonprescription loperamide (Imodium) (see Diarrhea).

■ For steatorrhea, consider pancreatic enzyme tablets with each meal (see Pancreatitis).

■ For postgastrectomy patient at risk for dumping syndrome, recommend avoidance of sweets, large fluid volumes (especially those rich in sugar), and lying down after meals (see Diarrhea).

Constipation

■ When likely to occur from narcotic use for pain control, institute prophylactic measures:
  • High-fiber diet;
  • Good fluid intake (≥2 L/day);

- Stool softeners (e.g., dioctyl sodium sulfosuccinate);
- Gentle laxative qhs (e.g., 15 mL milk of magnesia).

■ Rule out obstruction of lower intestinal tract or ileus before instituting laxative Rx.

■ Check for and correct hypokalemia and hypercalcemia.

Malignant Ascites

■ Rule out ovarian cancer as source if etiology unknown.

■ Treat etiologically.

■ Treat symptomatically only if causing intolerable discomfort.

■ Consider therapeutic paracentesis, performing large-volume paracentesis while taking care to preserve intravascular volume.

■ Remove 4–6 L of ascitic fluid slowly over 60–90 mins.

■ Infuse albumin simultaneously only if severely hypoalbuminemic.

■ If possible, avoid reliance on peritoneal-venous shunting (see Cirrhosis and Chronic Liver Failure).

■ Consider shunting only if
- life expectancy >3 mos;
- ascetic fluid viscous, not loculated, and nonbloody; and
- fluid rapidly reaccumulates despite repeated paracentesis and medical Rx.

■ Avoid intra-abdominal instillation of chemotherapeutic agents, radio-isotopes, sclerosing drugs, and irritants.

Peritoneal Implants, Bowel Obstruction, and Fistulas

■ Refer for consideration of surgical bypass or regional surgical resection ("debulking") if peritoneal implants coalesce into large mass lesions causing obstruction.

■ Proceed only when there is hope of prolonging meaningful survival (e.g., indolent malignancy with single localized point of obstruction).

■ For pelvic implants leading to fistulous communication with bladder or skin, refer for consideration of local surgical excision or radiation Rx.

Obstructive Jaundice

■ Refer to appropriately skilled interventionist for consideration of endoscopic or percutaneous placement of biliary stent.

■ Consider radiation Rx for palliation of obstructive jaundice caused by radiosensitive tumor (e.g., breast cancer, lymphoma) in porta hepatis.

Other Complications

Spinal Cord Compression

■ Promptly obtain plain films of spine in all cancer patients with new-onset back pain.

■ If radiographic findings are abnormal or if new neurologic deficits are noted, immediately hospitalize and order gadolinium-enhanced spinal MRI.

■ If MRI is unavailable, order CT with myelography using water-soluble contrast; before injecting dye, withdraw several cc CSF and send for cytology, cell count, and protein and glucose determinations.

■ Obtain prompt neurologic and oncologic consultations.

■ Begin high-dose corticosteroids (e.g., 4 mg dexamethasone q6h).

■ Obtain prompt surgical and radiation oncology consultations.

- Choose surgical decompression if neurologic function deteriorates rapidly.
- Consider radiation Rx in patients with myeloma, lymphoma, or SCLC.
- Consider chemotherapy for multifocal obstructing disease.

Meningeal Carcinomatosis
- Perform lumbar puncture to confirm; look for malignant cells in CSF.
- Refer to oncologist to help choose among corticosteroids, irradiation, and intrathecal administration of cytotoxic agents.

Cardiac Tamponade
- If suspected (pulsus paradoxus, narrowed pulse pressure, inspiratory distention of neck veins, friction rub), urgently hospitalize and obtain cardiac U/S.
- Refer for pericardiocentesis; send fluid for cytologic, hematologic, and chemical analyses.

Hypercoagulability/Bleeding
- Consider acute disseminated intravascular coagulation (DIC) when there is bleeding and prolongations in PT, PTT, and thrombin time, and low platelet count.
- Immediately hospitalize, send blood to check for fibrin split products, and check peripheral smear for microangiopathic changes (schistocytes).
- Treat with platelet and plasma transfusions followed by definitive Rx for underlying malignancy.
- Consider chronic DIC if there is thrombotic end-organ damage and thrombosis. Treat underlying cancer.

Superior Vena Cava Syndrome
- Consider if there is asymptomatic, unexplained distention of neck veins, especially if followed by swelling of face, neck, and upper extremities, plethora, shortness of breath, and persistent headache.
- Check for right superior mediastinal or hilar mass on CXR.
- Obtain biopsy when result will alter Rx [e.g., if small cell carcinoma or lymphoma, then chemotherapy indicated (see Hodgkin's Disease; Lung Cancer; Non-Hodgkin's Lymphoma)].
- Obtain urgent radiotherapy and oncology consultations to help design Rx program and choose between radiation and chemotherapy.
- Consider diuretics and corticosteroids for temporary symptomatic control.
- No role for heparin.

Hypercalcemia
- See also Hypercalcemia.
- Decide whether Rx is appropriate, especially if late stage of illness.
- Hospitalize if Rx appropriate.
- Start with vigorous rehydration with IV saline.
- Follow with furosemide to accelerate saline diuresis.
- Add daily calcitonin injection.
- Consider corticosteroids in myeloma, lymphoma, and metastatic breast cancer.
- For long-term control, begin bisphosphonate Rx (e.g., pamidronate).
- Treat underlying tumor if possible, recognizing that prognosis is poor and life expectancy limited.

Fever in the Setting of Neutropenia (<500 cells/mL)
- Monitor absolute neutrophil count.
- View patients with fever as infected until proved otherwise, with bacterial infection (often gram-negative) as most likely etiology, but also viral, fungal, and parasitic causes in patients with leukemia or on long-term steroids or broad-spectrum antibiotics.
- In absence of usual symptoms and signs of infection, suspect bacteremia and pneumonitis.
- Promptly hospitalize, regardless of whether additional signs of infection are present (mortality 18–40% within first 48 hrs).
- Obtain cultures of urine, sputum, blood, and material from any suspected site (e.g., CSF).
- If blood cultures negative but there is suspicion of mycobacterial or fungal infection, proceed with liver and bone marrow biopsies with cultures, and test for cryptococcal antigen (see Fever).
- Consider G-CSF for prophylaxis.
- In absence of identified pathogen, begin broad-spectrum antibiotic Rx:
  - Third-generation cephalosporin (e.g., ceftazidime); or
  - Semisynthetic penicillin (e.g., imipenem).
  - Add aminoglycoside when Pseudomonas infection is concern.

Malignant Pleural Effusion
- Consider Rx if respiration impaired; optimal Rx is systemic Rx of underlying malignancy (see Lung Cancer).
- Avoid repeated thoracentesis; ineffective and associated with considerable morbidity.
- Obtain surgical consultation for placement of indwelling chest tube for several days, followed by instillation of sclerosing agent (e.g., tetracycline).

Thrombocytopenia and Bleeding
- See Bleeding Problems

Paraneoplastic Syndromes

Due to Ectopic Hormone Production
- Cushing's syndrome
  - From ACTH production in 5% of patients with SCLC; late-stage occurrence.
  - Characterized by increased pigmentation, recalcitrant hypokalemia, impaired resistance to infection, and sometimes virilization.
  - Treat hypokalemia with spironolactone and large doses of supplemental potassium.
  - Consider metabolic inhibitors of adrenal hormone synthesis (aminoglutethimide, metyrapone, mitotane).
- Syndrome of inappropriate secretion of ADH
  - Causes hyponatremia and renal sodium wasting; urine osmolality inappropriately elevated; leads to confusion and disorientation.
  - Restrict intake of free water.
  - Inhibit ADH with lithium carbonate or demeclocycline.
  - Avoid infusions of hypertonic saline solution and diuretics.
  - Treat underlying tumor.
- Ectopic production of PTH-related protein (see Hypercalcemia).

- Hyperthyroidism and acute thyrotoxicosis
  - Treat underlying tumor, which makes hCG (which functions as TSH); e.g., choriocarcinoma.
  - Try beta-adrenergic blocking agents.
- Gynecomastia (see Gynecomastia).
- Fasting hypoglycemia (see Hypoglycemia).

Immunologically Mediated Paraneoplastic Syndromes
- Myasthenic (Eaton-Lambert) syndrome
  - With SCLC.
  - Proximal muscle weakness of limbs; resembles myasthenia, but EEG shows facilitation and increasing evoked muscle potential.
  - Treat with guanidine.
  - Avoid anticholinesterases used to treat myasthenia.
- Subacute cerebellar degeneration
  - With SCLC and ovarian and breast cancers.
  - Treat underlying cancer.
- Peripheral neuropathy
  - Symmetric sensory neuropathy; in advanced malignant disease.
  - Treat underlying cancer if appropriate.

Paraneoplastic Syndromes of Unknown Etiology
- Hypertrophic pulmonary osteoarthropathy
  - If exquisitely painful, consider removal of chest tumor.
- Hyperpyrexia and tumor-related fever
  - With hepatic metastases, typically from colon cancer; also with Hodgkin's disease.
  - Control fever with NSAIDs.
- Nephrotic syndrome
  - With Hodgkin's disease; massive edema with proteinuria and hypoalbuminemia.
  - Treat underlying malignancy.

Cutaneous Paraneoplastic Syndromes
- Hyperpigmentation or melanosis associated with ACTH-producing tumors.
- Necrotizing erythema with glucagon-secreting malignancies of pancreas.
- Proliferation of seborrheic keratoses with internal malignancy.
- Acanthosis nigricans or freckling and hyperpigmentation in axillary folds with intestinal cancer.
- Acquired ichthyosis with lymphomas.
- Treat underlying tumor.

CHRONIC CANCER PAIN

- Carefully assess each pain complaint; patients may have multiple pains with multiple origins and mechanisms.
- Attempt to diagnose each underlying cause, because specific causes respond best to specific Rx. In particular, be alert for bone pain, neuropathic pain, and cord compression.
- Use stepped approach for analgesic use as outlined by the WHO analgesic ladder (see below), but individualize analgesic Rx for each patient.
- Treat chronic cancer pain with around-the-clock (not prn) dosing, supplemented by prn ("rescue") doses for breakthrough pain.

- Use simplest route of administration, most convenient dosage schedule, and least invasive pain management measures. Oral Rx is preferred.
- Consider adding simple nonpharmacologic modalities, such as heat or cold application, massage, relaxation techniques, and guided imagery, which can complement appropriate analgesic regimens.
- For pain caused by severe localized disease, consider tumor-specific Rx (e.g., radiation, surgery, chemotherapy).
- Reassess frequently and at regular intervals, especially when pain worsens and after medication changes have been made.
- Treat patient worry in addition to discomfort; psychological support contributes greatly to effective pain control.

Mild to Moderate Pain

- Begin with acetaminophen, aspirin, or an NSAID:
  - Acetaminophen, up to 650 mg q4h or 975 mg q6h
  - Aspirin, up to 650 mg q4h or 975 mg q6h
  - Choline magnesium trisalicylate (Trilisate), 750–1,500 mg tid
  - Salsalate (Disalcid), 750–1,500 mg tid
  - Ibuprofen (Motrin, Advil), 600 mg q6h
  - Naproxen (Naprosyn, Aleve), 250–500 mg bid
  - Ketorolac (Toradol), 10 PO mg q6h; 30 mg IM q6h (up to 5 days)
  - Celecoxib (Celebrex), 100–200 mg bid
  - Rofecoxib (Vioxx), 12.5–25 mg/day
- Adapted from Jacox A, Carr DB, Payne R, et al. Management of cancer pain. Clinical practice guideline No. 9 AHCPR Publication No. 94-0592. Rockville, MD: Agency for Health Care Policy and Research, U.S. Department of Health and Human Services, Public Health Service, March 1994.

Moderate to Severe Pain

- When pain persists or increases, add weak opioid or low dosage of stronger opioid.
- For severe pain, treat with higher dosages of opioids or stronger opioid preparation.
- Initiate opioid Rx by quickly establishing necessary opioid dose. Do this by titrating with short-acting preparation, increasing each dose by 25–50% until patient achieves satisfactory pain control.
- Once effective dose established, switch to long-acting preparation (e.g., MS Contin, OxyContin, Oramorph SR, Duragesic patch).
- Use highest opioid dose necessary to achieve effective pain relief.
- Treat breakthrough pain with doses of short-acting opioid equal to 10–20% of total 24-hr opioid dose and give q2–4h prn.
- Minimize adverse effects of opioid use by periodically retitrating and prescribing laxatives to prevent severe constipation.
- Address common misunderstandings about addiction to minimize underdosing.
- If patient develops tolerance to one opioid, consider switching to another.
- Use equianalgesic doses when switching between different opioids and routes:
  - Morphine
    - MSIR tablets or capsules, 15 mg, 30 mg

- MSIR "soluble" tablets, 10 mg, 15 mg, 30 mg
- Roxanol (elixir), 10/5 mL, 20/5 mL, 100/5 mL
- MS Contin, 15 mg, 30 mg, 60 mg, 100 mg, 200 mg
- Oramorph SR, 15 mg, 30 mg, 60 mg, 100 mg
- Hydromorphone
  - Dilaudid, generic, 2 mg, 4 mg, 8 mg
- Codeine
  - Codeine sulfate tablets, 15 mg, 30 mg, 60 mg
- Codeine with acetaminophen
  - Tylenol (No. 2, No. 3, No. 4), 15 mg, 30 mg, 60 mg, respectively
- Codeine with aspirin
  - Empirin (No. 3, No. 4), 30 mg, 60 mg, respectively
- Hydrocodone with acetaminophen
  - Lortab, 2.5 mg, 5 mg, 7.5 mg, 10 mg
  - Lorcet, 5 mg, 7.5 mg, 10 mg
  - Vicodin, 5 mg, 7.5 mg
- Oxycodone
  - Roxicodone, 5 mg
  - OxyContin, 10 mg, 20 mg, 40 mg, 80 mg
- Oxycodone with acetaminophen
  - Percocet, Roxicet, Tylox, generic, 5 mg
- Oxycodone with aspirin
  - Percodan, 5 mg
- Levorphanol
  - Levo-Dromoran, generic, 2 mg
- Methadone
  - Dolophine, generic, 5 mg, 10 mg

Adapted from Weissman DE, Dahl JL, Dinndorf PA. Handbook of cancer pain management. Madison, Wisconsin Cancer Pain Initiative. 1996, with permission.

Severe Neuropathic or Bone Pain/Adjuvant Agents

■ For neuropathic pain, consider adjuvant agent, such as tricyclic antidepressant, anticonvulsant, psychostimulant, or glucocorticosteroid, including

- Amitriptyline (Elavil), 10–150 mg qhs
- Nortriptyline (Pamelor), 10–150 mg qhs
- Carbamazepine (Tegretol), 100–800 mg bid
- Gabapentin (Neurontin), 100–400 mg tid
- Phenytoin (Dilantin), 300–500 mg/d
- Dextroamphetamine (Dexedrine), 5–10 mg/d bid
- Methylphenidate (Ritalin), 2.5–15.0 mg qd-bid
- Dexamethasone (Decadron), 4–96 mg bid-qid
- Prednisone, 10–100 mg/d bid

Adapted from Jacox A, Carr DB, Payne R, et al. Management of cancer pain. Clinical practice guideline No. 9. AHCPR Publication No. 94-0592. Rockville, MD: Agency for Health Care Policy and Research, U.S. Department of Health and Human Services, Public Health Service, March 1994.

■ For bone pain: consider bisphosphonate Rx: alendronate (Fosamax), 10 mg/day.

Refractory Pain

■ When pain does not respond to Rx, reevaluate role of psychosocial factors, consider whether pain is neuropathic, and seek help from pain specialists.

- For poorly controlled pain or problematic side effects, consider referral for nerve block or placement of epidural catheter.

PSYCHOLOGICAL SUPPORT

Giving Bad News

- In communicating Dx, do not avoid words such as cancer and malignant tumor at outset of interview, although constant repetition of terms is usually unnecessary.
- Keep patients and families well informed to help alleviate hopelessness and feeling of lost control.
- Provide full and frequent reports of patient's status and prognosis.
- Be accurate without destroying all hope.
- Omit the term fatal in discussions of prognosis because it implies little hope of control.
- Redirect patient toward realistic therapeutic approaches and reinforce living instead of dying.
- When informed of incurable malignancy, patient and family may want to know how much time is left. Avoid indicating a specific period of time, because apt to be inaccurate.

Dealing with Misconceptions and Dysfunctional Defense Mechanisms

- Promptly address common patient misconceptions, such as certainty of death, intractable pain, and erosive, disfiguring disease.
- Recognize and respond to common defense mechanisms (denial, hostility, rejection of loved ones, regression, or even withdrawal) with patience and understanding.
- When denial is mild, reinforce remarks by repeatedly presenting facts and providing objective and tangible evidence.
- When denial is extreme and functioning as crude psychological defense mechanism, avoid constant onslaught of evidence and consider psychiatric consultation instead.
- When hostility is expressed, recognize it as a defensive reaction and do not respond personally. Allow response to run natural course without withdrawing support.
- When regression is infantile or more than transient, mitigate by assuming a more parental role of being supportive yet firm.
- When withdrawal is evident, directly confront patient and encourage setting of goals (e.g., ambulation, planning trips, visiting friends).
- Help family cope with dysfunctional patient responses and with any guilt that may arise.

Support during Treatment

- Inquire into patient's concerns and fears and offer realistic appraisal to minimize unnecessary anguish ("demythologizing").
- Provide detailed patient ed to cushion stress of entering Rx; allow patient to intellectualize disease and its Rx; provide detailed explanation of effect of Rx on tumor and potential side effects.
- Consider support groups and meditation techniques to facilitate patient's coping with stresses of cancer Rx.

BIBLIOGRAPHY

■ For the current annotated bibliography on cancer, see the print edition of *Primary Care Medicine*, 4th edition, Chapters 86–92, or www.LWWmedicine.com.

Cervical Cancer

SCREENING AND/OR PREVENTION

- High prevalence, long mean duration of asymptomatic detec   disease, and availability of highly specific screening test make cervical cancer screening important task for PCPs.
- Known risk factors, including early sexual activity and high number of sexual partners, allow selection of high-risk patients and populations.
- Because of long duration of preinvasive detec   disease in women of reproductive age, annual screening in absence of specific risk factors may be unnecessary. You may use 2 screens with short interval (e.g., 1 yr) to reduce number of false-negatives. Lengthen interval between subsequent screens for low-risk individuals. Presence of risk factors, particularly in menopausal or postmenopausal patients, may be indication for more frequent (i.e., yearly) screening.
- Annual Pap smears after 2 negative smears 6 mos apart is recommended strategy for women with HIV. Benefits for women with only 1–2 yrs life expectancy due to late-stage HIV infection are modest.
- Cytologic smear positive for cancer or high-grade squamous intraepithelial lesion is indication for referral to gynecologist for further evaluation, including appropriate biopsies.
- Nongynecologist can further evaluate smears suggestive of reactive or reparative changes or mild dysplasia. If concurrent infection is evident, repeat smear after specific infection Rx. If no infection present, repeat smear after 3- to 6-month interval. Refer women with repeatedly abnormal smears for colposcopy or biopsy.
- Cease screening after age 65 in women with Hx of regularly obtained negative smears, but perform screen if not done regularly before age 65 or if smear has been abnormal.

MANAGEMENT

- Oncologists and gynecologists usually provide Rx of women with genital tract cancer, but primary physician should assume ongoing responsibility for patient counseling and monitoring and management of medical problems.
- Early stages of cervical carcinoma are curable. For earliest tumors, conization need not interfere with subsequent childbearing.

BIBLIOGRAPHY

- For the current annotated bibliography on cervical cancer, see the print edition of *Primary Care Medicine*, 4th edition, Chapters 107 and 123, or www.LWWmedicine.com.

SCREENING AND/OR PREVENTION

TEST SELECTION AND FREQUENCY OF SCREENING

- Most authorities recommend that all patients, including those at normal risk, be screened with annual fecal occult blood test (FOBT) + periodic sigmoidoscopy or colonoscopy, depending on the estimated risk for colorectal cancer (CRC).
- To guide screening, annually reassess patient's risk by reviewing family Hx for CRC and larger (>1 cm) adenomas in first-degree relatives, and medical Hx for CRC, larger adenomas, and ulcerative colitis with pancolonic involvement.
  - For high-risk persons (i.e., ulcerative pancolitis for >10 yrs, familial adenomatous polyposis, or hereditary nonpolyposis colon cancer): refer to gastroenterologist for surveillance colonoscopy.
  - For intermediate- to high-risk persons [i.e., those with personal Hx of CRC or larger (>1 cm) adenomatous polyps]: obtain follow-up colonoscopy approximately q3yrs.
  - For intermediate-risk persons (i.e., those with strong family Hx of CRC, larger adenomas in first-degree relative aged <60, or >1 affected first-degree relative): begin screening at age 40 with colonoscopy approximately once q5yrs.
  - For lower intermediate-risk persons [i.e., those with one first-degree relative with CRC or polyps diagnosed after age 60, or with personal Hx of a smaller (<1 cm) adenomatous polyp]: begin screening at age 40 with annual FOBT and flexible sigmoidoscopy q5yrs.
- For average-risk patients (i.e., those with no risk factors other than age): begin screening with annual FOBT at age 50 and flexible sigmoidoscopy q5yrs.
- Because cost-effectiveness of endoscopic screening remains to be fully determined, review with reluctant patient benefits and risks of available screening strategies and plan individualized approach.

TEST PERFORMANCE

- Perform FOBT by instructing patient to obtain 2 samples on each of 3 days during which dietary peroxidases and rare red meat are restricted.
- Follow any positive FOBT result with colonoscopy or combination of sigmoidoscopy + air-contrast barium enema (preferable to repeating any positive test obtained on undefined diet).
- Order colonoscopy in any patient with larger polyp, multiple smaller polyps, or polyp with tubulovillous or villous histology found on screening sigmoidoscopy.
- Substitute rigid sigmoidoscopy for flexible sigmoidoscopy if latter is unavailable (see *Primary Care Medicine*, 4th edition, Chapter 56 appendix).

PREVENTION

- Recommend regular physical activity and dietary habits that ensure RDA of folic acid and calcium, but do not insist on high-fiber diet or megadose vitamin supplements.
- Data are intriguing but insufficient at present to recommend HRT or NSAIDs for prevention.

Management of Colorectal Polyps

- Submit all polyps for histologic exam to detect those with potential for malignant transformation (villous adenomas, tubular adenomas, and mixed tubulovillous adenomas). Hyperplastic polyps require no additional action.
- Proceed to colonoscopy for full exam of colon and cecum in all patients with polyp found on sigmoidoscopy with potential for malignant transformation, especially if polyp has tubulovillous or villous histology, patient age >65, positive family Hx of CRC, or >1 distal adenoma.
- Perform first follow-up study in 3 yrs, then q5yrs if first study is normal.
- Refer to GI consultant for consideration of regular colonoscopic surveillance as alternative to prophylactic colectomy in persons with hereditary nonpolyposis CRC mutations discovered through genetic screening.
- Recommend prophylactic colectomy to patients with familial adenomatous polyposis.

WORKUP

- Obtain colonoscopy in patient suspected of CRC (e.g., because of guaiac-positive stools, rectal bleeding, unexplained iron-deficiency anemia, or change in bowel habits). If unavailable, proceed to combination of flexible sigmoidoscopy plus barium enema (air contrast).
- For patients with cancer or polyp in rectosigmoid, perform preoperative exam of entire colon up to cecum for detection of synchronous tumors.
- Obtain preoperative baseline CEA level to facilitate postoperative monitoring.
- Stage patient according to findings at surgery and pathologic exam (see below); ask for detailed exam of draining lymph nodes in patients with stage B (stage II) disease, including molecular testing for micrometastasis. There is no need for preoperative liver scanning or CT, because results do not affect decision to remove tumor unless there is rectal cancer, in which case obtain CT or MRI of pelvis to determine extent of rectal cancer and candidacy for surgery.
- Base survival probabilities predominantly on basis of surgical and pathologic staging (see Table 76-1 in *Primary Care Medicine*, 4th edition).

MANAGEMENT

SURGERY

- Refer to surgery for curative and palliative procedures.
- For colon cancer, colectomy is procedure of choice, with adequate amounts of bowel on both sides of lesion removed to avoid cutting into intramural lymphatics that may contain cancerous cells.

- Consider temporary diverting colostomy in patients presenting with obstruction; follow later with reanastomosis.
- Consider salvage surgery, often with curative intent, for resectable recurrence of tumor (e.g., in abdomen, lung, or liver).
- For resectable rectal cancer, refer for abdominoperineal resection aided by adjuvant radiation Rx.
- For patients with small exophytic tumors in lower third of rectum, consider alternatives to abdominoperineal resection: local excision, fulguration, and intrarectal radiation Rx.

RADIATION

- Consider adjuvant radiation Rx in patients with rectal cancer that has penetrated bowel wall; it reduces risk of local recurrence and improves survival.
- For patients with extensive local disease, consider preoperative irradiation.
- For those at high risk for recurrence (stage B2 or C), consider postoperative radiotherapy; it may permit anterior resection with primary anastomosis in patients who would otherwise require colostomy.

CHEMOTHERAPY

- Consider postoperative levamisole and 5-FU in patients with stage C colon cancers.
- For patients with advanced unresectable disease, 5-FU remains only option; leucovorin increases response rate modestly but does not enhance survival.
- No benefit from high-dose vitamin C or immunotherapy.

MONITORING

- Arrange regular follow-up because of risk of new polyps, new primary tumors, or appearance of early, surgically curable metastasis to abdomen, lung, or liver.
- Monitor symptoms (weight loss, fatigue, change in bowel habits), PE (especially chest and abdomen), and alkaline phosphatase (rises with infiltration of liver).
- Repeat colonoscopy beginning 6 mos after surgery and q24–36mos if no polyps are found and q6mos if they are.
- If colonoscopy is unavailable or cannot reach cecum, order air-contrast barium enema and sigmoidoscopy as substitute.
- Monitor CXR q6mos for first 12–48 mos.
- Follow serum CEA after initial resection, checking determinations q6mos for first 2 yrs, provided that CEA was elevated before surgery and fell to low levels within 2–4 wks after surgery.
- If CEA rises ≥30%/mo from its postop level, proceed to search for curable recurrent disease in abdomen, liver, and lung.
- Consider periodic U/S or CT to check for early liver metastasis. MRI does not appear to offer advantages over CT.

SUPPORTIVE THERAPY

- Provide careful and detailed counseling and patient ed pre- and postop for patients requiring temporary or permanent colostomy.

- Make use of ostomy groups and stoma nurses to complement patient-doctor relationship.
- For patients with unresectable disease, meet with patient and family to address obvious but difficult questions regarding prognosis and Rx, and formulate personalized plan that maximizes patient's quality of life, comfort, and dignity. Also consider addressing elements necessary to complete advance directive.

BIBLIOGRAPHY

- For the current annotated bibliography on colorectal cancer, see the print edition of *Primary Care Medicine*, 4th edition, Chapters 56 and 76, or www.LWWmedicine.com.

Endometrial Cancer

SCREENING AND/OR PREVENTION

- Endometrial carcinoma is source of substantial M&M, with lifetime cumulative incidence of 3%. Well-defined risk factors include older age (most occurring in sixth and seventh decades), breast and/or colon cancer, obesity and glucose intolerance, and estrogens (including both clinical syndromes of ovarian estrogen excess and postmenopausal use of exogenous estrogens).
- Postmenopausal bleeding is most common presentation; prevalence of cancer is 10–70%, with higher rates among women whose bleeding began after longer span of yrs since menopause.
- Initiate prompt diagnostic workup, with transvaginal ultrasound (U/S) perhaps preceding endometrial biopsy in patients with postmenopausal bleeding.
- In absence of symptoms, screening for endometrial cancer with cytological exam of cells aspirated from vaginal pool, cervical os, or endometrial cavity has not been demonstrated to be effective.
- Transvaginal U/S of endometrial thickening with subsequent curettage for abnormalities may be advisable for high-risk women, including those on unopposed estrogen Rx for menopause (rarely advised for women with intact uteri) or tamoxifen for breast cancer.
- You can reduce risk associated with postmenopausal ERT by adding progesterone to HRT program (see Fertility Control).

MANAGEMENT

- Oncologists and gynecologists usually provide Rx of women with genital tract cancer, but primary physician should assume ongoing responsibility for patient counseling and monitoring and management of medical problems.
- Patients with stage I or stage II endometrial cancer are curable when treated with hysterectomy/bilateral salpingo-oophorectomy + irradiation. Adding radiation Rx is especially useful in stage II disease.

BIBLIOGRAPHY

- For the current annotated bibliography on endometrial cancer, see the print edition of *Primary Care Medicine*, 4th edition, Chapters 109 and 123, or www.LWWmedicine.com.

Esophageal Cancer

SCREENING AND/OR PREVENTION

- Advise smoking cessation and reduction of excess alcohol intake (see Alcohol Abuse; Smoking Cessation).
- Obtain surveillance endoscopy + biopsy in high-risk patients (e.g., those with Barrett's esophagus; see Heartburn and Reflux).
- Consider chronic acid-suppression Rx (e.g., PPIs) for patients with severe chronic reflux, although long-term efficacy remains unproved.

WORKUP

- Consider endoscopy and biopsy for patients with new-onset odynophagia, worsening dysphagia, or long-standing severe heartburn (especially if heavy drinker or smoker).
- Institute program of regular surveillance endoscopy and biopsy for those found to have metaplastic change indicative of Barrett's esophagus, and refer for possible surgical resection those who show dysplastic change (see Heartburn and Reflux).
- Once Dx is made, begin staging by checking for supraclavicular adenopathy and hepatomegaly.
- Obtain CT or MRI of chest and upper abdomen to assess for mediastinal invasion.
- Consider endoscopic ultrasound to determine depth of invasion.
- Use T1 and T2 designations for disease confined to esophageal wall; T3 refers to invasion through wall, and T4 indicates metastatic disease.

MANAGEMENT

- Sustain good nutrition; recommend pureed diets and liquid diet supplements; consider hyperalimentation as temporary means in patients with potential for meaningful survival.
- For patients with early-stage disease, refer to surgery for primary Rx; best candidates are those with disease confined to mucosa and those with severe dysplasia or carcinoma in situ.
- For patients with more advanced disease, obtain multidisciplinary consultation, exploring appropriateness of radiation Rx and even preoperative chemotherapy in addition to surgery.
- For palliation, consider surgery to reestablish swallowing ability; most successful in patients with disease confined to distal esophagus.
- For persons with locally advanced unresectable disease, consider radiation Rx, sometimes with chemotherapy (e.g., cisplatin and 5-FU) to allow use of lower radiation doses.
- Consider laser Rx for palliation in patients too ill to undergo surgery or radiation.

■ For dysphagic patients too ill for surgery yet in need of palliation, obtain consultation for endoscopic esophageal dilatation and polyvinyl stent placement; gastrostomy may be of help for nutrition but provides no symptomatic relief from disabling dysphagia.

BIBLIOGRAPHY

■ For the current annotated bibliography on esophageal cancer, see the print edition of *Primary Care Medicine*, 4th edition, Chapter 76, or www.LWWmedicine.com.

Gastric Cancer

SCREENING AND/OR PREVENTION

- Despite significant downward trend in incidence, gastric cancer remains disease of high M&M.
- Yearly analysis of stool for occult blood is indicated in all adult patients. Analysis is especially important for those with Hx of pernicious anemia, atrophic gastritis, *H. pylori* infection, or other gastric pathology.
- Consider early detection through endoscopic or radiologic screening only in high-risk populations (e.g., in Japan).
- Value of gastric cytology, endoscopy, and contrast studies as routine procedures in high-risk patients is unproved. They are diagnostic procedures and should generally be reserved for symptomatic patients or patients with occult blood demonstrated by stool analysis.
- Prevent exposure of young children to spoiled food; role of *H. pylori* screening and eradication is not established.

WORKUP

- Proceed with endoscopy + brushings and biopsy in patients aged >45 who have any of these risk factors: unexplained iron deficiency anemia; asymptomatic guaiac stool test positivity; epigastric discomfort; gastric ulceration; recurrent nausea, vomiting, anorexia, and weight loss; or lack of response healing after 6 wks of ulcer Rx (see Peptic Ulcer Disease).

MANAGEMENT

- For cure and palliation, refer for surgery as primary mode of management, except for patients with linitis plastica.
- Provide patient ed regarding importance of small frequent feedings and use of high-calorie supplements.
- Consider chemotherapy (e.g., 5-FU) as sole Rx mode in patients with metastatic disease; role of adjuvant chemotherapy after surgical resection remains unconfirmed.
- For gastric lymphomas, refer for chemotherapy after gastrectomy (see Lymphoma). Do not refer for radiation Rx because gastric adenocarcinomas and gastric lymphomas are not radiosensitive.
- Monitor by symptoms and not by routine testing for potential metastatic sites, because only palliative therapeutic options exist for advanced disease.

BIBLIOGRAPHY

- For the current annotated bibliography on gastric cancer, see the print edition of *Primary Care Medicine*, 4th edition, Chapters 55 and 76, or www.LWWmedicine.com.

Hodgkin's Disease

DIFFERENTIAL DIAGNOSIS

- See Lymphadenopathy.

WORKUP

- See Lymphadenopathy.

STAGING

- Stage I: Confined to single node-bearing area
- Stage II: Confined to 2 contiguous node-bearing areas on 1 side of diaphragm
- Stage III: In nodal areas on both sides of diaphragm
- Stage IV: Visceral lesions (liver, lung) not in contiguity with nodes
- Special categories
  - E: Visceral extranodal disease in contiguity with nodes (e.g., lung mass extending out from hilum)
  - B: Symptoms of fever, weight loss, or night sweats

Staging procedures

- Ascertain presence of fever, night sweats, or weight loss (B symptoms).
- Carefully palpate all lymph nodes and assess liver and spleen size.
- Obtain CXR for all patients.
- Follow with chest CT if CXR suggests hilar or mediastinal disease or if CXR is negative and chest CT findings would alter Rx or prognosis.
- Obtain abdominal CT for information on retroperitoneal lymph nodes and evidence of disease below the diaphragm (MRI offers no advantage over CT and costs more).
- Consider lymphangiography for complementary information about structure of retroperitoneal nodes; most useful to identify lymph nodes for removal in patients with clinical stage I or II disease without B symptoms who are scheduled for laparotomy.
- Order bone marrow biopsy in patients with systemic symptoms or clinical stage IIB disease and beyond; multiple biopsies are necessary to avoid sampling error; marrow aspiration is insufficient.
- Omit laparotomy if bone marrow biopsy is positive (stage IV).
- Consider laparotomy (with wedge biopsy of liver, splenectomy, and exam of contiguous lymph node chains) when results will change Rx; most useful in asymptomatic patients with clinical stage I or II disease who are being considered for radiotherapy alone.
- Administer pneumococcal immunization before splenectomy.
- Consider laparoscopy with liver biopsy for identifying liver involvement in patients with high probability of disease below diaphragm (e.g., those with B symptoms).

- In sum: for patients with clinical stage I or II disease, obtain CXR and abdominal and chest CTs + lymphangiography, followed by staging laparotomy to be sure there is no disease below diaphragm; extent of disease must be well documented.
- For patients with B symptoms, limit staging to laparoscopy and bone marrow biopsy; positive result obviates need for laparotomy.
- Consider monitoring additional prognostic factors for persons with advanced disease (i.e., stages III and IV), including albumin <4.0 g/dL, hemoglobin <10.5 g/dL, male gender, age >45, WBC count >15,000/mm^3, and lymphocytopenia (<600 cells/mL or <8% of WBCs).
- Consider assessment of biologic factors with possible prognostic value, including CD30, number of activated cytotoxic T cells, presence of CD15 in biopsy specimens, and presence of IL-16.

MANAGEMENT

BASIC PRINCIPLES

- Base Rx decisions predominantly on pathologic staging (which includes biopsy).
- Refer to oncologist skilled and experienced in management of Hodgkin's disease for design and implementation of Rx program. Information provided here to serve as guide to primary care physician and to aid in monitoring.

GUIDELINES BY STAGE

Stages I and II

- Radiation is Rx of choice.
- For stages IA and IIA disease, local and extended-field radiotherapy to contiguous node-bearing areas and adjacent regions.
- For stages IB and IIB, total nodal radiation Rx.
- For large mediastinal mass, chemotherapy + radiation or substituted for radiation if patient does not respond or relapses.
- Monitor for radiation side effects [gum disease and increased risks of thyroid cancer (20-yr latency), hypothyroidism (50%), radiation pneumonitis (6–20%), accelerated CAD, second solid tumor (incidence,1%/yr), and leukemia (with high-dose Rx to bone marrow)].

Stages III and IV

- Combination chemotherapy is cornerstone of Rx.
- Basic programs: mustargen, oncovin, prednisone, procarbazine (MOPP); or doxorubicin (Adriamycin), bleomycin, vinblastine, dacarbazine (ABVD).
- Combination and hybrid regimens used to address tumor resistance and drug toxicity.
- Chemotherapy administered for 6 mos, at which time restaging is carried out; in absence of residual disease, Rx is discontinued. No benefit is derived from "maintenance program."
- Radiation sometimes used for stage III1A disease program.

- Monitor closely for severe emesis, bone marrow suppression with increased susceptibility to infection, and neuropathy; also for late-onset cancer (e.g., leukemia).
- If MOPP is to be used, consider sperm banking before therapy; incidence of permanent sterility less with ABVD.
- Administer polyvalent pneumococcal vaccine before splenectomy, but if not done, administer after surgery and ≤10 days before chemotherapy.

RELAPSES

- Non–cross-resistant regimen, such as ABVD, used in place of or in some form of combination with original program.
- Autologous bone marrow transplantation followed by retreatment in drug-resistant patients.

MONITORING

- Periodically examine involved nodes and extranodal and visceral sites.
- Follow CXR for mediastinal involvement.
- Continue monitoring for ≥36 mos after completion of Rx, especially in patients with stage I disease.
- Consider gallium scanning for mediastinal monitoring.
- Consider abdominal CT to help detect late disease.
- Provide careful late follow-up even after 3 yrs because response to retreatment is good.

PATIENT EDUCATION AND INDICATIONS
FOR CONSULTATION

- Without raising false hopes, review 5-yr survival rates and the high percentage of patients disease-free after 10 yrs.
- Advise patients who have undergone splenectomy of importance of polyvalent pneumococcal vaccination.
- Review risk of permanent sterility with chemotherapy and advise pre-therapy sperm storage.
- Counsel young women (age <26) that they are capable of bearing phenotypically normal children.
- Once Dx is confirmed and clinical staging is complete, refer to oncologist for planning pathologic staging and Rx program.
- During initial Rx, follow closely with oncologist, helping to coordinate care and provide support.

BIBLIOGRAPHY

- For the current annotated bibliography on Hodgkin's Disease, see the print edition of *Primary Care Medicine*, 4th edition, Chapter 84, or www.LWWmedicine.com.

SCREENING AND/OR PREVENTION

- Lung cancer is major cause of M&M, especially among men. Incidence is increasing among women.
- Smoking is overwhelming risk factor for lung cancer. Occupational exposures also relevant.
- Little is known about presymptomatic natural Hx of lung cancer. It is presumed to be highly variable. The 5-yr survival despite all forms of Rx is 5–10%. Survival is slightly better when asymptomatic lesion is detected.
- Cytologic exam of the sputum and CXR are complementary diagnostic tests. Neither is sensitive or specific enough to serve as screening test, however.
- Large-scale early detection programs have demonstrated little benefit. Such efforts to improve prognosis have been thwarted by usually rapid course of lung cancer, characteristics of patients at risk, and relative insensitivity of available tests.

DIFFERENTIAL DIAGNOSIS

- Most forms of lung cancer are minimally responsive to Rx, although important exceptions exist. PCP must be knowledgeable about Rx options, including how they depend on cancer type and stage, and their effects on survival and quality of life.
- Common types of bronchogenic carcinoma are squamous cell, adenocarcinoma, large cell, and SCLC. All except SCLC share similar natural Hx and response to Rx. Consequently, lung cancers are often classified as NSCLC and SCLC.
- Central endobronchial lesions may produce symptoms early in course of illness. Hemoptysis, cough, sputum production, and localized wheeze are symptoms reported by 7–10% of patients. Occasionally systemic syndromes such as hypertrophic osteoarthropathy (see Clubbing), peripheral neuropathy, or inappropriate secretion of antidiuretic hormone may precede other evidence of disease [see Cancer (General)].
- Symptoms of advanced disease include anorexia, weight loss, nausea and vomiting, hoarseness (recurrent laryngeal nerve involvement), pleuritic chest pain, bone pain, and neurologic deficits.
- Most frequent sites of metastasis include local or regional lymph nodes within chest (25–45%), liver (30–45%), bone and bone marrow (20–40%), and CNS (20–35%).

WORKUP

LAB STUDIES

- CXR is primary diagnostic modality; appearance of lesion and doubling time are helpful in distinguishing benign from malignant disease. Finding calcified nodule can be helpful, especially if pattern of calcification is eccentric (see Solitary Pulmonary Nodule).

- Chest CT confirms presence of suspected lung mass and clarifies pattern of any calcium. CT has become critical to staging by determining presence and extent of hilar and mediastinal node involvement.
- Sputum cytology may provide evidence of lung cancer and even cell type. Presence of pulmonary histiocytes indicates adequate specimen. Negative cytologic exam does not rule out cancer, especially in patients with peripheral lesions.
- Use of fiberoptic bronchoscopy with washings, brushings, or forceps biopsy enhances cytologic testing. Complication rate is low in experienced hands.
- On occasion, transbronchial biopsy is means of establishing Dx (e.g., in suspected alveolar cell carcinoma; see Sarcoidosis). Risk for pneumothorax is 5%.
- With peripheral lesions, percutaneous transthoracic fine-needle biopsy, usually guided by CT or chest fluoroscopy, has proved accurate in lung cancer Dx. Sensitivity and specificity depend in part on adequacy of specimen and pathologist skill.
- For patients unable to tolerate any degree of pneumothorax, controlled thoracotomy may be preferable to needle aspiration.
- Scalene node biopsy indicated when peripheral nodes are enlarged; it can save patient extensive testing for Dx and staging.

STAGING

Non–Small Cell Lung Carcinoma

- Clinical course of NSCLC depends on surgical pathologic stage. Perform staging to determine prognosis and Rx and to assess tumor resectability.
- Perform CXR and chest CT with contrast, but negative CT result does not rule out microscopic spread. Patients with ipsilateral nodal disease may still be surgical candidates, but contralateral involvement of regional nodes is contraindication. For that reason, many surgeons advise mediastinoscopy before thoracotomy. Transthoracic and transbronchial needle aspiration biopsies are alternatives in some centers.
- MRI is superior to CT for judging chest wall involvement and disease in superior sulcus. Although symptomatic metastasis to head and bone is relatively common, routine use of head CT and bone scanning is wasteful unless there is clinical evidence of disease [see Cancer (General)].

Small Cell Lung Carcinoma

- Because SCLC prognosis is more independent of anatomic distribution at time of Dx, goal of staging is to distinguish between disease limited to hemithorax of origin and regional nodes and disease that is more extensive.
- Perform marrow biopsy; invasion is present in 25% of patients. CT of common sites of metastatic disease (e.g., brain) may also be useful.

MANAGEMENT

OVERALL APPROACH

- PCP should be able to recognize and promptly respond to complications of NSCLC and SCLC (including superior vena cava syndrome and malignant pleural effusion for both types, and tumor humoral syndromes for SCLC) as well as Rx complications.

- Realistic assessment of prognosis and pros and cons of Rx is essential for effective decision making by patient and family. Elicit and respect patient's preferences and willingness to undergo Rx.

NON–SMALL CELL LUNG CARCINOMA

- Surgical resection for possible cure is performed in 35–45% of patients with NSCLC, but only 60% have successful resection. Of these, 5-yr survival is 25–40%.
- Radiation for cure of NSCLC is disappointing. It is more effective at achieving local control. Chemotherapy added to surgery or radical radiation Rx produces 13% relative (4–5% absolute) 5-yr mortality reduction.
- For >60% of patients with inoperable disease, distant metastases occur regardless of local control and usually determine clinical course.
- Chemotherapy toxicity (usually cisplatin based) can be disabling. Most patients who experience it do not consider best estimate of median survival benefit (3 mos) sufficient to justify use. Discuss with patient this trade-off between harms and benefits.

SMALL CELL LUNG CARCINOMA

- Extremely sensitive to chemotherapy and radiation. Patients with limited-stage disease receive both, whereas those with disseminated disease receive chemotherapy alone. Surgery has no role.
- Use of reduced-dose etoposide + cisplatin regimen after course of 3-drug Rx (cyclophosphamide, doxorubicin, vincristine) has improved survival and reduced marrow suppression. Shorter courses of Rx (≤4–6 mos) are standard; longer courses are without additional benefit. In elderly, single-dose etoposide appears to provide up to 80% of response without significant compromise of survival.

BIBLIOGRAPHY

- For the current annotated bibliography on lung cancer, see the print edition of *Primary Care Medicine*, 4th edition, Chapters 37 and 53, or www.LWWmedicine.com.

Non-Hodgkin's Lymphoma

DIFFERENTIAL DIAGNOSIS

- See Lymphadenopathy.

WORKUP

- See Lymphadenopathy.

STAGING

- Examine all node-bearing areas carefully, including epitrochlear nodes, Waldeyer's ring, and preauricular area.
- Note any liver or spleen enlargement.
- Obtain CXR and chest and abdominal (including pelvis) CTs.
- Consider lymphangiography if CT is unavailable; staging laparotomy unnecessary.
- Examine peripheral smear and obtain multiple bone marrow samplings (aspirate + biopsy).
- Base remainder of staging workup on clinical or histopathologic findings.
- For high-grade histologic pattern, no further workup needed because advanced disease almost certain.
- For marrow involvement, lymphoblastic histology, young age, or HIV infection, obtain lumbar puncture to check for CNS spread.
- Consider GI endoscopy if there is intermediate-grade disease involving Waldeyer's ring.

GRADING OF DISEASE

- Histology is major determinant of grading.
  - Low-grade lymphoma
  - Small lymphocytic
  - Follicular, small cleaved cell
  - Follicular, mixed, small cleaved cell
  - Intermediate-grade lymphoma
  - Follicular, predominantly large cell
  - Diffuse small cleaved cell
  - Diffuse mixed, small, large cell
  - Diffuse large cell, cleaved/noncleaved
  - High-grade lymphoma
  - Diffuse large cell; immunoblastic
  - Lymphoblastic
  - Small noncleaved cell (Burkitt's, non-Burkitt's)

Adapted from Rosenberg SA. National Cancer Institute–sponsored study of classifications of non-Hodgkin lymphomas: summary and description of a working formulation for clinical usuage. Cancer 1980;45:2188, with permission.

MANAGEMENT

BASIC PRINCIPLES

- Grade and, to somewhat lesser degree, stage are key determinants of response to Rx and prognosis and basis for Rx decisions.
- Other predictors of outcome include absence of bulky disease, minimal extranodal disease, absence of B symptoms, young age, and female gender.
- Refer to oncologist for design and implementation of Rx program.
- Chemotherapy is predominant mode of Rx, administered as single agent or as complex multidrug regimen.
- Radiation used for localized disease.

TREATMENT GUIDELINES

Low-Grade (Indolent) Disease

- Most forms of Rx produce responses and remissions, but relapse is common after 2 yrs.
- Remission after retreatment is rule, but cure is rare.
- Benefit of aggressive chemotherapy vs watchful waiting remains to be demonstrated.
- Median survival is about 10 yrs.
- Investigational Rx: aggressive chemotherapy + radiation, followed by autologous bone marrow transplantation (ABMT) in selected patients who relapse; also, IFN-α + combination chemotherapy.

Intermediate-Grade (Aggressive) Disease

- For localized disease: combination chemotherapy [e.g., with cyclophosphamide, hydroxydaunomycin, vincristine (Oncovin), and prednisone (CHOP)] with or without local radiation; 5-yr disease-free in 85–95%.
- Predictors of poor outcome: advancing age, B symptoms, marrow involvement, elevations in LDH, large abdominal mass, and multiple extranodal sites.
- For lack of response or relapse: non–cross-resistant drugs (e.g., bleomycin and doxorubicin).
- For advanced-stage disease: aggressive combination chemotherapy (80% remission rate; long-term survival in up to 70%); high-level *BCL-2* oncogene associated with poor prognosis.
- For relapse, high-dose chemotherapy and ABMT.

For High-Grade (Highly Aggressive) Disease

- For patients with symptomatic or rapidly progressive disease: intensive multidrug chemotherapy, often with radiation Rx.
- Refer to tumor burden, LDH, *p53* gene mutations, and IL-6 levels to gauge likelihood of response.
- For diffuse large cell disease: high-dose chemotherapy with ABMT.
- For lymphoblastic and some Burkitt's lymphomas: acute leukemia regimens.
- Response rates with multidrug Rx: 95%; median survival >2 yrs; cure rates: 20–40%.
- Investigational Rx: monoclonal antibodies, ABMT, and IFN.

MONITORING THERAPY

- Monitor for bone marrow suppression [see Cancer (General)].
- Repeat exam for relapse (within 12–18 mos) usually in areas of previous disease.
- Watch for neurologic symptoms in those with predisposition to CNS spread (see above).

PATIENT EDUCATION

- Provide accurate assessment of prognosis after careful histologic study and staging have been carried out. Often, prognosis is far better than patient's fearful expectations.
- Review possible adverse effects of Rx (e.g., sterility, infection).
- Note experimental nature of Rx for which data on long-term outcomes is lacking.
- Monitor response and adverse effects, maintain continuity, and provide psychological support.

INDICATIONS FOR REFERRAL

- Refer early in course of illness, when Dx is first suspected.
- Work closely with oncologist experienced in lymphoma, who should select and conduct Rx.

BIBLIOGRAPHY

- For the current annotated bibliography on non-Hodgkin's lymphoma, see the print edition of *Primary Care Medicine*, 4th edition, Chapter 84, or www.LWWmedicine.com.

Oral Cancer

SCREENING AND/OR PREVENTION

- Incorporate screening for oral cancer into routine health maintenance exam of all patients.
- Review medical Hx for smoking, drinking, smokeless tobacco use (major risk factors) and maintain high index of suspicion if positive.
- Check Hx for mucosal sore or ulceration that does not heal within 1–2 wks.
- Perform thorough visual and manual exam of lips and oral cavity.
- View with suspicion any atrophic or hyperplastic areas of oral mucosa, particularly if red or white (erythroplasia or leukoplakia) and lasting >2 wks after cessation of smoking, drinking, and irritant exposure.
- If found, eliminate any source of presumed mechanical irritation (e.g., poorly fitting dentures, jagged tooth, acute aspirin burn) and follow clinical healing of mucosal wound over short time.
- Note any swelling beneath normal-appearing oral mucosa (commonly benign due to infection, bony exostosis, or mucus retention phenomena, but may represent neoplasm of minor salivary glands or other submucosal structures).
- Refer for immediate biopsy patients with deeply ulcerative or fungating lesions.
- Refer for biopsy any red or white lesion that persists for 2 wks after initial recognition and elimination of irritating agents.
- Do not rely on exfoliative cytology or *in vivo* staining with toluidine blue in lieu of biopsy.

BIBLIOGRAPHY

- For the current annotated bibliography on oral cancer, see the print edition of *Primary Care Medicine*, 4th edition, Chapter 211, or www.LWWmedicine.com.

Ovarian Cancer

SCREENING AND/OR PREVENTION

- Ovarian carcinoma is hard to detect in early stages. Advise women at very high risk (i.e., those with family Hx of hereditary disease and mutation of *BRCA* genes) of prophylactic approaches. Options include regular CA 125 screening and ultrasound (U/S), prophylactic oophorectomy, and oral contraceptive Rx.
- Women from families with genetic predisposition to ovarian cancer are at high risk and should have annual CA 125 screening and U/S beginning at age 35. Women carrying *BRCA1* mutation are at higher risk than those with *BRCA2* mutation; semiannual screening beginning at earlier age (e.g., 25) may be advisable.
- Women with family Hx of sporadic ovarian cancer may benefit from CA 125 screening, but because of low predictive value and morbidity associated with further diagnostic evaluation, routine screening is not recommended.
- Advise women of potential benefits and harms of screening. Similarly, routine screening is not recommended for pre- and postmenopausal women without family Hx of ovarian cancer.
- Advise women of childbearing age of ovarian cancer risk reduction afforded by oral contraceptive use. This may be especially important for women with family Hx or genetic predisposition.
- Apprise women of potential slight increase in breast cancer risk associated with current use of oral contraceptives, but likely that benefit of ovarian cancer risk reduction outweighs potential harm.

WORKUP

- See Abdominal Pain; Menstrual or Pelvic Pain

MANAGEMENT

- Oncologists and gynecologists usually provide Rx of women with genital tract cancer, but primary physician should assume ongoing responsibility for patient counseling and monitoring and management of medical problems.
- Although tumor is responsive to cancer Rx, its bulk and spread limit results. Cure is still limited. Major advance in chemotherapy has been achieved with combination regimen of cisplatin + paclitaxel.

BIBLIOGRAPHY

- For the current annotated bibliography on ovarian cancer, see the print edition of *Primary Care Medicine*, 4th edition, Chapters 108 and 123, or www.LWWmedicine.com.

Pancreatic Cancer

WORKUP

- Begin with abdominal ultrasound (U/S) or CT in patients with suspected disease (see Abdominal Pain).
- When you identify distinct pancreatic mass, obtain percutaneous FNAB guided by direct U/S or CT visualization.
- For patients with mass at pancreaticobiliary junction, order endoscopic retrograde cholangiopancreatography with pancreatogram and cytologic sampling.
- Reserve serum tumor markers for monitoring.
- To stage, use CT with contrast as staging procedure of choice (especially for visualizing tumor, liver, and lymph node metastases), complemented by laparoscopy (for undetected peritoneal or omental metastases) and angiography (for vascular invasion) to assess resectability.
- Consider endoscopic U/S with transendoscopic FNA, to determine spread beyond pancreatic capsule and local nodal involvement.

MANAGEMENT

- Refer for consideration of curative surgery (Whipple procedure, pancreatoduodenectomy) only patients with relatively small lesions confined to head of pancreas; make referral only to surgeons able to perform operation with <5% mortality. Regional pancreatectomy or total pancreatectomy provides no survival benefit.
- Carefully individualize decision to subject patient with pancreatic cancer to major operation with high degree of operative mortality and only modest chances for substantially improved survival; 5-yr survival rates are best in patients with small (≤2 cm) tumors, approaching 30% at centers with surgical expertise in performing operation.
- For palliation, consider biliary bypass and endoscopic stent placement for patients with biliary obstruction, and surgical or percutaneous ablation of celiac ganglion for relief from intractable pain.
- Consider radiation Rx for patients with localized but unresectable disease; when used with 5-FU Rx, it prolongs survival modestly; consider radiation also for control of intractable retroperitoneal pain.
- Consider gemcitabine chemotherapy for unresectable disease and refractory pain.
- For those with pancreatectomy, prescribe insulin Rx (20–30 U/day) + pancreatic enzyme preparations.

BIBLIOGRAPHY

- For the current annotated bibliography on pancreatic cancer, see the print edition of *Primary Care Medicine*, 4th edition, Chapter 76, or www.LWWmedicine.com.

Prostate Cancer

SCREENING AND/OR PREVENTION

- Evidence on digital rectal exam (DRE) screening for prostate cancer is conflicting. Many clinicians, however, simply consider DRE part of thorough PE of older men.
- If prostatic abnormality identified on DRE in younger patient or older patient without significant comorbid disease who would be eligible for curative Rx, make urologic referral for biopsy.
- Consider prostate-specific antigen (PSA) measurement at age 50 (and perhaps at age 40 among men at higher than average risk, such as those with positive family Hx). Because there is no evidence that screening reduces long-term mortality, it is optional.
- Normal PSA result does not exclude cancer in presence of palpable abnormality.
- Patients should understand pros and cons of screening before undergoing test.
- When to proceed to biopsy is controversial; PSA threshold of 4 ng/mL is commonly used.
- Screening periodicity has not been established, but repeating PSA measurement q1–2yrs is reasonable (use longer interval when initial PSA level is lower).
- Early detection efforts are not indicated for men with life expectancy <10 yrs.
- Routine transrectal ultrasound is no longer recommended as primary screening test; its main role is in evaluation of abnormalities found on DRE or PSA measurement.

WORKUP

OVERALL STRATEGY

- Give men with prostate cancer opportunity to learn explicit quantitative estimates of prognosis based on disease stage at time of Dx, histologic grade of tumor (Gleason score), and PSA level.
- PSA levels provide useful prognostic information. Level >15 ng/mL (Hybritech assay) suggest extension through capsule or into seminal vesicles. PSA level <20 ng/mL greatly reduces likelihood of bony involvement and obviates need for bone scan.
- Pelvic and abdominal CT to assess pelvic and retroperitoneal lymph node involvement is insufficiently sensitive to justify its use.

GLEASON SCORE

- Prostate cancers are scored according to Gleason system on scale of 2–10. More disrupted and undifferentiated normal glandular architecture means higher grade of tumor and poorer prognosis.
- Men with Gleason score 2–4 rarely die of prostate cancer in ensuing 15 yrs regardless of age at Dx.

- For men with Gleason score 8–10, prognosis is much worse, with 15-yr case fatality rates ≥80%.
- Cancers with Gleason score 5 confer prognosis similar to that of Gleason score 2–4.
- Gleason 7 score is similar to Gleason 8–10.
- Prognosis for men with Gleason 6 score is intermediate.

MANAGEMENT

- Most elderly patients with cancer detected during prostatectomy for Rx of BPH and low-grade histology need no Rx because survival is unaffected by disease. Patients with ≥10 yrs life expectancy should consider curative Rx.
- Advise most patients with early stage disease that Rx options include radiation (external beam, brachytherapy, or combination), radical prostatectomy (± attempt to preserve neurovascular bundles and thereby preserve sexual function), or delayed endocrine Rx.
- Patients should appreciate that Rx choice depends heavily on preferences regarding uncertain comparative benefits and rates of side effects including impotence and incontinence.
- Offer men with symptomatic metastatic disease hormonal Rx, which may include orchiectomy or LH-RH agonists ± antiandrogen.
- Antiandrogen agents (e.g., flutamide, bicalutamide) block effects of testosterone at receptor level, which makes them useful for countering adrenal androgen secretion and surge that accompanies early LH-RH agonist Rx. Do not use as monotherapy because they increase LH release that eventually stimulates sufficient testosterone secretion to overcome their blocking effect.
- When initial hormonal monotherapy fails, flutamide is sometimes considered. Responses average 6 mos and occur in only about 20% of patients.
- Hydrocortisone, aminoglutethimide, and ketoconazole have been used to suppress adrenal androgen production. Under investigation are 5-α-reductase inhibitors (e.g., finasteride), which block peripheral conversion of testosterone to its more active metabolite dihydroxytestosterone.
- External beam radiation is effective means of palliation for patients with bone pain. It can prevent fracture and is used in cases of impending spinal cord compression [see Cancer (General)].
- Chemotherapy has been disappointing, with no agent altering survival. Response rates are <20%.
- Serum PSA determination is best means of monitoring response to Rx. PSA half-life of 48 hrs allows it to reflect quickly changes in tumor activity and mass.

BIBLIOGRAPHY

- For the current annotated bibliography on prostate cancer, see the print edition of *Primary Care Medicine*, 4th edition, Chapters 126 and 143, or www.LWWmedicine.com.

Renal Cell Carcinoma (Hypernephroma)

WORKUP

- High index of suspicion necessary to make early Dx of renal cell carcinoma. Hematuria in setting of normochromic, normocytic anemia and markedly elevated ESR are suggestive, as is triad of fever, elevated ESR, and increased α_1-globulin.
- If suspicion remains high, begin radiologic evaluation with IV pyelography. If mass is found, determine whether it is cystic (and therefore most likely benign) or solid.
- Renal ultrasonography + CT or MRI helps determine local extent of disease, including perinephric involvement, renal vein obstruction, and spread to retroperitoneal nodes.

MANAGEMENT

- Tumor confined to kidney is curable. When it extends beyond Gerota's capsule, prognosis is poor. Hormonal Rx (progesterone and androgens) have produced responses in some patients, but without prolonging survival.
- Minority of patients have partial or complete responses to IFN, IL-2, or both, but response is rarely durable.

BIBLIOGRAPHY

- For the current annotated bibliography on renal cell carcinoma (hypernephroma), see the print edition of *Primary Care Medicine*, 4th edition, Chapter 143, or www.LWWmedicine.com.

Skin Cancer

SCREENING AND/OR PREVENTION

SCREENING

- Check skin of all patients carefully on every periodic health mainte-
  nance exam; screening for skin cancer represents one of the best
  examples of early detection leading to improved outcome.
- Monitor most closely and most frequently patients with Hx of arsenic
  exposure, previous radiation Rx, radiation dermatitis, heavy sun exposure, or Hx of skin cancer.
- Examine for hallmarks of a potentially dysplastic or malignant pigmented lesion:
  - Asymmetry of lesion
  - Border irregularities
  - Color variegation
  - Diameter >6 mm
- Look for features of actinic keratosis, precursor of squamous cell carcinoma: raised, scaly, rough lesion in sun-exposed area.
- Recognize Bowen's disease, the carcinoma-in-situ stage of squamous
  cell carcinoma: chronic, asymptomatic, nonhealing, erythematous
  patch with some crusting and sharp but irregular borders, even cutaneous horn.
- Check for invasive squamous cell carcinoma: asymptomatic flesh-
  colored nodule with crusting ± cutaneous horn and ulceration.
- Look for signs of typical basal cell carcinoma: translucent papule with
  telangiectasia and subsequent development of central ulceration giving
  borders pearly raised appearance. Also, when finding isolated
  erythematous plaque with irregular scaly border, consider superficial
  spreading basal cell disease.
- If any doubt exists about whether skin lesion is benign, perform or
  arrange for biopsy of lesion.
- Emphasize importance of self-exam and prompt reporting of any suspicious lesion.
- Teach patients to report any new, slowly growing, nodular or papular
  lesion that is flesh-colored or translucent, particularly if there is any
  bleeding, ulceration, or horn formation. Areas of maximum solar exposure are at greatest risk.
- Ask patients to report any pigmented lesion with irregular border or
  color variation, especially blue, gray, or black. Any growth in pigmented lesion or color change should also arouse suspicion.

PREVENTION

- Advise all fair-skinned persons who sunburn easily and those with evidence of solar damage or skin cancer to avoid sun exposure between
  11:00 A.M. and 2:30 P.M., during which 70% of exposure to harmful UV
  radiation occurs.

■ Recommend that all patients wear protective clothing and use broad-spectrum sunscreen on sun-exposed areas. Sunscreen preparation should effectively block UVA and UVB radiation and have SPF ≥15 and preferably 30.

BIBLIOGRAPHY

■ For the current annotated bibliography on skin cancer, see the print edition of *Primary Care Medicine*, 4th edition, Chapter 177, or www.LWWmedicine.com.

Testicular Cancer

WORKUP

- Presume any solid, nontransilluminating, painless testicular mass in young men to be primary testicular cancer until proved otherwise. If testicular ultrasonography confirms testicular mass, obtain prompt urologic consultation for consideration of surgical removal of involved testicle.
- Staging begins with orchiectomy findings and proceeds to CXR and chest CT for metastatic disease of chest, and to abdominal CT for assessment of retroperitoneal lymph nodes.
- Circulating tumor markers also provide means to detect occult disease. hCG β-subunit is always elevated in choriocarcinoma and in about half of other nonseminomatous germ cell tumors (rarely elevated in pure seminoma, but several seminomatous cases have mixed disease and elevated hCG). α-Fetoprotein is produced by about 80% of patients with embryonal cell cancer. Both markers also provide excellent means of monitoring response to Rx (see below).

MANAGEMENT

- Treat stage I seminomatous tumors with inguinal orchiectomy, which may precede adjuvant retroperitoneal node irradiation. Cure rate is close to 100%. Patients who relapse are candidates for combination chemotherapy, which is extremely effective (see below). Also treat patients with stage IIA disease with retroperitoneal radiation. Cure rates are still close to 100% at this stage. Treat patients with stage IIB and stage III disease with cisplatin-based chemotherapy. Cure rates are >90%.
- Treat stages I and IIA nonseminomatous tumors with surgery only. Surgical cure rates average 95% when lymph node dissection shows no regional disease. Patients with stage IIB disease have high probability of relapse and are candidates for chemotherapy, as are patients with stage III disease.
- Multiple-agent chemotherapy based on cisplatin represents important breakthrough in testicular cancer Rx. Even patients with distant metastatic disease now have high probability of cure.
- Close monitoring of response to Rx is essential. Use hCG and α-fetoprotein levels to detect subclinical relapse and lack of Rx response. Patients having isolated elevations in tumor markers as sole manifestation of relapse have nearly 100% chance of cure when treated promptly with chemotherapy.

BIBLIOGRAPHY

- For the current annotated bibliography on testicular cancer, see the print edition of *Primary Care Medicine*, 4th edition, Chapter 143, or www.LWWmedicine.com.

Thyroid Nodules and Thyroid Cancer

SCREENING AND/OR PREVENTION

- Check for risk factors (especially childhood neck irradiation, exposure to high levels of environmental radiation, and positive family Hx of thyroid cancer; also age <40, male gender).
- In high-risk patients, perform yearly thyroid exam, checking for nodularity.
- Consider periodic thyroid ultrasound (U/S) of very-high-risk patients.
- Obtain needle biopsy if new solitary nodule is identified.

DIFFERENTIAL DIAGNOSIS

SOLITARY

- Benign adenoma: solid or mixed cystic and solid; most euthyroid and responsive to TSH; those >3 cm may become autonomous and present as hot nodule on scan.
- Cancer:
  - Papillary or mixed: single hard nodule; local adenopathy; cold on scan; slow-growing; metastasizes very late.
  - Follicular: same as papillary or mixed, although metastasizes earlier; some cystic.
  - Medullary: may be familial; multiple endocrine neoplasia; calcitonin elevated; cold nodule.
  - Lymphoma: primary cancer arises in patients with chronic lymphocytic thyroiditis; prominent regional nodes.

MULTINODULAR

- Hashimoto's thyroiditis: multinodular, rubbery gland; antithyroid antibodies; one-third hypothyroid; heterogeneous uptake; TSH responsive.
- Multinodular goiter: multiple nodules, enlarged gland; heterogeneous uptake on scan with some areas of decreased or absent uptake; clinically euthyroid, although some with mild decrease in TSH; autonomous gland.
- Cancer:
  - Thyroid: (see above).
  - Lymphoma: may arise in Hashimoto's gland.

WORKUP

HISTORY

- Elicit Hx of nodule.
- Check for cancer risk factors (neck irradiation in childhood, exposure to excessive environmental radiation, positive family Hx of thyroid cancer, age <40, male gender).

- Ask about symptoms suggestive of local compression or invasion (hoarseness, dysphagia, and tracheal wheezing).
- Note risk factors for nonmalignant goiter [family Hx of goiter, residence in iodine-deficient area, presence of goiter, intake of goitrogens (e.g., lithium, turnips, beets)].
- Check for symptoms of hypo- or hyperthyroidism.

PHYSICAL EXAM

- Focus on gland and adjacent lymph nodes.
- Note overall size, consistency, and number and size of nodules; determine whether single or multinodular.
- Be especially suspicious of solitary hard nodule that is irregular and fixed (does not move with swallowing).
- Check adjacent lymph nodes, especially those on same side as nodule.
- Check vocal cords of patients with hoarseness.

LAB STUDIES

Single Nodule

- Consider thyroid U/S to confirm nodule is solitary, but do not use cystic appearance of nodule to rule out malignancy, because 7% of solitary cystic lesions are malignant, as are 12% of mixed nodules.
- Order FNAB as test of choice for initial evaluation of euthyroid patient with single thyroid nodule.
- Refer to physician skilled in performing FNAB and to pathologist experienced in interpreting thyroid cytology.
- Be sure cystic lesion drains completely, and obtain samples from residual mass.
- If cytology is malignant, refer to surgery for removal.
- If cytology benign, observe for 1 yr and perform follow-up thyroid U/S.
- If reading is suspicious, obtain radionuclide scan to determine nodule uptake.
- Consider radionuclide scanning as supplementary test performed after FNAB in patients with suspicious or "indeterminate" cytology to help determine need for surgical excision.
- If nodule is hot on radionuclide scan, omit surgery.
- If nodule in patient with suspicious cytology is warm or cold on scan, proceed to surgical excision.
- Refer patients with suspicious or indeterminate lesions for consideration of surgical excision of nodule if malignancy not ruled out by other means (e.g., radionuclide scan).
- Check TSH level.
- Check antimicrosomal antibodies if gland multinodular.
- Consider ESR in setting of acutely tender gland.
- Obtain serum calcitonin determination if strong family Hx of thyroid cancer.
- If follow-up thyroid U/S of initially benign nodule indicates increase in nodule size, repeat biopsy.
- If nodule enlarging yet benign on repeat biopsy, treat with levothyroxine suppressive Rx (see below) and repeat U/S in 1 yr.

- If nodule stops enlarging on suppressive Rx, continue and reassess by U/S annually.
- If size is increasing despite suppressive Rx, refer for surgical removal.
- If following patients expectantly, instruct them to call promptly if they note change in size, lymphadenopathy, pain, dysphagia, or hoarseness.

Multinodular Goiter

- Omit initial biopsy unless there are risk factors for cancer (neck irradiation, cervical adenopathy, rapid growth of single nodule in otherwise stable gland, or onset of recurrent laryngeal nerve palsy).
- Obtain antithyroid antibody determination because most cases represent Hashimoto's thyroiditis.
- Consider FNAB of gland in presence of enlarging, tender goiter, cervical adenopathy, or goiter markedly enlarging on thyroid hormone suppression.

Benign Adenonoma

- Determine whether it is functioning autonomously.
- Follow without further workup if <2 cm.
- If >3 cm, perform serial radionuclide scans, checking for response to stimulation by TRH or suppression by thyroid hormone.
- Observe smaller low-risk lesions rather than refer for ablation.
- Annually determine nodular size and hormonal output.
- Scan q5yrs to see if suppression of extranodular tissue is increasing (sign of impending toxicity).
- Also check size (>3 cm), rise in serum T_3 to ULN, and decreasing responsiveness to stimulation or suppression.

"Incidentaloma"

- Usually found on U/S scanning for other reasons.
- Observe as long as patient has no risk factors for thyroid cancer and lesion diameter is <1.5 cm.
- Biopsy unnecessary, but follow up carefully.
- Proceed to biopsy if lesion >1.5 cm, prior head or neck irradiation, strongly positive family Hx of thyroid cancer, or U/S findings suggestive of malignancy at outset.

MANAGEMENT

BENIGN SOLITARY NODULE (CLINICALLY EUTHYROID)

- Consider low-dose suppressive Rx with levothyroxine (sufficient to reduce TSH level to low but not undetectable levels) if deemed desirable and safe to inhibit nodule growth and decrease its size.
- Begin with small doses (e.g., 0.05 mg/day) and increase gradually until TSH declines to about 0.3 mU/L (required dosage 0.10–0.15 mg/day).
- Avoid further TSH suppression, because of risk of side effects (e.g., T_4-induced osteoporosis; see Hypothyroidism).
- Use with great caution in the elderly and those with underlying coronary disease (see Hyperthyroidism).

- Alternatively, observe nodule for 1 yr after initial biopsy, recheck size by U/S, perform another biopsy on any nodule that appears to be enlarging, and if nodule is benign, institute modest suppressive Rx to halt enlargement and achieve size reduction.
- If nodule continues to enlarge, refer for surgical removal.
- If nodule responds to suppressive Rx, continue levothyroxine and check nodule size at regular intervals.

NONTOXIC MULTINODULAR GOITER

- Not responsive to suppressive Rx.
- For very large, bothersome cysts, consider surgical removal, but aspirate smaller ones as necessary to rule out malignancy (incidence about 1%) and to increase comfort and improve appearance.

TOXIC NODULES AND AUTONOMOUSLY FUNCTIONING SOLITARY ADENOMAS

- Advise avoiding substances with high iodine concentrations (medications, kelp, radiographic contrast media) because at high risk for precipitating thyrotoxicosis; if contrast study necessary, start on beta blocker 10 days before study.
- Consider for ablative Rx especially if nodule diameter >3 cm, serum T_3 level at ULN, and nodule increasingly unresponsive to T_4 suppression.
- Choose between surgery and radioiodine; obtain consultation.
- Consider surgery if skilled thyroid surgeon available; best candidates are young patients.
- Consider radioiodine for elderly; monitor for development of posttreatment hypothyroidism (see Hyperthyroidism).
- Alternatively, consider watchful waiting, as long as patient has no risk factors for thyroid cancer and lesion is <1.5 cm; careful follow-up essential.

BIBLIOGRAPHY

- For the current annotated bibliography on thyroid nodules and thyroid cancer, see the print edition of *Primary Care Medicine*, 4th edition, Chapters 94 and 95, or www.LWWmedicine.com.

Tumor of Unknown Origin

DIFFERENTIAL DIAGNOSIS

TREATABLE MALIGNANCIES THAT MAY PRESENT AS TUMOR OF UNKNOWN ORIGIN

- Potentially curable, even when metastatic
  - Gestational trophoblastic tumors
  - Germ cell cancer, gonadal (e.g., testicular carcinoma)
  - Hodgkin's disease
  - Non-Hodgkin's lymphoma
  - Squamous cell carcinoma of oropharynx
  - Poorly differentiated carcinoma of neuroendocrine type (presents with poorly differentiated or undifferentiated histology)
  - Poorly differentiated carcinoma of extragonadal germ cell origin
- Very responsive to Rx, although incurable when metastatic
  - Prostate cancer
  - Breast cancer
  - Small-cell lung carcinoma (SCLC)
  - Ovarian carcinoma
  - Endometrial cancer
  - Thyroid cancer
  - Poorly differentiated carcinoma of neuroendocrine type (presents with poorly differentiated or undifferentiated histology)
  - Poorly differentiated carcinoma of extragonadal germ cell origin (presents with poorly differentiated or undifferentiated histology)
  - Peritoneal carcinomatosis (presents with poorly differentiated or undifferentiated histology)

ORIGIN OF TREATABLE METASTATIC DISEASE BY SITE OF PRESENTATION

- Lung and mediastinum
  - Lung (small-cell)
  - Breast
  - Hodgkin's disease
  - Extragonadal germ cell
  - Neuroendocrine
  - Germ cell (testicular)
- Bone
  - Osteoblastic lesions
    - Prostate
    - Lung (small-cell)
    - Hodgkin's disease
  - Osteolytic or mixed lesions
    - Breast
- Liver
  - Breast
  - Lung (small-cell)
  - Colon

- Brain
  - Breast
  - Lung (small-cell)
  - Lymphoma
- Bone marrow
  - Breast
  - Lung (small-cell)
  - Prostate
- Lymph nodes
  - High cervical
    - Squamous cell cancer
    - Hodgkin's disease, lymphoma
    - Neuroendocrine
  - Axillary
    - Breast (ipsilateral)
    - Lymphoma
    - Lung (small-cell)
  - Inguinal
    - Prostate
    - Ovary
    - Endometrium
    - Lymphoma
  - Retroperitoneal
    - Hodgkin's disease
    - Testes
    - Prostate
    - Ovarian
    - Neuroendocrine
    - Extragonadal germ cell

WORKUP

GENERAL STRATEGY

- Search for treatable disease (see above).
- Once metastatic lesion identified, omit testing other potential sites of metastasis because tumor is already staged sufficiently.
- Examine for detection of treatable malignant disease (i.e., breast, uterus, ovaries, prostate, testicles, lymph nodes, colon).
- Obtain imaging studies pertinent to detecting treatable cancers [e.g., mammography for breast cancer, ultrasound (U/S) for testicular or prostatic cancer, CT for ovarian disease].
- Consider pertinent serologic markers [e.g., PSA, alpha fetoprotein (AFP), hCG β-subunit].
- Obtain thorough histologic assessment by tissue biopsy from metastatic site, including immunohistochemical, electron microscopic, and receptor studies; cytologic sampling is usually insufficient.

HISTOLOGIC DIAGNOSIS

- Ascertain cell type (adenocarcinoma, lymphoma, SCLC, sarcoma, squamous cell carcinoma, melanoma, undifferentiated).

- Check special stains (e.g., mucin for prostate, kidney).
- Request immunohistochemical staining when undifferentiated carcinoma encountered, testing for diagnostically important intracellular substances, such as PSA and prostatic acid phosphatase for prostate cancer, serum AFP and hCG for germ cell tumors, and substances suggestive of lymphoma and melanoma.
- When immunohistochemistry is inconclusive, consider electron microscopy to help classify cell origin as epithelial, mesenchymal, mesothelial, or melanocytic and to subclassify it.
- Other studies: estrogen and progesterone receptors, cytogenetic studies, PCR testing for DNA sequences.

WORKUP FOR COMMON TREATABLE CANCERS PRESENTING AS TUMOR OF UNKNOWN ORIGIN

- Squamous cell, nasopharynx, oropharynx: PE (nodule, plaque), CT or MRI, blind biopsy.
- Lymphoma: PE (adenopathy), immunohistochemical stains.
- Ovarian cancer: PE (ascites or mass), pelvic CT or MRI, serum AFP and hCG levels, peritoneal implants.
- Prostate cancer: PE (nodule), PSA level, prostate U/S, immunohistochemical stains.
- Breast cancer: PE (breast nodule), receptor studies.
- Testicular cancer: PE (testicular nodule), U/S, serum AFP and hCG levels.
- Extragonadal germ cell: PE (adenopathy), CT (lung cancer nodules, mediastinal mass, retroperitoneal mass), immunohistochemical studies, serum AFP and hCG levels.
- Neuroendocrine: PE (adenopathy), chest and abdominal CT (carcinoma, retroperitoneal nodes, mediastinal nodes), electron microscopy.

PULMONARY NODULES, PLEURAL EFFUSIONS, AND MEDIASTINAL MASSES

- Assess for small cell, neuroendocrine, and extragonadal germ cell cancers and lymphoma.
- Obtain open biopsy (procedure of choice); subject specimen to electron microscopy and immunohistochemical studies.
- For pleural effusions, obtain pleural biopsy and aspiration (see Pleural Effusions); check immunohistochemical, receptor, and mammographic studies.
- For symptomatic mediastinal disease (almost invariably due to primary lung cancer, metastatic breast cancer, or lymphoma, all of which respond to local radiation Rx), proceed directly to Rx; no immediate need for extensive evaluation for primary tumor.
- For silent mediastinal disease, check for neuroendocrine and extragonadal germ cell cancers (see above).

OSSEOUS METASTASIS

- Biopsy bony lesion if tissue is not obtainable elsewhere. If bony lesion is difficult to sample, consider bone marrow biopsy at iliac crest as reasonable alternative, or obtain bone scan to identify other sites of tumor that may be more easily biopsied.

- Note appearance of lesion on plain film to determine whether it is lytic, blastic, or mixed, which can help focus differential Dx.
- Tumors of lung and kidney (usually not very treatable) prove to be most common sources of skeletal metastases of unknown cause.

LIVER METASTASIS

- Once metastatic adenocarcinoma identified in liver, further testing to identify primary tumor is usually unwarranted because few are sufficiently responsive to justify workup [exception is colon cancer if resectable (see Colorectal Cancer)].

ASCITES

- In men, search for primary tumor unwarranted because malignant ascites most likely derives from pancreas, stomach, or colon involving peritoneal surface.
- In women, check for ovarian cancer by pelvic U/S, CT, or MRI, and obtain serum CA 125, hCG, and AFP levels as well as immunohistochemical study of tumor.

HIGH CERVICAL LYMPHADENOPATHY

- Perform careful exam of nasopharynx, oral cavity (including base of tongue), and larynx as well as detailed exam of all lymph nodes.
- Obtain CT or MRI of deeper submucosal and neck structures.
- If node biopsy reveals squamous cell or epidermoid histology but no primary tumor is evident, consider blind biopsies of areas likely to harbor nasopharyngeal tumor (base of tongue, nasopharynx).
- If histopathology is adenocarcinoma, then sinuses or salivary glands may be primary source; perform careful PE supplemented by CT or MRI.
- If histologic studies indicate lymphoma or Hodgkin's disease, proceed to formal staging (see Hodgkin's Disease; Non-Hodgkin's Lymphoma).

AXILLARY ADENOPATHY

- Perform detailed breast exam and mammography.
- Consider estrogen and progesterone receptor assays on nodal tissue obtained from axilla.
- Obtain immunohistochemical study for markers of lymphoma.
- If histology indicates small cell disease, order chest CT.

INGUINAL ADENOPATHY

- Check for local disease and lymphoma; perform careful pelvic and anorectal exams.
- Obtain detailed pathologic study, including immunohistochemical and receptor studies of biopsied tissue.
- Order pelvic U/S.
- If inguinal node biopsy identifies lymphoma, proceed to formal staging (see Hodgkin's Disease; Non-Hodgkin's Lymphoma).

RETROPERITONEAL MASS

- Because incidentally discovered retroperitoneal mass is likely to represent advanced-stage lymphoma or metastatic prostate, germ cell, or ovarian cancer, search for more accessible biopsy site.

- Examine peripheral nodes, prostate and testicles in men, and pelvic organs in women.
- Order U/S of prostate and testicles in men and of ovaries in women.
- Check AFP, hCG β-subunit, and PSA levels.

BRAIN

- Focus on breast, small cell, and lymphomatous disease.
- Brain biopsy is usually unnecessary unless peripheral tissue is unavailable.
- If you order brain biopsy, conduct detailed immunohistochemical and receptor studies.

BONE MARROW INVASION

- When pancytopenia or myelophthisic picture with leukoerythroblastic changes encountered, consider marrow invasion.
- Confirm by bone marrow biopsy (see Anemia).
- In marrow exam, check for clusters of malignant cells, which may help in identification.
- Once presence confirmed, search for the treatable etiologies.

MANAGEMENT

COMMON CANCERS AND THEIR RESPONSE RATE (%) TO THERAPY

- Responsive
  - Breast: 40–60
  - Ovary: 60–70
  - Prostate: 60–70
  - Head, neck: 50–70
  - Testicular: 80–100
  - Lymphoma: 80
  - Lung (small-cell): 80
- Marginally responsive
  - Neurosecretory: 30–50
  - Sarcoma: 30
  - Colon, other GI tumors: 10–15
  - Melanoma: 10–15
  - Hepatoma: 20
- Unresponsive
  - Renal
  - Lung (non-SCLC)
  - Brain

GENERAL STRATEGY

- Treat as etiologically as possible by focusing on identification of treatable cancers.
- When primary tumor remains unknown (as in substantial proportion of cases), consider choice between empiric Rx and watchful waiting.
- Discuss with patient and family uncertain benefit of empiric Rx and its likely adverse effects and minimal chance of long-term effect.
- Consider for empiric Rx only symptomatic patients.

EMPIRIC TREATMENT

- Initiate only in conjunction with oncologic consultation.
- Two basic approaches to empiric Rx:
  - Using "broad-spectrum" chemotherapy [e.g., doxorubicin (Adriamycin) and mitomycin C], potent agents with high potential for toxicity; monitor marrow for suppression; halt Rx after 2 courses if no response.
  - Treating most likely treatable tumor, judged by cell type, age, sex, and site (see above).
- For undifferentiated cell type, treat for lymphoma and germ cell neoplasms.
- For adenocarcinoma in men, treat for metastatic prostate cancer (see Prostate Cancer).
- For adenocarcinoma in women, treat for ovarian or breast cancer (see Breast Cancer; Ovarian Cancer).
- For high cervical adenopathy and epidermoid or squamous cell histology, consider radiation with or without node dissection.
- For adenocarcinoma of inguinal node without known primary tumor, consider local radiation Rx bilaterally if blind biopsy shows no evidence of anal or prostatic lesion.
- For palliation of localized symptomatic disease that involves bone, mediastinum, or lymph nodes, consider local irradiation. In absence of symptoms, monitor bony metastasis unless you can identify definitively responsive tumor, such as prostate or breast cancer.

PATIENT EDUCATION AND INDICATIONS FOR REFERRAL

- Assemble max support for patient when delivering news of metastatic cancer of unknown origin.
- Provide modicum of hope in presenting plan to search strategically for treatable/curable disease.
- Share plan and its rationale with patient and family; goals are to (1) provide hope and sense of control over difficult situation, and (2) reduce irrational pressure to "find the cause" at all costs.
- When search for treatable disease proves unrevealing, refer to oncologist for help in addressing issue of empiric Rx. Experienced and wise oncologist can be of great help to patient and family.
- For patients suspected of having metastatic lesion of spinal cord, urgently admit for prompt Rx [see Cancer (General)].

BIBLIOGRAPHY

- For the current annotated bibliography on tumor of unknown origin, see the print edition of *Primary Care Medicine*, 4th edition, Chapter 85, or www.LWWmedicine.com.

Vaginal Cancer

SCREENING AND/OR PREVENTION

- One million women are at risk for genital tract abnormalities, including clear cell adenocarcinoma, because of *in utero* exposure to DES or other synthetic estrogens.
- Risk of malignancy among exposed women is low, but because of significant M&M associated with these tumors, careful case finding and evaluation are indicated.
- Because routine screening procedures such as Pap smear are inadequate, PCP must identify patients at risk using careful Hx if they are to receive proper evaluation and counseling.
- Promptly examine exposed daughters with symptoms such as vaginal discharge or bleeding regardless of age. Asymptomatic daughters with exposure Hx should have initial evaluation at age 14, with subsequent yearly exams.
- More frequent exams advised when extensive epithelial changes are present. When possible, gynecologist experienced in colposcopy should perform exams.

MANAGEMENT

- Oncologists and gynecologists usually provide Rx of women with genital tract cancer, but primary physician should assume ongoing responsibility for patient counseling and monitoring and management of medical problems.
- Vaginal carcinoma is relatively rare. Prior irradiation may be predisposing factor. Most lesions appear on posterior wall and in upper third of vaginal vault. Careful observation during pelvic exam and referral for biopsy are PCP responsibilities.

BIBLIOGRAPHY

- For the current annotated bibliography on vaginal cancer, see the print edition of *Primary Care Medicine*, 4th edition, Chapters 110 and 123, or www.LWWmedicine.com.

Vulvar Cancer

DIFFERENTIAL DIAGNOSIS

- Vulvar carcinoma presents as mass or growth, vulvar pruritus, or bleeding. About 20% are asymptomatic. Best means of early Dx is high index of suspicion, especially in women with HSV or HPV infections.

MANAGEMENT

- Oncologists and gynecologists usually provide Rx of women with genital tract cancer, but primary physician should assume ongoing responsibility for patient counseling and monitoring and management of medical problems.
- Surgical excision is Rx of choice. Cure rates >90% are achievable for localized disease <2 cm in greatest dimension. Radiation Rx is used for unresectable disease.

BIBLIOGRAPHY

- For the current annotated bibliography on vulvar cancer, see the print edition of *Primary Care Medicine*, 4th edition, Chapter 123, or www.LWWmedicine.com.

Endocrinologic Problems

DIFFERENTIAL DIAGNOSIS

- Solute diuresis
  - Diabetes mellitus
  - Diuretics
- Water diuresis
  - Diabetes insipidus (DI)
    - Central
    - Idiopathic
    - Trauma
    - Tumor (local or metastatic to sellar region)
    - Granulomatous disease (sarcoidosis, tuberculosis)
    - Postsurgical (removal of pituitary adenoma)
    - Vascular (Sheehan's syndrome, old stroke)
    - Nephrogenic
    - Drugs (amphotericin, demeclocycline, lithium)
    - Tubulointerstitial disease (pyelonephritis, polycystic kidney disease, sickle cell disease, obstructive uropathy)
    - Metabolic (hypercalcemia, hypokalemia)
  - Primary polydipsias
    - Psychogenic (schizophrenia)
    - CNS disease (multiple sclerosis)
    - Idiopathic

WORKUP

TRUE POLYURIA OR JUST URINARY FREQUENCY?

- Ascertain whether there is frequent voiding of large volumes of dilute (colorless or pale) urine both day and night or just frequent voiding of small volumes of concentrated urine.
- If uncertainty remains, perform 24-hr urine collection to confirm true polyuria (volume >3 L).

IF TRUE POLYURIA, IS THIS WATER DIURESIS OR SOLUTE DIURESIS?

- Measure urine osmolality to differentiate water diuresis (<250 mOsm/L) from solute diuresis (>350 mOsm/L).
- If osmolality falls between two boundaries, calculate total solute excretion (urine volume/day × average urine concentration); if <1,200 mOsm/day, water diuresis likely.
- If solute diuresis suspected, check urine for glucose and electrolytes for confirmation.

IF A WATER DIURESIS, IS THIS DIABETES INSIPIDUS OR PRIMARY POLYDIPSIA?

- Consider clinical context: known renal tubulointerstitial disease or drug use (nephrogenic DI); manifestations of pituitary disease, CNS cancer, or granulomatous disease (central mechanism); mental illness (primary polydipsia).

- Measure serum osmolality. If >290 mOsm/L in context of inappropriately dilute urine (osmolality <275 mOsm/L), consider DI. If low, consider primary polydipsia.
- If reliable assay for measurement of serum vasopressin (ADH) is available (not widely), consider ordering when confusion persists.
- When cause remains uncertain and in absence of reliable measure of ADH, consider admitting patient for trial of desmopressin (DDAVP, an ADH analogue) under supervision of endocrinologist and close monitoring of fluid intake and excretion.

IF DIABETES INSIPIDUS, CENTRAL OR RENAL?

- Confirm central DI if in response to DDAVP there is 50% decrease in urine volume, increase in urine osmolality, and return of serum osmolality toward normal.
- Confirm renal DI if no response to DDAVP; refer for renal consultation.
- If central DI strongly suspected, obtain gadolinium-enhanced MRI. CT is reasonable alternative if MRI unavailable or cost is issue, but less sensitive than MRI for detection of important pathology.
- Refer for further assessment of hypothalamic-pituitary axis if MRI shows mass lesion.

DEFINITELY PRIMARY POLYDIPSIA?

- Consider primary polydipsia if DDAVP decreases polyuria and increases urine osmolality (monitor closely for fall in serum osmolality to subnormal levels and hyponatremia).
- Consider inpatient water restriction test for confirmation (all parameters return to normal) in patients with low normal or low serum osmolality, polyuria, low urine osmolality, and concurrent psychiatric disease.
- Conduct in carefully supervised inpatient setting because dehydration testing can be dangerous for patients with other causes of water diuresis.
- Supervised water restriction also necessary because patients with primary polydipsia tend to be psychotic and drink surreptitiously.

MANAGEMENT

- For symptomatic relief of central DI, consider DDAVP nasal spray taken qhs to eliminate nocturnal polyuria; adjust dose to allow normal amounts of daytime urination.
- Alternatively, consider drugs that enhance ADH secretion (carbamazepine, chlorpropamide, clofibrate).
- Consider thiazide-like diuretic (e.g., indapamide) for symptomatic relief of DI (enhanced proximal resorption of sodium and water due to distal diuretic effect).
- Consider NSAIDs for nephrogenic DI.
- Arrange formal psychiatric workup for patient with primary polydipsia.

BIBLIOGRAPHY

■ For the current annotated bibliography on diabetes insipidus, see the print edition of *Primary Care Medicine*, 4th edition, Chapter 101, or www.LWWmedicine.com.

Diabetes Mellitus

SCREENING AND/OR PREVENTION

- Screen asymptomatic patients at increased risk for DM (family Hx of diabetes in twin, sibling, or parent; obesity; gestational diabetes; Hx of impaired glucose tolerance).
- Use fasting glucose determination; fasting test is preferred since it is most sensitive of methods appropriate for asymptomatic adult populations when threshold for positive test is glucose >126 mg/dL.
- For patients with fasting glucose >126 mg/dL, proceed to confirmatory testing for presence of any of 3 diagnostic glucose abnormalities found on 2 separate days:
  - Fasting plasma glucose >126 mg/dL
  - Random plasma glucose >200 mg/dL in person with diabetic symptoms
  - 2-hr postprandial plasma glucose level >200 mg/dL after administration of equivalent of 75-g glucose load

MANAGEMENT

ALL PATIENTS

- Treat hyperglycemia aggressively. Attempt to normalize blood glucose; goal is HbA1C concentration <7.0% and fasting glucose level <126 mg/dL.
- Emphasize importance of maintaining ideal body weight. For obese patients, institute caloric restriction without compromising regularity of meal timing.
- Prescribe regular aerobic exercise.
- Prescribe balanced diet that achieves reduction in calories and saturated fat.
- Diagnose and aggressively treat all major additional atherosclerotic risk factors (see Cardiovascular Rehabilitation; Hypercholesterolemia; Hypertension; Smoking Cessation).
- Teach diabetic patients, (especially those on insulin Rx) how to monitor glycemic control daily with home blood glucose determinations.
- Assess long-term glucose control with HbA1C measurements 3–4 times/yr.
- Carefully investigate causes of worsening hyperglycemia:
  - Inadequate dose
  - Increased caloric intake
  - Failure to take insulin properly
  - Occult infection (especially urinary tract)
  - Coronary ischemia
  - Severe emotional stress
  - Corticosteroid use
  - Somogyi phenomenon

- Insulin resistance
- Growth hormone surge in early morning

- Regularly perform comprehensive Hx, PE, and selected lab studies (BUN, creatinine, urinalysis, lipid profile) for complications (e.g., CAD, nephropathy, cerebrovascular disease, peripheral vascular disease, neuropathy, and retinopathy).
- Closely monitor urinalysys and renal function for earliest signs of diabetic renal injury (e.g., microalbuminuria, microscopic hematuria, rising BUN and creatine).
- At first sign of renal impairment, tighten glycemic control and prescribe angiotensin blockage, either with ACE inhibitor or angiotensin-receptor blocker.
- Also institute angiotensin blockage for patients with concurrent HTN.
- Consider prophylactic angiotensin blockade for all diabetics, especially those who are middle-aged.
- When serum creatinine level reaches 3 mg/dL, obtain nephrology consultation regarding candidacy for dialysis or transplantation.
- Exercise caution in use of iodinated contrast agents, especially in setting of renal impairment.
- Refer all patients for annual diabetic eye exam to check for proliferative retinopathic changes (see Diabetic Retinopathy).
- Emphasize foot care to diabetic patients with neuropathy or vascular insufficiency. Arrange regular podiatric care for such patients.
- Perform careful perioperative assessment of diabetic patients undergoing surgery. Pay particular attention to worsening hyperglycemia and diligently observe for infection and occult CAD, particularly in those with evidence of microvascular disease.
- Consider including well-trained nurse, nurse practitioner, or physician assistant in long-term management program to complement and support physician efforts at achieving glycemic control.

TYPE 1 DIABETES MELLITUS PATIENTS

- Consider early institution of intensive insulin Rx to achieve very tight control (HbA1C 6–7%), especially for highly motivated patients willing to perform multiple daily glucose determinations and self-administer insulin according to results of tests.
- Consider less intensive insulin Rx or infusion pump technology for those unable to carry out intensive insulin regimen.
- For those attempting intensive insulin Rx
  - start with modest dose of long-acting insulin, such as Ultralente or new long-acting preparations as they become available, administered once/day in evening; start with dose of 15 U and increase in 2-U increments based on fasting glucose determinations;
  - begin program of short-acting insulin, such as regular (CZI) or Semilente, started at 5 U administered 30–45 mins ac and adjusted according to results of postprandial home glucose measurements;
  - prescribe human recombinant insulin for newly treated diabetics to minimize risks for insulin allergy, insulin resistance, and antibody development;
  - consider prescribing insulin lispro (or another fast-onset, very short-acting insulin), administered 10–15 mins ac, to patients achieving

tight control but bothered by frequent hypoglycemic episodes or inconvenience of standard regimen of regular insulin.

- For those unable to carry out intensive insulin program
  - begin bid insulin regimen with intermediate-acting insulin (e.g., NPH or Lente), administered before breakfast and before evening meal for basal coverage, mixed with short-acting insulin (e.g., CZI, Semilente) for prandial control;
  - adjust doses according to fasting and 4 P.M. glucose determinations;
  - teach importance of regular caloric intake and regular spacing of meals to match peak insulin effects and activity schedules.

TYPE 2 DIABETES MELLITUS PATIENTS

- Emphasize weight reduction to ideal body weight as cornerstone of Rx for type 2 DM. Composition of diet is less important, but diet should have high ratio of polyunsaturated to saturated fat and contain cholesterol and complex carbohydrates. Diets low in protein may be beneficial in averting diabetic nephropathy (see Sexual Dysfunction).
- Prescribe practical program of regular exercise that fits patient's lifestyle; suggest ≥30 mins of exercise qod (see Exercise).
- Continue exercise for its own sake, independent of any effect it may have on weight.
- If after 4–8 wks of diet and exercise mild to moderate glucose intolerance persists (fasting glucose <240 mg/dL), then in addition to diet and exercise,
  - begin oral Rx with second-generation sulfonylurea (e.g., 2.5 mg glyburide; 5 mg glipizide; or 1 mg glimepiride) or biguanide (e.g., 500 mg metformin bid, with breakfast and evening meal). Choose metformin if patient is obese;
  - increase oral agent dose q1–2wks prn. Consider bid dosing for glyburide and glipizide to maximize control or once-daily dosing of sustained-release glipizide. Advance until patient achieves glycemic goals or reaches max dose (20 mg/day for glyburide and glipizide; 8 mg/day for glimepiride);
  - if after 4–8 wks of monotherapy patient has not achieved glycemic goals, add second oral agent from different class (e.g., metformin if a sulfonylurea used first and vice versa) or add small dose of intermediate-acting insulin taken qhs (e.g., 10 U NPH). If sulfonylurea was starting drug, reduce sulfonylurea dose to avoid risk for prolonged hypoglycemia;
  - if after 4–8 wks of 2-drug oral agent Rx patient has not achieved control, consider adding dose of intermediate insulin qhs (e.g., 10 U of NPH) or third oral agent (e.g., a thiazolidinedione or acarbose);
  - If adding thiazolidinediones (e.g., pioglitazone, rosiglitazone), start with low dose (for pioglitazone, 15 mg/day; for rosiglitazone, 2 mg/day), and monitor liver function (ALT) monthly for at least first several mos, halting Rx at first sign of persistent elevation. Until thiazolidinediones are proved hepatically safe, consider them only if all other attempts to date have not achieved reasonable glycemic control and patient is reliable, free of underlying liver disease, and willing to have close monitoring of liver function tests;
  - if program of insulin supplementation considered, be aware that initially supplementing oral agent Rx with small qhs dose of insulin may suffice but usually latter stages of type 2 DM require insulin as main-

stay of Rx, supplemented by thiazolidinedione (e.g., pioglitazone, rosiglitazone) or metformin to reduce insulin resistance and keep dose manageable.

■ If after 4–8 wks of diet and exercise patient has not achieved Rx goals and is very symptomatic or manifests moderate to severe glucose intolerance (fasting glucose >240 mg/dL), then
  • begin insulin Rx with intermediate-acting insulin preparation (Lente or NPH) at modest once-daily dose (e.g., 10 U before breakfast);
  • specify human recombinant insulin for newly treated diabetic patients to minimize risks for insulin allergy, insulin resistance, and antibody development;
  • advance insulin program according to glucose monitoring results with reference to target levels;
  • if high doses of insulin, poor control, and weight gain become problems, consider adding metformin to insulin program to improve tissue responsiveness and reduce insulin requirements and weight gain. Thiazolidinediones can also improve insulin responsiveness and control, but do not halt weight gain.

BIBLIOGRAPHY

■ For the current annotated bibliography on diabetes mellitus, see the print edition of *Primary Care Medicine*, 4th edition, Chapters 93 and 102, or www.LWWmedicine.com.

Galactorrhea and Hyperprolactinemia

DIFFERENTIAL DIAGNOSIS

- Normoprolactinemic galactorrhea
  - Local breast stimulation/irritation (suckling, trauma, inflammation)
  - Oral contraceptive use
  - Recent pregnancy
  - Idiopathic (? transient elevation in prolactin from stress, breast stimulation)
- Hyperprolactinemic galactorrhea
  - Impairment of hypothalamic pituitary inhibition
  - Drugs (haloperidol, heroin, methyldopa, metoclopramide, phenothiazines, reserpine)
  - Lesions of pituitary stalk (nonfunctioning sellar tumors, infarction)
  - Hypothalamic disease (craniopharyngioma, infiltrative disease, infarction)
- Overproduction by pituitary adenoma
  - Prolactinoma
  - Hypothyroidism (simulates adenoma by TRH stimulation of lactotrope cells)
- Idiopathic
  - ? Microadenoma undetectable by neuroimaging
  - ? Stress, trauma, breast stimulation

WORKUP

HISTORY

- Inquire into menstrual pattern, recent pregnancy, infertility, medications, change in libido, symptoms of hypothyroidism, breast stimulation, chest trauma, and presence of headache or visual complaints.
- Review drug use, particularly oral contraceptives and drugs that block central dopaminergic transmission (e.g., phenothiazines, haloperidol, metoclopramide, and, less commonly, reserpine, methyldopa, isoniazid, and imipramine).

PHYSICAL EXAM

- Check breasts to be sure discharge is milky and not caused by local breast disease.
- Perform visual field testing and funduscopic exam.
- Note any signs of hypothyroidism on exam (see Hypothyroidism).

LAB STUDIES

- Measure TSH in patients with suspected thyroid disease.
- Measure serum prolactin concentration and ensure maximum accuracy by performing test in morning using small catheter placed 1 hr before drawing sample and with patient resting during this time.

- Obtain neuroimaging of sellar region if prolactin level is elevated in absence of obvious explanation (e.g., medication, pregnancy). Gadolinium-enhanced MRI is procedure of choice; CT is reasonable alternative if MRI unavailable.
- Order formal visual field testing in all patients with sellar mass or visual symptoms.
- Follow expectantly with annual prolactin determinations galactorrheic woman with normal prolactin and regular menses.

MANAGEMENT

NO EVIDENCE OF MASS LESION

- Reassure and follow expectantly patients with normal periods and normal prolactin levels; no Rx required.
- Discontinue or try to reduce medication dose in those with galactorrhea secondary to dopaminergic-blocking drug.
- Correct underlying hypothyroidism (see Hypothyroidism).
- Treat symptomatic patients with idiopathic disease (galactorrhea, abnormal periods, elevated prolactin, normal MRI findings, no other evident disease) as if they have microadenoma (see below).

PROLACTINOMA

For Microadenomas (Diameter <10 mm)

- Consider watchful waiting, especially if patient not bothered by symptoms; obtain endocrinologic consultation.
- In such patients monitor prolactin levels regularly and repeat MRI periodically.
- Consider dopaminergic agonist bromocriptine for patients with stable microadenomas who are bothered by menstrual irregularities, severe galactorrhea, and infertility, or concerned about osteoporosis risk.
- Prescribe continuous bromocriptine (initially 2.5–10 mg/day; lower doses for maintenance), maintaining Rx for 2 yrs followed by trial of cessation.
- Consider oral contraceptive Rx as alternative to bromocriptine when pregnancy is not desired.

For Macroadenomas

- Begin with bromocriptine (initially 5–20 mg/day; for maintenance, 0.625–10 mg/day).
- Treat indefinitely.
- Refer for surgical consideration patients with rapidly progressing vision loss or symptoms refractory to bromocriptine Rx, but advise patient that recurrence rate is high after surgery. Radiation Rx is sometimes considered.

PATIENT EDUCATION AND INDICATIONS FOR REFERRAL

- Provide accurate information, moral support, and close follow-up.
- Reassure by explaining very favorable prognosis for vast majority of patients with microadenomas and excellent response of most prolactinomas to bromocriptine.

- Inform patients with concurrent amenorrhea and interest in pregnancy that numerous options for induction of fertility are available and may be pursued according to patient's wishes.
- Obtain endocrinology consultation when there is macroadenoma, suspected pituitary neoplasm other than prolactinoma, lack of response to bromocriptine, vision loss, or desire to become pregnant.

BIBLIOGRAPHY

- For the current annotated bibliography on galactorrhea and hyperprolactinemia, see the print edition of *Primary Care Medicine*, 4th edition, Chapter 100, or www.LWWmedicine.com.

Glucocorticoid Therapy

MANAGEMENT

PRINCIPLES OF USE

- Prescribe corticosteroids only when maximal doses of other forms of Rx have proved insufficient and when therapeutic benefit outweighs risks of steroid use.
- Try to minimize required steroid dose by attempting to add steroid Rx to ongoing Rx program and tapering to lowest dose possible.
- Try to minimize duration of steroid Rx or at least duration of high-dose Rx.

SELECTION OF PREPARATION

- In setting of active autoimmune or inflammatory disease, initiate full-strength program of daily glucocorticoid Rx with prednisone (40–60 mg/day, or prednisolone in cases of hepatocellular failure).
- When patient needs urgent replacement Rx for adrenal cortical insufficiency, use IV hydrocortisone (see below).
- To minimize risk for hypothalamic-pituitary-adrenal (HPA) suppression, avoid routinely prescribing long-acting preparations,
- Reserve long-acting preparations (e.g., dexamethasone) for testing HPA axis and for rare patient who needs very-high-dose, sustained-action Rx (e.g., increased ICP).
- Commonly used glucocorticoids (minimum doses in mg)
  - Short acting
    - Cortisol (hydrocortisone), 20
    - Cortisone, 25
    - Methylprednisolone, 4
    - Prednisolone, 5
    - Prednisone, 5
  - Intermediate acting
    - Triamcinolone, 4
  - Long acting
    - Betamethasone, 0.60
    - Dexamethasone, 0.75

DOSING

- Advise patients that steroid absorption is not impaired if taken with food.
- To minimize HPA suppression, schedule entire dose for morning if possible, and continue for shortest possible time.
- Try initiating qod Rx when symptoms are not severe and condition is not one with an absolute requirement for daily Rx (i.e., temporal arteritis, pemphigus vulgaris, severe inflammatory bowel disease).

TAPERING THERAPY

- Once control is achieved, taper to lowest dose that maintains control and terminate if possible.

- Conduct tapering empirically; monitor patient for disease activity and evidence of adrenal insufficiency (postural hypotension, GI upset, fatigue, muscle weakness, hypoglycemia).
- Base rate of tapering on disease activity and appearance of steroid withdrawal or adrenal insufficiency.
- For brief courses of corticosteroid Rx (<7–14 days), taper rapidly over 7–10 days to full cessation, provided that disease activity remains quiescent.
- When patient requires longer courses of Rx, taper more slowly, reducing dose in 10-mg steps when dose >40 mg/day and in 5-mg steps when <40 mg/day.
- Once dosage is reduced to 5 mg prednisone qod, stop Rx or switch to 5-mg hydrocortisone or 1-mg prednisone tabs and reduce in decrements of 2.5 mg hydrocortisone or 1 mg prednisone.

ALTERNATE-DAY THERAPY

- If tapering unsuccessful or patient needs prolonged Rx, ascertain and maintain lowest effective dose and try switching to qod regimen.
- When switching to qod Rx, begin by modestly reducing second day's dose and adding that amount to first day's dose to maintain same total dose. If dose is >40 mg/day, reduce it on alternate day by equivalent of 10 mg prednisone, and by 5 mg if dose is <40 mg/day. When <20 mg/day, decrement is 2.5 mg.
- Determine interval between dose changes empirically based on patient's clinical status.
- Attain end point of switching when patient takes previous entire 2-day dose once qod.
- If withdrawal symptoms are problematic on qod Rx, a small morning dose of hydrocortisone (10–20 mg) given on off day may help alleviate symptoms without prolonging HPA suppression.

MANAGING HYPOTHALAMIC-PITUITARY-ADRENAL SUPPRESSION

- When HPA responsiveness is in question, perform cosyntropin stimulation test. Administer 250 µg parenterally and measure serum cortisol immediately before, 30 mins, and 60 mins after administration.
- Because 9–12 mos of HPA suppression may begin after as little as 2–4 wks of 20–30 mg/day prednisone, advise patients taking daily pharmacologic doses to supplement steroid intake when under stress or experiencing acute illness.
- In setting of injury, surgery, or inability to take medication PO, prescribe parenteral hydrocortisone or equivalent. Total daily stress dose is 100–400 mg hydrocortisone in divided doses q6–8h.
- Provide prepackaged syringe containing 4 mg dexamethasone for IM emergency use.

STEROID-INDUCED OSTEOPOROSIS

- To prevent or treat steroid-induced osteoporosis, begin by measuring vertebral bone density.
- If patient is markedly osteoporotic, prescribe 5 mg/day alendronate; if patient is postmenopausal, prescribe 10 mg/day. Instruct patient regarding proper intake of alendronate to minimize risk for esophageal irritation (see Osteoporosis).

■ Alternatively, consider ERT with calcium and vitamin D supplementation for menopausal women taking corticosteroids if degree of osteoporosis is not severe and risk for steroid-induced disease is small (see Osteoporosis).

BIBLIOGRAPHY

■ For the current annotated bibliography on glucocorticoid therapy, see the print edition of *Primary Care Medicine*, 4th edition, Chapter 105, or www.LWWmedicine.com.

Gynecomastia

DIFFERENTIAL DIAGNOSIS

- Inhibition of androgen effect
  - Spironolactone (at high doses only)
  - Cimetidine (common at high doses)
  - Flutamide
  - Decreased androgen availability secondary to increased binding or conversion
  - Cirrhosis (very common)
  - Hyperthyroidism (uncommon, except with thyrotoxicosis)
- Decreased androgen synthesis
  - Testicular failure, primary (Klinefelter's syndrome) or secondary (orchiectomy, cancer drugs, ketoconazole)
  - Increased estrogen synthesis or estrogen effect
  - Estrogen-secreting tumor of testis or adrenal gland (very rare)
  - Klinefelter's syndrome (about 15% of pubertal cases)
  - Ectopic hCG-secreting tumor of testis, lung, colon, pancreas (rare)
  - Digitalis (uncommon)
  - Exogenous estrogen (dose-related)
- Increased availability of estrogen substrate
  - Androgen-producing tumor (rare)
  - Exogenous androgen (common)
  - CHF (common)
  - Physiologic
  - Puberty
  - Recovery from chronic illness or starvation
  - Old age

WORKUP

HISTORY

- Note onset, location, duration, and course.
- Inquire into drug use, including chronic alcoholism and use of cimetidine, spironolactone, flutamide, digitalis, ketoconazole, or exogenous estrogens or androgens (including androstenedione by adolescents and body builders).
- Check for symptoms of hyperthyroidism, heart failure, and hepatocellular failure.
- Ask about changes in libido, skin, voice, testicles, and hair quality and distribution.
- Note any weight loss, chronic cough, hemoptysis, change in bowel habits, headaches, or visual field disturbances.

PHYSICAL EXAM

- Look at skin for signs of hepatocellular failure (jaundice, spider angiomas, ecchymoses, pallor, palmar erythema) and hyperthyroidism (warm, sweaty skin and fine hair).

- Check eyes for exophthalmos and neck for goiter.
- During breast exam, distinguish glandular texture of true gynecomastia from fatty consistency of breast enlargement related to obesity and nodularity of carcinoma; note any asymmetry and nodules; carefully palpate axillary nodes.
- Checks for signs of heart failure and cirrhosis; note any abdominal masses and test stool for occult blood.
- Examine testicles for atrophy and nodules.
- If onset at puberty, check for features of Klinefelter's syndrome (arm span > height; small, firm testes; absence of secondary sex characteristics).

LAB STUDIES

- Refer for breast biopsy if breast enlargement is unilateral and eccentric, or if there is localized firmness or nodularity or axillary adenopathy.
- Refer for testicular evaluation if testicular nodule found (see Scrotal Pain, Masses, and Swelling).
- If etiology remains elusive after Hx and PE, order measurements of gonadotropins (LH and FSH).
  - If gonadotropins high:
    - Check serum β-hCG subunit levels for ectopic hCG production; if found, begin search for responsible tumor.
    - Obtain buccal smear and examine for chromatin positivity (Barr bodies) if suspicious of Klinefelter's syndrome; if smear negative, consider primary testicular failure.
  - If gonadotropins low:
    - Repeat questioning about exogenous steroid use.
    - Check levels of free testosterone and estradiol; for best results, pool 3 samples taken 15 mins apart.
  - If serum estrogens elevated, consider adrenal cancer and Leydig's cell tumor of testes.
  - If gonadotropins and sex hormone levels normal, reassure patient and follow expectantly with periodic reevaluation.

MANAGEMENT

PATIENT EDUCATION

- Inform patient that gynecomastia may resolve after its cause resolves; however, gynecomastia attributable to alcoholic liver disease or Klinefelter's syndrome is unlikely to respond.
- Specifically reassure patient with benign etiology that condition is not reflection of loss of maleness or carcinomatous process.
- Counsel adolescents against using androstenedione for body building and athletic performance (see Adolescents).
- Deal with any pain, irritation, or social problems sympathetically.

INDICATIONS FOR REFERRAL

- Refer when considering symptomatic Rx, be it medical or surgical.
- Consider mastectomy for patients who are bothered by breast enlargement, but only after elucidating underlying cause.

- Consider experimental use of antiestrogen tamoxifen in reducing breast size in patients with painful gynecomastia.
- When etiology found that also reduces potency, discuss and address specifically with patient.
- Consult with endocrinologist when Klinefelter's syndrome is suspected; include discussion of risk of carcinomatous degeneration in gynecomastia.
- Consult with endocrinologist when ectopic hCG production or autonomous sex hormone production is under consideration (low gonadotropin levels).

BIBLIOGRAPHY

- For the current annotated bibliography on gynecomastia, see the print edition of *Primary Care Medicine*, 4th edition, Chapter 99, or www.LWWmedicine.com.

Hirsutism

DIFFERENTIAL DIAGNOSIS

CAUSES OF HIRSUTISM

- Hirsutism without virilization
  - Idiopathic
  - Late-onset congenital adrenal hyperplasia
  - Cushing's syndrome (ACTH-induced)
  - Polycystic ovary disease
  - Insulin resistance/obesity
  - Drugs: anabolic steroids, danazol, diazoxide, glucocorticoids, minoxidil, phenytoin
- Hirsutism with virilization
  - Ovarian hyperthecosis
  - Ovarian neoplasms
  - Adrenal neoplasms, especially adrenal carcinoma

WORKUP

HISTORY

- Identify those likely to have important underlying endocrine disease.
- Inquire into virilization (voice change, temporal hair recession, increased muscle mass, acne), rapid progression (particularly sudden increase in hair growth after age 25), amenorrhea or menstrual changes, and galactorrhea.
- Note any new onset of HTN in setting of hirsutism.
- Take detailed drug Hx, making special note of anabolic steroids, oral contraceptives, danazol, phenytoin, corticosteroids, minoxidil, cyclosporine, diazoxide.
- Inquire into any daily or regular use of nonprescription sex hormone precursors, such as androstenedione.
- Check for Southern European or Mediterranean ancestry in conjunction with hirsutism of similar degree in mother, grandmothers, aunts, and sisters.

PHYSICAL EXAM

- Note any new growth of terminal hair, especially on upper abdomen, sternum, upper back, and shoulders, and distinguish from that on face, lower abdomen, and areolae.
- Check for temporal and vertical scalp hair loss, deep voice, acne, increase in muscle mass, and clitoromegaly.
- Examine for signs of Cushing's syndrome (centripetal obesity, muscle wasting with myopathy, and violaceous striae).
- Perform careful pelvic exam in patients with oligomenorrhea to check for bilaterally enlarged cystic ovaries.

- Examine women with virilization and amenorrhea for palpable adrenal or ovarian neoplasm.

LAB STUDIES

General

- Limit cost by performing workup according to whether patient has idiopathic or familial, oligomenorrheic/amenorrheic, cushingoid, or virilizing forms of hirsutism based on Hx and PE findings.

Idiopathic and Familial Types

- Lab testing unnecessary.

Oligomenorrheic/Amenorrheic Disease

- Order pelvic ultrasonography (U/S).
- Measure serum testosterone, particularly unbound testosterone; because testosterone secretion is episodic, obtain 3 serum samples taken 15 mins apart and pool them.
- Check ratio of LH to FSH.
- If no evidence of polycystic disease, evaluate for late-onset congenital adrenal hyperplasia (most often 21-hydroxylase deficiency) by performing ACTH stimulation test and measuring plasma 17-hydroxyprogesterone 30–60 mins after IV administration of 1 ampule (25 µg) cosyntropin.
- Obtain prolactin determination, especially if galactorrhea is present; if elevated, proceed to MRI scanning of hypothalamic/pituitary region.

Cushingoid Appearance

- Screen with 24-hr urinary free cortisol determination or overnight dexamethasone suppression test.
- If 24-hr urinary free cortisol is elevated or elevated cortisol is not suppressed by dexamethasone, perform more extensive dexamethasone testing to determine likelihood and cause of Cushing's syndrome.
- Check urinary 17-ketosteroids if concerned clinically about adrenocortical carcinoma.

Virilization

- Measure serum testosterone and urinary 17-ketosteroids.
- If serum testosterone level >200 ng/dL, consider masculinizing ovarian or adrenal neoplasms.
- Check adrenal hormonal production by measuring DHEA sulfate; if >800 µg/dL, consider adrenal tumor.
- Obtain U/S or CT if ovarian or adrenal tumor suspected.

MANAGEMENT

SUPPORTIVE MEASURES AND COSMETIC MANIPULATIONS

- Provide reassurance to patients free of significant endocrine disease, emphasizing that hirsutism does not impair sexuality or fertility.
- Educate adolescents of adverse cosmetic and developmental consequences of taking exogenous sex hormone precursors such as androstenedione to enhance athletic performance; address "unnatural" effects of taking "natural" supplements.

- Consider cosmetic manipulations (e.g., bleaching dark terminal hair with 6% hydrogen peroxide solution or commercially available cream, epilation with tweezers or hot wax, chemical depilation, electrolysis) for women concerned about appearance.

SUPPRESSION OF OVARIAN AND ADRENAL ANDROGEN OVERPRODUCTION

- Recommend program of weight reduction if obese.
- Prescribe preparations containing ≥35 μg ethinyl estradiol or 50 μg mestranol to reduce androgen levels.
- Choose formulation with least androgenic of progestins, such as norethindrone (1 mg) or ethynodiol acetate.
- If hormonal and clinical responses determined at 3 mos are inadequate, prescribe oral contraceptive containing larger amounts of estrogen; use with caution if at all in persons with relative contraindications to oral contraceptives (see Fertility Control).
- Advise that decrease in hirsutism may not be evident for 3–6 mos.
- In partial congenital adrenal hyperplasia, consider suppressing adrenal androgens by prescribing 1 mg dexamethasone qhs. Consider qod corticosteroid Rx to reduce risk of adverse effects. Monitor 17-hydroxyprogesterone concentration.

ANTAGONIZING TESTOSTERONE AT TARGET TISSUE

- Consider spironolactone as adjunct to oral contraceptives in patients with severe polycystic ovary disease; begin with 50 mg bid taken on days 4–22 of each menstrual cycle; monitor over 3-mo period, but observe for menstrual disturbances. High doses contraindicated in women of childbearing age (teratogenic).
- If spironolactone contraindicated, consider cimetidine as less potent alternative.
- Watch for reports on efficacy and safety of flutamide and finasteride.

INDICATIONS FOR REFERRAL

- Refer women with virilization and elevated testosterone levels to a gynecologist or endocrinologist for consideration of virilizing tumor.
- Refer to fertility specialist for consideration of clomiphene Rx if polycystic ovary syndrome is present and infertility is an issue; evaluation for endometrial hyperplasia with endometrial biopsy is also appropriate.
- Hyperprolactinemia with sellar mass seen on MRI scan necessitates referral to those skilled in its management.
- Refer patients with Cushing's syndrome for endocrinologic evaluation of pituitary, adrenal, or ectopic origin.

BIBLIOGRAPHY

- For the current annotated bibliography on hirsutism, see the print edition of *Primary Care Medicine*, 4th edition, Chapter 98, or www.LWWmedicine.com.

Hypercalcemia

DIFFERENTIAL DIAGNOSIS

- Hyperparathyroidism
- Malignancy
- Sarcoidosis
- Hyperthyroidism
- Addison's disease
- Excess vitamin D and calcium
- MEN syndrome
- Hypocalciuric hypercalcemia

WORKUP

GENERAL STRATEGY

- Confirm hypercalcemia by repeating calcium determination in conjunction with serum albumin level.

HISTORY

- Even if asymptomatic, check for subtle degrees of fatigue, weakness, lethargy, arthralgias, nonspecific GI complaints, impairment of intellectual performance, and depression.
- Note any HTN, gout, pseudogout, and nephrolithiasis.
- Pursue symptoms of underlying malignancy (breast, lung, myeloma).
- Review intake of antacids, food additives, and health food preparations for excessive ingestion of vitamin D or calcium.
- Note symptoms of hyperthyroidism (see Hyperthyroidism) and renal dysfunction.

PHYSICAL EXAM

- Search for signs of malignancy (breast mass, lymphadenopathy, bone tenderness) and sarcoidosis (lymph node enlargement, abnormalities on lung exam).

LAB STUDIES

- After confirming hypercalcemia and in absence of obvious cause, obtain serum PTH determination.
- If PTH markedly elevated, hyperparathyroidism is confirmed; check electrolytes and fasting phosphate concentrations (for fasting hypophosphatemia and mild hyperchloremic metabolic acidosis of hyperparathyroidism).
- Obtain alkaline phosphatase to detect increased osteoblastic activity (hyperparathyroidism, malignancy, Paget's disease).
- If PTH low or absent, work up for malignancy and sarcoidosis.

- Check hematocrit, ESR, and globulin levels; if suspicion high for multiple myeloma (low hematocrit, high globulin and ESR), order serum immunoelectrophoresis (± urine immunoelectrophoresis).
- Consider CXR for hilar adenopathy or pulmonary parenchymal abnormalities indicative of sarcoidosis. If found, obtain an angiotensin-converting enzyme level (see Asthma).
- If sarcoidosis under consideration, obtain diffusing capacity and perform hydrocortisone suppression study (40 mg tid × 10 days); if histologic confirmation needed, refer for bronchoscopy or mediastinoscopy.
- If metastatic cancer a consideration, order bone scan.
- Consider bone films for suspected metastatic lesions and to detect subperiosteal resorption specific for hyperparathyroidism.
- If PTH not elevated, check 24-hr urinary calcium excretion to rule out familial hypocalciuric hypercalcemia (must be ≥80–100 mg/day).
- Check TSH if Hx suggestive; if undetectable, obtain total T_3 by radioimmunoassay.
- Measure serum cortisol after cosyntropin (Cortrosyn) stimulation testing if Hx suggestive of Addison's disease.
- For suspected hypervitaminosis D, check 1,25-dihydroxyvitamin D_3 level.

MANAGEMENT

HYPERPARATHYROIDISM

- Choose between definitive surgery and expectant medical management.
- Base decision in part on severity of hypercalcemia and degree and risk of bone loss. Obtain bone densitometry (see Osteoporosis) with measurements made in proximal wrist (cortical bone).

Surgery

- Consider for surgical cure hyperparathyroid persons (especially women) who are young or middle-aged and who must anticipate synergistic effects of menopausal bone loss; also consider those who will not tolerate close long-term monitoring required with medical Rx.
- Refer only to surgeons experienced in complexities of parathyroid surgery, not only for cure of potential hyperplasia and discovery of parathyroid adenoma in unusual location but also for prevention of complications of recurrent laryngeal nerve injury and hypoparathyroidism.
- If surgery chosen, localize parathyroid adenoma by ultrasonography and Tc 99m sestamibi scanning. Reserve selective angiography or venous sampling for patients unresponsive to surgical exploration by experienced parathyroid surgeon.

Indications for Surgery

- Marked elevation of serum calcium, usually >12.5 mg/dL
- Hx of life-threatening hypercalcemia
- Reduced creatinine clearance
- Presence of kidney stones detected by abdominal radiography
- Markedly elevated 24-hr urine calcium excretion

- Substantially reduced bone mass determined by direct measurement
- Medical surveillance neither desirable nor suitable:
  - Patient is young (age <50)
  - Patient requests surgery
  - Consistent follow-up is unlikely
  - Coexistent illness complicates management

  Adapted from Proceedings of the NIH Consensus Development Conference on Diagnosis and Management of Asymptomatic Primary Hyperparathyroidism. J Bone Miner Res 1991;6[Suppl 1–2]:S1.

Medical Therapy

- For truly asymptomatic patients without significant bone loss, consider close follow-up and medical management as alternative to surgery (only 25% chance of disease progression), but only on condition that patient cooperates with biannual serum calcium determinations and annual measurements of urinary calcium excretion and BMD.
- Carefully review prognosis with all patients and emphasize importance of close long-term follow-up for those choosing medical Rx.
- Prescribe HRT (see Menopause) to postmenopausal patients.
- In women with family or personal Hx of breast cancer, prescribe tamoxifen in lieu of HRT.
- Stress importance of preventing dehydration and remaining physically active.
- In patients with moderate hypophosphatemia, begin 250–500 mg neutral phosphate qid if bothered by fatigue, weakness, or kidney stones.
- Administer phosphate cautiously in cases of renal insufficiency (risk of calcium deposition in skeletal and extraskeletal sites).
- Avoid diuretics, such as furosemide or bumetanide, that increase renal calcium excretion and cause dehydration, increasing risk of stone formation; however, consider thiazides to limit hypercalciuria and renal stones.
- No role for calcitonin or bisphosphonates.
- Increase dietary calcium intake to 1.0–1.5 g/day as long as there is no associated nephrolithiasis or increased levels of 1,25-dihydroxyvitamin D_3.
- Recommend fluid intake of ≥2 L/day and advise reporting any illness that might lead to dehydration (and worsening hypercalcemia).

HYPERCALCEMIA OF MALIGNANCY

- See Cancer.

BIBLIOGRAPHY

- For the current annotated bibliography on hypercalcemia, see the print edition of *Primary Care Medicine*, 4th edition, Chapter 96, or www.LWWmedicine.com.

Hyperthyroidism

DIFFERENTIAL DIAGNOSIS

- Autonomous hormone production
  - Toxic multinodular goiter
  - Toxic adenoma
- Increased hormone release
  - Subacute thyroiditis
  - Lymphocytic (Hashimoto's) thyroiditis
  - Iodide exposure
- Increased glandular stimulation (stimulant)
  - Graves' disease (TSAb)
  - Functioning pituitary adenoma (TSH)
  - Choriocarcinoma (hCG)
- Exogenous hormone intake
  - Intake of >20 µg/day levothyroxine
- Extraglandular production
  - Struma ovarii
  - Metastatic thyroid cancer

WORKUP

HISTORY

- Inquire into goiter, thyroid nodule, use of iodides or thyroid hormone, eye changes, recent pregnancy or viral illness, and known ovarian, pituitary, or thyroid neoplasm.
- Include in review of systems a search for symptoms of pituitary tumor (see Galactorrhea and Hyperprolactinemia).

PHYSICAL EXAM

- Focus on thyroid gland, checking overall size and nodularity.
  - Diffusely enlarged, nontender gland suggests Graves' disease.
  - In rare instances, TSH-secreting tumor may cause diffuse glandular stimulation.
  - Bruit may accompany diffusely enlarged gland of Graves' disease.
  - Exquisitely tender, diffusely enlarged gland in context of viral illness points to subacute thyroiditis.
  - Gland in lymphocytic thyroiditis is nontender and diffusely but only modestly enlarged.
  - Small gland indicates extrathyroidal hormone source.
  - Multinodularity is consistent with toxic multinodular goiter and also occurs in patients with Hashimoto's thyroiditis.
  - Otherwise atrophic gland with single nodule, especially if diameter >3 cm, strongly suggests toxic adenoma.

- Note extrathyroidal findings, which may be diagnostically significant:
  - True proptosis (eye protrusion >20 mm from orbital bone) is hallmark of Graves' disease.
  - Pretibial myxedema, same.
  - Lid lag and stare are nonspecific consequences of hyperthyroidism and may simulate proptosis.
- Check neck nodes for adenopathy. Painless cervical lymphadenopathy may signal thyroid malignancy.
- Pelvic exam and visual field testing are important to check for ovarian and pituitary sources.

LAB STUDIES

- Consider radionuclide thyroid scan to help determine cause when clinical picture remains uncertain.
  - Toxic adenoma is characterized by hot nodule with little uptake by rest of gland.
  - Uptake is low in patients with thyroiditis, exogenous hormone intake, extraglandular hormone production, and iodide exposure.
  - Uptake is diffusely increased in patients with Graves' disease or functioning pituitary adenoma.
- Consider testing for antithyroid antibodies (including those directed against microsomal peroxidase) when Hashimoto's thyroiditis is under consideration, but be aware that they are also increased in Graves' disease, limiting their diagnostic utility in hyperthyroidism.
- Obtain serum thyroglobulin determination when surreptitious intake of thyroid hormone is suspected. Exogenous hormone use results in suppression of thyroglobulin synthesis.
- Consider whole-body scanning only when concerned about extrathyroidal hormone synthesis (struma ovarii or metastasis from thyroid malignancy).
- Obtain a screening bone density study in postmenopausal hyperthyroid patients (see Osteoporosis).

MANAGEMENT

SYMPTOMATIC CONTROL AND PREVENTION OF OSTEOPOROTIC FRACTURES

- For prompt control of adrenergic symptoms of hyperthyroidism, regardless of underlying cause, start Rx immediately with a beta-blocking agent (e.g., propranolol, 80 mg/day; or atenolol, 50 mg/day).
- Increase dose daily until symptoms are controlled. Use with caution in patients with preexisting heart failure unrelated to thyroid disease.
- Treat all postmenopausal hyperthyroid women found to be osteopenic by bone density testing. Risk of fracture is increased, especially in areas of cortical bone (hip, wrist) (see Osteoporosis).

GRAVES' DISEASE

Antithyroid Medication

- For nonpregnant young and middle-aged patients with Graves' disease, start methimazole (20–30 mg/day) in addition to beta blocker program.

- Continue both for 4–8 wks, then taper beta blocker as antithyroid agent takes effect.
- Adjust antithyroid drug dose according to clinical status and thyroid indices (TSH, free T_4).
- Use lowest possible dose that maintains biochemical and biologic control. Monitor closely to avoid hypothyroidism.
- Monitor WBC count if patient is taking >30 mg/day methimazole or if patient is elderly.
- If condition responds, continue antithyroid Rx for 12–24 mos.
- Measure TSAb at 12 mos: If absent and patient appears to be in remission clinically and biochemically, try discontinuing Rx. If relapse occurs, consider resuming antithyroid Rx for 12 more mos or radioiodine Rx.
- For pregnant patient with Graves' disease, consider antithyroid drug Rx, but obtain endocrinologic consultation before initiating Rx. PTU is preferred (starting dose: 100 mg tid) and can also be given to patient eager to breast-feed. Fully explain risks of Rx and be sure patient understands. Careful monitoring of thyroid status in mother and baby is essential. Maintain pregnant patient's free T_4 levels near ULN; monitor TSH closely.
- For all patients taking antithyroid medication, consider monitoring WBC count q2–4wks during first 4 mos of Rx, then q4–6mos. Stop Rx if neutrophil count is <1,500/mL. Risk for agranulocytosis and need for close monitoring are greatest in elderly patients and those taking PTU or >30 mg/day methimazole.

Radioiodine Therapy

- Consider iodine 131 Rx for elderly patients with Graves' disease and other patients with Graves' disease who are not or cannot be maintained with antithyroid drugs (relapse, agranulocytosis).
- Continue beta-blockade for 2–3 mos necessary for radioiodine to exert full effect.
- Monitor TSH for evidence of hypothyroidism 3–6 mos after Rx onset and q3–6mos thereafter; correct promptly by starting thyroid replacement Rx before hypothyroidism develops.

Surgical Therapy

- Refer for surgical consideration patients with neck obstruction, major cosmetic concern, or noncompliance in taking antithyroid medication.
- Also consider surgery when antithyroid drug Rx is ineffective or contraindicated. Young patients do particularly well.
- If contemplating surgery, continue antithyroid or beta-blocking Rx up to moment of surgery.
- Monitor for postoperative hyperthyroidism.

GRAVES' OPHTHALMOPATHY

- For patients with severe symptomatic ophthalmopathy, obtain prompt endocrinologic consultation. Options include very-high-dose systemic glucocorticoids (120–150 mg/day prednisone), local steroid injection, surgical decompression, and radiation Rx.
- For patients with mild to moderate ophthalmopathy, minimize risk for worsening eye disease by avoiding posttreatment hypothyroidism.

- Consider systemic daily steroid Rx for prophylaxis of posttreatment exacerbation for patients who begin radioiodine Rx with moderately severe eye changes already established (e.g., prednisone, 20–40 mg/day for 1 mo, then taper to full cessation during next 8 wks).
- For periorbital edema, advise elevating head of bed, and prescribe mild diuretic (e.g., hycrochlorothiazide, 50 mg/day).
- Prescribe methylcellulose drops to prevent corneal drying (see Exophthalmos).

SOLITARY TOXIC NODULE

- Refer for radioiodine Rx.

THYROIDITIS-INDUCED HYPERTHYROIDISM

- Treat patients with transient hyperthyroidism associated with thyroiditis symptomatically with beta-blockade until condition resolves.

BIBLIOGRAPHY

- For the current annotated bibliography on hyperthyroidism, see the print edition of *Primary Care Medicine*, 4th edition, Chapter 103, or www.LWWmedicine.com.

Hypoglycemia

DIFFERENTIAL DIAGNOSIS

IMPORTANT CAUSES OF HYPOGLYCEMIA

- Patient looks healthy/insulin-related
  - Excessively tight diabetic control with insulin or sulfonylurea Rx
  - Factitious hypoglycemia induced by surreptitious insulin administration
  - Sulfonylurea overdose
  - Insulinoma
  - Intense exercise
  - Prior gastric surgery
  - Early type 2 diabetes mellitus
- Patient looks ill/non–insulin-related
  - End-stage renal disease
  - End-stage liver disease
  - HIV infection, severe
  - Pituitary failure
  - Alcohol binge, severe, with little food intake
  - Hepatic dysfunction secondary to severe CHF, sepsis, infiltrative disease
  - IGF-II production by malignancy (most patients are ill)
- Patient looks ill/drug-related
  - Pentamidine for *P. carinii* pneumonia
  - Salicylates in renal failure
  - Propoxyphene in renal failure
  - TMP-SMX in renal failure
  - Quinine in cerebral malaria

WORKUP

OVERALL STRATEGY

- Confirming true hypoglycemia
  - Measure blood glucose at time of symptoms to confirm that patient with low blood glucose or "hypoglycemic" symptoms actually has true hypoglycemia (no need for glucose tolerance test).
  - Finger-stick method most convenient; venous sample more accurate at low glucose levels.
  - Note type of symptoms and concurrent blood glucose level.
  - Confirm true hypoglycemia if following criteria are met (Whipple's triad):
    - Symptoms consistent with neuroglycopenia (blurred or double vision, confusion, odd behavior, lethargy) or adrenergic stimulation (anxiety, tremulousness, headache, palpitations, sweats), +
    - Low blood glucose concentration (<50 mg/dL, 2.8 mmol/L) at time of symptoms, +
    - Relief of symptoms when glucose level returns to normal.
  - Eliminate from consideration patients with blood glucose level >50 mg/dL at time of symptoms.

- Eliminate from consideration patients without symptoms even in presence of low blood glucose level.
- Avoid labeling patients hypoglycemic if they do not fulfill criteria; consider alternative explanations for symptoms, including anxiety disorders, depression, and hyperthyroidism.

HISTORY

- Determine first whether condition is insulin-related.
- Review use of insulin and sulfonylurea agents (other agents for Rx of hyperglycemia do not alone confer risk for hypoglycemia).
- Have high index of suspicion for surreptitious insulin or sulfonylurea use in persons with vocational Hx of medical or paramedical work.
- Note relation of symptoms to meals.
  - If postprandial, check for Hx of type 2 DM or gastric surgery.
  - If onset within 1–2 hrs after eating and Hx of gastric surgery, consider rapid emptying as underlying pathophysiology.
  - If symptoms begin 3–5 hrs after eating, check for risk factors and symptoms of DM and consider early type 2 disease.
  - Check for fasting non–insulin-related causes by inquiring into recent binge drinking in absence of food intake, end-stage liver or kidney disease, adrenal insufficiency, marked hypopituitarism, and Hx of malignancy.
  - If symptoms occur after exercise or fasting, consider insulinoma, especially if accompanied by neuroglycopenic symptoms (blurred vision, diplopia, sweats, confusion, poor memory).
  - If insulinoma suspected, also check for symptoms of hypercalcemia (see Hypercalcemia) due to concurrent hyperparathyroidism from underlying MEN.

PHYSICAL EXAM

- Note any postural hypotension, alcohol on breath, needle marks at common insulin injection sites, signs of hepatocellular failure (see Cirrhosis and Chronic Liver Failure), hyperpigmentation, visual field defects, abdominal mass, ascites, upper abdominal surgical scar, any neurologic deficits.

LAB STUDIES

- Differentiate between insulin-related and non–insulin-related causes, and if insulin-related, between endogenous and exogenous causes.
- Obtain concurrent measurements of serum insulin, C-peptide (formed as proinsulin and split during endogenous synthesis), and glucose at time of symptoms.
- Perform overnight fast to elicit hypoglycemia and make possible simultaneous serum determinations.
- Consider exercise after overnight fasting to promote fall in serum glucose and elicit symptoms.
- Consider insulin-related cause if levels of insulin inappropriately high and glucose low (insulin to glucose ratio >0.3).
- Consider exogenous insulin source if insulin level high and C-peptide level low.
- Consider insulinoma and surreptitious sulfonylurea use if insulin and C-peptide levels elevated (>6–10 mg/mL and >0.2–0.4 nmol/ml, respectively).

- Rule out surreptitious sulfonylurea use by testing urine or serum sample for sulfonylurea.
- When insulinoma suspected, consider C-peptide suppression test (insulin infused during 1 hr and C-peptide levels obtained); failure to suppress C-peptide formation strongly suggests insulinoma.
- Attempt preoperative localization of suspected insulinoma by pancreatic ultrasonography (U/S) or CT; more definitive is direct pancreatic palpation at time of surgery, guided by intraoperative U/S.
- In patients with non–insulin-dependent hypoglycemia, assess need for additional studies based on clinical context [e.g., obtain cortisol and ACTH determinations if hypopituitarism or adrenal insufficiency is suspected clinically (see Diabetes Insipidus); for suspected tumor-induced hypoglycemia, consider IGF-II determination, but responsible tumor is usually already evident].

MANAGEMENT

- Treat underlying cause (e.g., remove insulinoma, debulk tumor producing IGF-II, arrange for psychotherapy for self-destructive behavior, adjust DM Rx regimen; see Diabetes Mellitus).
- For postprandial hypoglycemia (e.g., after gastric surgery), recommend frequent small feedings (6/day) and high-protein, low-carbohydrate diets.
- Consider anticholinergic Rx (e.g., 7.5 mg propantheline ac) to delay gastric emptying, a beta blocker (e.g., 10 mg propranolol ac), administration of pectin, and in refractory severe cases, reversal of 10-cm segment of jejunum.
- For patients with postprandial symptoms without hypoglycemia (i.e., those previously diagnosed with functional reactive hypoglycemia), consider similar measures as for those with true postprandial hypoglycemia.

PATIENT EDUCATION

- Take seriously patients who seek medical attention because of fear of "hypoglycemia," but once Dx has been ruled out, provide specific reassurance by responding to patient concerns, and then refocus attention to other possible causes.
- Reassure patients with "functional reactive hypoglycemia" (glucose levels normal during symptoms) that the symptoms are "real," but not related to low blood glucose or disturbances in glucose homeostasis; recommend simple dietary measures (see above).
- Respond to requests for glucose tolerance testing with information about its lack of specificity.
- Inform patients with suspected insulinoma that almost all cases are benign and that tumor removal is curative, with little risk for relapse or recurrence.

INDICATIONS FOR ADMISSION AND REFERRAL

- Promptly refer fasting hypoglycemia patient with suspected insulinoma (at risk for profound fall in serum glucose) to endocrinologist and surgeon familiar with treating condition.

- Admit to hospital immediately for glucose infusion and detailed evaluation any hypoglycemic patient with severe symptoms (seizure, mental confusion).
- Avoid routine referral of patients with postprandial symptoms for glucose tolerance testing.

BIBLIOGRAPHY

- For the current annotated bibliography on hypoglycemia, see the print edition of *Primary Care Medicine*, 4th edition, Chapter 97, or www.LWWmedicine.com.

Hypothyroidism

SCREENING AND/OR PREVENTION

- Consider TSH screening for women aged >50 (especially if hyperlipidemic or complaining of fatigue); admit to geriatric units persons with Hashimoto's thyroiditis, recent radioiodine or external neck irradiation, or recent thyroid surgery, and patients with mental dysfunction.
- Stop exogenous thyroid or antithyroid medication if reason for use is unclear; recheck TSH level 4–6 wks after Rx stops.
- Confirm Dx of hypothyroidism with TSH and free T_4 or free T_4 index determinations.
- If patient appears clinically and biochemically hypothyroid but TSH is not appropriately elevated, test for pituitary insufficiency.

DIFFERENTIAL DIAGNOSIS

- Primary hypothyroidism
  - Hashimoto's thyroiditis
  - Postpartum disease (transient)
  - Postirradiation disease
  - Subtotal thyroidectomy
  - Subacute thyroiditis (transient)
  - Antithyroid drugs (lithium, paraaminosalicylic acid, PTU, methimazole, iodide excess)
  - Iodide deficiency
  - Infiltrative disease (hemochromatosis, amyloidosis, scleroderma)
  - Biosynthetic defect, hereditary
- Secondary hypothyroidism
  - Pituitary macroadenoma
  - Empty sella syndrome
  - Infarction
  - Infiltrative disease (e.g., sarcoidosis)
  - Surgery or radiation-induced injury

WORKUP

HISTORY

- Check for possible etiologic factors, such as iodine 131 exposure, neck irradiation, recent viral infection, use of medications with antithyroid activity (lithium, excess iodide), residence in area of iodide deficiency, subtotal thyroidectomy, pituitary surgery or irradiation, and recent pregnancy.

PHYSICAL EXAM

- Look carefully at thyroid gland for size, consistency, and nodularity:
  - Exquisitely tender gland suggests subacute thyroiditis.

- Nontender, diffusely enlarged gland is seen in early Hashimoto's disease, iodide deficiency, and congenital biosynthetic defects, and after childbirth.
- Rubbery, multinodular goiter suggests more advanced Hashimoto's thyroiditis.
- When you suspect secondary hypothyroidism, check BP for postural hypotension and visual fields for deficits.

LAB STUDIES

- Obtain TSH, free T_4 (or free T_4 index), and total T_3 determinations to confirm Dx of hypothyroidism and differentiate primary from secondary disease.
- For suspected primary disease, check antimicrosomal antibody titer (presence of antibodies strongly suggests Hashimoto's thyroiditis).
- Obtain CBC and vitamin B_{12} determination in those with suspected Hashimoto's disease.
- For suspected secondary disease, obtain neuroimaging of the pituitary-hypothalamic region; MRI with gadolinium is the test of choice; CT of sella (with contrast) is reasonable alternative if MRI unavailable.
- In patients with sellar mass lesion, consider serum LH, FSH, ACTH, and prolactin levels (see Diabetes Insipidus; Galactorrhea and Hyperprolactinemia).
- Obtain lipid profile (see Hypercholesterolemia) in all hypothyroid patients because it is likely to be abnormal and require attention.

MANAGEMENT

PRIMARY HYPOTHYROIDISM

- If taking drug with potential antithyroid effect (e.g., iodides, paraaminosalicylic acid, lithium), stop or reduce dose.
- Begin thyroid replacement with levothyroxine, the thyroid replacement preparation of choice; select and stay with particular manufacturer's preparation. Use of desiccated thyroid and sole use of T_3 preparations not recommended.
- Base initial dose on patient age and weight, severity and duration of hypothyroidism, and presence of underlying heart disease. Be particularly cautious and use small starting doses in presence of underlying coronary disease. In general, consider 50 μg qam in young, otherwise healthy patients and 25 μg qam in older patients.
- Monitor initial Rx by checking symptoms and measuring TSH 4 wks after onset of Rx. Goal is normalization of TSH, but be aware that TSH level may initially require several mos to normalize despite adequate thyroid hormone replacement.
- Allow 4–6 wks for new dose to take full effect before considering another dose increase. Average levothyroxine replacement dose for most adults is 100–125 μg/day; for the elderly, average dose is 20% less.
- If TSH still elevated and symptoms of hypothyroidism continue, increase L-thyroxine dose in increments of 25–50 μg q30d; lower increment is appropriate for elderly patients and those with heart disease.

- If patient is clinically euthyroid but TSH still elevated, continue same dose and repeat TSH determination in 4–8 wks.
- Avoid excessive doses of replacement Rx (TSH <0.5 mU/L) because of risk for inducing osteoporosis and adverse cardiac effects.
- If TSH becomes abnormally low, check for symptoms suggestive of excessive replacement Rx (e.g., tremor, angina, palpitations, nervousness) and obtain free T_4 (or free T_4 index).
- Once proper dose achieved, monitor Rx q6–12mos with TSH determination.
- Patients with neuropsychiatric symptoms clearly referable to hypothyroidism may benefit from trial of mixed replacement Rx, in which T_3 is used with levothyroxine in ratio of 1:4, substituting 12.5μg of T_3 for 50 μg of total levothyroxine dose. Patients with major depression should be considered for antidepressants Rx (see Depression) if thyroid hormone replacement is not helping.
- Patients with mild to moderate hypothyroidism and underlying coronary disease need not receive replacement Rx before urgent surgery, but careful planning of anesthesia is necessary.

SECONDARY HYPOTHYROIDISM

- Perform ACTH stimulation test to assess adrenal reserve. If low, give cortisone acetate before prescribing thyroid replacement.
- Replace thyroid hormone as for primary hypothyroidism.
- Monitor Rx by following clinical signs and free T_4.

PATIENT EDUCATION

- Instruct patient and family on importance of continuing replacement Rx indefinitely and watching for symptoms and signs of recurring hypothyroidism. Suggest patients measure and record their weight regularly and report any unexplained change of ≥5 lbs.
- Warn hypothyroid patients of the danger of increasing their medication too rapidly or taking more than is prescribed.
- Advise euthyroid patients taking thyroid replacement for fatigue or weight loss of dangers inherent in such Rx and recommend cessation.

BIBLIOGRAPHY

- For the current annotated bibliography on hypothyroidism, see the print edition of *Primary Care Medicine*, 4th edition, Chapter 104, or www.LWWmedicine.com.

Gynecologic Problems

Breast Masses and Nipple Discharge

DIFFERENTIAL DIAGNOSIS

- Breast masses
  - Malignancy
  - Benign tumor (fibroadenoma)
  - Mastitis
  - Fat necrosis
  - Hematoma
  - Ductal ectasia
- Nipple discharge
  - Lactescent
    - Prolactinoma
    - Hypothyroidism
    - Medication
    - Breast stimulation
    - Chest wall irritation
    - Physiologic
  - Bloody
    - Intraductal carcinoma
    - Benign papilloma
    - Paget's disease of the nipple
  - Yellow or brown
    - Fibrocystic disease
    - Cyst communicating with duct
    - Ductal ectasia
    - Mastitis
    - Breast abscess

WORKUP

PHYSICAL EXAM

Breast Mass

- Reexamine young women with diffusely lumpy and fibrous breasts several times in menstrual cycle. Persistent solitary or dominant nodule requires biopsy.
- Examine lymph nodes in all patients with breast lump, which may provide important supporting evidence for malignancy, especially if there is otherwise unexplained adenopathy in ipsilateral axilla.

Nipple Discharge

- Perform careful breast exam that includes careful palpation; note whether discharge is unilateral or bilateral, spontaneous or expressible, and localized to 1 or many ducts.
- If unilateral and expressed from single duct, note quadrant of breast from which it seems to be coming. Examine for masses and adenopathy.

LAB STUDIES

Breast Mass

- Mammography may provide useful diagnostic information, but because of 10% false-negative rate, negative mammogram does not obviate need for biopsy.
- Ultrasonography useful in distinguishing cystic from solid masses and in guiding needle aspiration.
- Needle aspiration of cystic and solid masses obtains adequate specimens in 60–85% of cases. Among adequate samples, sensitivity is 80% and specificity 99%.
- Cystic lesions that resolve with aspiration, have negative cytology, and do not recur require only follow-up exams and mammograms. Exceptions are cystic lesions with serosanguinous fluid, which should excised.
- Solid lesions with suspicious or negative cytology require biopsy.
- Because of limited sensitivity of needle aspiration, many women may prefer more definitive approaches, including excisional biopsy. Discuss advantages and disadvantages of alternative approaches when surgical referral is made.

Nipple Discharge

- Test expressed fluid for occult blood.
- Mammography can be useful. When no apparent benign explanation, refer to surgeon experienced in evaluating breast disease.

MANAGEMENT

- Women with breast mass or discharge have legitimate concern about breast cancer. PCP can reassure many by learning proportion of patients with these presentations that prove to have cancer: 5–20% for women with dominant breast mass, and 5–10% for those with unilateral nipple discharge. Prompt, efficient evaluation is essential to good patient care.

BIBLIOGRAPHY

- For the current annotated bibliography on breast masses and nipple discharge, see the print edition of *Primary Care Medicine*, 4th edition, Chapter 113, or www.LWWmedicine.com.

MANAGEMENT

OVERALL APPROACH

- Inform women who practice "natural" birth control methods, including various approaches to rhythm method and withdrawal, of likelihood of pregnancy (e.g., 1 pregnancy/2 yrs) and reasons for failure.
- Patient ed and nonjudgmental counseling are critical to decision making.

BARRIER METHODS

- Barrier methods, including condoms (male and female), diaphragms, and cervical caps, are inexpensive, safe, and up to 95% effective when properly used. Male condom with nonoxynol 9 spermicide has added advantage of protection against HIV, chlamydia, gonococci, HSV, and possibly HPV.
- Spermicidal creams, jellies, and foams are difficult to use effectively if patients use them without barrier devices.
- IUDs confer sevenfold and threefold increased risks of PID in nulliparous and multiparous women, respectively. This has implications for subsequent tubal infertility. IUDs are most suitable for multiparous women and nulliparous women in monogamous relationships and at lower risk of STDs. Apprise nulliparous women of risks.
- IUDs are highly effective. Women should be aware of possibility of spontaneous expulsion, especially during first yr and if nulliparous.

ORAL CONTRACEPTIVES

- Use effectiveness of oral contraceptive pills exceeds that of barrier methods, spermicides, and IUDs. There are dozens of different preparations. PCP should become familiar with 4–5 products to prescribe in clinical situations and their absolute and relative contraindications.
- Combination preparations are most commonly used oral contraceptives in U.S. To minimize cardiovascular risks and side effects, favor pills with lowest effective estrogen dose (20–35 µg ethinyl estradiol) and lowest possible progestin dosage, respectively.
- Women with Hx of premenstrual breast engorgement and soreness, cyclic weight gain, or heavy periods might do better with preparations containing low estrogen and progestin with minimal estrogenic effect (e.g., Necon 0.5/35, a generic preparation with norethindrone, 0.5 mg/ ethinyl estradiol, 35 µg; or Ovcon with ethinyl estradiol, 35 µg/norethindrone, 0.4 mg).
- For women with acne or hirsutism, give preparation with low androgenic progestin, such as desogestrel or norgestimate.
- These lower-dose agents have higher rates of spotting, breakthrough bleeding, and amenorrhea as well as greater risk of pregnancy. Regimens with longer hormone cycles and biphasic and triphasic formulations have been developed to lower these rates.
- Progesterone-only pills are suitable for women who should not take estrogens because of lactation, complex migraine headaches, thromboembolic disease, or smoking after age 35.

- Carefully explain adverse effects of oral contraceptives that underlie absolute and relative contraindications and place them in context by comparing to risks associated with unintended pregnancy, whether carried to term or terminated.

Contraindications of Oral Contraceptives

- Absolute contraindications
  - Thromboembolic disorders, cardiovascular disease, thrombophlebitis, or past Hx of these conditions or others that predispose to them
  - Markedly impaired liver function from severe hepatitis, alcoholism, etc.
  - Known or suspected estrogen-dependent neoplasm (cancers of breast, endometrium, etc.)
  - Undiagnosed genital bleeding
  - Known or suspected pregnancy
- Relative contraindications
  - Migraine headache
  - HTN
  - Familial hyperlipidemia
  - Epilepsy
  - Uterine leiomyoma
  - Hx of idiopathic obstructive jaundice of pregnancy
  - Smoking ≥ half a pack/day
  - DM
  - Severe heart disease
  - Patient unreliability
  - Age >35

OTHER METHODS

- Levonorgestrel can be surgically implanted in slender Silastic tubes (Norplant). Released continuously at very low levels for 5 yrs, it suppresses ovulation and achieves cumulative pregnancy rates of 0.6–4%. Alternative is q3mo injections of medroxyprogesterone acetate (Depo-Provera), 150 mg during first 5 days of cycle.
- Postcoital contraception is 97–99% effective if started within 12–24 hrs of unprotected intercourse. Regimens include
  - estrogen/progestin [ethinyl estradiol, 100 μg + levonorgestrel, 1.0 mg (e.g., 2 Ovral tablets)] repeated in 12 hrs;
  - high-dose estrogen (ethinyl estradiol, 0.5 mg) bid × 5 days;
  - progestin only (levonorgestrel, 0.75 mg) repeated in 12 hrs; or
  - mifepristone (600 mg, single dose).

STERILIZATION

- Vasectomy is safest and simplest means of sterilization. Advise men to use alternative methods of birth control for 3 mos after vasectomy, when semen analysis should confirm azoospermia. Because only one-third of men who undergo reanastomosis father children, patients should consider vasectomy irreversible.
- Tubal sterilization can be performed through small laparotomy, vaginally, or laparoscopically. Avoid vaginal approach during postpartum period. As with vasectomy, patients should consider tubal sterilization irreversible.

BIBLIOGRAPHY

■ For the current annotated bibliography on fertility control, see the print edition of *Primary Care Medicine*, 4th edition, Chapter 119, or www.LWWmedicine.com.

DIFFERENTIAL DIAGNOSIS

MEN

- Most causes of male infertility are associated with azoospermia or oligospermia.

Important Causes of Male Infertility

- Hypothalamic/pituitary
  - Prolactinoma
- Idiopathic
  - Drugs (e.g., alcohol, marijuana)
- Testicular
  - Klinefelter's syndrome
  - Sertoli-cell-only syndrome
  - Irradiation
  - Adult mumps
  - Alkylating agents
- Anatomic/functional
  - Obstruction of epididymis or vas
  - Impotence
  - Retrograde ejaculation
  - Infection
  - Antisperm antibodies
  - Idiopathic defects in sperm quantity or quality

WOMEN

- Most common causes of female infertility are disorders of ovulation, which account for as many as 40% of cases. Tubal obstruction due to past infection (and therefore preventable) or inflammation account for 25%. Uterine and vaginal pathology, including infection, account for others.

Important Causes of Female Infertility

- Hypothalamic/pituitary
  - Hypothalamic dysfunction
  - Polycystic ovary syndrome
  - Prolactinoma
- Ovarian
  - Primary failure (e.g., premature menopause)
  - Irradiation
- Tubal
  - Pelvic inflammatory disease
  - Endometriosis
  - Adhesions
- Uterine
  - Fibroids
  - Scarring (Asherman's syndrome)
  - Anatomic abnormalities

- Cervical
  - Poor mucus quality
  - Infection
  - Anatomic abnormalities

WORKUP

HISTORY

- Both partners may have impaired fertility. Interpersonal problems, including those related to difficulty conceiving, may contribute. Empathic, supportive, nonjudgmental exploration of marital relationship is essential; it is often best done by interviewing couple together (to observe their interactions) and each partner separately.

Men

- Inquire into drug and medication use (marijuana, alcohol, antihypertensive agents), urethral discharge, headache and other symptoms of pituitary tumor, past Hx of radiation Rx or cancer chemotherapy, mumps, toxin exposure, and systemic illnesses (especially DM with associated retrograde ejaculation).
- Sexual Hx that reviews marital relationship, sexual techniques, erectile function, and frequency of intercourse is also important.

Women

- Focus on menstrual and reproductive Hx, including any abortions, complicated deliveries, curettages, menstrual irregularities, or episodes of amenorrhea.
- Lifelong Hx of menstrual irregularities suggests polycystic ovary syndrome, especially if accompanied by hirsutism and obesity.
- Note situational or emotional stress, marked weight loss, or excess exercise, because they can lead to hypothalamic dysfunction and impairment of ovulation (see Secondary Amenorrhea; Vaginal Bleeding).
- Checking for symptoms of hypothyroidism (see Hypothyroidism), hyperprolactinemia and Cushing's syndrome (see Galactorrhea and Hyperprolactinemia), and androgen excess (see Hirsutism) may yield clues of conditions that can impair hypothalamic function.
- Inquiry into headaches, visual field disturbances, galactorrhea, symptoms of pituitary insufficiency (see Galactorrhea and Hyperprolactinemia), and Hx of postpartum hemorrhage helps to screen for sella turcica lesion.
- Checking for Hx or symptoms of PID (vaginal discharge, pelvic pain, fever, dyspareunia) is also essential. Any malignant disease Hx is important to note, especially if Rx included irradiation or alkylating agents.
- Obtain detailed psychosocial Hx that reviews pertinent details of marital relationship and sexual activity. Loss of libido may signify psychosocial or hormonal dysfunction.

PHYSICAL EXAM

Men

- Note general appearance and signs of diminished androgenization (decreased body hair, gynecomastia, eunuchoid proportions).

- Examine scrotum for testicular size, presence of varicocele, hypospadias, and absent vas deferens. Soft, small testes (<4 cm in longest diameter) are consistent with primary testicular failure and pituitary-hypothalamic insufficiency.
- Perform Valsalva maneuver while patient is standing to help reveal small varicocele.
- Observe urethra for discharge, and prostate and seminal vesicles for tenderness and other signs of infection.
- If you suspect pituitary condition, visual field testing by confrontation might reveal important field defect; normal study does not rule out mass lesion.
- Testing deep tendon reflexes may uncover delay in relaxation suggestive of hypothyroidism (see Hypothyroidism).

Women

- Check for obesity, excessive weight loss, hirsutism, cushingoid appearance, stigmata of hypothyroidism (see Hypothyroidism), visual field disturbances, and goiter.
- Pelvic exam is important to note any ovarian, uterine, or adnexal masses, thickening, or tenderness. Cervical exam should include check for erosions, discharge, polyps, masses, scarring, and pain on cervical motion.
- Examine hirsute patients for clitoromegaly.

LAB STUDIES

Men

- Perform semen analysis. Quantitative analysis includes number of sperm/mL semen (counts >20 million/mL are normal) and semen volume (<1.5 mL may be inadequate to buffer vaginal acidity).
- Patients with normal counts should have qualitative studies of sperm (motility, morphology, cervical mucus interaction), although these studies are often more useful for identifying infertile individual than for defining Rx. In normal persons, counts for motile forms and spermatozoa with oval heads are >50%.
- Those with azoospermia or oligospermia should have LH, FSH, and testosterone measures. Proper sampling technique is important to avoid misleading results. Pool 3 serum samples drawn 20 mins apart.
  - High concentrations of gonadotropins and low or low-normal testosterone suggest primary gonadal problem.
  - Low gonadotropins and low testosterone characterize pituitary-hypothalamic etiology.
  - Normal FSH, testosterone, and testicular size in patient with azoospermia suggests obstruction.
  - Normal hormone and gonadotropin concentrations in setting of oligospermia are characteristic of patients with varicocele or idiopathic disease.
  - Small testes, gynecomastia, elevated FSH, and reduced testosterone suggest Klinefelter's syndrome. Confirm Dx using buccal smear that shows extra chromatin of Barr body.
- In those with suspected pituitary disease, obtain prolactin level and head CT. Elevated prolactin in setting of normal CT may be due to drug-induced problem, but repeat CT in 6 mos to be sure that early tumor has not been missed.

- Utility of more elaborate studies (e.g., antisperm antibodies, sperm-cervical mucus interaction, penetration testing) is best determined by infertility specialist.

Women

- To determine whether ovulation is taking place, women should monitor for rise in basal body temp, indicating ovulation, or have serum progesterone measured on days 21–23 of cycle. Endometrial biopsy may also be useful but is more expensive and more painful and may remove long-awaited pregnancy.
- Those without temp rise or with progesterone level <10 ng/ml are likely anovulatory and should have serum prolactin, FSH, and LH measures.
- Exam within 2–12 hrs of coitus with ≥5 motile sperm found in cervical mucus indicates competent partner. Also examine mucus for viscosity (stretching to 6 cm is normal) and "ferning," manifestations of estrogen effect.
- If after Hx, PE, postcoital test, and serum progesterone, it appears that tubal or uterine disease may be responsible for infertility, consider hysterosalpingography and laparoscopy. Choice of test should be made by gynecologist experienced in evaluation of infertility.

MANAGEMENT

- Specialists generally treat infertility, but PCPs play critical role in helping patients understand its causes and their options for achieving pregnancy.
- Men or women with hypothalamic dysfunction should be referred to reproductive endocrinologists. Refer those with structural problems to urologist or gynecologist.
- Evident psychosocial problems require careful listening, explanation, and selective referral.
- Education and reassurance is appropriate for couples who have not conceived after trying for 1 yr and who are younger than late thirties, unless there is evidence for endocrinopathy, tumor, genitourinary tract infection, anatomic disorder, or contributing interpersonal problems. Older couples and those who will not be reassured should have further evaluation.

BIBLIOGRAPHY

- For the current annotated bibliography on infertility, see the print edition of *Primary Care Medicine*, 4th edition, Chapter 120, or www.LWWmedicine.com.

MANAGEMENT

OVERALL APPROACH

■ Decisions about Rx of postmenopausal changes require careful weighing and thorough discussion of risks and benefits. Elicit and address postmenopausal woman's preferences and concerns when designing program.

HOT FLASHES

■ Consider oral estrogen at lowest dose necessary (often as little as 0.3 mg/day conjugated estrogens).

■ Regularly reevaluate need for continued Rx. If patient has intact uterus and requires indefinite Rx, consider adding progestin to program (see below).

ATROPHIC VAGINITIS

■ With severe dysuria or unacceptable dyspareunia, prescribe topical estrogen (e.g., conjugated estrogen cream) applied 1–2 times/wk. Systemic absorption occurs, but its effect is uncertain. Avoid prolonged daily use because of risk of endometrial stimulation. In instances of painful coitus only, advise trial of water-soluble lubricant, especially if there is desire to avoid estrogen exposure.

DEPRESSION

■ Treat with supportive psychotherapy and/or standard antidepressant drug regimen (see Depression); HRT does not substitute for this Rx.

OSTEOPOROSIS PROPHYLAXIS

■ Explain need for long-term Rx and its risks. For those at increased risk of osteoporosis and willing to undergo indefinite Rx, initiate oral HRT (see below) at onset of menopause. Continue for ≥10 yrs and indefinitely if possible. Incorporate 1.5 g/day calcium, consider vitamin D supplementation in elderly, and prescribe weight-bearing aerobic exercise program.

■ Consider bisphosphonate Rx as alternative to indefinite hormone supplementation, particularly in patient with prior vertebral compression fracture (see Osteoporosis). HRT cannot replace lost bone; it is not Rx for reversing established osteoporosis. For women without increased risk of osteoporosis, you may reasonably delay HRT until age 60.

PROPHYLAXIS OF CARDIOVASCULAR DISEASE

■ Do not initiate oral HRT specifically for cardiovascular risk reduction. Consider possible long-term risk reduction along with other benefits and harms when making decision.

■ Among women already taking HRT, it need not be discontinued because of concerns about possible increase in cardiovascular risk. Incorporate appropriate diet, exercise, and pharmacologic measures pertinent to patient's major risk factors (see Exercise; Hypercholesterolemia; Hypertension; Stable Angina).

ORAL HORMONE REPLACEMENT REGIMENS

- For woman with intact uterus, treat with continuous daily estrogen combined with low-dose progestin (e.g., 0.625 mg/day conjugated estrogens + 2.5–5 mg/day medroxyprogesterone acetate or equivalent), or continuous estrogen + cyclic progestin (e.g., 0.625 mg/day conjugated estrogens + 5–10 mg/day of medroxyprogesterone acetate added on 10–14 consecutive days of month). Base choice on desirability and acceptability of periodic vaginal bleeding.
- For women with hysterectomies, treat with continuous estrogen Rx (e.g., 0.625 mg/day conjugated estrogens). No benefit to adding progestin.

BIBLIOGRAPHY

- For the current annotated bibliography on menopause, see the print edition of *Primary Care Medicine*, 4th edition, Chapter 118, or www.LWWmedicine.com.

DIFFERENTIAL DIAGNOSIS

GENERAL CONSIDERATIONS

- PCP should approach etiologic Dx of pelvic pain by first considering whether symptoms are acute, recurrent, or chronic and, if recurrent, whether related or unrelated to menstruation.

IMPORTANT CAUSES OF PELVIC PAIN

- Acute pain
  - Pelvic inflammatory disease
  - Ectopic pregnancy with rupture
  - Torsion of fallopian tube, ovary, or ovarian cyst
  - Ruptured ovarian cyst
  - Extrapelvic disease (e.g., appendicitis)
- Recurrent pain with menstruation
  - Primary dysmenorrhea
  - Secondary dysmenorrhea
  - Endometriosis
  - Adenomyosis
  - Chronic PID
  - IUDs
- Recurrent pain unrelated to menstruation
  - Mittelschmerz
  - Leaking ovarian cysts
  - Nongynecologic pathology: adhesions, irritable bowel disease, functional bowel
- Chronic pain
  - Benign neoplasms
  - Malignancy
  - Enigmatic or psychogenic pain

WORKUP

- Approach to acute pelvic pain requires some urgency. Vital signs, including rectal temp and postural changes in BP and pulse, are essential. PE should check for signs of peritoneal irritation (rigidity, percussion tenderness, rebound), presence of bowel sounds, cervical motion tenderness, or abnormal masses. Lab evaluation should include CBC, differential, ESR, urinalysis, and serum hCG β-subunit pregnancy test.
- Hospitalize patients with high fever, orthostatic signs, or acute abdomen, even if lab results are unavailable. Further PE and lab studies should focus on causes that warrant early intervention.
- Refer immediately to gynecologist patients with ruptured ectopic pregnancy, torsion of fallopian tube or ovary, or ruptured ovarian cyst with evidence of significant rapid bleeding.

- Even if situation is urgent, several historical facts can help establish Dx. Ask about any delay in menstrual period, dyspareunia, IUD use, shaking chills, abnormal vaginal discharge or bleeding, recent abortion, and location and radiation of pain.
- Generalized severe pain indicates possible peritoneal involvement, especially with rigid abdomen and absent bowel sounds. Unilateral pain suggests local tubal or ovarian problem; bilateral pain indicates PID or diffuse pelvic irritation.
- Elicit symptoms of constipation, nausea, vomiting, diarrhea, flank pain, and dysuria to rule out nongynecologic etiologies such as appendicitis, acute pyelonephritis, or urethral stone.
- If pain is chronic or recurrent, obtain more detailed Hx during office visit, including relationship of pain to menstrual cycle and complete menstrual and obstetric Hx. Note onset, quality, and radiation of pain and any exacerbating or ameliorating factors.
- Perform detailed pelvic and rectal exams to look for adnexal thickening, cervical discharge, uterine masses, fixation of any structures, ovarian masses, and focal tenderness.
- Lab tests should include serum hCG, CBC, ESR, urinalysis, and culture of cervix and rectum for gonorrhea and chlamydia. If you find a mass, perform ultrasound (possibly with transvaginal probe) to confirm finding, better localize mass, and distinguish solid from cystic lesion.
- Laparoscopy or dilation and curettage may be necessary to establish Dx.

MANAGEMENT

- Treat patients with PID as outpatients if they are nontoxic and reliable. Antibiotics should cover *N. gonorrhea* and *C. trachomatis* (see Vaginal Discharge).
- Pain with menstruation in absence of pelvic pathology is primary dysmenorrhea. Treat with lower-dose OTC NSAIDs. Oral contraceptives are also helpful.
- Treat PMS with low-dose antidepressants (e.g., an SSRI) limited to luteal phase of menstrual cycle. Alprazolam has also been shown effective. Leuprolide, a GnRH agonist, has been used to suppress ovarian hormones and eliminate symptoms in some women.
- Systematic review suggests that vitamin B_6 in doses up to 100 mg/day is effective. Less evidence supports calcium supplementation at 1,200 mg/day. Exercise and elimination of xanthines, alcohol, and salt have limited effect. NSAIDs are ineffective for PMS.
- Refer women with endometriosis and other causes of secondary dysmenorrhea to gynecologist for Rx.
- Chronic pelvic pain requires coordination of psychological, behavioral, and medical Rx. PCP is well positioned for this role. Consider tricyclic antidepressants.

BIBLIOGRAPHY

- For the current annotated bibliography on menstrual or pelvic pain, see the print edition of *Primary Care Medicine*, 4th edition, Chapter 116, or www.LWWmedicine.com.

Secondary Amenorrhea

DIFFERENTIAL DIAGNOSIS

GENERAL CONSIDERATIONS

- Missed periods may raise concerns about pregnancy or menopause that PCP must address.
- Rule out possible pregnancy using serum hCG β-subunit determination. Sensitivity of urine hCG-precipitation slide test can be as low as 70%. Negative tests therefore require follow-up testing.
- Secondary amenorrhea (cessation of menses ≥3 mos after previously normal cycles) suggests disturbance at level of hypothalamus, pituitary, ovaries, or uterus that may require further evaluation.
- Hypothalamic dysfunction accounts for 30% of cases of secondary amenorrhea, usually due to disorder of GnRH release causing loss of LH surge and failure to ovulate. This in turn is usually due to marked weight loss (<70% ideal, as in anorexia nervosa and other eating disorders; see Eating Disorders), severe emotional upset, or excessive exercise (competitive athletes). Situational anxiety and moderate weight loss can be sufficient cause.
- Other causes include excess endogenous cortisol, androgens, and prolactin. Prolactin excess may be related to hypothyroidism. Amenorrhea can last 6 mos after cessation of oral contraceptives.
- Pituitary disease, mostly prolactinomas, which also cause galactorrhea and infertility, account for 15% of cases of secondary amenorrhea. Other pituitary lesions include pituitary necrosis and granulomatous disease.
- Ovarian failure produces amenorrhea along with marked estrogen deficiency and elevations of LH and FSH. Its premature occurrence, accounting for roughly 15% of secondary amenorrhea cases, is due to autoimmune disease, radiation Rx, or chemotherapy with alkylating agents. Polycystic ovary syndrome, which produces hirsutism, anovulation, and oligomenorrhea or amenorrhea, accounts for 30% of cases.
- Uterine causes of amenorrhea, including endometrial or cervical scarring, account for 5%.

CAUSES OF SECONDARY AMENORRHEA

- Hypothalamic dysfunction
  - Mild
    - Situational stress
    - Dieting
    - Concurrent illness
    - Increased exercise
    - Drugs (phenothiazines, oral contraceptives)
    - Idiopathic
  - Marked
    - Anorexia nervosa with severe weight loss
    - Serious emotional stress or psychopathology
    - Serious concurrent illness

- Competitive distance running
- Excess androgen, prolactin, or cortisol
- Idiopathic

■ Pituitary disease

- Prolactinoma
- Other pituitary neoplasm
- Empty sella syndrome
- Pituitary infarction (Sheehan's syndrome)
- Granulomatous disease (sarcoidosis)

■ Ovarian

- Menopause
- Polycystic ovary syndrome (may have hypothalamic etiology)
- Premature ovarian failure (idiopathic, autoimmune disease, radiation Rx, chemotherapy, endometriosis, oophoritis)
- FSH resistance

■ Uterine

- Obliteration of uterine cavity by intrauterine scarring and synechiae formation: Asherman's syndrome (overly vigorous curettage, septic abortion, radiation)
- Cervical scarring with resultant os closure

■ Endocrinopathies

- Thyroid disease
- Cushing's syndrome
- Hyperandrogenism

■ Pregnancy

WORKUP

HISTORY

■ Obtain detailed menstrual Hx and circumstances of amenorrhea. Note age of menarche, character of normal cycles, timing of missed periods, and prior pregnancies or abortions.

■ Psychosocial Hx may provide evidence for hypothalamic amenorrhea and should include inquiry into situational stresses (job, school, family, friends), emotional problems, excessive dieting, bulimia, marked weight loss, and heavy physical training. Nutritional imbalance including severe dietary fat restriction may be relevant.

■ Carefully review oral contraceptive use and intake of other medications such as antipsychotics.

■ Review of systems should include check for hot flashes, skin changes of hypothyroidism (see Hypothyroidism), hirsutism, headache, visual disturbances, thyroid enlargement, breast changes or lactescent nipple discharge, change in libido, and change in muscle mass or body habitus.

■ Several patterns are suggestive. Amenorrhea in context of marked weight loss suggests anorexia nervosa (see Eating Disorders). If periods were irregular before onset of amenorrhea, anovulatory bleeding was probably occurring and one of its etiologies is likely (see Vaginal Bleeding).

■ Amenorrhea accompanied by galactorrhea is strongly suggestive of hyperprolactinemia, which may be due to prolactinoma, destructive lesion of sella, or hypothyroidism (see Galactorrhea and Hyperpro-lactinemia).

- Hx of irregular periods since menarche with obesity and hirsutism raises probability of polycystic ovary syndrome. Rapid onset of amenorrhea, hirsutism, and frank virilization suggests androgen-producing neoplasm, usually of adrenal or ovarian origin.

PHYSICAL EXAM

- Observe patient's general appearance, noting low body weight, marked obesity, hirsutism, virilization (see Hirsutism), and Cushing's syndrome.
- Examine integument for signs of hypothyroidism (see Hypothyroidism) and adrenal disease, vision for visual field defects, and breasts for lactescent nipple discharge.
- On pelvic exam, note any clitoromegaly, atrophy of vaginal mucosa, scarring of cervical os, ovarian or adnexal masses, and uterine enlargement or masses.

LAB STUDIES

- Hx and PE often suggest Dx. Rule out pregnancy. Reassure and follow women with apparent mild hypothalamic dysfunction or menopause. Bimonthly 5-day courses of medroxyprogesterone (10 mg/day) induce shedding of proliferative endometrium in those with chronic amenorrhea.
- Galactorrhea is indication for prolactin testing. Evaluate others for presence or absence of withdrawal bleeding after single 100-mg IM dose of progesterone or 5 days of oral medroxyprogesterone (10 mg/day).
- Women who have withdrawal bleeding should have serum LH measurement: low or normal indicates mild hypothalamic dysfunction; persistently high levels indicate polycystic ovary syndrome.
- For women without withdrawal bleeding but with Hx suggesting uterine scarring, give course of conjugated estrogens (1.25 mg/day × 21 day) followed by 5-day course of medroxyprogesterone (10 mg/day). Continued absence of bleeding confirms uterine disease.
- Most women with absence of bleeding on progesterone trial should have serum FSH measured: high level suggests ovarian failure (confirmed by low serum estradiol level); low or normal level followed by normal prolactin level suggests severe hypothalamic dysfunction that may warrant measurement of androgens and cortisol if etiology is not evident from Hx and PE; low or normal level followed by high prolactin level suggests pituitary disease and warrants CT or MRI and TSH determination.

MANAGEMENT

- Refer women with polycystic ovary syndrome who want to restore fertility for consultation and consideration of ovarian wedge resections, clomiphene administration, or GnRH analogues. When fertility is not immediate concern, oral contraceptives inhibit gonadotropin release and ovarian androgen production. Spironolactone (50–150 mg/day × days 1–25), as well as finasteride and flutamide, are alternatives.
- Refer women with confirmed uterine disease to gynecologist.

■ Severe hypothalamic dysfunction requires Rx of underlying cause (e.g., weight gain or decrease in extreme exercise levels for those with anorexia or extreme weight loss). Consider HRT (conjugated estrogens 0.625–1.250 mg/day on days 1–25 and medroxyprogesterone 10 mg/day × 12 days starting on day 15) to prevent osteoporosis in those with chronic amenorrhea.

■ Women with ovarian failure should receive estrogen/progesterone replacement Rx as described above.

■ Refer women with hyperprolactinemia or other forms of pituitary disease for endocrine consultation, which may include consideration of medical or surgical Rx as well as HRT.

■ Regardless of etiology, patient ed and explanation is critical for women with secondary amenorrhea, especially those concerned about fertility.

BIBLIOGRAPHY

■ For the current annotated bibliography on secondary amenorrhea, see the print edition of *Primary Care Medicine*, 4th edition, Chapter 112, or www.LWWmedicine.com.

Unplanned Pregnancy

MANAGEMENT

- When women present with unintended and unwanted pregnancy, PCP should serve as knowledgeable source of information about community resources for prenatal care, abortion, and adoption.
- Refer patient to another provider if your beliefs interfere with objective counseling.
- Inform women considering surgical abortion that when performed appropriately it is safe, with lower death rates than those from pregnancy across all age groups.
- Surgical termination is safest when performed earlier in gestation. Risk increases with gestational age, maternal age, and higher parity.
- Assessment before surgical termination should include pregnancy testing, urinalysis, CBC, blood type and Rh factor determination, syphilis serologies, gonorrhea and chlamydia testing, and Pap smear. Consider HIV testing and ultrasonography.
- Advise women that major complications of surgical abortion, including uterine perforation, hemorrhage, and infection, occur in 1/1,000 procedures. Minor complications, including infection, cervical stenosis, cervical tear, and bleeding or incomplete abortion requiring resuctioning, occur in 8/1,000 procedures. Complication rates increase with gestational age.
- Address contraception before or immediately after surgical termination of pregnancy. After procedure, advise women to avoid intercourse, douching, or tampons for 1–2 wks.
- Women concerned about subsequent childbearing should know that single first-trimester vacuum aspiration procedure does not increase risk for infertility, miscarriage, ectopic pregnancy, stillbirth, or major pregnancy- or delivery-associated complication. Effect of multiple abortions on future childbearing is uncertain.
- Advise women who are <7 wks pregnant that therapeutic abortion induced by mifepristone, usually followed by progesterone administration, is safe and effective alternative.
- Placing child for adoption is alternative for woman who believes it impossible to raise child and prefers to avoid abortion. Keeping child may emerge as realistic option if problematic social situation is amenable to change.

BIBLIOGRAPHY

- For the current annotated bibliography on unplanned pregnancy, see the print edition of *Primary Care Medicine*, 4th edition, Chapter 121, or www.LWWmedicine.com.

Vaginal Bleeding

DIFFERENTIAL DIAGNOSIS

GENERAL CONSIDERATIONS

- Vaginal bleeding that occurs at inappropriate times (<21 or >36 days after last period) or in excessive amounts (clots lasting >7 days) has very different implications depending on patient age and stage of reproductive function.
- In premenopausal women, PCP must distinguish between anovulatory and ovulatory bleeding.
- Ovulatory bleeding, characterized by menorrhagia or by intermenstrual bleeding, is usually caused by endometrial or cervical lesions. Evaluate promptly to rule out cervical or endometrial cancer.
- Anovulatory bleeding, characterized by metrorrhagia, is usually manifestation of hypothalamic-pituitary-ovarian axis dysfunction and is common in yrs after puberty and before menopause and with situational stress, excessive exercise, or weight loss. Usually self-limiting; when not, test for excess androgen (including polycystic ovary syndrome), prolactin, or cortisol, and hypothyroidism.
- In postmenopausal women, bleeding indicates endometrial, cervical, or vaginal pathology; evaluate promptly.
- In pregnant women, vaginal bleeding may indicate ectopic pregnancy, failing pregnancy, or retained products of gestation (following abortion). Prompt gynecologic evaluation and consideration of hospitalization indicated.

CAUSES OF ABNORMAL VAGINAL BLEEDING

- Ovulatory bleeding
  - Normal variant
    - Mittelschmerz
  - Anatomic lesion
    - Uterine fibroids
    - Cervical disease (inflammation, polyp, cancer)
    - Endometrial carcinoma
    - PID
    - IUD
  - Concurrent disease
    - Bleeding diathesis
    - Foreign body
- Anovulatory bleeding
  - Hypothalamic dysfunction
    - Puberty
    - Perimenopausal state
    - Situational stress, excessive exercise, weight loss
    - Excess androgen, prolactin, cortisol; hypothyroidism
    - Polycystic ovary syndrome
  - Oral contraceptive use
    - Inadequate estrogen dose

- Postmenopausal bleeding
  - Endometrial pathology
    - Fibroid
    - Cancer
    - Polyp
  - Cervical pathology
    - Cancer
    - Polyp
    - Erosion
  - Vaginal pathology
    - Atrophic vaginitis
- Pregnancy
  - Ectopic pregnancy
  - Postabortion (retained products of gestation)
  - Failing pregnancy

WORKUP

HISTORY

Overall Considerations

- Most important part of Hx is patient's normal menstrual cycle (duration, frequency, intensity) and how current bleeding pattern compares.
- In patients of childbearing age, inquire into unprotected intercourse and symptoms of pregnancy (breast engorgement, morning sickness, cessation of normal menses).
- Although intensity of bleeding (e.g., by number of pads or tampons used) is more useful for management than for Dx, new onset of clots or duration of >7 days argues for abnormal bleeding.

Ovulatory Bleeding

- Ovulatory etiology likely if menstrual regularity persists despite increase in intensity or duration of flow or onset of intermenstrual staining. Presence of premenstrual symptoms such as breast engorgement, pelvic cramping, fluid retention, and mood swings support this Dx.
- Ask about symptoms of bleeding diathesis and medicines that inhibit normal clotting (see Bleeding Problems). Check for dyspareunia, postcoital bleeding, vaginal discharge, pelvic pain, fever, trauma, and IUD use. Review risk factors for endometrial carcinoma (see Endometrial Cancer).

Anovulatory Bleeding

- Suggested by absence of above symptoms + complete irregularity of menstrual periods, especially if accompanied by months of amenorrhea.
- Ask about important precipitants, such as emotional stress, weight loss, exercise, and chronic illness.
- In adolescent girls, check for Hx of irregular periods since onset of menarche.
- Ask about oral contraceptive use, noting estrogen dose and Hx of breakthrough bleeding.
- In perimenopausal women, menstrual irregularity and skipping of periods suggest functional etiology, but do not rule out cancer.

- Symptoms of hirsutism and virilization (see Hirsutism) and Hx of infertility suggest androgen excess.
- Lifelong Hx of irregular menses, hirsutism, infertility, and obesity suggests polycystic ovary syndrome.
- Inquire into galactorrhea and development of cushingoid appearance, and check for prolactin and cortisol excess.
- Note any symptoms of hypothyroidism (see Hypothyroidism) and iron deficiency (see Anemia).

Postmenopausal Bleeding

- Take any Hx of bleeding, even minor staining, as evidence of possible malignancy, but inquiry into symptomatic atrophic vaginitis and uterine prolapse may provide useful clues.

PHYSICAL EXAM

- Check all patients for postural signs of significant intravascular volume depletion.
- Careful speculum and bimanual pelvic exams are essential, noting any vaginal or cervical erosions, uterine or adnexal masses, focal tenderness, or purulent or bloody discharge.
- Check for signs of pregnancy (engorged breasts, pigmented areolae, bluish cervix, enlarged uterus) in women of reproductive age.
- For suspected ovulatory bleeding, focus on pelvic exam but also check for signs of bleeding diathesis (petechiae, ecchymoses, splenic enlargement).
- For suspected anovulatory bleeding, examine for hirsutism, virilization, cushingoid appearance, milky nipple discharge, goiter, dry skin, coarse hair, and "hung-up" reflexes. Visual field testing indicated if large pituitary adenoma suspected. Presence of hirsutism or virilization necessitates thorough pelvic and abdominal exams for ovarian or adrenal masses.
- In postmenopausal women, note friability of vaginal mucosa and cervix and presence of any uterine or adnexal masses.

LAB STUDIES

Overall Considerations

- Test for pregnancy all women of reproductive age with abnormal vaginal bleeding. Serum hCG β-subunit is most sensitive (see Secondary Amenorrhea).

Ovulatory Bleeding

- Perform pelvic exam with Pap smear and perhaps cervical culture. Cervical culture for gonorrhea and other pathogenic organisms necessary in patients with pain on motion of cervix and adnexal tenderness (see Vaginal Discharge); elevated ESR suggests pelvic inflammation.
- Transvaginal ultrasound (U/S) may be necessary with subsequent dilation and curettage for abnormalities.
- Endometrial sampling is central to evaluation when noninvasive evaluation is unrevealing. Contraindicated in presence of cervical stenosis, infection, or pregnancy.
- Consider bleeding diathesis, especially platelet abnormalities.

Anovulatory Bleeding

- No additional studies necessary when etiology evident (e.g., situational stress, puberty, chronic illness, marked weight loss).
- When hirsutism or virilization evident, serum testosterone is best test. Rapid onset of these signs or serum testosterone >600 nmol/L suggests functioning adrenal or ovarian neoplasm. 17-Hydroxyprogesterone determination can facilitate Dx.
- If FSH >40 IU/mL, ovarian failure imminent.
- An LH:FSH ratio >2:1 indicates polycystic ovary syndrome.
- Fasting serum insulin level is indicated in patients with elevated testosterone (>350 nmol/L, 100 ng/mL). Fasting insulin level >180 pmol/L suggests insulin resistance.

Postmenopausal Bleeding

- Conduct noninvasive study for pelvic pathology as above.
- Transvaginal U/S may reveal abnormal thickening of endometrium or fibroids. Because of high prevalence of endometrial cancer in this age group, particularly those whose bleeding occurs long after menopause, endometrial sampling or dilation and curettage may be indicated if U/S findings are normal.

MANAGEMENT

- Hospitalize women with heavy bleeding and signs of intravascular volume depletion.
- Progestin usually controls moderate acute anovulatory bleeding within 24–48 hrs [oral medroxyprogesterone (Provera), 10 mg/day × 10 days, or single injection of progesterone (100 mg IM)].
- Chronic anovulatory bleeding responds to medroxyprogesterone during last 10–12 days of menstrual cycle. Continued bleeding on this regimen is indication for dilation and curettage. When necessary, you can achieve maintenance hormonal Rx using estrogen-progestin oral contraceptive (see Fertility Control). When patient wants to become pregnant, refer for consideration of clomiphene Rx.
- NSAIDs may reduce anovulatory bleeding and can be used with oral contraceptives. Danazol is effective but has androgenic side effects.
- In perimenopausal women, begin Rx of anovulatory bleeding with monthly medroxyprogesterone (10 mg/day × 10–12 days) after you have adequately evaluated possibility of serious structural cause. Oral contraceptives are alternative for nonsmokers without cardiovascular risk factors.
- Consideration of surgical options including endometrial ablation and hysterectomy may be appropriate when medical Rx fails to control chronic bleeding. Maintain supportive role in decision making, adequately informing patients about harms and benefits of surgical intervention. Especially important that women approaching menopause appreciate that symptoms will diminish over time with "watchful waiting" and symptomatic Rx.

BIBLIOGRAPHY

■ For the current annotated bibliography on abnormal vaginal bleeding, see the print edition of *Primary Care Medicine*, 4th edition, Chapter 111, or www.LWWmedicine.com.

Vaginal Discharge

DIFFERENTIAL DIAGNOSIS

GENERAL CONSIDERATIONS

- Among premenopausal women, most common cause of abnormal vaginal discharge is infection. Most common infections are bacterial vaginosis, candidiasis, and *Trichomonas*. Among postmenopausal women, atrophic vaginitis is most common cause. Hx and PE including exam of discharge should focus on these likely causes.

- Dx of bacterial vaginosis is made by presence of 3 of these criteria: vaginal pH >4.5; thin, white, homogenous discharge; positive amine test; and clue cells on saline wet prep.

- Trichomoniasis occurs in about 3 million women annually. *T. vaginalis*, a small, mobile protozoan, is usually sexually transmitted but can survive in hot tubs, tap water, and chlorinated swimming pools, so sexual contact may not be only mode of transmission. Symptoms include vaginal discharge, pruritus, dyspareunia (caused by vulvar edema), dysuria, urinary frequency, and abdominal pain. Vaginal discharge may be minimal or abundant, frothy, and foul smelling. Signs and symptoms alone are insufficient to make Dx. Sensitivity of wet-mount prep for trichomonads is 25%.

- With candidiasis, discharge is often thick and white. Symptoms are rapid in onset occurring shortly before menstruation.

- Cytolytic vaginosis is caused by overgrowth of lactobacilli and possibly other bacteria, with cytolysis of vaginal epithelium and frothy white discharge.

COMMON CAUSES OF VAGINAL DISCHARGE

- Infectious
  - Bacterial vaginosis
  - Vulvovaginal candidiasis
  - *T. vaginitis*
  - Mucopurulent cervicitis (*C. trachomatis*)
  - Gonorrhea
  - Condyloma acuminata
  - Herpesvirus type 2
  - Cytolytic vaginosis
- Normal discharge secondary to hormonal changes
  - Physiologic leukorrhea (midcycle cervical mucus/postintercourse)
  - Atrophic vaginitis
- Other
  - Chemical/allergic vaginitis, foreign body
  - Desquamative inflammatory vaginitis (erosive lichen planus)
  - Chronic cervicitis
  - Cervical ectropion
  - Cervical polyps
  - Cervical and endometrial cancer
  - Collagen vascular diseases

WORKUP

HISTORY

- Hx should include onset, appearance, amount, and odor (if any) of discharge, and associated symptoms. Note relation of discharge to phase of menstrual cycle, coitus, and use of medication (especially antibiotics). Details about associated symptoms, such as dysuria, pruritus, pain, dyspareunia, and skin rash, provide additional information.
- Asking patient for detailed sexual Hx will aid in understanding whether she is at risk for infections. Ask about exposure to STDs and whether patient's partner has penile discharge or lesion.
- Review known allergies in conjunction with use of spermicides and douches. Ask about use of foreign bodies and bubble baths, soaps, or genital deodorants.
- Consider Hx of previous vaginal infection, DM, or recent use of antibiotics or corticosteroids in search for alterations in vaginal flora or host defenses.
- Inquire about self-Rx, because OTC antifungal medication is now readily available. Women with chronic or recurrent discharge also turn to wide range of alternative Rx, including oral and vaginal acidophilus pills, oral and vaginal yogurt, and douches with vinegar and boric acid. These self-remedies may complicate Dx and management.

PHYSICAL EXAM

- Inspect vulva and vaginal canal for evidence of lesions, discharge, erythema, atrophy, or prolapse. During speculum exam, look at cervical surface for lesions, erosion, erythema, or friability.
- Color, consistency, pH, and odor of discharge can provide useful clues to etiology.
- On bimanual exam, check for tenderness on cervical motion and for adnexal and uterine masses.

LAB STUDIES

- Wet-mount exam of discharge is simple and potentially diagnostic. Test pH and examine slide before sample dries. Sample pH for *Trichomonas* is usually >5.0.
- Saline wet mount from patients with bacterial vaginosis characteristically shows few polymorphonuclear neutrophils and many (>20%) clue cells. Two additional diagnostic criteria for bacterial vaginosis are sample pH >4.5 and positive amine test (presence of "fishy odor" after adding potassium hydroxide to sample).
- In suspected candidal infection, adding potassium hydroxide to sample dissolves most cellular material except for filamentous hyphae and budding forms of *Candida* (sensitivity, 40–80%). Gram's stain has higher sensitivity. Vaginal pH is closer to normal.
- Wet smear of discharge in suspected cytolytic vaginosis should show few WBCs; no *Trichomonas*, clue cells, or filamentous hyphae; and increased lactobacilli with evidence of epithelial cytolysis and pH close to normal.
- When you suspect gonorrhea and chlamydia, Gram's stain of discharge can yield additional information (see Chlamydial Infection; Gonorrhea).

Presence of >10 WBCs/oil-immersion field distinguishes chlamydia from other types of cervicitis. Follow up suspicion of chlamydial infection with direct immunofluorescent staining or culture.

- CBC is indicated if pelvic pain or dysuria is present. Obtain urinalysis to check for pyuria and bacteriuria, especially with dysuria or flank pain.

- Women with poorly controlled and, occasionally, new-onset DM may have persistent or recurrent yeast infections; fasting blood sugar may be useful.

- Perform Pap smear, recognizing that it may be abnormal in presence of inflammation (see Cervical Cancer). In patients with obvious infection, deferring Pap test until after vaginitis or cervicitis Rx may be reasonable. Pap testing and probably colposcopy are indicated with chronic inflammation of cervix, however.

MANAGEMENT

- Most effective Rx for bacterial vaginosis is metronidazole, 500 mg PO bid × 7 days. Single dose of 2 g metronidazole is also effective, less likely to lead to secondary yeast infections, and generally recommended for Rx during pregnancy. Instruct patients to avoid alcohol while taking drug because of disulfiram-like effects.

- Rx with metronidazole intravaginal gel 0.75% bid × 5 days is equally effective with fewer systemic side effects but is more expensive than oral metronidazole regimens. Disadvantage may be mitigated by recent evidence that once-daily dosing with gel × 5 days is as effective as bid dosing. Oral (300 mg bid × 7 days) or topical (2% cream vaginally qhs × 7 days) clindamycin is alternative when there is contraindication to metronidazole.

- First-line Rx for candidiasis is OTC topical miconazole (Monistat), clotrimazole (Mycelex), and butoconazole (Femstat), generally for 3–7 days. These agents often provide symptomatic relief within 2 days, but encourage patients to complete Rx course (3–7 days).

- Nystatin is also effective when used for 7–14 days. Reserve prescription regimens for women who do not improve with OTC regimens. Terconazole (Terazol; 0.4% cream × 7 days, 0.8% for 3 days, or 80-mg suppository for 3 days) may be more effective against *C. glabrata*. One-day oral regimens include fluconazole, 150 mg; or itraconazole, 200 mg.

- For recurrent vulvovaginal candidiasis, 100 mg/day ketoconazole × 6 mos has been used, but hepatotoxicity is a concern. Fluconazole, 150 mg weekly or monthly, is alternative with less hepatotoxicity. When infection is related to menstruation, 100-mg clotrimazole vaginal suppositories for several nights preceding menstruation, or 200 mg ketoconazole orally bid × 5–7 days beginning before menstruation, are alternatives.

- Metronidazole is Rx of choice for trichomoniasis. Most effective if administered orally in dosage of 500 mg bid × 7 days, with cure rates up to 95%. One-time oral dose of 2 g is less effective (80–88%) but has better compliance rates. Efficacy for single-dose Rx is increased if you treat male partner. Recommended Rx for recurrent *T. vaginalis* infections is additional 1-wk Rx with metronidazole (500 mg bid) and, if symptoms persist, 2 g/day × 3–5 days. Instruct patients to avoid alcohol while taking drug because of disulfiram-like effects.

- For cytolytic vaginosis, prescribe sodium bicarbonate douches 2–3 times/wk and then 1–2 times/wk prn. Douching solution should include 30–60 g sodium bicarbonate to 1 L warm water.

- Mucopurulent cervicitis results from chlamydia and responds to doxycycline (100 mg bid × 7 days) or erythromycin (500 mg tid × 7 days), with Rx of partner and follow-up culture 1 wk after completed Rx.

- Treat atrophic vaginitis with estrogen cream. Daily use for 1–2 wks followed with Rx for 1–2 days for occasional symptom control is recommended. Oral conjugated estrogens are less effective for vaginal symptoms.

- Refer for colposcopy and biopsy women with suspicious cervical or vaginal lesions, especially with erosions and ulcerations that do not clear with Rx of known pathogen.

- Provide patient ed about normal responses to hormone changes, measures to avoid infection and irritation, and importance of completing prescribed course of Rx.

BIBLIOGRAPHY

- For the current annotated bibliography on vaginal discharge, see the print edition of *Primary Care Medicine*, 4th edition, Chapter 117, or www.LWWmedicine.com.

Vulvar Pruritus

DIFFERENTIAL DIAGNOSIS

GENERAL CONSIDERATIONS

- Age provides significant cue to cause. Infections, chemical irritants, and allergic reactions are common in young and older women. Atrophic vaginitis, dermatoses, and carcinoma become concerns with advancing age.

CAUSES OF VULVAR PRURITUS

- Infections
  - *Candida*
  - *Trichomonas*
  - Bacterial vaginosis
  - Hidradenitis suppurativa
  - Herpes simplex
  - HPV
  - Dermatophytes
  - Scabies
- Dermatoses
  - Lichen sclerosus
  - Lichen simplex chronicus
  - Lichen planus (erosive vaginitis)
  - Psoriasis
  - Seborrheic dermatitis
- Low estrogen states: atrophic vaginitis
  - Postpartum
  - Postmenopausal
- Premalignant/malignant conditions
  - Vulvar intraepithelial neoplasia
  - Squamous cell carcinoma
  - Adenocarcinoma
- Irritants
  - Contact dermatitis

WORKUP

HISTORY

- Inquire about vaginal discharge, skin rashes, urinary incontinence, vulvar lesions, and other sites of itching. Identify possible irritants and allergies, such as creams, soaps, bubble baths, vaginal deodorants, douches, and contraceptive foams.
- Sexual Hx or presence of genital itching in partners or roommates may suggest infection or infestation.
- Information related to duration of problem and responses to prior Rx can be useful.

- Ascertain presence of ulceration or nodule that has persisted or grown. Obtain Hx of HPV- or HSV-associated lesions or abnormal Pap smears.

PHYSICAL EXAM

- Inspect vulva and perineal skin for macules, papules, scaling, erythema, ulcerations, pigmented lesions, hypopigmentation, excoriation, rash, lice, and mites. Close look at hair shaft may reveal lice eggs (nits), which are pathognomonic of infestation (see Scabies and Pediculosis).
- Speculum exam identifies vaginitis or discharge (see Vaginal Discharge). Palpate inguinal nodes.

LAB STUDIES

- Obtain smear of discharge for identification of organism and urinalysis for glycosuria.
- Refer women with persistent suspicious vulvar lesions to dermatologist or gynecologist for biopsy.

MANAGEMENT

- Atrophic vaginitis responds well to topical estrogen cream (see Menopause). Occasionally, patient may use antihistamine at night to relieve itching and break itch/scratch cycle. In cases in which etiology is known, short-term use of steroid creams may reduce inflammation.
- Patient should stop self-Rx with potential irritants. Educate women about factors that contribute to vulvar irritation, including excessive hygiene or moisture (secondary to tight-fitting jeans, panty hose, nylon underwear, or exercise clothes). Teach them to use hand mirror to inspect vulva, looking for moles, changes in pigmentation, warts, ulcers, and sores.

BIBLIOGRAPHY

- For the current annotated bibliography on vulvar pruritus, see the print edition of *Primary Care Medicine*, 4th edition, Chapter 114, or www.LWWmedicine.com.

Genitourinary Problems

Benign Prostatic Hyperplasia

MANAGEMENT

- PCP should objectively assess severity of lower urinary tract symptoms and determine their effect on patient's quality of life.
- All patients with symptoms likely caused by BPH should have baseline creatinine determination and urinalysis.
- Routine urinary tract imaging is unnecessary. Upper tract imaging, preferably by ultrasonography, is indicated if hydronephrosis is concern (large postvoid residual urine volume or elevated creatinine level).
- Urine flow rate measurement may be useful when symptomatology is confusing or ambiguous; it helps identify patients who have symptoms but little evidence of obstruction (peak flow rates >15 mL/s).
- Make patients aware of possible coexistence of prostate cancer and BPH and availability of further evaluation, including PSA screening. Impact of early detection on prostate cancer mortality is doubtful in men with life expectancy <10 yrs.
- Follow most patients expectantly unless evidence of hydronephrosis, recurrent or persistent infection, or deterioration in renal function is present. Such complications warrant prompt surgical attention. Patients should avoid nighttime fluids and drugs that affect lower urinary tract function.
- Selective alpha $_1$ blocker Rx (doxazosin, prazosin, terazosin, tamsulosin) can provide symptomatic relief for some patients.
- 5-α-Reductase inhibitor finasteride may be worth considering in persons with larger prostate glands (reflected by baseline PSA levels >3.2 ng/mL), primarily to reduce future risk for acute retention or surgery. It is less effective than alpha blocker Rx in reducing lower urinary tract symptoms in short run.
- Elective urologic consultation is indicated when Dx is confusing or when, despite medical Rx, quality of life is sufficiently compromised to warrant consideration of operation to achieve symptomatic relief.
- Less invasive Rx for BPH provide increased array of Rx options in coming years, but prostatectomy remains standard for long-term symptom relief.

BIBLIOGRAPHY

- For the current annotated bibliography on benign prostatic hyperplasia, see the print edition of *Primary Care Medicine*, 4th edition, Chapter 138, or www.LWWmedicine.com.

Chlamydial Infection

SCREENING AND/OR PREVENTION

- Screening for chlamydial genitourinary infection is worthwhile, but universal screening is not recommended in most primary care practices because prevalence of asymptomatic infection in that setting is likely below threshold of cost-effective universal screening.
- In settings with very high prevalence (e.g., >10%), universal screening deserves consideration.
- Antigen testing becomes cost-effective among patients whose pretest risk is >7%. Culturing becomes cost-effective among patients whose pretest risk is >14%. DNA-based PCR testing lowers prevalence threshold for cost-effective screening.
- Selective screening is recommended based on clinical estimate of risk for chlamydial infection.
- Because prevalence of chlamydial infection among sexually active girls and women aged <21 is high, and because risk for sterility resulting from subclinical infection is also high, annual screening of patients with or without symptoms has been recommended.
- CDC recommends annual screening for women aged 20–24 if either major risk factor for chlamydial infection is present: (1) lack of barrier contraception, or (2) new or multiple partners in preceding 3 mos. Also screen women aged >24 with both risk factors.
- Screen for chlamydial infection all men presenting with urethral discharge and all women with mucopurulent cervicitis.
- Partner notification and Rx, by provider or patient referral, is critical to interrupt cycle of reinfection by asymptomatic partners.
- Although antigen testing of cervical or urethral swab is least expensive screening method, DNA-based PCR is recommended as testing method of choice, especially in settings of lower prevalence, because its sensitivity is superior and it allows testing of urine in addition to cervical specimens, which lowers prevalence threshold at which screening is cost-effective.
- Urge all young women who do not desire pregnancy to insist on condom use during intercourse.

MANAGEMENT

- For urethritis or cervicitis without PID, single 1-g dose of azithromycin is Rx of choice. Alternatives are 7-day courses of doxycycline (100 mg bid), tetracycline (500 mg qid), or erythromycin (500 mg qid).

BIBLIOGRAPHY

- For the current annotated bibliography on chlamydial infection, see the print edition of *Primary Care Medicine*, 4th edition, Chapter 125, or www.LWWmedicine.com.

DIFFERENTIAL DIAGNOSIS

IN WOMEN

- Organisms other than *N. gonorrhoeae* capable of producing genital infections include *Chlamydia*, *Gardnerella*, *Trichomonas*, and *Candida* (see Vaginal Discharge).
- Differential Dx of gonococcal salpingitis and peritonitis mainly encompasses causes of nongonococcal PID (see Menstrual or Pelvic Pain), but other conditions, such as appendicitis, ectopic pregnancy, hemorrhagic ovarian cysts, and endometriosis, can produce similar clinical findings and often require urgent Rx very different from that of PID.

IN MEN

- Causes of NGU enter differential Dx (see Urethritis in Men). Also consider gonococcal infection among causes of pharyngitis (see Pharyngitis) and proctitis (see Anorectal Complaints).

WORKUP

HISTORY

- Dx of gonorrhea requires high index of suspicion and sexual Hx.

PHYSICAL EXAM

- PE findings in men with urethritis are usually normal except for purulent urethral discharge.
- In asymptomatic women, PE findings are normal, but cervicitis may produce cervical inflammation, discharge, and marked cervical tenderness. Adnexal tenderness and fullness are signs of salpingitis and may be unilateral or bilateral in women with gonorrhea. Tubal abscesses may be suspected because of palpable mass, and rebound tenderness is sign of pelvic peritonitis.
- PID caused by organisms other than gonococcus may present similarly. Clinical features favoring gonococcus include purulent cervical discharge, onset early in menstrual cycle, no Hx of PID, and exposure to male partner with urethritis.

LAB STUDIES

- Gram's stain of urethral discharge can be highly reliable diagnostic tool. Sensitivity of Gram's stain is >95% in symptomatic men but declines to 50–60% in those with asymptomatic urethral infection. Gram's stains are much less reliable in cervical, rectal, and pharyngeal infections.
- Cultures confirming Dx of gonorrhea are mandatory in both sexes. *N. gonorrhoeae* is fragile and fastidious organism that requires special lab handling.

- Gonococcus is readily killed by drying; plate all cultures promptly. Modified Thayer-Martin medium at room temperature is preferred for specimens obtained from genital, anal, or pharyngeal sites; storage of cultures in carbon dioxide atmosphere recommended.
- In men, cultures of anterior urethra suffice unless you suspect homosexual contacts, in which case cultures of anal canal and pharynx are also indicated.
- In women, culture endocervix by inserting swab into cervical os through speculum lubricated only with water. In all women, rectal cultures are indicated because rectal infection can result simply through direct spread from genital tract.
- If pharyngitis suspected, throat culture is mandatory.
- If acute arthritis present, obtain joint fluid by arthrocentesis and evaluate with cell counts, Gram's stain, and culture.
- Blood cultures are indicated in patients with fever, skin lesions, and tenosynovitis or arthritis.

MANAGEMENT

UNCOMPLICATED GONORRHEA (INCLUDING URETHRAL, CERVICAL, AND RECTAL INFECTION)

- Prescribe ceftriaxone (125 mg IM once), cefixime (400 mg PO once), ciprofloxacin (500 mg PO once), or ofloxacin (400 mg PO once) + azithromycin (1 g PO once) or doxycycline (100 mg bid × 7 days).
- Prescribe spectinomycin (2 g IM once) for patients allergic to β-lactam antibiotics (i.e., cephalosporins and penicillins) or who cannot take fluoroquinolones (e.g., pregnant women).
- Prescribe erythromycin base (500 mg qid × 7 days) for patients who cannot take doxycycline (e.g., pregnant women and allergic patients).

DISSEMINATED GONOCOCCAL INFECTION

- Hospitalize initially and begin ceftriaxone (1 g IV or IM q24h × 7 days).
- Treat with higher doses for more prolonged period if meningitis, endocarditis, or osteomyelitis is present.
- Treat with spectinomycin (2 g IM q12h × 7 days) those who are allergic to β-lactam antibiotics.
- Discharge those who respond well to initial 1–2 days of parenteral Rx, provided they return daily for IM ceftriaxone or complete 1 wk of oral Rx with ciprofloxacin (500 mg bid).
- Treat also for chlamydial infection, as in uncomplicated disease.

BIBLIOGRAPHY

- For the current annotated bibliography on gonorrhea, see the print edition of *Primary Care Medicine*, 4th edition, Chapter 137, or www.LWWmedicine.com.

Hematuria

DIFFERENTIAL DIAGNOSIS

MICROSCOPIC HEMATURIA

- Definitions of significant hematuria are necessarily arbitrary. Nonetheless >8 RBCs/HPF is reasonable cutoff for separating likelihood of benign cause from that of potentially serious disease.
- Microscopic hematuria discovered on routine urinalysis may have harmless etiology, especially in asymptomatic, otherwise healthy, young patients. Fever, strenuous exercise, and distance running are among harmless causes of microscopic hematuria in these patients.
- Most commonly associated with infection and benign prostatic hypertrophy.
- Prevalence of serious underlying disease (e.g., cancer, polycystic disease) in community-based study of asymptomatic microscopic hematuria is 0.1%, compared to 10% in referred populations.
- Population-based studies indicate that 1–5% of children and adults have microhematuria on routine urinalysis; <2% of these patients have serious and treatable urinary tract disease. Incidence of urinary tract cancers rises dramatically with age and is >2 times higher in men.
- Normal repeat urinalysis in healthy young person requires no further investigation other than follow-up urinalysis in 1–2 mos. In older patients further evaluation is necessary even if repeat urinalysis is negative.
- Dx in 500 referred cases of asymptomatic microscopic hematuria (% patients)
  - Kidneys (6.2)
    - Calculus (3.4)
    - Cyst (1.2)
    - Hydronephrosis (0.6)
    - Tumor (0.4)
    - Others (0.6)
  - Ureters (0.8)
    - Calculus (0.4)
    - Ureterocele (0.4)
    - Bladder (8.6)
    - Infection (6.6)
    - Tumor (1.8)
    - Others (0.2)
  - Prostate (23.6)
    - BPH (23.6)
  - Urethra (23.4)
    - Infection (21.2)
    - Calculus (1.8)
    - Others (0.4)
  - Essential hematuria (44.0)

From Greene LF, O'Shaughnessy EJ Jr, Hendricks ED. Study of 500 patients with asymptomatic microhematuria. JAMA 1956;161:610, with permission.

GROSS HEMATURIA

- Most commonly associated with infections and neoplasms; requires thorough investigation.
- Dx in 1,000 referred cases of gross hematuria (% patients)
  - Kidneys (15.0)
    - Tumor (3.5)
    - Infection (3.0)
    - Calculus (2.7)
    - Obstruction (1.5)
    - Others (2.3)
  - Ureters (6.5)
    - Calculus (5.3)
    - Tumor (0.7)
    - Others (0.5)
  - Bladder (39.5)
    - Infection (22.0)
    - Tumor (14.9)
    - Others (2.6)
  - Prostate (23.6)
    - BPH (12.5)
    - Infection (9.0)
    - Tumor (2.1)
  - Urethra (4.3)
    - Stricture (1.7)
    - Calculus (1.3)
    - Others (1.3)
  - Essential hematuria (8.5)

From Lee LW, Davis E, et al. Gross urinary hemorrhage: a symptom, not a disease. JAMA 1953;153:782, with permission.

WORKUP

HISTORY

- Hx is important in narrowing scope of workup. With Hx of trauma, direct attention to possible renal, ureteral, or urethral injury. Massive hematuria is usually associated with bladder neoplasm, benign prostatic hyperplasia, or trauma. Passage of large, bulky clots implicates bladder as source, whereas long, shoestring-shaped clots suggest ureteral origin.
- Hx of analgesic excess makes analgesic nephropathy possible.
- With Hx of nephritis, consider chronic nephritis as cause of hematuria. Family Hx of renal diseases may suggest polycystic kidney disease or hereditary nephritis.
- Benign familial hematuria is inherited in pattern consistent with autosomal dominant transmission; checking for hematuria in relatives may avoid extensive workup in otherwise healthy-appearing patients.
- Harmless, self-limited forms of microscopic hematuria are suggested by recent Hx of strenuous exercise, distance running, or minor febrile illness.

PHYSICAL EXAM

- Check for fever, HTN, rash, purpura, petechiae, friction rub, heart murmur, or joint swelling. Presence of HTN suggests renal parenchymal disease.

- Examine abdomen for enlargement of one or both kidneys, liver, or spleen.
- Thorough exam of prostate in men and pelvis in women is essential.

LAB STUDIES

- Examine urine sediment for clues to etiology, including WBCs and bacteria (cystitis), WBC casts (pyelonephritis or interstitial nephritis), and RBC casts (glomerulonephritis). Urine specimen for culture is indicated when pyuria is noted (see Urinary Tract Infection). It should include culture for acid-fast bacillus if sterile pyuria and hematuria persist.
- Perform three-glass test (see Prostatitis) to attempt to identify bleeding site. Initial hematuria is usually associated with anterior urethral lesions, such as stenosis and urethritis. Terminal hematuria usually arises from lesion in posterior urethra, bladder neck, or trigone. Total hematuria is associated with lesions at level of bladder or above.
- Check renal function in suspected renal parenchymal disease. With renal colic, strain urine to detect calculi or papillae. Send 3 first-void morning urine specimens for cytology in patients aged >40. Normal findings on cytology do not rule out malignancy (see Bladder Cancer); cystoscopy is usually indicated. If these tests do not define cause of hematuria, perform IV pyelogram with tomograms.
- Obtain postvoid film to assess amount of postvoid residual urine, which can help estimate degree of bladder neck obstruction. Ultrasound, body CT, and MRI are useful to differentiate solid mass from cystic lesion.
- Renal angiography is reserved for evaluation of possible renal trauma, suspected renal masses, and possible arteriovenous malformations.
- In patients aged >50, proceed to cystoscopy if less invasive measures have not determined cause of hematuria (see Bladder Cancer). Procedure is particularly useful during periods of active bleeding.
- Refer patients with evidence of glomerulonephritis to nephrologist for consideration of renal biopsy, which is indicated only to establish Dx that will affect Rx selection (see Proteinuria).
- When thorough workup does not reveal cause, patient is said to have essential hematuria. Long-term prognosis is excellent.

BIBLIOGRAPHY

- For the current annotated bibliography on hematuria, see the print edition of *Primary Care Medicine*, 4th edition, Chapter 129, or www.LWWmedicine.com.

Incontinence and Lower Urinary Tract Dysfunction

DIFFERENTIAL DIAGNOSIS

GENERAL CONSIDERATIONS

- Causes of incontinence are best classified by mechanisms, each of which has characteristic presentation: detrusor instability (frequent episodes of urgency with loss of small volumes), stress incontinence (triggered by straining), reflex incontinence (Hx of spinal cord injury or neurological deficit), overflow incontinence (frequent loss of small volumes with Hx of obstructive symptoms), and functional incontinence (physically or mentally impaired patient).

IMPORTANT CAUSES OF INCONTINENCE

- Detrusor instability
  - Bladder infection
  - Chronic cystitis
  - CNS disease (dementia, stroke)
  - Detrusor hyperreflexia
  - Detrusor hypertrophy
  - Irradiation
- Stress incontinence
  - Aging
  - Autonomic neuropathy
  - Estrogen deficiency
  - Pelvic laxity
  - Perineal injury
  - Urologic surgery
- Reflex incontinence
  - Disk herniation
  - Multiple sclerosis
  - Spinal cord disease
  - Tumor
- Overflow incontinence
  - Diabetes mellitus (DM)
  - Medications
  - Outflow obstruction
  - Peripheral neuropathy
  - Sacral cord lesion
  - Tabes dorsalis
  - Vitamin B_{12} deficiency
- Functional incontinence
  - Acute illness
  - Medications
  - Psychiatric disease

WORKUP

HISTORY

- Focus on circumstances, precipitants, timing, frequency, and volume of urine loss, presence of warning symptoms, and intactness of perineal and bladder sensation.
- When Hx is incomplete, ask patient or family to keep diary of events and contributing factors (time of urination; estimate of volume; symptoms associated with each void, such as leakage; and any precipitating events, such as laughing or coughing).
- Question patient and family about medications, especially those with anticholinergic, α- and β-adrenergic blocking, tranquilizing, or diuretic effects (e.g., tricyclic antidepressants, major and minor tranquilizers, decongestants, and antihypertensives). Note any excessive use of coffee, tea, or alcohol.
- Ask patients with isolated urinary frequency about increased thirst, which is consistent with DM and diabetes insipidus (DI). Compulsive water drinkers with psychogenic polydipsia may deny intake of water but do not report nocturia (symptom of DM and DI). Sudden onset of intense thirst for ice water is suggestive of DI.

PHYSICAL EXAM

- Note general appearance and any lack of personal hygiene.
- Urogenital exam should include suprapubic palpation and percussion of bladder after voiding to detect distention and masses.
- Check rectum for impaction or prostatic enlargement in men.
- Examine women with stress incontinence in lithotomy position. Note pelvic motion and continence during cough or Valsalva's maneuver.
- Check vaginal mucosa for atrophic changes (red, thin mucosa with watery discharge) indicative of inadequate estrogen. Perform bimanual exam, noting any uterine or adnexal masses.
- Test for stress incontinence with bladder full unless problem is severe and requires little provocation. Focus assessment of neurologic control of voiding on integrity of autonomic reflex arc by checking bulbocavernosus reflex or anal sphincter control.

LAB STUDIES

- Urinalysis and several chemistry studies (BUN, creatinine, and glucose) are appropriate for most patients.
- Urine culture may be indicated to exclude concurrent infection.
- Pelvic ultrasonography offers noninvasive method of assessing postvoid residual when you suspect outflow obstruction or detrusor failure. Straight catheterization after voiding is alternative. Volume >50 mL is abnormal.
- Cystometrogram is rarely needed but can help to sort out complicated mixed conditions.
- Measuring urine flow rates provides information on outflow obstruction and aids in monitoring progression of obstruction.
- Check patients with polyuria for glycosuria, hypercalcemia, and hypokalemia. Those with normal levels should have urine-concentrating ability tested by measuring urine osmolality after 8 hrs of fluid

restriction (usually overnight). Normal persons and those with psychogenic polydipsia can concentrate urine to >700 mOsm/L after 8 hrs fluid restriction. Inability to concentrate requires further testing, including measurement of serum osmolality before and after water restriction and parenteral administration of ADH. Direct measurement of ADH may be helpful (see Diabetes Insipidus).

MANAGEMENT

GENERAL MEASURES

- Restrict fluid loads, coffee, tea, and alcohol.
- Limit use of diuretics; if they are necessary, give them in morning.
- Give anticholinergic drugs for nonurologic purposes with care and in lowest possible dosages.
- Avoid use of indwelling catheters because of risk for infection, exacerbation of detrusor instability, and leakage.
- Avoid use of condom catheters, except for short, well-supervised periods.
- Advise use of adsorbent pad for patients with refractory symptoms and recommend that they change it frequently to prevent skin breakdown.
- If long-term indwelling catheterization is unavoidable, catheter should be inserted only by trained personnel under aseptic conditions, drained with bag always below patient's bladder, manipulated as little as possible, irrigated only if flow is reduced, changed if blocked, and removed if upper UTI infection is suspected.
- Antibiotic prophylaxis is not recommended.

DRUGS USED TO TREAT INCONTINENCE

- Detrusor instability
  - Imipramine hydrochloride (Tofranil): 10–25 mg qd–qid
  - Oxybutynin chloride (Ditropan): 2.5–5.0 mg tid
  - Tolterodine (Detrol): 1–2 mg bid
  - Detrusor atony
  - Bethanechol chloride (Urecholine); 5–25 mg bid–qid
  - Prazosin (Minipress): 1–5 mg bid–qid
  - Doxazosin (Cardura): 2–8 mg/day
  - Terazosin (Hytrin): 1–10 mg/day
  - Tamsulosin (Flomax): 0.4 mg qd–bid
- Sphincter incompetency
  - Imipramine hydrochloride (Tofranil): 10–25 mg qd–qid
  - Estrogen cream: (Premarin; in women) qd initially then 2–3 times/wk
  - Phenylpropanolamine: 25 mg qd–qid
- Reflex incontinence
  - Prazosin (Minipress): 1–5 mg bid–qid
  - Doxazosin (Cardura): 2–8 mg/day
  - Terazosin (Hytrin): 1–10 mg/day
  - Tamsulosin (Flomax): 0.4 mg qd–bid

FOR DETRUSOR INSTABILITY (URGE INCONTINENCE)

- Teach patient to void at regular, frequent intervals. Patients can learn to suppress urge to void by contracting pelvic muscles and then relaxing them slowly or by engaging in distracting activities (such as mathematical calculations or conversations). Over time, they can increase intervals. Sometimes, merely keeping voiding diary improves urinary control.

- Provide bedside commode or urinal for patient.
- Initiate trial of tricyclic agent, such as imipramine (10–100 mg/day in divided doses).
- Initiate trial of agent with smooth-muscle relaxant and anticholinergic properties, such as oxybutynin (2.5–5 mg tid). Lower doses can be effective in elderly, avoiding untoward CNS side effects and intolerable dry mouth. Selective bladder smooth-muscle relaxant tolterodine (1–2 mg bid) has fewer side effects than oxybutynin and may be better tolerated.

FOR DETRUSOR ATONY (OVERFLOW INCONTINENCE)

- For acute and chronic obstruction, place indwelling catheter or repeatedly catheterize patient to decompress bladder.
- If this does not restore bladder function, teach patient to void while performing Credé's maneuver (suprapubic external compression) or Valsalva's maneuver.
- Add alpha blocker such as prazosin (2–20 mg/day in divided doses), doxazosin (2–8 mg/day), terazosin (1–10 mg/day), or tamsulosin (0.4–0.8 mg/day) to reduce sphincter resistance.
- Add bethanechol (25–125 mg/day in divided doses) to augment bladder contraction.
- Monitor effects of these agents by checking postvoid residuals; patients with residual >300 mL require repeated sterile catheterization on intermittent basis (bid–qid).

FOR SPHINCTER INCOMPETENCE (STRESS INCONTINENCE)

- Instruct male patients to exercise by voluntarily contracting anal sphincter slowly 15 times/day or bid.
- Instruct female patients in Kegel exercises.
- For female patients with evidence of atrophic vaginitis, prescribe topical estrogen cream. Patient should apply daily for first 3 wks, then 2–3 times/wk thereafter to maintain sufficient estrogen to restore internal sphincter and urethral tone in postmenopausal women. Continuous use may increase risk for uterine cancer in women with intact uteri. Concurrent use of progestin eliminates this risk (see Menopause).
- Prescribe α-adrenergic agonist phenylpropanolamine (50–100 mg/day in divided doses) for patients who need more than exercises. This agent is especially useful for weakened pelvic muscles and after surgical instrumentation of urethra. It is found in most OTC cold remedies, but do not give to patients with HTN.
- Try course of imipramine (10–100 mg/day in divided doses) for those with bladder irritability and stress incontinence.
- Pessaries come in variety of shapes and can improve continence. Patient must change and clean them regularly.
- Penile clamp may be necessary in men who do not respond to other measures. Careful monitoring and competent patient are necessary.

REFLEX INCONTINENCE

- In patient with bladder-sphincter dyssynergy, try pharmacologically decompressing bladder by giving prazosin (2–20 mg/day in divided doses), doxazosin (2–8 mg/day), terazosin (1–10 mg/day), or tamsulosin (0.4–0.8 mg/day).
- Consider agent used for detrusor instability (see above). Patient may require sphincterotomy to ensure bladder emptying.

FOR FUNCTIONAL INCONTINENCE

- Prime effort is to ease patient's access to urinal, bedpan, or commode. Bedside placement is obvious solution. For more disabled patients, consider regular use of absorbent diapers, frequent straight catheterization, or (rarely) condom or indwelling catheterization.

INDICATIONS FOR REFERRAL

- Promptly refer incontinent patients with suspected cord lesion or other neurologic injury.
- Urologic referral is needed in cases of outflow tract obstruction, especially if severe enough to cause hypotonic bladder and large postvoid residual (>100 mL). Risk for ureteral reflux and hydronephrosis makes definitive Rx essential.
- Women with refractory stress incontinence are candidates for reconstructive surgery; refer to surgeon experiences in correcting pelvic incompetence.

BIBLIOGRAPHY

- For the current annotated bibliography on incontinence and lower urinary tract dysfunction, see the print edition of *Primary Care Medicine*, 4th edition, Chapter 134, or www.LWWmedicine.com.

Nephrolithiasis

DIFFERENTIAL DIAGNOSIS

GENERAL CONSIDERATIONS

- Two-thirds of all renal calculi are composed of calcium oxalate or calcium oxalate + calcium phosphate. Stones of pure uric acid and those of struvite or magnesium ammonium each account for about 10%. Cystine, xanthine, and silicate stones occur infrequently. In many instances, stone formation is manifestation of systemic disease.

IMPORTANT CONDITIONS ASSOCIATED WITH NEPHROLITHIASIS

- Calcium stones
  - Increased GI calcium absorption
    - Primary hyperparathyroidism
    - Sarcoidosis
    - Vitamin D excess
    - Milk-alkali syndrome
    - Idiopathic nephrolithiasis
    - Increased bone calcium resorption
    - Primary hyperparathyroidism
    - Neoplastic disorders
    - Immobilization
    - Distal renal tubular acidosis
  - Renal calcium leak
    - Idiopathic hypercalciuria
  - Hyperoxaluria
    - Small-bowel disease
    - Enzymatic deficiency
    - Pyridoxine deficiency
    - Increased ingestion
- Magnesium ammonium phosphate stones
  - Alkaline environment
    - UTI caused by urea-splitting organism
- Uric acid stones
  - Increased uric acid production
    - Primary gout
    - Secondary gout (myeloproliferative disorder, chemotherapy)
- Cystine stones
  - Inherited disorder for amino acid transport
- Xanthine stones
  - Xanthine oxidase deficiency
  - Use of xanthine oxidase inhibitor

WORKUP

OVERALL STRATEGY

- Knowledge of stone composition is essential to rational management of patient with recurrent nephrolithiasis. Obtaining stone for chemical analysis is single most valuable element of evaluation.

HISTORY

- When stone is unavailable for analysis, clinical Hx can be helpful in evaluation. Obtain patient age at onset of nephrolithiasis because metabolic disorders such as hyperoxaluria, cystinuria, xanthinuria, and renal tubular acidosis are often associated with stones at early age; idiopathic calcareous nephrolithiasis and primary hyperparathyroidism commonly develop after age 30.
- Sex of patient is helpful; idiopathic nephrolithiasis is common in males, whereas primary hyperparathyroidism is more common in females.
- Hx of stones is invaluable if composition has been previously determined. Note any Hx of systemic illness (e.g., sarcoidosis or cancer) and any UTIs.
- Family Hx of nephrolithiasis increases risk for stone disease and may suggest hereditary metabolic disorder.
- Take dietary Hx to rule out excessive protein, oxalate, or calcium intake. Consuming apple and grapefruit juice has been associated with increased risk for stone formation. Alcoholic beverage consumption is associated with decreased risk.
- Check for use of drugs that promote stone formation. Medications that result in increased risk for stone formation include vitamins A, C, and D; loop diuretics; acetazolamide; ammonium chloride; calcium-containing medications; alkali; and antacids. Medications may increase urinary calcium concentrations (vitamin D, loop diuretics, calcium-containing medications, ammonium chloride), alter urinary pH (acetazolamide, ammonium chloride, and alkali), or decrease urinary concentrations of inhibitors (ammonium chloride, absorbable antacids, and alkali can decrease urinary citrate concentration).

PHYSICAL EXAM

- PE is unrevealing in most cases, but check patient for evidence of systemic disease, such as sarcoidosis (lymphadenopathy, organomegaly) or cancer (adenopathy, breast mass, and so forth).

LAB STUDIES

- Lab evaluation should include urinalysis to determine pH, and exam of urinary sediment for crystals. Alkaline pH suggests infection with urea-splitting organisms and struvite formation. Urine culture is needed.
- Obtain serum to determine calcium, uric acid, BUN, and creatinine levels, and collect 24-hr urine for creatinine, calcium, uric acid, and oxalate determinations.
- Repeat determinations of fasting serum calcium and phosphorus are necessary in suspected primary hyperparathyroidism. Obtain serum albumin determination at same time because 40–45% of serum calcium is protein bound. Confirm Dx by obtaining simultaneous PTH determination, which should reveal inappropriately elevated level (see Hypercalcemia).

- If clinical presentation suggests rare cause of nephrolithiasis, such as cystinuria or xanthinuria, send special 24-hr collections of urine for study.
- Radiographic evaluation includes plain film of kidneys, ureter, and bladder, and IV pyelogram.

MANAGEMENT

OVERALL APPROACH

- Preventive Rx is indicated in all patients with nephrolithiasis. Maintaining dilute urine using vigorous fluid Rx around the clock is beneficial in all forms of nephrolithiasis. High fluid intake has been associated with 40% reduction in recurrence risk.

CALCIUM STONES

- Patients with calcium stones can reduce recurrence by restricting dietary protein and sodium. Some benefit from dietary oxalate restriction. Evidence does not support dietary calcium restriction.
- Evaluate patients with recurrent stone formation despite dietary restriction for underlying systemic conditions before initiating drug Rx. Thiazides [e.g., hydrochlorothiazide (50 mg/day)] reduces stone formation.
- Patients with hyperuricosuria benefit from protein restriction and allopurinol. Studies in patients with no identifiable metabolic disorder have demonstrated reduction in new stone formation when patients receive thiazide and allopurinol.

MAGNESIUM AMMONIUM PHOSPHATE STONES

- Acidification of urine with ascorbic acid, along with prolonged (often ≥2 mos) course of appropriate antibiotic Rx to eradicate any Proteus UTI, is essential to prevent struvite stone recurrence.

URIC ACID STONES

- Advise patients with uric acid stones to maintain copious urine flow. Advise allopurinol Rx and alkalinization of urine with 100–150 mEq sodium bicarbonate q24h in divided doses.

CYSTINE STONES

- Copious urine flow and urinary pH >7.5 are important in preventing and dissolving cystine stones. D-penicillamine has also been shown effective, but patient may experience significant side effects.

XANTHINE STONES

- For patients with xanthine stones, limitation of dietary purines, maintenance of urine flow, and maintenance of very high urine pH (>7.6) may reduce recurrence rates.

BIBLIOGRAPHY

- For the current annotated bibliography on nephrolithiasis, see the print edition of *Primary Care Medicine*, 4th edition, Chapter 135, or www.LWWmedicine.com.

Prostatitis

DIFFERENTIAL DIAGNOSIS

ACUTE PROSTATITIS

- Readily evident by clinical presentation and exquisitely tender prostate found on rectal exam.

CHRONIC PROSTATITIS

- Often resembles other common forms of urinary outflow tract obstruction, such as BPH (see Benign Prostatic Hyperplasia), prostatic carcinoma (see Prostate Cancer), and urethral stricture (see Incontinence and Lower Urinary Tract Dysfunction).
- Lower urinary tract irritative symptoms associated with chronic prostatitis may accompany urethritis (see Urethritis in Men), bladder carcinoma (see Bladder Cancer), sphincter dyssynergy, and neurogenic bladder (see Incontinence and Lower Urinary Tract Dysfunction).

WORKUP

HISTORY

Acute Prostatitis

- Check for acute onset of fever, perineal pain, dysuria, and diminished urine flow. Urethral discharge is sometimes reported.

Chronic Prostatitis

- Inquire into recurrent perineal, back, or testicular discomfort, dribbling, slow stream, dysuria, and hematospermia.

PHYSICAL EXAM

Acute Prostatitis

- On rectal exam, prostate is exquisitely tender.
- Exam should proceed cautiously to avoid precipitating bacteremia.
- If symptoms of urinary outflow obstruction are present, check abdomen for bladder distention.

Chronic Prostatitis

- Prostate is enlarged, boggy, and sometimes tender on exam.

LAB STUDIES

Acute Prostatitis

- Obtain Gram's stain and culture of expressed prostatic secretions or VB3 (postmassage urine) and treat immediately.

Chronic Prostatitis

- Document infectious organism and presence of prostatic inflammation with sequential urinary culturing and expressed prostatic secretion exam or with premassage/postmassage test.

MANAGEMENT

ACUTE PROSTATITIS

- For nontoxic patient, oral antibiotic Rx is sufficient. Prescribe TMP-SMX DS (160 mg TMP, 800 mg SMX bid), ciprofloxacin (500 mg bid), or levofloxacin (500 mg/day) for 4 wks. Amoxicillin (500 mg tid), doxycycline (100 mg bid), and carbenicillin indanyl sodium (1 g qid) are reasonable alternatives, all given for 4 wks.

CHRONIC PROSTATITIS

- Treat with prolonged course of antibiotics, such as TMP-SMX DS (160/ 800 mg bid) for 8–12 wks, or ciprofloxacin (500 mg bid) or levofloxacin (500 mg/day) for 4 wks. Latter 2 are considerably more expensive.
- After Rx, follow closely for return of infection. Second course of antibiotics with same or alternative drug for up to 12 wks may be necessary in partially responsive infections. For patients who do not respond initially, prescribe 12-wk course of doxycycline (100 mg bid), erythromycin (500 mg qid), or carbenicillin indanyl sodium (1 g qid).
- Schedule return 1–2 wks after completion of Rx to assess effects of Rx by checking expressed prostatic secretions or VB3 (postmassage urine specimen).
- Prescribe peripheral alpha blocker such as doxazosin (2–8 mg/day), terazosin (2–10 mg/day), or tamsulosin (0.4–0.8 mg/day) with initiation of antibiotic Rx. Continue as long as patient derives benefit.

BIBLIOGRAPHY

- For the current annotated bibliography on prostatitis, see the print edition of *Primary Care Medicine*, 4th edition, Chapter 139, or www.LWWmedicine.com.

Proteinuria

DIFFERENTIAL DIAGNOSIS

GENERAL CONSIDERATIONS

- Excretion of urinary protein >150 mg/24 hrs is clinically significant proteinuria. Causes range from benign conditions, such as exercise and orthostatic proteinuria, to glomerulonephritis with rapidly deteriorating renal function. When proteinuria is found on routine urinalysis, determine whether it is significant, and if so, search noninvasively for treatable underlying conditions, and identify patients who require referral for renal biopsy.
- Proteinuria can be transiently or persistently asymptomatic or symptomatic.

PRESENTATIONS OF PROTEINURIA

- Asymptomatic-transient
  - Exercise
  - Upright posture
  - Lower urinary tract disease (e.g. infection)
  - Fever (occasionally)
  - Congestive heart failure (occasionally)
- Asymptomatic-persistent
  - Idiopathic
  - Fixed postural type
  - Mild glomerular injury
  - Mild tubular injury
- Symptomatic
  - Glomerular disease
  - Severe tubular disease (see below)

IMPORTANT CAUSES OF PROTEINURIA

- Idiopathic glomerular injury
  - Membranous nephropathy
  - Minimal change disease
  - Focal and segmental glomerulosclerosis
  - Membranoproliferative glomerulonephritis
- Secondary glomerular injury
  - Diabetes mellitus (DM)
  - Light-chain disease
  - Amyloidosis
  - Systemic lupus erythematosus
  - Infection (endocarditis, malaria, syphilis, hepatitis B)
  - Non-Hodgkin's lymphoma
  - Hodgkin's disease
  - Drug hypersensitivity
  - Hepatitis B
  - Cancer (lung, colon, breast)

- Nephrotoxins (gold, other heavy metals, high-dose captopril, penicillamine)
- Heroin
- HIV infection
- Mechanical (renal vein thrombosis, inferior vena cava obstruction)
- Pregnancy (preeclampsia)

TUBULAR DISORDERS ASSOCIATED WITH PROTEINURIA

- Analgesic abuse
- Pyelonephritis
- Fanconi's syndrome
- Cadmium and mercury poisoning
- Balkan nephropathy
- Lowe syndrome
- Hepatolenticular degeneration

WORKUP

HISTORY

- Focus on risk factors for glomerular disease, including long-standing DM, SLE, paraproteinemia, infectious disease (HIV infection, malaria, syphilis, endocarditis), medications (gold, penicillamine, NSAIDs, antibiotics, high-dose ACE inhibitors), hepatitis B, toxin exposure (heavy metals, heroin), allergen exposure (bee sting, serum sickness), and malignancy (lymphoma, Hodgkin's disease, cancer of breast, lung, or colon).
- Seek risk factors for tubular disorders, including analgesic abuse (especially with phenacetin-containing compounds), heavy metal exposure, family Hx of proteinuria, and Hx of pyelonephritis.

PHYSICAL EXAM

- Check BP. HTN is poor prognostic sign, raising specter of significant renal impairment.
- Check patient for vasculitic skin changes, other rashes, retinopathy, lymphadenopathy, signs of right-sided heart failure and constrictive physiology, abdominal masses, organomegaly, stool positive for occult blood on guaiac testing, prostatic enlargement, peripheral edema, and joint inflammation.

LAB STUDIES

- Perform repeat urinalysis when proteinuria is detected by dipstick. Dipstick test detects albumin concentrations >30 mg/dL.
- Single negative test does not rule out intermittent proteinuria (e.g., orthostatic proteinuria) or protein other than albumin (e.g., light chains in myeloma). False-positive dipstick reactions can be seen in patients who are dehydrated, have gross hematuria, or are receiving large doses of nafcillin or cephalosporins.
- On sediment exam search for RBC casts (indicating glomerulonephritis), WBC casts (pyelonephritis and interstitial nephritis), and oval fat bodies (lipiduria in patients with nephrotic syndrome).

- Quantify confirmation of proteinuria with 24-hr urine collection. In addition to urinary albumin, note urine creatinine to assess for adequacy of collection.
- Creatinine clearance is best determination of renal function; it approximates glomerular filtration rate. Obtain simultaneous serum creatinine and 24-hr urine collection for urinary creatinine levels. Random measurements of BUN or serum creatinine are less accurate than clearance determination but are useful for following patient once you know creatinine clearance.
- CBC identifies any anemia resulting from severe subacute or chronic renal insufficiency.
- Serum albumin level is worth monitoring because it correlates inversely with severity of proteinuria.
- Protein selectivity index is useful for Dx and Rx in patients with nephrotic syndrome. Proteinuria is selective when urine contains large amounts of low-molecular-weight proteins. High degree of selectivity in patients with nephrotic syndrome suggests minimal change disease, which is responsive to corticosteroids.
- Use radiographic exam of kidneys, ureters, and bladder to judge kidney size, which may help elucidate etiology (e.g., small, shrunken kidneys suggest significant chronic bilateral disease). Renal ultrasonography may be more accurate and informative; it can detect cystic disease, mass lesions, and obstruction.
- IV pyelography is indicated when considering chronic pyelonephritis. It also provides estimate of individual kidney function based on how well each concentrates and excretes contrast material. When creatinine clearance is reduced >75%, kidneys may not concentrate contrast medium sufficiently for visualization. Contrast-induced acute renal failure is risk in patients with preexisting renal disease, especially those with DM or multiple myeloma.
- Kidney biopsy deserves consideration when treatable disease remains possible but cause remains elusive despite clinical and lab evaluations.

MANAGEMENT

ASYMPTOMATIC PROTEINURIA

- Reassure patients with transient proteinuria; Rx is unwarranted. Patients with idiopathic and fixed orthostatic forms of proteinuria that occur as isolated findings without other associated abnormalities have been found to have excellent prognosis in prospective studies with 5–20 yrs of follow-up.
- Follow expectantly asymptomatic patients with persistent isolated proteinuria. They are at greater risk for eventual development of renal impairment and should be followed with annual checks of BP, urine, BUN, and creatinine.

SYMPTOMATIC PROTEINURIA/NEPHROTIC SYNDROME

- Patients with marked proteinuria due to systemic disease are best helped by treating underlying condition.
- ACE inhibitors (see Hypertension) help reduce albumin loss and preserve renal function, presumably by limiting hyperfiltration.

- Sodium restriction and judicious use of loop and distally acting diuretics are helpful in nephrotic syndrome.
- Modest dietary protein restriction (approximately 1 g/kg/day) may be of benefit in slowing course of patients with progressive renal disease. Patients for whom protein restriction is prescribed require close nutritional follow-up to ensure adequate nitrogen balance.
- All nephrotic patients should receive pneumococcal and influenza vaccines.
- In idiopathic nephrotic syndrome, Rx depends on renal pathology defined by biopsy.

BIBLIOGRAPHY

- For the current annotated bibliography on proteinuria, see the print edition of *Primary Care Medicine*, 4th edition, Chapter 130, or www.LWWmedicine.com.

Renal Failure

WORKUP

HISTORY

- Monitor for fatigue, shortness of breath, bleeding problems, and edema.

PHYSICAL EXAM

- Monitor BP closely for development of HTN.
- Check for pallor, signs of bleeding, pleural effusion, and pleuropericarditis.

LAB STUDIES

- Follow BUN, creatinine, serum albumin, calcium phosphate, and electrolytes. Also monitor CBC and urinalysis.
- Consider CXR, if signs of pleural effusion or pleural rub noted on PE.
- Obtain ECG if pericardial friction rub noted on PE.

MANAGEMENT

- PCP often responsible for initial conservative management, including interventions that delay disease progression.
- Additional objectives are to prevent or minimize complications of uremia, monitor disease progression, and judge when referral to nephrologist is indicated for consideration of dialysis or transplantation.
- Conservative management of renal failure can prolong survival and preserve quality of life by compensating for excretory, regulatory, and endocrine kidney functions. Goals of Rx are to reduce symptoms, slow progression, and avoid preventable complications.
- Consider initiating ACE inhibitor Rx (e.g., 25 mg captopril bid–tid) early in course of renal failure, especially in patients with DM, but also in those with nondiabetic renal disease. HTN is not Rx prerequisite.
- Exert caution with ACE inhibitor use in setting of acute dehydration. Monitor BP, renal function, and serum potassium regularly. Omit in persons with bilateral renal artery stenosis.
- Restrict protein intake to 0.5 g high-quality protein/kg/day if patient is symptomatic or acidotic, and to 0.5–0.75 g/kg/day if BUN level >75 mg/dL but patient is asymptomatic. Maintain calorie intake at 40–50 cal/kg/day.
- Fluid restriction is unnecessary with mild to moderate renal insufficiency unless patient also has HTN or CHF. Restrict fluids only in presence of oliguria. Intake should equal urine output and insensible losses.
- ACE inhibitors are Rx of choice for HTN, especially in those with DM or marked proteinuria and also in those with nondiabetic renal disease. Angiotensin receptor blockers are reasonable alternative to ACE inhibitors in type 2 DM. Calcium channel blockers also delay onset of nephropathy

in patients with type 1 DM. Base choice of agent on cost and convenience (e.g., 25 mg captopril tid); monitor renal function. Other alternatives include alpha and beta blockers and vasodilators (see Hypertension). Attempt to achieve lowest BP possible in patients with marked proteinuria.

- Salt restriction is unnecessary with mild to moderate renal insufficiency. In patients with HTN or CHF, salt restriction to 2 g sodium/day may be necessary. Restrict sodium in presence of oliguria or CHF.

- For hypokalemic patients, administer potassium supplements in low doses and check levels frequently, especially in oliguric patients. Do not maintain potassium supplementation indefinitely. Avoid potassium-sparing diuretics in patients with moderate renal insufficiency. Treat potassium levels >6 mEq/L and admit if ECG changes accompany levels >6.5 mEq/L. Best Rx for mild chronic hyperkalemia are exchange resins such as sodium polystyrene sulfonate (Kayexalate) PO or instilled as enema in sorbitol. Kayexalate exchanges sodium ion for potassium ion; therefore, be alert to possible sodium and volume overload.

- Correct hyperphosphatemia with calcium citrate (667 mg tid ac). Symptomatic or severe hypocalcemia despite normalization of serum phosphate requires calcium supplements (e.g., 600 mg calcium carbonate bid), vitamin D in pharmacologic doses (e.g., calcitriol, 0.25 mg/day), or both.

- Treat acidosis if serum bicarbonate concentration <15 mEq/L. Remove external acid load. Treat acidosis with 600 mg sodium bicarbonate bid initially, and titrate bicarbonate to 16–20 mEq/L. Follow serum potassium and calcium levels during acidosis Rx because both may fall.

- Treat hyperuricemia only if symptomatic gout develops; use allopurinol (see Gout).

- Treat anemia with 1,000–6,000 U erythropoietin SQ 3 times/wk; monitor hemoglobin, hematocrit, reticulocyte count, and serum ferritin. Avoid antiplatelet drugs. Give 325 mg oral ferrous sulfate/day to patients with iron deficiency. Transfuse for high-output failure or angina. Avoid unnecessary bloodwork and injections.

- Treat CHF with salt restriction. Add furosemide if CHF persists. Add metolazone (2.5–5 mg) if refractory fluid overload is present; monitor renal function and electrolytes closely. Consider using ACE inhibitor (e.g., start with 12.5–25 mg captopril bid–tid); monitor renal function closely. Digoxin can be used, but monitor levels frequently.

- Minimize uremic symptoms (itching, hiccups, nausea) by reducing dietary protein intake. Prescribe 5–10 mg prochlorperazine PO qid for nausea. Treat itching topically with menthol or phenol lotion or trial of capsaicin cream; cholestyramine and UV light have also been used successfully (see Pruritus).

- If dietary Rx becomes intolerable or ineffective, consider dialysis or transplantation. Referral to nephrologist is necessary.

BIBLIOGRAPHY

- For the current annotated bibliography on renal failure, see the print edition of *Primary Care Medicine*, 4th edition, Chapter 142, or www.LWWmedicine.com.

Scrotal Pain, Masses, and Swelling

DIFFERENTIAL DIAGNOSIS

- When men present with scrotal problems, PCP must promptly recognize torsion and epididymitis and differentiate benign masses from those suggesting malignancy, which require referral for urologic evaluation.
- Consider firm, tender masses of acute onset in afebrile young men to represent torsion until proved otherwise. Dx is supported by finding testicle with horizontal lie on uninvolved side.
- Other causes of acute painful swelling are epididymitis, mumps orchitis, and hemorrhage into testicular cancer.
- In men aged <35, painful swelling may be due to epididymitis, which occurs as consequence of gonococcal, chlamydial, or Ureaplasma infection. May be accompanied by symptoms of urethritis (dysuria, discharge).
- In older men, cause is more likely prostatitis, recent urinary instrumentation, or structural lesion.
- Testicular cancer presents as hard, heavy, firm, nontender mass that does not transilluminate. Although usually painless, about 20% cause some discomfort in scrotum, and patient may report frank pain and tenderness, especially after hemorrhage into tumor.
- Cystic scrotal masses include hydroceles, epididymal cysts, and spermatoceles. They are slow growing and painless collections of fluid or sperm.
- Varicoceles have "bag of worms" appearance and almost always appear on left side.

WORKUP

HISTORY

- Inquire into acuteness of symptoms, duration, clinical course, tenderness, recent trauma, urethral discharge, dysuria, fever, inguinal herniation, and concurrent infection (e.g., mumps, gonorrhea, prostatitis). Complaint of scrotal heaviness is common but nonspecific, found in conditions ranging from tumor to hydrocele and epididymitis.
- Note patient's age; testicular cancer is disease of men aged <40, and torsion is most common among adolescents and young men.
- Hx of undescended testicle raises possibility of testicular cancer. Do not dismiss vague abdominal, back, or chest complaints because they may herald onset of metastatic testicular cancer.
- Recurrent episodes in young men suggest torsion.
- Flank pain, abdominal pain, prostatitis, or known extratesticular cancer suggests extrascrotal source, especially in absence of scrotal pathology on physical exam.

PHYSICAL EXAM

- During inspection, note any erythema, masses, hernias, or varices. Normal testicle is freely movable and uniform in consistency. Check for abnormalities that may provide clues to disease on involved side, such as horizontally oriented "bell clapper" mobility in person at risk for torsion.

- Identify scrotal structures and examine for tenderness, warmth, swelling, and nodularity. If mass or nodule is found, determine whether it is testicular or extratesticular, solid or cystic. Examine inguinal canal for hernia.

- Transillumination with penlight in darkened room is necessary to help determine whether lesion is cystic or solid. Cystic lesions usually allow light transmission, although bloody exudate may not.

- Mass that appears extratesticular and cystic is most likely benign (spermatocele, cyst of epididymis, or hydrocele). If it is hard and does not transilluminate, or patient reports steady growth, consider tumor and refer for urologic evaluation, even if mass appears extratesticular.

- If testicular tumor suspected, check supraclavicular lymph nodes, chest, and abdomen because >50% present with metastatic disease. (Inguinal adenopathy does not suggest testicular cancer because testicular lymphatics drain into para-aortic nodes. Scrotal nontesticular lymphatics drain into inguinal nodes.) Examine breasts for gynecomastia.

- Tender scrotum in absence of mass, redness, increased warmth, or swelling should trigger check for extrascrotal pathology. Examine abdomen for signs of appendicitis, aneurysm, and inguinal hernia; check prostate and flanks for tenderness.

LAB STUDIES

- If you note mass, or uncertainty persists, testicular ultrasonography (U/S) is helpful in determining whether lesion is testicular or extratesticular, solid or cystic. Measurement of hCG and α-fetoprotein levels more useful for monitoring testicular cancer than for Dx (see Bladder Cancer; Prostate Cancer; Renal Cell Carcinoma; and Testicular Cancer), but marked elevation is suggestive. Sensitivity is low; negative study does not rule out cancer.

- If you suspect metastatic disease, perform CXR and abdominal CT as part of staging process.

- Urinalysis is helpful for detection of pyuria or bacteriuria in cases suggesting infection. Perform semen analysis only when infertility is concurrent complaint.

- Right-sided varicocele or suddenly appearing left-sided varicocele requires further evaluation because of possibility of venous obstruction or renal carcinoma. In such cases, IV pyelogram or renal U/S is indicated.

- When you suspect extrascrotal pathology, direct workup appropriately (see Abdominal Pain; Prostatitis).

MANAGEMENT

- Acutely painful, swollen testicle requires urgent assessment because if testicular torsion is present, permanent damage may occur if Rx does not begin ≤4 hrs of onset. Urgent urologic consultation is necessary to determine need to explore scrotum.

- Teaching testicular self-exam might help shorten or eliminate delay in presentation common in patients with testicular carcinoma.

- Reassure patient with clearly extratesticular, transilluminating scrotal lesion that cancer is virtually ruled out and that no further cancer evaluation is necessary other than periodic follow-up exam.
- Patient with solid testicular mass needs prompt referral to urologist regardless of whether mass is tender.
- Refer patients with varicoceles that do not decrease in size when patient lies down, are painful, or are associated with infertility.
- Surgical Rx is unnecessary for most hydroceles and cystic lesions except to relieve discomfort or difficulty with intercourse. Do not aspirate hydroceles. When indicated, surgery does not compromise fertility or sexual function.
- Refer patient with scrotal mass representing inguinal hernia to general surgeon if hernia is not easily reducible.

BIBLIOGRAPHY

- For the current annotated bibliography on scrotal pain, masses, and swelling, see the print edition of *Primary Care Medicine*, 4th edition, Chapter 131, or www.LWWmedicine.com.

Sexually Transmitted Diseases

MANAGEMENT

OVERALL APPROACH

- See also Chlamydial Infection; Gonorrhea; Herpes Simplex; HIV-1 Infection; Scabies and Pediculosis; Syphilis; Warts.

CHANCROID AND GRANULOMA INGUINALE

- Chancroid, endemic in some areas of U.S., is caused by gram-negative *H. ducreyi*. It typically produces painful genital ulcers often accompanied by regional adenopathy. Azithromycin (1 g PO) or ceftriaxone (250 mg IM), both given as single dose, are Rx of choice.
- Painless, slowly progressive genital ulcers characterize granuloma inguinale, caused by gram-negative *D. granulomatis*. TMP-SMX DS bid, or 100 mg doxycycline bid, both for 21 days, are Rx of choice.

LYMPHOGRANULOMA VENEREUM

- Microorganism belonging to *Chlamydia* group of obligate intracellular parasites causes lymphogranuloma venereum. Inguinal nodes enlarge and may suppurate to produce chronic draining sinuses. Scarring and lymphatic obstruction may result. Doxycycline (100 mg bid × 21 days) is Rx of choice. Alternative is 21-day course of erythromycin (500 mg qid).

BIBLIOGRAPHY

- For the current annotated bibliography on sexually transmitted diseases, see the print edition of *Primary Care Medicine*, 4th edition, Chapter 141, or www.LWWmedicine.com.

Syphilis

SCREENING AND/OR PREVENTION

- After decades of decline, syphilis is becoming more common, especially among IV drug abusers, urban poor, and HIV-infected persons.
- Screening for latent disease is simple, and late manifestations of syphilis are entirely preventable by early Rx.
- Many patients have been screened routinely at time of marriage, during prenatal care, before giving blood, or on hospital admission. Frequent screening is unnecessary, but document nonreactivity of sexually active persons, particularly those with multiple sex partners, at 5-yr intervals.
- Special indications for screening include exposure to or infection with other STDs, pregnancy, IV drug abuse, and HIV infection.
- Counsel all patients with syphilis about HIV infection and advise them to accept HIV testing.
- Nontreponemal tests such as RPR or VDRL are appropriate for screening because of their sensitivity and simplicity. Reserve MHA-TP or other treponemal tests for confirming Dx suspected on basis of clinical presentation or positive nontreponemal test results.

WORKUP

HISTORY AND PHYSICAL EXAM

- Check for
  - Hallmark of primary syphilis: chancre occurring at site of inoculation about 3 wks after exposure.
  - Secondary syphilis: systemic disease that appears about 2 mos after infection and is characterized by flulike syndrome, generalized lymphadenopathy, and skin eruption.
  - Latent syphilis: Untreated patient who becomes asymptomatic after experiencing manifestations of primary or secondary disease.
- Check for forms of tertiary syphilis
  - Cardiovascular syphilis: characterized by aneurysmal dilation of ascending aorta and aortic insufficiency.
  - Neurosyphilis: may be asymptomatic or may present as general paresis with disorders of intellect and personality, or as tabes dorsalis, with ataxic gait, impaired pain and temperature sensation, autonomic dysfunction, and hypoactive reflexes.
  - Gummas: isolated, slowly progressive, destructive granulomatous lesions of skin, bone, liver, or other organs.
- Be aware of risk for congenital syphilis due to transplacental transmission of spirochetes during second or third trimester.

LAB STUDIES

- *T. pallidum* cannot be cultured *in vitro*, but experienced observers can make syphilis Dx by direct visualization of treponema from chancre using darkfield or fluorescent microscopy. Dx usually depends on clinical features and serologic testing.

■ Most widely used serologic tests for syphilis include VDRL, Hinton, and RPR tests. These are excellent, but false-positive rate is as high as 30%, often as result of unrelated infections or inflammatory diseases that produce hyperglobulinemia.

■ More specific serologic tests use treponemal antigens and can distinguish true-positive from false-positive results. Most frequently used treponemal test is MHA-TP test.

MANAGEMENT

■ Rx for early syphilis (primary, secondary, early latent stages) is 1 dose of 2.4 million U benzathine penicillin IM. Penicillin-allergic patients should receive 500 mg oral tetracycline qid for 14 days, or 100 mg doxycycline bid for 14 days. Doxycycline and tetracycline are contraindicated in pregnancy.

■ Rx for syphilis of >1 yr in duration (latent, tertiary, or unknown duration) is 2.4 million U benzathine penicillin IM/wk × 3 consecutive wks. Penicillin-allergic patients should receive 500 mg oral tetracycline qid × 28 days, or 100 mg doxycycline bid × 28 days.

■ Treat neurosyphilis with 18–24 million U aqueous penicillin G IV, divided q4h, × 14 days. Some experts recommend 1 dose of 2.4 million U benzathine penicillin IM after IV Rx. After Rx, reexamine CSF q6mos until findings are normal.

■ HIV infection may increase risk for neurosyphilis, but CSF abnormalities are common in HIV-infected patients, and their presence is of uncertain significance. Consider lumbar puncture. No data suggest that syphilis Rx regimens prescribed for HIV-negative patients will be less effective in HIV-positive patients. Monitor HIV-infected patients closely after Rx.

■ Always treat syphilis in pregnancy and neurosyphilis with penicillin. Desensitize penicillin-allergic patients if necessary.

■ Jarisch-Herxheimer reaction, often with headache and myalgia, may occur within first 24 hrs after syphilis Rx, especially in early syphilis. Warn patients of this possibility, but do not delay Rx.

■ Report all cases of syphilis to appropriate public health authorities so that case finding can be performed. Screen syphilis patients for other STDs, including HIV infection, chlamydial infection, and gonorrhea (see Chlamydial Infection; Gonorrhea; HIV-1 Infection), and counsel about HIV infection and safe sex practices.

BIBLIOGRAPHY

■ For the current annotated bibliography on syphilis, see the print edition of *Primary Care Medicine*, 4th edition, Chapters 124 and 141, or www.LWWmedicine.com.

Urethritis in Men

DIFFERENTIAL DIAGNOSIS

- Differential Dx of penile discharge is divided into gonococcal and non-gonococcal etiologies, with NGU accounting for majority of cases.
- Among causes of NGU are chlamydial, *Ureaplasma*, and trichomonal infections of urethra; Reiter's syndrome; prostatitis; and urethral malignancy. Chlamydial disease responsible for about half of NGU cases. Pathogen remains unidentified in up to one-third of cases. Occasionally, urethral infection with HSV or HPV may be responsible for problem.

WORKUP

HISTORY

- Inquire into number of sexual partners during past few months and use or nonuse of barrier contraception.
- Check for symptoms of prostatitis, gonorrheal infection, and Reiter's syndrome and for reports of penile warts, HSV infection, and sexual contact with partner with trichomonal infection.

PHYSICAL EXAM

- Take temp and examine for signs of gonococcemia and Reiter's syndrome. Also check urethral meatus for herpetic lesions and warts, and testes and prostate for signs of epididymitis and prostatitis, respectively.

LAB STUDIES

- Obtain urethral swab for Gram's stain and for plating onto Thayer-Martin medium for culture of *N. gonorrhoeae*.
- Obtain second swabbing for chlamydial antigen detection by direct fluorescent antibody staining or enzyme immunoassay.
- Alternatively, send second swab for DNA amplification testing, which is more sensitive and specific.
- Test female partners of NGU patients; if testing is unavailable, treat empirically for presumptive chlamydial infection. Also test male homosexual partners, but do not treat empirically.
- When routine cultures and Gram's stains are not diagnostic and empiric trial of Rx for NGU is unsuccessful (see below), reevaluate and consider culturing for *Ureaplasma* or trichomonads.

MANAGEMENT

- Treat all patients with NGU for chlamydial infection regardless of whether *Chlamydia* is definitively identified, because information often helps improve compliance, facilitate counseling, and guide care if symptoms persist.

- Treat NGU initially with doxycycline (100 mg bid for 7 days) or azithromycin (1 g orally in single dose).
- Treat documented NGU recurrences with erythromycin (500 mg qid × 3 wks).
- If you find *Trichomonas* in relapsed patients, metronidazole Rx (2 g as single dose or 250 mg tid × 1 wk) may prove useful.

BIBLIOGRAPHY

- For the current annotated bibliography on urethritis in men, see the print edition of *Primary Care Medicine*, 4th edition, Chapter 136, or www.LWWmedicine.com.

Urinary Tract Infection

SCREENING AND/OR PREVENTION

- Rx is moderately effective in short term, but because of high rates of spontaneous recurrence and resolution, likelihood that bacteriuria will be noted with longer follow-up is not significantly influenced by short-term Rx.
- Symptomatic infections are generally not prevented by Rx of asymptomatic bacteriuria in nonpregnant women.
- Although association exists between bacteriuria and renal abnormalities, no evidence suggests etiologic relationship. Furthermore, there is no evidence that infection Rx in absence of urinary tract abnormalities prevents progressive renal disease.
- Screening for asymptomatic bacteriuria is recommended only in selected high-risk populations, including
  - pregnant women;
  - elderly men with clinical prostatism or other urologic abnormalities, before and after required instrumentation;
  - all patients recently catheterized; and
  - patients with known renal calculi or other structural abnormalities of urinary tract.
- Screening with reagent strips is insufficiently sensitive for high-risk patients likely to benefit from detection and Rx.
- Screening of pregnant women should include urine culture.

DIFFERENTIAL DIAGNOSIS

IN WOMEN

- About 20–30% of women have UTI in their lifetime, and 40% of women with 1 infection have recurrence. PCPs must respond to clinical syndromes ranging from acute urethral syndrome to pyelonephritis with efficient evaluation and effective Rx.
- About 10–15% of women with symptoms suggesting UTI have acute urethral syndrome (symptomatic abacteriuria). About 70% have some degree of pyuria (>2–5 WBCs/HPF in centrifuged sample) and true infection, with bacterial counts <100,000 organisms/mL or with *C. trachomatis*. Remaining 30% have no pyuria and no infection. Cause of their dysuria is unknown.
- Symptomatic bacteriuria, in form of cystitis or pyelonephritis, is most common of clinical syndromes. Cystitis usually presents primarily as frequency, urgency, dysuria, and bacteriuria.
- Pyelonephritis is usually associated with fever, flank pain, and systemic symptoms such as nausea and vomiting. Distinguishing between them can be difficult.

IN MEN

- Helpful to distinguish among UTIs by patient age. UTI in young men usually represents urethritis or introduction of bacteria through instrumentation (e.g., bladder catheterization for surgery). At times, congenital anomaly of urinary tract is responsible, although presentation is usually at earlier age. Patients who respond fully to 7-day course of antibiotics are unlikely to have serious underlying pathology.
- Test young patients with acute urethral symptoms for chlamydial infection.
- Increase in rate of UTI that occurs in men aged 50–65 parallels increase in prostate size that occurs with gland hyperplasia. Enlargement leads to bladder outflow tract obstruction, and postvoid residual develops in bladder.
- Among elderly men with further prostatic enlargement, postvoid residual and infection risk continue to rise. Use of condom or urethral catheters, urinary incontinence, and Hx of UTI are other risk factors for UTI in this age group.

WORKUP

HISTORY

In Women

- Evaluate acutely ill patients with fever, flank pain, and systemic symptoms for possible urinary tract obstruction and superimposed infection. Question about Hx of DM, sickle cell anemia, and excessive analgesic use, which pose higher risk for renal papillary necrosis and subsequent obstruction by sloughed papillae. Hx of renal calculi is cause for concern in this setting.
- Patient with any of these risk factors who appears toxic (high temp, prostration) and restless on exam and who has marked tenderness in costovertebral angle requires immediate urologic evaluation to rule out obstruction.
- Infection behind obstruction constitutes medical and urologic emergency.
- Question acutely dysuric women about vaginal discharge, external irritation on urination, and pain on intercourse to differentiate vaginal causes of dysuria from those referable to urinary tract.
- Also take sexual Hx to identify risk factors for chlamydial urethritis, including new sexual partners, partner with penile discharge or recent urethritis, mucoid vaginal discharge, or gradual onset of symptoms. Elicit Hx of gonorrhea or exposure to gonorrhea.

In Men

- Complaints of dysuria, frequency, and urgency have predictive value of about 75% for UTI. Acute onset of hesitancy, nocturia, slow stream, and dribbling have predictive value of about 33%. No symptoms differentiate upper from lower UTI, with possible exception of fever (rare in men with lower tract disease).

PHYSICAL EXAM

In Women

- Take temp, then percuss costovertebral angle to test for tenderness, and palpate suprapubic region to detect discomfort and distention.
- On pelvic exam note any urethral discharge, vaginal erythema, discharge, or atrophy, and cervical discharge, erosion, vesicles, or tenderness on motion.

In Men

- Take temp and perform genitourinary tract exam. Examine urethral meatus for erythema and discharge; testes and epididymides for tenderness and swelling; and prostate for enlargement, nodularity, and pain on palpation.
- In suspected acute prostatitis, palpate gently to avoid causing bacteremia.
- Check abdomen for suprapubic distention and tenderness in costovertebral angles.

LAB STUDIES

In Women

- Urinalysis and Gram's stain of unspun urine are often diagnostic. Instruct women to use clean-voided technique to minimize contamination from vaginal and labial sources. Elderly patients may need assistance. When you suspect repeated contamination, you can perform straight catheterization of bladder with relatively little risk.
- Examining urine promptly minimizes artifactual findings. Finding pyuria (>25 WBCs/HPF in spun sediment) indicates UTI and predicts response to antibiotic Rx. Absence of pyuria suggests vaginal cause for dysuria or noninfectious variant of acute urethral syndrome.
- Presence of 1 organism on HPF exam of Gram's-stained unspun sample represents clinically significant bacteriuria (>100,000 organisms/mL).
- In dysuria without complications you can reserve urine culture for patients with recurrence or Hx of multiple episodes.
- Acute severe symptoms warrant urine culture and, with fever and chills, blood cultures.
- Reserve IV pyelography, excretory urography, and cystoscopy for those with suspected anatomic abnormalities (e.g., onset of UTIs in childhood) or those with likely obstruction or developing renal insufficiency.

In Men

- Unlike women, men require urine culture because of wider range of causative agents and their less-predictable drug sensitivities. Dx of UTI is justified on isolation of pure culture of 1,000 CFU/mL urine. Culture that grows <1,000 CFU/mL or ≥3 organisms (without 1 being predominant) suggests contamination.
- Examine spun and unspun urine specimens. Examine spun sediment for WBC casts (indicative of pyelonephritis) and pus, and perform Gram's stain to identify predominant organism, if present. Perform Gram's stain of unspun urine; finding 1 organism or WBC/HPF has sensitivity of 85% for UTI and specificity of 60%, about same as those of other rapid diagnostic methods.

- Obtain culture specimens from patients with indwelling catheter by cleansing side port of catheter with povidone-iodine and drawing urine through needle attached to sterile syringe. Culture is positive for organisms when ≥100 CFU/mL are present. Most patients with indwelling catheters have positive cultures.

- Obtain culture specimen from incontinent patient without resorting to catheterization by cleansing glans penis with povidone-iodine solution, applying fresh condom catheter and drainage system, and collecting first voided specimen in drainage bag within 2 hrs. Study is positive if >100,000 CFU/mL are present; lesser growth represents contamination.

- Straight catheterization and direct bladder aspiration are alternative methods of obtaining specimen in incontinent patients. The former carries slight risk of inducing a bacteremia (see Bacterial Endocarditis); skill is necessary in latter procedure.

- Some UTIs or their causes may compromise renal function. BUN and creatinine are reasonable determinations. WBC count usually contributes little to Dx but may provide confirmatory evidence in patient who appears toxic.

- Reserve IV pyelogram for those with recurrent infection, suspected upper tract obstruction, or pyelonephritis.

- In elderly patient with recurrent UTI, residual volume assessment helps identify risk factors for recurrence. Volume >50 mL is abnormal. IV pyelogram also provides estimate of residual volume. Whether reduction in residual volume by Rx of bladder outlet obstruction reduces risks and morbidity of UTI is still undetermined.

- Persistence of symptoms or quick relapse suggest refractory infection. Prostatic involvement (about half of instances), obstruction, anatomic anomaly, or functional disease may be responsible, necessitating repeated urine culture and consideration of IV pyelogram, 3-glass testing, and prolonged course of Rx (6–12 wks) with antibiotic that penetrates prostate and is active against resistant organisms. Fluoroquinolone antibiotics recommended in this setting (e.g., 400 mg norfloxacin bid).

- Differentiating upper from lower UTI is helpful because of implications for clinical course and Rx. Instrumentation (ureteral catheterization, bladder washout) is only proved method for making determination. Best available test has been response to initial course of antibiotics.

- STDs may present with urethral symptoms and mimic UTI. Test for chlamydial infection young patients with acute urethral symptoms, even if unaccompanied by discharge (see Chlamydial Infection; Urethritis).

MANAGEMENT

FOR WOMEN

- Hospitalize women, especially if elderly, with high fever, chills, flank pain, costovertebral angle tenderness, nausea, and vomiting; they may have upper UTI or bloodstream infection.

- Ampicillin + gentamicin is time-honored choice for serious UTI, providing effective, low-cost coverage. Expensive alternatives for initial Rx include imipenem/cilastatin, ciprofloxacin, and ceftriaxone.

- When culture and sensitivity results become available, revise regimen to provide more focused coverage.

- Urosepsis requires 2–3 wks of IV antibiotics. Treat pyelonephritis without bloodstream invasion parenterally until fever resolves, then with oral antibiotics to complete 14-day course.

- Patients with pyuria respond to single-dose antibiotic Rx with TMP-SMX (1 single-strength tab bid for 10 days) or doxycycline (100 mg bid × 10 days). Those without pyuria do not respond to antibiotics. Symptomatic Rx with fluids and urinary analgesics such as phenazopyridine (Pyridium) can be effective.

- Treat otherwise healthy women with uncomplicated pyelonephritis entirely on outpatient basis with 10–14 days of oral antibiotics provided that they are reliable, can take fluids, are not seriously immunocompromised, and have no obstruction.

- Base choice of initial Rx on Gram's stain findings. For infection with gram-negative rods, TMP-SMX or fluoroquinolone (e.g., ciprofloxacin, norfloxacin) is reasonable. Gram-positive cocci seen on urine Gram's stain suggest enterococci and *S. saprophyticus*, which are best treated with amoxicillin.

- Women with mild to moderate symptoms usually have cystitis and respond well to short course of oral antibiotics. With gram-negative rods on Gram's stain, TMP-SMX or amoxicillin is recommended. For patients allergic to sulfa drugs and penicillin, fluoroquinolone (e.g., ciprofloxacin) is effective alternative. For gram-positive cocci, amoxicillin is drug of choice.

- Recurrent infections are characteristic of some patients, especially sexually active women, women with host defenses compromised by underlying systemic illness or residual urine in bladder, women with upper UTIs, and pregnant women.

- Recurrences may be (1) relapses, in which antimicrobial Rx suppresses original organism, which reappears when antibiotic stops; or (2) reinfections, in which antimicrobial Rx eliminates original organism and new bacterial strain causes recurrent infection. Approximately 80% of recurrences represent reinfection.

- Recurrences in sexually active women are most often reinfections. Prophylaxis at time of intercourse with single-tablet Rx minimizes UTI frequency and severity. Patient-initiated 1- or 3-day courses of standard antibiotic Rx for uncomplicated UTI at first sign of symptomatic infection also are effective for women with recurrent infection.

- In postmenopausal women, topical vaginal estrogens can prevent recurrent infection by returning vaginal flora to premenopausal composition with few Enterobacteriaceae.

- For very elderly patients with recurrences due to bladder distention and postvoid residual urine, continuous prophylaxis with nightly TMP-SMX (one-half of 1 single-strength tab qhs) is more effective than regimens of sulfisoxazole or methenamine mandelate (Mandelamine) and ascorbic acid. Benefits of asymptomatic infection Rx in elderly patients are unclear.

- Rx of symptomatic UTI in pregnancy is recommended. Antibiotics safe for use in pregnancy include ampicillin, amoxicillin, and oral cephalosporins. Avoid fluoroquinolones in pregnant patients.

- Instruct women with UTIs about increasing fluid intake during symptomatic periods. Advise patients with UTIs temporally related to sexual intercourse to void after intercourse.

FOR MEN

- Treat symptomatic UTI in male patients. If you find gram-negative rods on Gram's stain, TMP-SMX double strength (1 tab bid × 7–10 days) usually suffices. If organisms are gram-positive cocci, amoxicillin (500 mg tid × 7–10 days) represents better choice.

- Test men with asymptomatic bacteriuria scheduled for surgery and requiring short-term urinary tract instrumentation and treat for infection preoperatively to avoid introduction of bacteria into upper urinary tract and bloodstream. This is especially important for patients scheduled to undergo urologic surgery or surgery that introduces foreign body. Fluoroquinolone antibiotics are usually appropriate, but culture and sensitivity results should determine antibiotic choice.

- Any UTI patient who appears toxic or obstructed requires immediate hospitalization. Urosepsis is potentially life-threatening complication of UTI that necessitates high-dose parenteral antibiotics and prompt evaluation and Rx.

BIBLIOGRAPHY

- For the current annotated bibliography on urinary tract infection, see the print edition of *Primary Care Medicine*, 4th edition, Chapters 127, 133, and 140, or www.LWWmedicine.com.

Musculoskeletal Problems

Asymptomatic Hyperuricemia

MANAGEMENT

- Do not treat without detailed consideration of costs and benefits. Cost of prophylactic Rx in patients who have never had gouty attack greatly exceeds cost of treating acute attack symptomatically, should it occur.
- Do consider prophylactic Rx in patients with frequent acute gouty attacks, because probability of recurrence is high and there is risk of joint injury from chronic gout (see Gout).
- Rx to prevent chronic tophaceous gout need not start until clinical evidence of gout develops.
- Do not institute urate-lowering Rx to prevent renal impairment, because risk of azotemia is very low, except in patients with myeloproliferative or lymphoproliferative disorders who are about to begin Rx. Degree of azotemia attributable to hyperuricemia is mild and clinically insignificant in most other instances.
- Risk for urolithiasis is sufficiently low to justify waiting for stone to develop before initiating prophylactic Rx unless patient has strong family Hx of nephrolithiasis. Avoid dehydration, however.
- Although hyperuricemia is associated with atherosclerotic disease, there is no known cardiovascular benefit from treating hyperuricemia *per se*.

BIBLIOGRAPHY

- For the current annotated bibliography on asymptomatic hyperuricemia, see the print edition of *Primary Care Medicine*, 4th edition, Chapter 155, or www.LWWmedicine.com.

Back Pain

DIFFERENTIAL DIAGNOSIS

- Conditions commonly presenting with sciatica
  - Disk herniation
  - Spinal stenosis
  - Compression fracture
  - Epidural abscess
  - Vertebral osteomyelitis (late)
  - Compression fracture
  - Intraspinal tumor
  - Spinal metastasis
  - Spondylolisthesis (occasionally)
- Conditions usually presenting without sciatica
  - Musculoligamentous strain
  - Ankylosing spondylitis
  - Spondylolisthesis
  - Depression
  - Vertebral osteomyelitis (early)
  - Epidural abscess (very early)
  - Retroperitoneal neoplasm

WORKUP

HISTORY

- In elucidating basic features of back pain (i.e., quality, location, onset, radiation), inquire specifically into symptoms potentially indicative of serious underlying disease (e.g., fever, progressive neurologic deficits, bilateral deficits, bladder dysfunction, saddle anesthesia, persistent pain unresponsive to bed rest).
- Note any Hx of recent injury or prior cancer as well as previous Rx for back problems, recent lumbar puncture, concurrent infection, and prolonged high-dose corticosteroid use.
- Check for morning stiffness in back relieved by activity (ankylosing spondylitis or other inflammatory conditions), worsening or onset of symptoms with standing or walking and relief with bending or sitting (spinal stenosis), and worsening with sitting, driving, or lifting (lumbar disk herniation).
- Ascertain impact of back pain on daily activities and, if complaints disproportionate to findings, emotional and social stressors and manifestations of depression (see Depression) and somatization disorder (see Somatization Disorders).

PHYSICAL EXAM

- Before back exam, check abdomen, rectum, groin, pelvis, and peripheral pulses for conditions that might mimic symptoms of spinal disease.

- Examine for fever, skin abscess, breast mass, pleural effusion, prostate nodule, lymphadenopathy, joint inflammation, and other signs of systemic or malignant disease that may affect spine.
- Measure thigh and calf circumferences to detect evidence of atrophy, and test joint motions of lower extremities.

Back Exam

- Perform with patient standing and back uncovered.
- Check for any abnormalities in symmetry, muscle bulk, posture, and spinal curvature.
- Assess flexibility, noting any muscle spasm or spinal segments that do not move freely.
- Describe what limits back motion.
- Palpate spine (tumor, infection, fracture, or disk herniation), sciatic notch (lower lumbar disk problems), and sacroiliac area (ankylosing spondylitis) for focal tenderness.
- Perform straight-leg raising (SLR) test (sensitive indicator of lower lumbar L5–S1 disk herniation) in supine position with passive lifting of patient's leg at heel while knee is fully extended on side of reported sciatica (ipsilateral SLR testing) and on opposite side (contralateral, or crossed SLR testing).
- Consider test positive if sciatica is reproduced as leg is elevated 30–70 degrees; specificity is greatest when symptoms develop early in test.
- Avoid confusing hamstring muscle tightness for positive test.
- Do not consider test positive if severe pain is reported on elevation and resistance occurs, yet patient can raise leg another 20–30 degrees when distracted.
- Dorsiflex ankle at end of elevation to enhance test sensitivity.
- Test higher lumbar (L2, L3, or L4) roots by flexing knee with patient lying in prone position.

Neurologic Exam

- Concentrate on areas suggested by Hx (e.g., territory of L5 and S1 roots in patient with sciatica).
- Test for S1 root function (L5–S1 disk) with tiptoe walking, plantar flexion against resistance, ankle deep tendon reflexes, and lateral foot sensation.
- Test for L5 root function (L4–5 disk) with heel walking (an imprecise test), dorsiflexion of ankle and big toe against resistance, and sensation on anterior medial dorsal foot.
- Test for upper lumbar disk lesion (L4 root) with knee deep tendon reflexes, quadriceps strength, and sensation about medial ankle.
- Assess sensory function by pinprick testing, limiting exam to several key distal dermatomal areas in feet (see Fig. 147-1 in *Primary Care Medicine*, 4th edition) and noting any asymmetry of response.
- Note any disturbances in strength or sensation that do not correspond to nerve root innervation patterns, inconsistency of responses to maneuvers, overreaction to palpation or passive movement, superficial or widespread tenderness, and pain on sham testing of spinal rotation (arms at sides while rotating hips). Three or more of these responses suggests considerable psychological overlay.

LAB STUDIES

- Avoid routine ordering of plain lumbosacral spine films.
- Reserve early radiography for clinical suspicion of
  - malignancy (patient age >50, focal persistent bone pain unrelieved by bed rest, Hx of malignancy);
  - compression fracture (prolonged corticosteroid Rx, postmenopausal woman, severe trauma, focal tenderness);
  - ankylosing spondylitis (young male, limited spinal motion, sacroiliac pain);
  - chronic osteomyelitis (low-grade fever, high ESR, focal tenderness);
  - major trauma;
  - major neurologic deficits;
  - back pain localized to high lumbar or thoracic region (compression fracture, metastatic tumor).
- Consider plain films for patients seeking compensation for back pain and for those who desire reassurance.
- Consider CT or MRI if severe symptoms persist for several wks despite conservative Rx and in suspected disk herniation or other surgically correctable disease.
- Choose MRI if visualization of entire spine or upper vertebrae desired (intraspinal tumor, disk herniation at upper level) or there is concern about osteomyelitis, epidural abscess, or cord compression.
- Limit MRI and CT to patients who are sufficiently symptomatic that surgical intervention must be considered or are suspected of having serious systemic disease.
- Reserve myelography (usually with CT) for patients with progressive neurologic deficits, especially those with findings suggestive of spinal cord injury (e.g., loss of sphincter control, bilateral numbness and weakness).
- Consider Tc bone scan for suspected osteomyelitis or metastatic disease (fever, weight loss, persistent back pain, Hx of malignancy, concurrent infection, markedly elevated ESR).
- Obtain immunoelectrophoresis of serum and urine for Bence-Jones protein for back pain in older person accompanied by unexplained anemia and very high ESR (? myeloma).
- Consider electromyography if needing further documentation of peripheral nerve deficits.

MANAGEMENT

ACUTE BACK PAIN

- Manage acute musculoligamentous strain, degenerative disk disease, and lumbar disk disease (with or without sciatica) conservatively.
- Encourage continuation of daily activity rather than bed rest.
- Recommend local application of heat, warm baths, and mild analgesic use.
- Use antiinflammatory agents in preference to narcotics, except for first 1–2 nights of symptoms.
- Avoid so-called muscle relaxants except to facilitate sleep.

- Recommend finding most comfortable position in bed (e.g., lying supine with pillows behind knees and low pillow for head; lying on side with hips and knees flexed).
- Avoid prolonged bed rest, even for patients with continuing pain and evidence of disk protrusion or extrusion.

Activity Prescription

- Prescribe walking for about 20 mins tid, interspersed with several hrs of bed rest for first 1–2 wks.
- Then ease patient into program of endurance exercises that may help prevent future back problems (see below).
- Educate patient about overall plan of gradual mobilization and resumption of normal activities, noting that pain is normal protective response to injury or inflammation.
- Use discomfort as guideline to determine pace at which to increase activity, but minor discomfort, stiffness, soreness, or mild aching should not interfere with progressive mobilization.
- Temporarily limit activity for several days if symptoms recur or marked pain develops related to specific activity or activity level.
- Halve activity if patient undertakes new or higher level of activity and pain increases within 24 hrs; then gradually increase.
- Encourage progress as rapidly as symptoms permit.

Exercises and Back Care

- Advise avoiding activities that cause pain and potentially injurious actions such as repetitive bending, heavy lifting, and shoveling snow.
- Prescribe physical Rx program designed to improve muscle strength and flexibility.
- Use instruction sheets to supplement office instruction.
- Avoid regular use of traction or braces in patients with disk herniation.
- Institute program of mild daily exercise with more vigorous endurance exercises 2–3 times/wk.
- Recommend brisk walking for 20 mins/day or bid, supplemented by swimming or stationary bicycling 2 times/wk for up to 30 mins.

Spinal Manipulation

- Consider for acute back pain only after ruling out root compression (by disk protrusion or extrusion or spinal stenosis) and other serious pathology.
- Avoid manipulation as Rx for chronic back pain (no evidence of benefit over placebo).

PERSISTENT PAIN OR WORSENING NEUROLOGIC DEFICITS

- Consider referral for surgery those with evidence of lumbar disk herniation who experience (1) persistent disabling root pain despite 4–6 wks comprehensive conservative Rx, (2) progressive neurologic deficits in lower extremities, or (3) disruption of bowel or bladder control.
- Refer for emergency disk excision (diskectomy) by open surgery patients with massive disk herniation causing cauda equina syndrome.
- Refer for elective diskectomy those with major progressive neurologic deficit, calcified disk, extruded disk fragments that are not in continuity

with disk space, or pain caused primarily by bony abnormalities rather than by disk herniation.

- Consider surgical referral for chronic disabling low back pain that persists after resolution of more acute symptoms and for frequent acute recurrences of severe back pain that patient cannot prevent by following careful back care program.
- Consider chymopapain disk injection for patients who do not require open procedure, although it is not indicated for backache alone.
- Counsel against acupuncture (no better than placebo) and chiropractic manipulation for chronic back pain (no prospective randomized data).
- Avoid other unproved or ineffective Rx, such as injecting facet joints with corticosteroids (no better than placebo), epidural injection for sciatica due to herniated nucleus pulposus, and transcutaneous electrical nerve stimulation.

CHRONIC REFRACTORY BACK PAIN IN THE ABSENCE OF ANATOMIC DEFICITS

- Identify and treat underlying psychopathology (depression, somatization).
- Avoid inappropriate tests, ineffective Rx, and unnecessary surgery. Arrange consultation with orthopedic surgeon or neurosurgeon experienced in back problems so that patient does not feel need to "shop around" for willing surgeon.
- Focus on preserving and enhancing patient's functional capacity and not on eliminating pain.
- Encourage patients to settle any pending legal matters quickly.
- Expedite any disability determination; arrange independent evaluation to avoid jeopardizing patient–doctor relationship.
- Avoid prolonged narcotic use unless objective basis for pain is identified and cannot be treated etiologically; consider substance abuse when patient with back pain but no objective pathology persistently requests narcotics (see Substance Abuse).
- Establish strong doctor–patient alliance and attend to underlying psychosocial issues.
- Keep patient functioning independently through cultivation of relationship and promulgation of activity and exercise program.
- Arrange regularly scheduled visits at intervals meaningful to patient.
- Provide detailed information about what has happened, what can be done, and what lies ahead. Review working differential when there is uncertainty.
- Reassure patients with disk herniation of generally favorable prognosis with conservative Rx and low risk of prolonged physical disability.
- Inform previously active patients that jogging, stationary cycling, and swimming are not only possible but often desirable, and that reemergence of mild to moderate discomfort with resumption of activity is expected and is not worrisome prognostic sign.
- Review symptoms of serious neurologic injury that would necessitate prompt reporting and hospital admission.
- Provide rationale and anatomic basis for back hygiene measures and exercises.

INDICATIONS FOR ADMISSION AND REFERRAL

- Urgently admit and refer if symptoms suggestive of cauda equina syndrome or cord compression develop (e.g., new bilateral neurologic deficits, urinary retention, sphincter incontinence, saddle anesthesia).
- Also promptly admit patients with acute vertebral collapse (risk of spinal instability), possible osteomyelitis, or epidural abscess. Obtain infectious disease consultation in latter two situations.
- Promptly refer patients with rapidly progressive neurologic deficits for neurologic and surgical consultations.
- Consider neurological consultation for surgical candidacy if back pain remains severe and intractable after 4–6 weeks of conservative Rx, or if important neurologic deficit develops (e.g., foot drop, gastrocnemius–soleus or quadriceps weakness).

BIBLIOGRAPHY

- For the current annotated bibliography on back pain, see the print edition of *Primary Care Medicine*, 4th edition, Chapter 147, or www.LWWmedicine.com.

Elbow, Wrist, and Hand Pain

WORKUP

GENERAL STRATEGY

- Try to localize symptoms for accurate Dx.
- Determine precise area of tenderness by careful palpation.
- Perform thorough functional exam for patient with hand problem (active and passive motions of wrist, digits, and thumb; sensory testing with light touch and pinprick; determination of specific flexor and extensor tendon function).
- Consider A-P and lateral radiographs when bony disease suspected; films of little value with tendinitis.
- Consider EMG and nerve conduction study for suspected peripheral nerve compression.

LATERAL EPICONDYLITIS ("TENNIS ELBOW")

- Check for Hx of pain on lateral aspect of elbow and repetitive injury from strong grasp during wrist extension (e.g., backhand strokes in tennis, constant knitting).
- Palpate for tenderness over lateral epicondyle, pain during resisted wrist extension with elbow extended, and reproduction of symptoms during resisted extension of elbow with forearm in pronation and wrist in palmar flexion.

MEDIAL EPICONDYLITIS ("GOLFER'S ELBOW")

- Inquire into possible contributing repetitive occupational and sporting activities (manual and household work, golf).
- Check for pain localized to region of medial epicondyle.
- Attempt to reproduce by forcefully extending elbow against resistance with forearm in supination and wrist in dorsiflexion.

OLECRANON BURSITIS

- Inquire into localized trauma or repetitive local pressure associated with occupation, and RA, gout, or sepsis.
- Note any Hx of antecedent trauma and cellulitis of skin, followed by localized swelling, redness, and tenderness about elbow.
- Check for contiguous skin break and cellulitis, and palpate for any painful swelling over posterior aspect of elbow.
- Examine for bursa swelling or fluctuance, and attempt to transilluminate.
- For suspected infection (e.g., contiguous soft tissue infection), aspirate fluid from bursa and send for Gram's stain, culture, WBC count, and glucose determination.

NERVE ENTRAPMENT SYNDROMES

- With suspected ulnar nerve compression, check for pain beneath medial epicondyle and numbness in fifth and lateral fourth fingers; note any intrinsic hand muscle weakness.

423

- For suspected posterior interosseous nerve compression, check for pain near lateral epicondyle (mimics tennis elbow) as well as pain reproduced by extension of middle finger against resistance.

ARTHRITIS

- Inquire into symptoms of rheumatoid disease.
- Examine for limitation of motion, swelling, and pain.
- Obtain radiographs to gauge extent of joint involvement if it will aid Dx and management.

SEPTIC ARTHRITIS

- Inquire into systemic symptoms and source of blood-borne infection.
- Note rapid onset of pain, diffuse joint swelling, and erythema.
- Check for underlying conditions (DM, steroid use, or RA).
- If sepsis suspected, perform arthrocentesis for Gram's stain and culture of joint fluid, WBC count, crystal exam, and glucose determination.

CARPAL TUNNEL SYNDROME

- Inquire into underlying hypothyroidism, inflammatory joint disease, osteoarthritis of wrist, recent trauma, and pregnancy.
- Check for characteristic symptoms (nocturnal hand and wrist pain and paresthesias) that are often relieved by shaking hand.
- Note any numbness affecting the middle or 3 radial fingers and occasionally thumb.
- Examine for altered sensitivity (first 3 fingers and radial side of fourth).
- Check thenar (base of thumb) muscle for atrophy.
- Attempt to elicit Tinel's sign (tapping over median nerve at wrist crease to produce "electric shocks" or paresthesias in median nerve distribution).
- Perform Phelan's test (maintain wrists in palmar flexion for 1 min to reproduce symptoms).
- Proceed to nerve conduction study and EMG only if you need objective confirmation (occupational claim) or if condition persists leading to numbness or weakness necessitating surgical consideration.
- Correlate clinical findings with neurophysiologic test results (high false-positive rate).

DE QUERVAIN'S TENOSYNOVITIS

- Inquire into pain exacerbated by use of thumb. Check for excessive repetitive work with hand, such as needlepoint, knitting, or peeling vegetables.
- Test by having patient, with wrist in ulnar deviation and palmar flexion, grasp thumb with adjacent digits (Finkelstein's test).

TRIGGER FINGER

- Inquire into snapping of digit (triggering) with use and locking or inability to extend proximal interphalangeal joint.
- Note any palpable thickening of flexor tendon at metacarpophalangeal joint level in palm.

GANGLION CYSTS

- Note cystic mass occurring in dorsum or radial volar surface of wrist.

MUCOUS CYSTS

- Inquire into underlying osteoarthritis of hands and check for characteristic findings.
- If in doubt, confirm with hand films (joint space narrowing, osteophytes).

OSTEOARTHRITIS

- Inquire into pain at carpometacarpal joint at base of thumb, often associated with decreased dexterity and diminished grip strength.
- Check for pain and crepitation on grasping thumb metacarpal and compressing it onto trapezium (grind test).
- If Dx in doubt, confirm with radiographic study (joint space narrowing, osteophytes, loose bodies).

RHEUMATOID ARTHRITIS

- See Rheumatoid Arthritis.

HAND INFECTIONS

- Note any redness, tenderness, or swelling about the fingernail (paronychia).
- Suspect closed compartment hand infection (felon) if pulp at distal tip of digit is swollen, exquisitely tender, and erythematous. Refer promptly to hand surgeon for incision, drainage, and administration of antibiotics.
- Suspect herpetic infection of fingertip if small vesicles present along pulp of fingertip.
- Promptly recognize and refer for hand surgical intervention patients with infectious flexor tenosynovitis (digit symmetrically swollen, painful along entire flexor sheath, flexed, and tender on passive extension of distal joint).

MANAGEMENT

GENERAL STRATEGY

- Treat acute nonspecific tenosynovitis and mild to moderate degenerative arthritis with antiinflammatory medication and simple splinting when appropriate.
- Refer to hand specialist patients with hand infection, fracture, nerve compression, or mass.

LATERAL EPICONDYLITIS ("TENNIS ELBOW")

- Begin symptomatic Rx with elbow rest and application of ice (if acute).
- Advise cessation or limitation of painful activity (racquet sports, handshake, forceful use of arm in hammering or unscrewing jars, and screwdriver use).
- Prescribe generic NSAID Rx (e.g., 375 mg naproxen bid, or 600 mg ibuprofen tid × 1–2 wks) for symptom relief.
- Consider local steroid injection only for refractory cases.
- Avoid repeated steroid injection (risk of tendon and fascial rupture).

- Consider referral to physical Rx to teach patients exercises that stretch and condition involved muscles. Discourage overemphasis on use of friction massage, ultrasound, and other alternative modalities.
- Recommend instruction for tennis players in proper stroking of shots with firm wrist and proper elbow positioning; forearm bands usually of limited value, but may allow play when mild pain is present.

MEDIAL EPICONDYLITIS ("GOLFER'S ELBOW")

- Rx is same as for lateral epicondylitis (see above).
- Also consider median and ulnar nerve entrapment syndromes, which may mimic this condition.

OLECRANON BURSITIS

- Treat with organism-specific parenteral antibiotics (*Staphylococcus* and *Streptococcus* most common organisms; occasionally *Pseudomonas*).
- Avoid aspiration unless infection is a concern.
- Provide antiinflammatory medication (e.g., naproxen, 500 mg bid) and sling + local protection to avoid pressure.

NERVE ENTRAPMENT SYNDROMES

- Treat ulnar nerve compression with avoidance of leaning on elbow and use of nighttime splint that holds elbow in extension; recommend use of protective pad during day.
- Refer entrapments accompanied by muscle atrophy that do not respond to simple measures.

RHEUMATOID ARTHRITIS

- Begin antiinflammatory Rx and consider disease-modifying program (see Rheumatoid Arthritis).

SEPTIC ARTHRITIS

- Treat confirmed infection with IV organism-specific antibiotics and consideration of operative débridement.

CARPAL TUNNEL SYNDROME

- Prescribe wrist splinting, control of any underlying systemic metabolic disorder, and occasional local injection of corticosteroids.
- Recommend wearing firm canvas or plaster wrist splint during sleep.
- Consider injection of corticosteroids (e.g., 0.5–1 mL dexamethasone + 1–2 mL lidocaine) directly into carpal tunnel if there is significant flexor tenosynovitis; refer if technique unfamiliar.
- Consider surgical intervention if symptoms persist >3 mos, if associated thenar muscle atrophy develops or if motor or sensory latencies on EMG and nerve conduction studies are extremely prolonged.

DE QUERVAIN'S TENOSYNOVITIS

- Prescribe oral NSAIDs (e.g., naproxen, 375 mg bid).
- Treat with splinting; order removable plaster or Orthoplast splint that holds wrist and thumb in slight dorsiflexion and radial deviation; have patient wear for 10–14 days except when bathing.
- Refer for hand surgical consultation and possible steroid injection if symptoms persist.

TRIGGER FINGER

- Treat with splinting, NSAIDs, and, if unsuccessful, corticosteroid injection.

GANGLION CYSTS

- Avoid Rx unless bothersome.
- If bothersome or Dx in doubt, consider aspiration with large-bore (16- or 19-ga) needle; recurrence rate is high even with steroid injection.
- Consider surgical Rx if cyst is painful, appearance is unsatisfactory, or exact nature of mass a concern.

OSTEOARTHRITIS

- Treat with NSAIDs and, if refractory, molded splint worn 4–6 hrs/day.
- Have splint custom made by trained occupational therapist, extending it beyond metacarpophalangeal joint but leaving wrist free (short opponens splint).

HAND INFECTIONS

- Treat infection around fingernail (paronychia) with warm soaks + antibiotics effective against gram-positive organisms. If infection spreads, refer for incision and drainage.
- For suspected closed compartment hand infection (felon), refer promptly to hand surgeon for incision, drainage, and administration of antibiotics.
- For herpetic infection of fingertip, no Rx necessary, but inform patient lesions are infectious until vesicles clear.
- Promptly refer for hand surgical intervention patients with infectious flexor tenosynovitis.
- For puncture wounds, particularly human bites, provide prompt and aggressive wound care, with puncture site left open and parenteral antibiotic Rx begun immediately.
- Consider penicillin for dog and cat bites (*P. multocida*; see Animal and Human Bites).

BIBLIOGRAPHY

- For the current annotated bibliography on elbow, wrist, and hand pain, see the print edition of *Primary Care Medicine*, 4th edition, Chapter 153, or www.LWWmedicine.com.

Fibromyalgia

DIFFERENTIAL DIAGNOSIS

- Myofascial syndromes
- Rheumatoid disease
- Polymyalgia rheumatica
- Ankylosing spondylitis
- Reiter's syndrome
- Chronic fatigue syndrome
- Lyme disease
- Polymyositis
- Depression
- Somatization disorder
- Hypertrophic osteoarthropathy

WORKUP

OVERALL STRATEGY

- Perform detailed Hx and PE with focus on fulfilling key American College of Rheumatology diagnostic criteria for fibromyalgia:
  - Hx of widespread pain (left and right sides of body, above and below waist, with axial skeletal involvement) for ≥3 mos.
  - Pain on digital palpation present in ≥11 of these 18 tender point sites (see Fig. 159-1 in *Primary Care Medicine*, 4th edition).
- Use Hx and PE to make Dx and rule out other similarly presenting etiologies (see above); reserve lab studies only to help rule out other conditions.
- Establish Dx firmly and rule out other concerns.

HISTORY

- Delineate location of pain and inquire into key associated features (fatigue, nonrefreshing sleep, and exacerbations associated with weather changes).
- Rule out other conditions by checking for somatic and affective symptoms of depression (see Depression) and hypothyroidism (see Hypothyroidism) and reviewing for complaints of frank arthritis, fever, rash, muscle weakness, and Hx of muscle injury.

PHYSICAL EXAM

- Examine skin, nails, mucous membranes, fundi, joints, spine, muscles, tendons, bones, and nervous system for evidence of rheumatoid disease, spondyloarthropathy, myopathy, osteoarthropathy, thyroid disease, and focal pathology.
- Perform mental status exam for signs of depression (see Depression).

- Carefully palpate characteristic 18 tender point sites (see above) using just enough pressure to cause blanching of examining fingertip. Perform with approximate force of 4 kg.
- Consider tender point "positive" when patient states that palpation was painful. Do not consider "tender" to be same as "painful."
- Note any elicitation of exaggerated tenderness or outright pain.
- Differentiate from trigger points (produce referred pain).

LAB STUDIES

- To rule out other mimicking conditions, order ANA determination (cognizant of high risk of false-positive with low pretest probability of SLE).
- Also obtain ESR, TSH, and creatine phosphokinase levels.
- Do not obtain Lyme titers unless patient has symptoms strongly suggestive of disease (residence in endemic area or deer tick exposure + rash, arthritis, neurologic complaints).
- Consider spinal and sacroiliac films when back pain is predominant symptom.
- When fatigue is primary complaint, consider additional testing (see Chronic Fatigue).

MANAGEMENT

- Stress principal goal of maintaining and enhancing functional capacity.
- Form effective patient–doctor relationship by
  - eliciting and responding to essential details of patient's illness and specific concerns;
  - performing directed PE pertinent to differential Dx and patient's concerns;
  - taking time at end of visit for focused but unhurried review of findings and their meaning.
- Address pain, fatigue, and any concurrent depression.
- Begin tricyclic antidepressant at low dose (e.g., amitriptyline, 10–25 mg qhs) or SSRI (e.g., paroxetine, 10 mg qam).
- Combine with program of family ed, aerobic exercise, relaxation training, and meditation.
- For additional pain control, consider analgesic tramadol or short-term use of benzodiazepine, but avoid prolonged tramadol or benzodiazepine use.
- Omit NSAIDs and systemic corticosteroids (no benefit).
- Omit injection of tender points.
- Advise that *S*-adenosyl-L-methionine (SAMe, a popular nonprescription derivative of methionine with purported antidepressant, analgesic, and antiinflammatory actions) gives only modest reductions in pain, depression, and number of tender points.
- Advise that acupuncture is of unproved benefit, as are biofeedback and hypnotherapy.
- Avoid empiric parenteral antibiotic Rx for Lyme disease; treat only in presence of hard evidence for condition (see Lyme Disease).
- For refractory complaints,

- conduct full psychosocial assessment, evaluating psychiatric, family, occupational, and social difficulties;
- give priority to any underlying psychosocial difficulties;
- consider cognitive-behavioral Rx to redirect focus from pain and disability toward restoration of function and full participation in daily life.

BIBLIOGRAPHY

■ For the current annotated bibliography on fibromyalgia, see the print edition of *Primary Care Medicine*, 4th edition, Chapter 159, or www.LWWmedicine.com.

DIFFERENTIAL DIAGNOSIS

COMMON CAUSES OF FOOT PAIN

- Digital deformities
  - Hammertoe
  - Claw toe
  - Mallet toe
- Forefoot pain
  - Great toe
    - Hallux valgus (bunion)
    - Hallux limitus/rigidus
    - Sesamoid disorders
  - Other structures
    - Tailor's bunion (bunionette)
    - Metatarsalgia
    - Morton's interdigital neuroma
    - Metatarsal stress fracture
- Hindfoot pain
  - Plantar
    - Plantar fasciitis
    - Infracalcaneal bursitis
    - Medial calcaneal nerve entrapment
    - Tarsal tunnel syndrome
    - Referred pain from subtalar arthritis or lumbosacral disk radiculopathy
  - Posterior
    - Posterior calcaneal bursitis
    - Exostosis ("pump bump")
    - Achilles tendinitis
    - Inflammatory arthritis

WORKUP

DIGITAL PROBLEMS

- Inquire into toe pain ± "corn" (clavus) and shoe-foot difficulties.
- Check for toe deformities (hammertoe, mallet toe, claw toe).

FOREFOOT PROBLEMS

First Metatarsophalangeal Joint

Medial Bunion

- Inquire into presence of bunion, its consequences (hammertoes, metatarsalgia), and shoe-foot incompatibilities.
- Note risk factors such as hyperpronation (flat feet) and inappropriate shoes (high heels, pointed toe box).

- Check for hallux valgus deformity and swollen tender bursa on dorso-medial aspect of first metatarsal head associated with irreducible lateral drift of the big toe.
- Obtain foot radiographs to detect underlying etiology (e.g., increased angle between first and second metatarsals due to RA).

Dorsal Bunion

- Inquire into loss of dorsiflexion of first MTP joint and a dorsal bunion associated with pain while walking or problems with shoe fitting.
- Note hallux limitus or hallux rigidus (marked pain and limited mobility of first MTP joint on dorsiflexion).
- Obtain foot radiographs to check for joint space narrowing, osteophytes, and sclerosis, and to differentiate from chronic gouty arthritis.

Sesamoid Disorders

- Inquire into Hx of excessive stress in this area (ballet or aerobic dancing, jogging).
- Note any localized pain and swelling at plantar aspect of first MTP joint.
- Check foot films, including sesamoid axial view, for fracture.

Lesser Metatarsophalangeal Joint

- Inquire into painful deformity in fifth metatarsal region with presence of bunionette; note any foot-shoe incompatibility.
- Check for tenderness on lateral aspect of fifth metatarsal head and local bursal swelling.
- Obtain foot films to check for primary defect (e.g., excessive angle between fourth and fifth metatarsals or enlarged fifth head).

Metatarsalgia

- Inquire into pain with weight bearing in vicinity of lesser metatarsal heads.
- Check for metatarsal tenderness to pressure, plantar protrusion (with patient lying prone), hypermobility of neighboring metatarsals, and callus directly beneath involved metatarsal.

Interdigital (Morton's) Neuroma

- Inquire into burning pain and cramping of third and fourth toes aggravated by wearing closed shoes and relieved by removing shoe and massaging forefoot.
- Check for Mulder's sign ("click" and reproduction of symptoms by compressing forefoot and pushing up in distal third intermetatarsal space).

Metatarsal Stress Fractures

- Inquire into sudden onset of pain in second or third metatarsal, usually in setting of increased foot stress and no prior difficulty.
- Palpate metatarsal shaft for tenderness over injury site.
- Note swelling (healing callus) 4–6 wks after injury.
- Consider bone scan for early Dx.

HINDFOOT PROBLEMS

Plantar Fasciitis

- Check for posterior heel pain with initial step after getting out of bed in the morning and diminishing as foot "stretches out," only to recur after periods of inactivity.

- Inquire into overuse syndromes (e.g., jogging).
- Note tenderness along medial plantar aspect of foot, approximately 3 finger breadths distal to posterior heel, increased by dorsiflexion of toes.
- Omit foot films (spurs usually incidental and unrelated).

Infracalcaneal Bursitis

- Inquire into focal pain in midplantar aspect of heel, increasing with weight bearing and more pronounced as day progresses.
- Elicit point tenderness in midportion of the calcaneus and note any localized warmth and swelling.

Proximal Nerve Entrapment

Medial Calcaneal Branch of Posterior Tibial Nerve
- Check for Hx of heel pain with proximal radiation upward toward region of tarsal tunnel beneath medial malleolus. Seek presence of Tinel's sign on exam.

Posterior Tibial Nerve
- Inquire into trauma (sprain, fracture), space-occupying lesion (varicosity, lipoma), or repetitive hyperpronation leading to paresthesias, dysesthesias, and nocturnal pain along plantar aspect of foot.

Radiculopathy (Herniated Lumbosacral Disk)

- Check for foot/heel pain associated with low back or buttock pain.
- Perform straight-leg raising test and examine for any motor, sensory, and deep tendon reflex deficits.

POSTERIOR HEEL PAIN

Bursitis

- Inquire into wearing inappropriate shoe with firm, unyielding heel counter.
- Note symptoms of systemic inflammatory conditions (RA, ankylosing spondylitis, and Reiter's syndrome).
- Review Hx for Achilles tendon injury.
- Check for focal tenderness on compression of heel cord just anterior to its attachment and with passive dorsal and plantar ankle flexion.

Exostosis

- Inquire into "pump bump" in young women, presenting as tender enlargement about lateral dorsal aspect of posterior calcaneus.
- Note pain aggravated by firm heel counter and thickened bursa over true exostosis.
- Check lateral radiograph to confirm.

Achilles Tendinitis

- Check for Hx of overuse, with discomfort worsened by athletic activity and subsequent swelling and stiffness.
- Note fusiform swelling and tenderness on palpation of tendon (often extending proximally).

FOOT DISORDERS ASSOCIATED WITH SYSTEMIC CONDITIONS

- Inquire into concurrent atherosclerotic vascular disease, DM, peripheral neuropathy, gout, and RA; examine and test accordingly.

RUNNER'S FOOT

- Check for hyperpronation (flat feet) and resultant medial knee pain felt after prolonged jogging.
- Note any rigid, cavus-type foot deformity and resultant complaints of leg, knee, and hip discomfort.

ANKLE DISORDERS

Ankle Sprain

- Inquire into causative event (running or walking over uneven surface), location of discomfort, and aggravating movements.
- For inversion injury, note Hx of inversion during plantar flexion and snap or tear heard or felt.
- Identify site and degree of injury by palpating anterior capsule and medial and lateral ligaments (see Fig. 154-2 in *Primary Care Medicine*, 4th edition).
- Note pain, ecchymosis, and swelling along involved ligaments with aggravation of symptoms with ankle inversion or eversion; be aware that complete ligamentous and capsular disruption may produce remarkably little edema because of extravasation into surrounding soft tissue.
- Assess severity of sprain: first degree (involving stretching of ligamentous fibers), second degree (involving tear of some portion of ligament with associated pain and swelling), and third degree (involving complete ligamentous separation).
- Perform anterior ankle draw sign (grasp distal tibia in 1 hand and calcaneus and heel in other hand, and slide entire foot forward, first with ankle in neutral position and then with 30-degree plantar flexion); >4-mm anterior shift indicates anterior/lateral ligamentous disruption. Simple strain does not result in joint instability.
- Note any joint instability with talar tilt (adduction of calcaneus; see Fig. 154-2 in *Primary Care Medicine*, 4th edition), producing gap between talus and malleolus on lateral aspect of ankle.
- Check ankle films if swelling or pain interferes with evaluation, especially in suspected moderate to severe injury; radiography can be performed after taping, icing, and elevation.
- Obtain A-P, lateral, and mortice views (A-P view with ankle in 20- to 30-degree internal rotation) + stress view (with local anesthesia, if necessary) to check for talar tilt (>15 degrees = suggestive; >25 degrees = diagnostic of lateral ligamentous injury).
- Consider referral for nerve block before x-ray if pain impairs determination of joint instability.

MANAGEMENT

DIGITAL PROBLEMS

- Recommend shoes that provide adequate room in toe box area.
- Refer to podiatrist or orthopedic specialist for digital splints if change in shoes is insufficient, and for consideration of surgery if Rx fails and patient is severely compromised.

FOREFOOT PROBLEMS

First Metatarsophalangeal Joint

Medial Bunion

- Recommend properly fitted shoes (commercial or custom made) and bunion shields, and refer for fitting of orthotic devices.
- Consider surgical intervention to correct structural deformity if refractory to conservative measures and pain incapacitating.

Dorsal Bunion

- Refer for fitting of orthotic device that limits stresses on joint and for shoe with extra depth and stiffened outer sole.
- Consider surgery [débridement of osteophytes (cheilectomy) or joint resection, replacement, or fusion] if conservative measures fail.

Sesamoid Disorders

- Recommend reduction in weight-bearing stresses in this area.
- Recommend stiff-soled, low-heeled shoe with full-length shank and soft innersole. Orthotic devices may be of additional help; consider orthotic fitting.

Lesser Metatarsophalangeal Joints

- Recommend alteration of shoe gear (i.e., wider or stretched); refer for surgical correction if necessary.

Metatarsalgia

- Disperse weight away from involved metatarsal using soft innersoles, molded shoes with innersoles, metatarsal bars, and orthotic devices.
- Refer for consideration of surgical intervention (metatarsal head resection) when there is deforming RA with dorsal dislocation of MTP joints.

Interdigital (Morton's) Neuroma

- Recommend use of wider shoes and refer for consideration of metatarsal bar, soft insoles, and orthotic devices.
- Prescribe NSAIDs and consider local anesthetic/steroid injection for persistent discomfort; refer for consideration of surgical excision if pain refractory.

Metatarsal Stress Fracture

- Recommend avoiding rigorous activities and wearing stiff-soled, low-heeled shoe.

HINDFOOT PROBLEMS

Plantar Fasciitis

- Recommend stretching exercises, activity modification, ice, NSAIDs, and heel cushion use.
- If unsuccessful, refer for consideration of cast immobilization and possibly steroid injections (used sparingly).

Infracalcaneal Bursitis

- Recommend ice, massage, NSAIDs, and soft heel pad with center punched out.
- If pain persistent and refractory, refer for steroid injection.

Proximal Nerve Entrapment

Medial Calcaneal Branch of Posterior Tibial Nerve
- Refer for local steroid injection and consideration of tarsal tunnel release.

Posterior Tibial Nerve
- Refer for Rx with orthotic devices and local steroid injections.

Radiculopathy (Herniated Lumbosacral Disk)

- Treat underlying disk disease (see Back Pain).

POSTERIOR HEEL PAIN

Bursitis

- Recommend ice application in first 24 hrs, followed by moist heat, NSAIDs, and rest.
- For chronic discomfort, refer for heel lift or orthotic device to control heel motion and for adjustments of heel counter of shoe.

Exostosis

- Treat with same Rx as for bursitis.
- Consider resection of posterior bony exostosis only for chronic incapacitating symptoms.

Achilles Tendinitis

- Recommend foot rest, heel lift, antiinflammatory agents, and heel cord stretching, and consider ultrasound and orthotic devices.

RUNNER'S FOOT

- For patients with hyperpronation arrange referral for molded orthotic device.
- If deformities found, arrange consultation for best approach.

ANKLE DISORDERS

Ankle Sprain

- Control swelling promptly (to minimize stretch and distention of joint leading to adhesions) with elastic bandage, ice pack or ice water (15–20 mins), and elevation. Repeat every few hrs.
- Use soft dressing or elastic bandage (ankle splint) for 1–2 wks to control swelling and provide stability, keeping ankle in neutral or slightly everted position to avoid tightening heel cord and other posterior structures.
- Allow partial weight bearing by use of crutch until pain subsides.
- Start non–weight-bearing exercises within 2–3 days of injury (active plantar flexion, dorsiflexion, toe flexion, inversion, eversion).
- Resume full weight bearing after pain subsides and swelling resolves.
- Recommend use of functional plastic "sprain brace."
- Postpone running for another 1–3 wks depending on injury severity.
- Advise taping before athletic activity to support lateral structures when there is contact, running, or jumping, particularly on uneven ground, and if there has been mild ligamentous laxity and repeated minor sprains.
- Instruct that tape strips be applied from medial aspect to lateral aspect of ankle (see Fig. 154-3 in *Primary Care Medicine*, 4th edition) to hold heel and ankle in eversion and provide support.

- Recommend exercises to strengthen ankle evertors, and use of high-laced leather supportive shoes.
- Refer promptly for cast immobilization if torn ligaments result in marked ankle instability.

BIBLIOGRAPHY

- For the current annotated bibliography on foot and ankle pain, see the print edition of *Primary Care Medicine*, 4th edition, Chapter 154, or www.LWWmedicine.com.

Giant Cell Arteritis

WORKUP

- Check for current American College of Rheumatology criteria:
  - Age at onset >50
  - New onset or new type of localized headache
  - Temporal artery tenderness or diminished pulse
  - ESR >50 mm/hr
  - Temporal artery biopsy specimen showing mononuclear infiltration or granulomatous infiltration with giant cells (negative first biopsy result does not rule out Dx)
- View presence of any 3 criteria as evidence for Dx of TA (sensitivity, 93.5%; specificity, 91.2%).
- If clinical suspicion high, corticosteroids can be started before biopsy as long as biopsy done within 1–2 wks.
- When possible, strive for histologic confirmation. However, biopsy unnecessary when it will have no effect on clinical decision making.
- Consider color duplex ultrasonography of temporal arteries as alternative or complement to temporal artery biopsy (key diagnostic finding: dark halo about vessel; sensitivity 73%, specificity 100%).
- Reserve arteriography (sensitive but nonspecific) to help define area to sample if first biopsy negative.

MANAGEMENT

- Begin Rx with daily high-dose glucocorticoids (e.g., prednisone, 40–60 mg qam).
- Consider prescribing IV methylprednisolone (100 mg q12h × 5 days) for patients with vision disturbances.
- Begin reducing initial dose once ESR has normalized (<40 mm/hr) and symptoms have cleared; aim for prednisone dose of 20–30 mg/day after 1–2 mos.
- Continue daily prednisone Rx, tapering as tolerated over 12–18 mos to minimum dose sufficient to keep ESR normal and patient symptom-free; prednisone dose <10 mg/day is often sufficient.
- Monitor symptoms and ESR to determine rate and extent of tapering permissible. Halt tapering if ESR rises or symptoms return.
- Continue daily steroids for 18–24 mos; consider trial of phasing-out Rx at that time and then q6–12mos.
- After cessation of Rx, monitor over next 12 mos for recurrence of symptoms and rise in ESR.
- Watch for development of aortic aneurysm.

BIBLIOGRAPHY

- For the current annotated bibliography on giant cell arteritis, see the print edition of *Primary Care Medicine*, 4th edition, Chapter 161, or www.LWWmedicine.com.

Gout

WORKUP

- See Asymptomatic Hyperuricemia; Monoarticular Arthritis

MANAGEMENT

ACUTE GOUT

- At first sign of acute gouty arthritis attack, begin generic NSAID (e.g., 500 mg naproxen tid).
- Continue full-dose Rx until symptoms resolve, then taper to cessation over 72 hrs. Advise patient that delay in starting Rx may impair response.
- For patients unable to take generic NSAIDs (e.g., Hx of peptic ulcer disease), consider COX-2 agent (see Peptic Ulcer Disease) or colchicine.
- For colchicine use, prescribe 0.6 mg qid, but warn that diarrhea and upper GI upset are likely during Rx; monitor CBC and hepatic and renal function. Avoid colchicine if underlying renal or hepatic insufficiency is present.
- For refractory cases of definite acute gout, consider 7- to 10-day course of PO corticosteroids; start with prednisone, 20–40 mg/day and taper as quickly as clinically possible. Intraarticular corticosteroid Rx is another option if oral Rx is not feasible and just 1 joint is involved.
- Provide extra supply of antiinflammatory Rx for prompt use in future episode.

INTERVAL GOUT

- Advise weight reduction (but not starvation diets) if patient is obese, and cessation of excess alcohol use; consider providing information on reduced purine diet if dietary events appear to precipitate attacks.
- Avoid drugs that raise serum uric acid (e.g., thiazides, loop diuretics, low-dose aspirin, and niacin).
- Determine with patient whether gouty attacks are sufficiently frequent and disabling to warrant prophylactic Rx. Once patient has 2 attacks/yr, long-term urate-lowering Rx becomes cost-effective.
- If patient is willing to take long-term urate-lowering Rx, determine whether allopurinol or uricosuric agent is best by
  - inquiring into any personal or family Hx of kidney stones or renal dysfunction,
  - measuring renal function (BUN, creatinine), and
  - determining 24-hr urinary uric acid excretion.

Allopurinol

- For patient who is excreting >1,000 mg/day of uric acid, has underlying azotemia, is at increased risk for nephrolithiasis, or is allergic or unresponsive to uricosuric Rx, begin allopurinol (started at 100 mg/day and increased to 200–300 mg/day over 4 wks).
- Adjust dose upward if response is inadequate. Reduce dose in setting of renal insufficiency and use cautiously, especially when patient is also taking diuretics or ampicillin.

- Stop at earliest sign of hypersensitivity reaction. Consider restarting at low dose if drug rash is mild, but monitor CBC and hepatic and renal function closely.
- Consider desensitization for patients who require allopurinol but who react with mild drug rash.

Uricosuric Agents

- Begin probenecid or sulfinpyrazone if patient has normal renal function, no risk for stone disease, and urate excretion <700 mg/day. Initiate Rx in small doses (e.g., 250 mg probenecid bid, or 50 mg sulfinpyrazone bid); at same time keep fluid intake large (2–3 L/day) to prevent precipitation of uric acid in urinary tract. Alkalinization of urine to pH 6.6 is desirable during first wk of Rx but is difficult to achieve; gram doses of sodium bicarbonate are required, supplemented by acetazolamide (250 mg) qhs.
- Advance uricosuric dose gradually to avoid triggering massive urate excretion. Max dose of sulfinpyrazone is 100 mg tid–qid; for probenecid, it is 500–1,000 mg bid–tid.
- Continue high fluid intake during early mos of Rx. Avoid concurrent use of aspirin because it inhibits urate excretion.

Monitoring and Concurrent Antiinflammatory Therapy

- Monitor serum uric acid concentration and treat to achieve level of <6.5 mg/dL, the initial concentration point of supersaturation.
- To reduce risk for attack of gout during first 3–6 mos of urate-lowering Rx, prescribe concurrent antiinflammatory prophylactic Rx with colchicine (0.6 mg qd–bid) or intermediate-acting NSAID (e.g., 250 mg naproxen qd–bid).
- Advise avoiding precipitants such as binge drinking, fasting, and very-low-calorie diets.

CHRONIC GOUTY ARTHRITIS

- Treat as for interval gout. Continue concurrent antiinflammatory Rx until all visible manifestations of uric acid deposits have resolved, which may take 6–12 mos.

RENAL COMPLICATIONS

- Pretreat cancer patients with allopurinol if large uric acid load is likely to result from chemotherapy.
- Advise marked reduction in lead exposure (e.g., home-distilled alcohol, industrial contact).
- Treat patients with urate nephrolithiasis or strong family Hx of kidney stones with allopurinol (300 mg/day) and hydration. Long-term efforts to alkalinize urine are impractical and need not be undertaken.
- Because risk for chronic renal failure from chronic hyperuricemia is nil, preventative long-term urate-lowering Rx is unnecessary.

BIBLIOGRAPHY

- For the current annotated bibliography on gout, see the print edition of *Primary Care Medicine*, 4th edition, Chapter 158, or www.LWWmedicine.com.

Hip Pain

DIFFERENTIAL DIAGNOSIS

- Degenerative joint disease
- Avascular necrosis of femoral head
- Bursitis
- Polymyalgia rheumatica
- Rheumatoid arthritis
- Ankylosing spondylitis
- Villonodular synovitis
- Referred pain
  - Herniated disk
  - Retroperitoneal tumor or abscess
  - Obturator or femoral hernia
- Aortoiliac insufficiency

WORKUP

HISTORY

- Ascertain onset, location, and radiation of pain as well as inciting and alleviating factors and presence of numbness or weakness.
- Inquire directly about trauma, involvement of other joints, morning stiffness, relation of pain to activity, response to rest, steroid or alcohol use, and current infection or fever.
- Note that stiffness itself is nonspecific (may occur with degenerative and rheumatoid etiologies); check response to continued activity (worsens in degenerative disease and lessens in RA).

PHYSICAL EXAM

- Examine for deformities (rheumatoid disease) and for fixed external rotation (fracture of femoral neck).
- Check gait and put hip through full range of passive motion to detect crepitus, limitation of movement, flexion contracture, muscle spasm, and guarding.
- Take particular note of any limitation or pain on internal rotation on hip (early sign of degenerative disease).
- Palpate joint and individual bursae for focal tenderness and swelling.
- Measure thigh circumference at fixed distance from bony reference point for atrophy (intrinsic hip disease).
- Palpate femoral pulses for diminution and auscultate for bruits.
- Examine pelvis and rectum for tumors, back for evidence of L1-2 or L2-3 disk herniation, and lower extremities for weakness, sensory loss, and reflexes.

LAB STUDIES

- Obtain plain films of hip with weight-bearing views to gauge extent of joint space narrowing in degenerative disease.
- Order sacroiliac and spine films if ankylosing spondylitis suspected.
- Check MRI for earliest detection of avascular necrosis of femoral head and stress fracture of femoral neck.
- Consider CBC, ESR, and RF determinations if considering rheumatoid disease.
- Aspirate suspected septic joint and send fluid for cell count, Gram's stain, and culture.

MANAGEMENT

DEGENERATIVE DISEASE

- Acutely, recommend daily periods of bed rest, analgesics (e.g., 500 mg acetaminophen qid), limitation of sitting, and crutch or cane support; no additional benefit from NSAIDs.
- Advise against spending large sums on glucosamine, chondroitin, and other expensive, unproved, nonprescription measures for osteoarthritis (see Osteoarthritis).
- After acute symptoms lessen, begin program of daily mild exercise (walking short distances as tolerated) preceded by acetaminophen, cane support if necessary, weight reduction if obese, and specific daily range-of-motion and strengthening exercises, preferably taught by physical therapist.
- Advise rest periods of 1 hr bid with local heat applied to hip if discomfort occurs after exercise.
- Suggest avoiding activities that specifically and markedly aggravate pain.
- Reemphasize importance of modest weight reduction if overweight and provide comprehensive program for weight reduction (see Overweight and Obesity).
- Consider surgical consultation if conservative measures do not control symptoms and patient desires to be active; need not delay indefinitely if symptoms are disabling.

BURSITIS

- Begin generic NSAID Rx (e.g., 500 mg naproxen bid × 1–2 wks) in conjunction with reduced activity.
- Advise commonsense measures (running only on flat surfaces, heel lift if legs not same length).
- Consider hip bursal steroid injection for relief of refractory severe focal pain.
- Refer to orthopedist or rheumatologist if unfamiliar with technique.

RHEUMATOID DISEASE

- Prescribe trial of low-dose steroids for suspected polymyalgia rheumatica (see Polymyalgia Rheumatica).
- Treat RA acutely with antiinflammatory drugs and select disease-modifying Rx (see Rheumatoid Arthritis).

HIP FRACTURE AND SEPTIC ARTHRITIS

■ Hospitalize immediately.

BIBLIOGRAPHY

■ For the current annotated bibliography on hip pain, see the print edition of *Primary Care Medicine*, 4th edition, Chapter 151, or www.LWWmedicine.com.

Knee Pain

DIFFERENTIAL DIAGNOSIS

- One knee only
  - Acute
    - Sprain
    - Strain
    - Acute gout
    - Meniscus tear
    - Early RA
    - Gonococcal arthritis
    - Septic arthritis
    - Reiter's syndrome
    - Bursitis
    - Pseudogout
    - Palindromic rheumatism
    - Ruptured Baker's cyst
    - Hemophilia
    - Sickle cell disease
    - Rheumatic fever
  - Chronic
    - Osteoarthritis
    - Baker's cyst
    - Chronic gout
    - Chondromalacia patella
    - Bursitis
    - Meniscal injuries
- One knee + other joints
  - See Monoarticular Arthritis; Polyarticular Complaints
- Symmetric involvement, knees only
  - Acute
    - RA
    - Juvenile RA
    - Early phase of other rheumatoid diseases
    - Trauma
  - Chronic
    - Osteoarthritis
    - Chondromalacia patellae
    - Bursitis
    - RA
    - Juvenile RA
    - Chronic gout
    - Neuropathic joints
    - Hemophilia
- Symmetric polyarthritis
  - See Polyarticular Complaints
- One knee + other joints
  - See Monoarticular Arthritis; Polyarticular Complaints

WORKUP

GENERAL STRATEGY

- Ascertain quality and location of pain, alleviating and aggravating factors, and associated symptoms such as swelling, redness, and warmth.
- Determine whether problem is acute or chronic, symmetric or asymmetric, and monoarticular or polyarticular (see above) and focus workup accordingly.

HISTORY

Acute Unilateral Knee Pain

- Inquire about trauma, jogging, swelling, pain on climbing stairs, concurrent fever, purulent vaginal or urethral discharge, rash, recent streptococcal infection or sore throat, heart murmur, morning stiffness, and urethritis or conjunctivitis.
- Note any Hx of gout, sickle cell disease, or hemophilia.
- For localized swelling, ascertain exact site.
- Take special note of knee locking (meniscal tear) or giving out (anterior cruciate disruption).

Chronic Unilateral Knee Pain

- Review previous or recurrent trauma (e.g., occupational).
- Check for pain associated with prolonged walking, standing, or climbing stairs; knee locking; crepitus; focal swelling; and recurrent acute episodes or exacerbations.

Acute Bilateral Knee Pain

- When both knees are involved acutely, inquire into symptoms of rheumatoid disease (see Polyarticular Complaints) and check for recent trauma.

Chronic Bilateral Knee Pain

- Same as for chronic unilateral knee pain, but include inquiry into rheumatoid symptoms (see Polyarticular Complaints).

Polyarticular Presentations

- When other joints are involved, inquire into symptoms of infectious and rheumatologic conditions.

PHYSICAL EXAM

- Perform complete PE when systemic illness a consideration.
- Examine skin and integument for rash, clubbing, psoriatic changes, rheumatoid nodules, pallor, alopecia, and tophi.
- Check conjunctivae for erythema and petechiae, oral cavity for aphthous ulcers, lymph nodes for enlargement, chest for signs of consolidation and effusion, heart for murmurs and rubs, abdomen for organomegaly and tenderness, pelvis for vaginal discharge and adnexal tenderness, urethra for discharge, and penis for balanitis.
- Evaluate all other joints and perform complete neurologic exam.
- Begin knee exam with inspection for distortion of normal contours and irregular bony prominences at joint margins.
- Check for muscle atrophy (measure knee, calf, and thigh circumferences) and note any effusion (increased knee circumference at midpa-

tella and distended, fluctuant capsule with fluid wave and ballotable patella).
- Palpate joint line for localized tenderness (meniscal tear).
- Perform McMurray and Apley tests for suspected meniscal injury (see Fig. 152-2 in *Primary Care Medicine*, 4th edition).
- Assess bursal regions for focal tenderness and swelling (bursitis).
- Check range of motion and collateral and cruciate ligaments for stability (apply mediolateral valgus-varus strain with knee in full extension and in 15–20 degrees of flexion) (see Fig. 152-3 in *Primary Care Medicine*, 4th edition).
- Test anterior cruciate ligament stability with anterior drawer test (with knee relaxed and flexed to about 25 degrees, gently pull tibia anteriorly while holding femur in fixed position, and note amount of anterior displacement of tibia relative to femur).

LAB STUDIES

- Obtain plain films of knee in cases of trauma (fracture) and suspected degenerative or chronic rheumatoid disease.
- Consider stress views if joint instability suspected and weight-bearing views for degree of joint obliteration.
- Reserve MRI for detection of serious meniscal and cruciate tears when clinical findings are insufficient to establish Dx and invasive diagnostic procedure would otherwise be necessary. Not indicated as routine test for soft tissue disease of knee.
- Aspirate joint for acute monoarticular effusion when there is need to differentiate infection from crystalline-induced disease; send fluid for Gram's stain and cultures, WBC count, differential, glucose level, and check for crystals (see Monoarticular Arthritis).
- With polyarticular presentations, test for inflammatory joint disease (see Polyarticular Complaints).
- Consider fiberoptic arthroscopy as gold standard for Dx of internal derangements of soft tissues of knee.

MANAGEMENT

FOR KNEE INJURY

- Restrict weight-bearing activities and recommend use of crutches.
- Prescribe knee brace.
- Allow only absolutely necessary walking and forbid kneeling, squatting, and stair climbing.
- Recommend aspirin in pharmacologic doses of 2–4 g/day or generic NSAID (e.g., naproxen, 375 mg bid; or ibuprofen, 400 mg tid).
- Begin rehabilitation once swelling subsides and painless full range of motion returns.
- Start with isometric quadriceps and hamstring exercises.
- Refer to orthopedic surgery if knee gives way or locks or if joint instability or internal derangement suspected; arthroscopy may be needed.

FOR CHRONIC KNEE PAIN OF OSTEOARTHRITIS

- Prescribe program of walking and resistance exercise in randomized trials.
- Choose non-narcotic analgesics such as acetaminophen over NSAIDs for control of chronic pain.
- Recommend against depending on chondroitin sulfate or glucosamine (effectiveness not demonstrated in well-designed studies).

BIBLIOGRAPHY

- For the current annotated bibliography on knee pain, see the print edition of *Primary Care Medicine*, 4th edition, Chapter 152, or www.LWWmedicine.com.

SCREENING AND/OR PREVENTION

- Teach patients basics of avoiding tick habitats, dressing properly, using DEET repellants safely, and removing ticks effectively.
- Advise complete and early tick removal, especially within the first 24–48 hrs (before transmission of *Borrelia*).
- Offer option of antibiotic prophylaxis to those with tick bite occurring in endemic region, prescribing single 200-mg dose of doxycycline to be taken within 72 hrs after tick bite.
- Consider vaccination only for persons with very high risk for infection (e.g., outdoor workers in highly endemic areas). Inform patient of limitations and risks of vaccine use:
  - Not fully protective;
  - Can compromise results of current serologic testing;
  - Long-term safety not established (? risk of antibody-induced arthritis).

DIFFERENTIAL DIAGNOSIS

- See Chronic Fatigue; Polyarticular Complaints.

WORKUP

OVERALL STRATEGY

- Make Dx of Lyme disease predominantly based on clinical presentation (e.g., erythema migrans, relapsing oligoarthritis, heart block, facial nerve palsy) and epidemiology (e.g., community incidence, outdoor exposure, tick bite).
- Use serologic testing only to supplement clinical Dx.

HISTORY

Early Disease/Acute Infection

- Focus on Hx and epidemiology to make Dx in early-stage disease, because antibody does not appear for several wks.
- Inquire about outdoor activity in wooded, brushy, or grassy area of endemic region.
- Check for Hx of tick bite (although not essential for Dx because springtime nymph tick very small and bite easily missed).
- Ask about onset of large erythematous lesion (erythema migrans) and any flulike illness occurring in spring or summer.

Disseminated Disease

- In addition to epidemiologic features, check Hx for new erythematous lesions (*secondary erythema migrans*), palpitations, near-syncope, stiff neck, facial weakness (may be bilateral), radicular pain, migratory musculoskeletal complaints, and later, frank oligoarticular arthritis, particularly of knee.

Late/Chronic Disease

■ Focus on musculoskeletal and neurologic symptoms.

PHYSICAL EXAM

Early Disease/Acute Infection

■ Examine for characteristic annular lesion of erythema migrans (pathognomonic; appears in 50–80% of cases).

Disseminated Disease

■ Check for multiple annular erythematous skin lesions of secondary erythema migrans, irregular pulse, nuchal rigidity, facial nerve palsy, and joint swelling with effusion.

■ Suspect early disseminated Lyme disease if lesions of secondary erythema migrans present.

Late/Chronic Disease

■ Check for chronic oligoarticular arthritis (particularly of knee), memory loss, spinal radicular pain, and distal paresthesias.

LAB STUDIES

Early Disease/Acute Infection

■ Avoid and discourage serologic testing if very early in course of illness because of increased risk for false-negative and false-positive results (too early to detect new antibody).

Disseminated Disease

■ Limit serologic testing to persons with at least intermediate (20–80%) pretest probability of Lyme disease (based on clinical presentation).

■ Consider 2-step approach to serologic testing to reduce false-positive rate:
  • ELISA
  • Western blot, if indeterminate or positive by ELISA

■ For patients with meningeal signs, consider lumbar puncture. Send CSF for antibody testing, cell count, differential, and chemistries. Most patients with CNS involvement have detectable antibody in CSF, pleocytosis, and elevated protein concentration. If uncertainty persists, consider (if available) PCR testing of CSF for *Borrelia* DNA.

■ If joint effusion present, perform arthrocentesis and send fluid for analysis (as for CSF). Consider subjecting joint fluid to PCR testing.

Late/Chronic Disease

■ Patients with findings suggesting encephalopathy should undergo lumbar puncture for antibody testing of CSF, cell count, and chemistries. Consider PCR testing of CSF. Confirm peripheral polyneuropathy with electrophysiologic study.

Concurrent Babesiosis

■ Make Dx by identifying parasite in RBCs on Giemsa-stained thin blood smear. Because you frequently cannot see parasites, test sensitivity is greatly decreased.

■ Indirect immunofluorescence is principal antibody study available; positive test result consists of 4-fold rise in titer and immunofluorescence persisting at 1:32 dilution.

■ PCR assays are very sensitive and highly specific but not widely available.

MANAGEMENT

OVERALL APPROACH

■ Treat empirically those persons with high pretest probability of Lyme disease (e.g., typical erythema migrans rash, endemic area).

■ Treat, but only after testing, those who present with intermediate pretest probability of Lyme disease and have positive serology.

■ Consider early prophylactic Rx (doxycycline, 200 mg, once) of asymptomatic persons who report tick bite while in hyperendemic areas. Alternatively, follow such persons closely and perform serologic testing if they develop symptoms and signs suggesting intermediate pretest probability of Lyme disease; treat those with positive test results.

■ Do not treat empirically persons with chronic nonspecific symptoms (e.g., chronic fatigue, arthralgias, confusion) and no epidemiologic or clinical findings characteristic of Lyme disease (e.g., no erythema migrans).

■ Avoid prolonged antibiotic programs if patients do not have symptomatic benefit after full standard course of Rx for acute Lyme disease.

■ For asymptomatic seropositivity, no Rx necessary.

■ Treat according to stage of disease and organ(s) involved.

ANTIBIOTIC THERAPY

Early Disease/Acute Infection

■ Prescribe
  • amoxicillin (500 mg tid for 3–4 wks); or
  • doxycycline (100 mg bid with meals for 3–4 wks); or
  • cefuroxime (500 mg bid for 3 wks).

■ Shorter courses (e.g., 2 wks) are reasonable for disease limited to 1 skin lesion.

■ Do not use a popular 1-wk azithromycin program because of increased risk for relapse.

■ For isolated facial nerve paralysis, use oral antibiotic program for 21–28 days.

Disseminated Disease

■ Treat according to organ(s) involved:
  • Meningitis, multiple neurologic deficits or severe cardiac manifestations:
    • Ceftriaxone (2 g/day IV for 2–4 wks); or
    • Penicillin G, 20 million U/day IV for 14–21 days.
  • Mild cardiac involvement (first-degree arteriovenous block only):
    • Oral doxycycline (100 mg bid) or amoxicillin (500 mg tid) for 4 wks.
  • Mild peripheral neuropathy or Lyme arthritis:
    • Amoxicillin + probenecid (500 mg tid) or doxycycline (100 mg bid) for 4 wks.
  • Severe neuropathy (e.g., radiculoneuropathy, peripheral neuropathy, encephalitis):
    • Ceftriaxone or penicillin (as for meningitis).

Late/Chronic Disease

■ Arthritis
  • Treat initially with same program of amoxicillin or doxycycline as for stage 2 joint disease.
  • If refractory, follow with
    • penicillin G, 20 million U/day IV × 14–28 days; or
    • ceftriaxone, 2 g/day IV × 14–28 days.
■ Encephalitis
  • Treat with ceftriaxone (2 g/day IV × 2–4 wks).

Pregnant Women

■ For localized early Lyme disease
  • Amoxicillin, 500 mg PO tid × 21 days
■ For disseminated early Lyme disease or any manifestation of late disease
  • Penicillin G, 20 million U/day IV × 14–21 days.

BIBLIOGRAPHY

■ For the current annotated bibliography on Lyme disease, see the print edition of *Primary Care Medicine*, 4th edition, Chapter 160, or www.LWWmedicine.com.

Monoarticular Arthritis

DIFFERENTIAL DIAGNOSIS

- Infection
  - Gonococcus
  - Gram-positive organisms (staphylococci, streptococci)
  - Gram-negative coliforms (compromised hosts)
  - Lyme disease
- Crystal-induced
  - Gout
  - Pseudogout
- Monoarticular presentations of polyarticular disease
  - Rheumatoid arthritis
  - Reiter's syndrome
  - Ankylosing spondylitis
  - Psoriatic arthritis
  - Arthritis of inflammatory bowel disease
  - Sarcoidosis
- Trauma/degenerative disease
  - Osteoarthritis

WORKUP

HISTORY

- Check first for clinical evidence of joint infection (requires immediate attention), and then examine for other forms of inflammatory disease and noninflammatory conditions.
- Inquire into onset, associated symptoms, location, risk factors, and concurrent illness.
- Note any report of skin lesions, vaginal or urethral discharge, back pain, exposure to gonorrhea, tick bites, DM, concurrent RA, joint prosthesis, immunosuppression, HIV infection, IV drug abuse, and previous trauma or gout.

PHYSICAL EXAM

- Examine all joints, note distribution of problem, and check for signs of inflammation.
- Differentiate inflammation of joint space from periarticular process.
- Take patient's temp (high fever suggests infection).
- Check integument for rash, splinter hemorrhages, manifestations of HIV disease (see HIV-1 Infection), needle tracks, tophi, rheumatoid nodules, pitting of nails and other psoriatic manifestations, erythema nodosum (seen with sarcoidosis and inflammatory bowel disease), and keratoderma blennorrhagicum and circinate balanitis of Reiter's syndrome.
- Examine eyes for conjunctivitis and iritis, fundi for signs of endocarditis, mouth for mucosal ulceration, and heart for murmurs.

- Check genitalia for signs of gonococcal urethritis and cervicitis (see Gonorrhea; Urethritis in Men).
- Examine spine for restriction of motion and focal tenderness; palpate sacroiliac joints for tenderness.

LAB STUDIES

- Avoid running standard battery of "arthritis tests." Instead, select tests according to these American College of Rheumatology guidelines:
  - If trauma or focal bone pain is present, first study should be radiography of the area.
  - If effusion or other signs of inflammation noted, proceed to joint aspiration with fluid cell count and differential to confirm presence of inflammation.
  - If no effusion or trauma present, test for trigger and tender points (see Fibromyalgia) to assess for tendinitis and fibromyalgia, respectively.

Examination of Joint Fluid

- Note appearance of joint fluid (turbid, bloody, clear and straw-colored, frankly purulent).
- Send fluid promptly for cell count and differential, and separate samples for glucose concentration and microscopic exam (crystals, Gram's stain) and for culture if initial fluid exam shows evidence of inflammation (WBC >2,000/mm^3; >75% neutrophils).
- If WBC >50,000/mm^3, consider gout and septic arthritis; ideally, perform crystal exam under polarizing lens; may be able to identify urate crystals under normal light.
- Be sure joint fluid is promptly plated onto proper media (including Thayer-Martin plates for detection of gonococci) in suspected infection.
- Retap joint to improve diagnostic yield of Gram's stain and culture if results of first arthrocentesis are negative but clinical suspicion remains high.

Other Tests

- Obtain CBC and ESR to help distinguish inflammatory from noninflammatory disease.
- If inflammatory joint fluid is sterile, proceed with workup for connective tissue disease (see Polyarticular Complaints), Lyme disease (see Lyme Disease), and sarcoidosis (see Sarcoidosis).
- If joint fluid is frankly bloody, determine PT, PTT, and platelet count to check for bleeding diathesis (see Bleeding Problems).
- If crystals are found, no need for serum uric acid or calcium determinations.
- Obtain blood cultures in suspected sepsis, and culture other possible foci of infection (skin lesions, urethral discharge, cervix).
- Consider subjecting joint fluid to PCR analysis for evidence of *B. burgdorferi* infection when late-stage Lyme disease is a real concern supported by clinical findings.

Serologic Studies

- Use only in specific instances and not as battery of routine tests.
- Test for HIV antibodies in suspected immune compromise or high-risk sexual behavior (see HIV-1 Infection).

- Consider testing for ANA and RF only with strong clinical suspicion of connective tissue disease; beware of high false-positive rate, especially in the elderly and persons with other inflammatory conditions (see Polyarticular Complaints).
- Avoid casual ordering of Lyme antibody titers; obtain only in cases with strongly supporting clinical and epidemiologic evidence for *Borrelia* infection (see Lyme Disease).

Radiography

- Consider plain films of joints in setting of trauma or focal bone pain.
- Avoid unnecessary MRI, but do consider it in suspected traumatic internal knee derangement and when management requires confirmation (see Knee Pain).
- In suspected osteomyelitis, proceed to bone scan or MRI.

MANAGEMENT

EMPIRIC THERAPY AND SYMPTOMATIC MEASURES

- If infection, trauma, and, less important, crystal-induced arthritis are ruled out, approach evaluation less hurriedly and manage expectantly.
- Until Dx is established, consider symptomatic measures: resting, immobilizing joint, and administering ice packs.
- Postpone empiric antiinflammatory Rx for ≥12–24 hrs if first arthrocentesis nondiagnostic, yet concern persists about infection (allows repeat arthrocentesis without altering joint fluid findings).
- If pain is unbearable and Dx is not yet established, prescribe analgesic without antiinflammatory effects (e.g., acetaminophen or codeine).
- After second negative arthrocentesis result in setting of joint inflammation, consider instituting antiinflammatory Rx even in absence of specific Dx, provided all cultures are negative and patient is at low risk for infection.
- Base more definitive Rx on underlying cause (see Gonorrhea; Gout; Lyme Disease; Osteoarthritis; Rheumatoid Arthritis).

INDICATIONS FOR REFERRAL AND ADMISSION

- Admit patient with septic arthritis for IV antibiotics and consultation with infectious disease specialist.
- When cause of acute monoarticular arthritis remains elusive and peripheral WBC count is very high, consult infectious disease specialist regarding further workup and appropriateness of empiric antibiotic Rx.
- Obtain rheumatologic consultation for more chronic case that defies Dx.

BIBLIOGRAPHY

- For the current annotated bibliography on monoarticular arthritis, see the print edition of *Primary Care Medicine*, 4th edition, Chapter 145, or www.LWWmedicine.com.

Muscle Cramps

DIFFERENTIAL DIAGNOSIS

- True cramps
  - Ordinary (nocturnal)
  - Heat-induced (volume depletion, hyponatremia)
  - Hemodialysis (volume and electrolyte shifts)
  - Lower motor neuron
  - Drug-induced (nifedipine, β-agonists)
- Dystonia
  - Occupational (writer's cramp)
- Tetany
  - Hypocalcemia
  - Hypomagnesemia
  - Respiratory alkalosis
  - Hypokalemia
- Contracture
  - McArdle's disease
  - Thyroid disease

  Adapted from McGee SR. Muscle cramps. Arch Intern Med 1990;150:511, with permission.

WORKUP

HISTORY

- Obtain detailed description of cramping, including setting in which episodes occur.
- Note nocturnal timing, concurrent hemodialysis, hypoglycemia, heavy sweating during prolonged exertion, use of calcium channel blockers or β-agonists.
- Check for onset with occupation-related fine motor activity and for life-long onset with exercise.
- Inquire into associated symptoms such as paresthesias, carpopedal spasm, weakness and fasciculations, and symptoms of thyroid disease.
- Take note of any cramping in calves brought on by walking.
- Review medications (e.g., potassium-wasting diuretics), and check for Hx of thyroidectomy (coincident removal of parathyroid glands).

PHYSICAL EXAM

- Check postural signs in suspected dehydration.
- Examine skin for signs of thyroid disease; neck for evidence of thyroidectomy; lower extremities for diminished or absent pulses, muscle wasting, and fasciculations; and nervous system for focal weakness and absent or abnormal deep tendon reflexes.
- If tetany suspected, try to elicit facial spasm of Trousseau's sign (by tapping facial nerve) or carpal spasm of Chvostek's sign (by inflating arm cuff above systolic pressure).

LAB STUDIES

- Avoid testing if complaint is nocturnal muscle cramps.
- Check serum glucose for hypoglycemia in diabetics taking insulin.
- Obtain determinations of serum sodium, BUN, and creatinine if severe dehydration and hyponatremia suspected.
- Determine sodium, potassium, calcium, albumin (to interpret calcium level), and magnesium levels in patients with possible tetany.
- Check TSH if thyroid disease a concern.
- Consider nerve conduction study for patient with fasciculations and possible lower motor neuron disease.

MANAGEMENT

ORDINARY CRAMPS

- Recommend passively stretching contracting muscle and gradually contracting opposing one (e.g., by simply walking around).
- Suggest massage of involved muscle.
- Teach prophylactic stretching of leg or foot to abort or prevent attacks (see Exercise), and avoidance of precipitating factors (e.g., ankle plantar flexion in bed).
- Consider quinine sulfate for patients bothered by nocturnal leg cramps; warn that higher than normal doses are needed (300–500 mg/day), which increases risk of serious side effects [nausea, vomiting, tinnitus, hearing loss, visual impairment, ventricular arrhythmias (QT prolongation), immune thrombocytopenia].
- Begin trial of quinine only after reviewing risks and benefits with patient; start with small doses (200–300 mg/day qhs) and monitor platelet count periodically; interrupt Rx and reassess after 2–4 wks.
- Advise against use of promoted agents that have no benefit (e.g., vitamin E).
- Prescribe replacement Rx for patients with ordinary cramps due to dehydration and sodium depletion.
- Rapidly expand volume (by infusing hypertonic dextrose or saline solution) in those with cramps due to hemodialysis.
- If hypoglycemia is responsible, adjust insulin regimen downward.
- Alter medical programs depending on β-agonists or calcium channel blockers.

OCCUPATIONAL CRAMPS

- Recommend rest and occupational aids.
- Consider minor tranquilizers only for short-term relief; avoid long-term use.
- Refer for consideration of botulinum toxin injection in disabling cases.

TETANY

- Arrange urgent hospital admission and careful parenteral correction of severe electrolyte disturbances.
- Consider prophylactic Rx for those with frequent or prolonged cramps but not for those with occasional cramps.

BIBLIOGRAPHY

■ For the current annotated bibliography on muscle cramps, see the print edition of *Primary Care Medicine*, 4th edition, Chapter 149, or www.LWWmedicine.com.

Neck Pain

DIFFERENTIAL DIAGNOSIS

- Musculoskeletal
  - Muscle strain
  - Muscle spasm
  - Cervical spondylosis
  - Cervical root compression
- Nonmusculoskeletal
  - Lymphadenopathy
  - Thyroiditis
  - Angina pectoris
  - Meningitis

WORKUP

HISTORY

- Check key Hx features, including precipitating events, aggravating and alleviating factors (particularly specific neck movements), area(s) of maximal tenderness, radiation of pain, presence of numbness or weakness in extremities, course, Hx of similar problems, and previous therapeutic efforts.
- Note any risk factors and symptoms of CAD.
- Inquire into feverishness and nuchal rigidity on flexion.

PHYSICAL EXAM

- Assess neck motions, including flexion-extension, left and right lateral flexion, and left and right rotation.
- Palpate neck for point of local tenderness (best indication of structure involved).
- Examine upper extremities for tendon reflexes, strength, sensation, range of motion, and pulses.
- Check for fever and meningeal signs.

LAB STUDIES

- Omit studies in clear-cut cases of nontraumatic neck strain.
- Obtain cervical spine films in traumatic neck strain (to rule out structural damage caused by hyperextension) and in suspected degenerative disease and ankylosing spondylitis.
- Order MRI if clinical evidence of root or cord compression; omit for assessment of degenerative disk disease if no neurologic compromise (specificity poor).
- Consider CT with myelography if MRI is indicated but unavailable or if surgery is contemplated.
- Consider bone scan or CT in suspected bony involvement by tumor; MRI if marrow invasion or cord compression suspected.

MANAGEMENT

MILD TO MODERATE STRAIN

- Recommend heat, ice, and gentle massage for muscle spasm.
- Prescribe generic NSAID preparation (e.g., aspirin, ibuprofen, naproxen).
- Supplement initially for several days with small dose of generic benzodiazepine (e.g., diazepam, 5 mg qhs); avoid prolonged benzodiazepine use.
- Teach range-of-motion and strengthening exercises.
- Consider short-term, qhs use of soft cervical collar to rest sore neck muscles; discourage prolonged wear (disuse atrophy).
- Avoid routine prescribing of so-called muscle relaxants (little more than sedatives; no advantage over short-term benzodiazepines; habituation potential).
- Avoid injecting anesthetic into tender body of muscle in spasm.

SEVERE STRAIN (E.G., HYPEREXTENSION INJURY)

- Limit use of cervical collar to periods of severe pain; eliminate use when pain eases (prolonged use counterproductive).
- Emphasize goals of returning neck function and range of motion; prescribe proper neck exercises and neck hygiene measures; advise quick settlement of any litigation.
- Advise against spinal manipulation (safety and efficacy not established; contraindicated when neurologic compromise or nerve root or cord impingement is possible).
- Advise that ultrasound (U/S) and diathermy are costly and of only modest short-term benefit at best.

DEGENERATIVE DISK DISEASE WITH RADICULOPATHY

- Provide detailed patient ed regarding neck hygiene and exercises; consider referral to seasoned physical therapist to provide teaching and supervision.
- Prescribe NSAID (e.g., generic ibuprofen or naproxen).
- Recommend continuous use of properly fitting cervical collar (holds neck in gentle flexion, the neutral position) to minimize root compression; continue round-the-clock use until pain disappears, then use only at times when added support may be helpful (nighttime, riding in car).
- Consider home cervical traction for severe, chronic, or recurrent neck pain caused by cervical spondylosis or disk herniation associated with radiculitis; prescribe bid for 20–30 mins using 6–10 lbs of weight.
- Instruct careful alignment of cervical traction apparatus (pull slightly forward at 20-degree angle) to follow natural line in neck (see Fig. 148-1 in *Primary Care Medicine*, 4th edition).
- Warn against spinal manipulation (contraindicated because of potential to worsen root or cord compression).
- Advise that U/S and diathermy treatments are harmless but of little proved benefit and probably no better than other means of delivering local heat to sore muscles.
- Consider neurologic consultation for surgical candidacy in refractory or clinically worsening disease with neurologic compromise.

INDICATIONS FOR ADMISSION AND REFERRAL

- Admit urgently if meningeal signs or coronary ischemia present.
- Obtain urgent neurosurgical consultation for any signs suggestive of cord injury (hyperreflexia, upturned toe, incontinence or retention, bilateral neurologic deficits).
- Obtain neurologic consultation as preliminary to referral for surgical intervention in patients with significant weakness in upper extremity and for intractable chronic pain unresponsive to conservative measures.
- Refer patient with persistent neck pain to skilled physical therapist to teach proper neck care and range-of-motion and neck-strengthening exercises. Avoid those who focus on application of physiotherapy (e.g., diathermy, U/S, spinal manipulation).

BIBLIOGRAPHY

- For the current annotated bibliography on neck pain, see the print edition of *Primary Care Medicine*, 4th edition, Chapter 148, or www.LWWmedicine.com.

Osteoarthritis

DIFFERENTIAL DIAGNOSIS

- See Monoarticular Arthritis; Polyarticular Complaints

WORKUP

- See Monoarticular Arthritis; Polyarticular Complaints

MANAGEMENT

EXERCISE, WEIGHT LOSS, AND PHYSICAL THERAPY

- Begin comprehensive, supervised exercise, weight loss, and patient ed programs for those with symptomatic hip or knee disease.
- If obese, emphasize importance and potential benefit of modest weight reduction. Customize program to patient's needs and capabilities. Obtain services of nutritionist to help support obese patient in weight reduction (see Overweight and Obesity).
- Inform patient that regular aerobic exercise is beneficial, and gentle walking, swimming, and stationary cycling are permitted.
- Provide referrals to physical and occupational therapists for design and implementation of comprehensive exercise and activity program.
- Emphasize programs that strengthen quadriceps and hip muscles, increase general conditioning, avoid excessive stress on affected joints, and ensure proper use of assist devices.
- Advise short period (1–2 days) of joint rest if severe hip or knee pain flares up, but continue isometric and non–weight-bearing exercises and avoid more prolonged inactivity. Limit joint stresses (e.g., stair climbing) and prescribe use of cane and other assist devices (e.g., railings, hand grips, elevated toilet seat).
- Consider use of heel lift if leg lengths are unequal, and use of shoe orthotic device if marked foot pronation is present. Check with orthopedist or podiatrist if uncertain.
- Advise bed rest followed by exercises to strengthen supporting musculature for patients with back pain. Corset or brace may help, but not in absence of exercise program (see Back Pain).
- For degenerative cervical spine disease, prescribe soft cervical collar with instructions to wear at all times, including nighttime and for as long as 4 wks. Consider cervical traction (see Neck Pain).

ANALGESICS

- Begin acetaminophen for pain control; prescribe up to 4 g/day.
- Consider NSAIDs (including aspirin) only for patients who do not respond to acetaminophen after full-dose trials.

- If NSAID Rx used, prescribe only low, analgesic doses (e.g., 325 mg enteric-coated aspirin tid, or 200 mg ibuprofen qid) unless patient's arthritis has inflammatory component.
- If gastritis or peptic ulcer disease prohibits standard NSAID use, consider selective COX-2 agent (e.g., 12.5–25 mg/day rofecoxib; see Peptic Ulcer Disease).
- Elicit and address sources of psychosocial distress.
- Avoid narcotic use except in setting of acute disabling exacerbation unresponsive to maximal doses of non-narcotic analgesics.
- Under such circumstances, consider no more than 1–2 days of Rx with codeine sulfate or oxycodone.

INDICATIONS FOR REFERRAL

- Refer for surgical consideration patients with refractory, incapacitating disease of major weight-bearing joint, provided patient is well motivated and healthy enough to tolerate surgery and engage in rehabilitation program (see Hip Pain; Knee Pain).

BIBLIOGRAPHY

- For the current annotated bibliography on osteoarthritis, see the print edition of *Primary Care Medicine*, 4th edition, Chapter 157, or www.LWWmedicine.com.

Osteoporosis

SCREENING AND/OR PREVENTION

GENERAL STRATEGY

- Although criteria for optimal patient selection remain to be defined, best available data and cost-effectiveness studies suggest that biannual screening should begin at menopause for women with major risk factor for osteoporosis and after age 65 for those with no risk factors.
- Order DEXA scanning of spine and femur for best screening measurement of BMD. DEXA study limited to forearm provides low-cost alternative, but is less sensitive.
- Screen all women aged >65 by DEXA scan.
- Obtain T- and Z-scores (T-score = number of standard deviations from mean BMD of young women; Z-score = number of standard deviations from mean BMD for age).
- Screening not recommended if results will not affect decision making (e.g., persons already taking medication for osteoporosis prevention, refusing it, or unable to take it).

RISK FACTORS FOR OSTEOPOROSIS

- Major
  - Hx of osteoporosis in first-degree relative
  - BMI <25th percentile (<22 kg/m^2)
  - Hx of fracture during adulthood
  - Current cigarette smoking
- Contributing
  - Lifelong inadequate intake of calcium
  - Caucasian race
  - Inadequate physical activity
  - Early menopause (age at onset <45)
  - Excessive alcohol intake

PREVENTION OF POSTMENOPAUSAL OSTEOPOROSIS

- Advise young women, especially if pregnant, to maintain daily dietary intake of $\geq 1–1.5$ g calcium and 400 IU vitamin D. Also encourage program of regular physical activity. Advise against smoking and alcohol excess.
- For perimenopausal and postmenopausal women, prescribe 30 mins weight-bearing exercise (e.g., walking, jogging, aerobics, dancing, tennis, weight lifting) ≥ 3 times/wk, total calcium intake of 1–1.5 g/day, and 400–800 IU/day vitamin D.
- If necessary, supplement diet with calcium carbonate tablets (least expensive) or calcium citrate (more expensive, slightly better tolerated) to achieve desired daily total; encourage supplement intake during meals and splitting of dose to maximize uptake and minimize GI upset and risk for kidney stones.

GLUCOCORTICOID-INDUCED OSTEOPOROSIS

- Consider program of osteoporosis prophylaxis in persons who require high-dose steroids (e.g., prednisone >20 mg/day) for at least several mos or lesser doses for longer periods.
- Give highest priority to those at greatest risk for osteoporosis (e.g., postmenopausal women; those with prior vertebral fracture).
- Consider DEXA determination of spinal BMD at start of Rx to determine pretreatment risk and establish baseline.
- For those at increased risk (e.g., T-score <−1.0 or postmenopausal), begin as follows:
  - Calcium and vitamin D supplementation (as detailed above) + 1 of these:
    - Alendronate: 5 mg qam (as detailed below) or 10 mg/day for late postmenopausal women not taking estrogen; or
    - Etidronate: 400 mg/day for 2 wks q3mos if alendronate not tolerated.
- Consider ERT if patient is in early menopause.

MANAGEMENT

POSTMENOPAUSAL OSTEOPOROSIS

T-Score >−1.0

- Continue calcium, vitamin D, and exercise; repeat bone density measurement in 1–2 yrs (depending on degree of osteoporosis risk).

T-Score between −1.0 and −2.5

- Begin more aggressive prevention program and avoid delaying Rx, because rate of bone loss is maximal during first few yrs after menopause.
- Help patient choose one of these (see Menopause):
  - HRT: conjugated *estrogen,* 0.625 mg/day, + medroxyprogesterone, 2.5–5 mg/day for woman with intact uterus;
  - Alternative HRT regimens (e.g., cyclic estrogen and progesterone; transdermal estrogen patch, 50 μg/day);
  - Raloxifene: 60 mg/day;
  - Alendronate: 5 mg qam on empty stomach with 8 oz water 30 mins before breakfast while remaining in upright position (to limit risk for esophageal ulceration).
- Continue Rx indefinitely unless replaced by Rx of nearly equal efficacy or complications develop.
- For those who refuse or cannot take such Rx but who might be candidates if osteoporotic risk increased further, monitor bone loss by DEXA scan q1–2yrs, and reconsider Rx if rate of loss is marked or T-score falls to <−2.5.

T-Score <−2.5

- For asymptomatic postmenopausal patients who have radiographic osteopenia or bone densitometry T-score <−2.5, begin as follows:
  - Calcium, vitamin D, and weight-bearing exercise (adjusted to minimize fracture risk) as detailed above, +1 of these:
  - Alendronate: 10 mg qam (as detailed above);

- Estrogen (as detailed above);
- Raloxifene: 60 mg/day;
- Calcitonin: 200 IU/day nasally alternating nostrils.

■ Continue Rx indefinitely unless replaced by Rx of nearly equal efficacy or complications develop.

OSTEOPOROTIC COMPRESSION FRACTURE

■ Treat initially with bed rest and analgesics.

■ When pain subsides, begin ambulation and mild exercise such as walking or swimming.

■ Recommend avoiding lifting and other weight-bearing stresses.

■ Strongly consider osteoporosis Rx (see above) if not already instituted.

■ Consider course of intranasal calcitonin (200 IU/day) for pain while marked discomfort persists.

■ Begin alendronate (10 mg/day) and continue indefinitely to reduce risk for recurrent fracture, or use etidronate (400 mg/day for 2 wks q3mos; no food 2 hrs before and after intake) if patient cannot use or tolerate alendronate.

■ Institute program of calcium and vitamin D supplementation as detailed above.

BIBLIOGRAPHY

■ For the current annotated bibliography on osteoporosis, see the print edition of *Primary Care Medicine*, 4th edition, Chapters 144 and 164, or www.LWWmedicine.com.

Paget's Disease

WORKUP

HISTORY AND PHYSICAL EXAM
- Check for focal bone pain, especially long bone and vertebrae.
- Note any bony deformity (skull, tibia, spine) and associated complications (e.g., fracture, hearing loss, cerebellar and long-tract signs).
- Check for resultant degenerative disease of the hip.

LAB STUDIES
- Test for hyperuricemia, elevations in bone-specific alkaline phosphatase and urinary pyridinoline.
- Obtain plain films of suspected areas of bony involvement.
- Consider radionuclide bone scan to identify increased uptake when changes not evident on plain film.

MANAGEMENT

- Follow asymptomatic patients yearly and expectantly and as long as they have no involvement of base of skull, spine, hip, knee, or lower extremity long bones; at annual visits, assess clinically and obtain alkaline phosphatase determination.
- For those with mild to moderate pain caused by localized bony involvement or secondary degenerative joint disease, prescribe acetaminophen (e.g., 300 mg qid), aspirin (325 mg tid), or another NSAID (e.g., ibuprofen, 400 mg tid prn; or naproxen, 500 mg up to bid prn) for short-term symptom relief.
- For all symptomatic patients and those with asymptomatic disease with bony involvement in potentially critical areas (base of skull, spine, hip, knee, or lower extremity long bone), obtain baseline plain films and alkaline phosphatase and urinary hydroxyproline measurements.
- Obtain 2 baseline alkaline phosphatase measurements and baseline skeletal radiograph or bone scan before starting Rx.
- Begin oral bisphosphonate Rx with second-generation preparation (e.g., alendronate, 40 mg/day; or risedronate, 30 mg/day).
- Specify that patient take each dose 30 mins before breakfast on empty stomach with ≥8 oz water and without lying down.
- Continue bisphosphonate Rx for standard Rx course (e.g., 6 mos for alendronate; 2 mos for risedronate) or until patient achieves clinical and biochemical remissions.
- Monitor alkaline phosphatase monthly until remission, then q6mos.
- Consider reinstituting Rx if symptoms recur or if alkaline phosphatase level rises to 20–30% above ULN.
- Consider IV pamidronate (30 mg/day) for patients with severe disease, especially those ill enough to require hospitalization.

- Consider parenteral calcitonin (100 MRC U/day SQ) to provide short-term relief for very symptomatic patients waiting for bisphosphonate Rx to take effect, especially if using etidronate.
- Once patient achieves clinical and biochemical remissions, reduce dose to 50 MRC units and continue Rx 3 times/wk.
- Follow serum alkaline phosphatase level monthly during Rx. Also monitor serum calcium level at outset. Routine repetition of radiologic procedures is unwarranted, but repeating radiography periodically may be helpful if patient has high-risk lesions (e.g., base of skull, lower extremity long bone). If you suspect fracture, another film is essential.
- Prescribe ≥2 L/day liquid, especially if patient is inactive. Advise patient to avoid immobilization and dehydration.
- Prescribe total calcium intake of 1.5–2 g/day and 800 IU/day vitamin D if patient is on parenteral or second-generation bisphosphonate Rx.
- Monitor serum calcium level if concerned about adequacy of calcium intake.

BIBLIOGRAPHY

- For the current annotated bibliography on Paget's disease, see the print edition of *Primary Care Medicine*, 4th edition, Chapter 162, or www.LWWmedicine.com.

Polyarticular Complaints

DIFFERENTIAL DIAGNOSIS

- Inflammatory joint disease
  - Rheumatoid arthritis
  - SLE
  - Scleroderma
  - Psoriatic arthritis
  - Reiter's syndrome
  - Ankylosing spondylitis
  - Polyarticular gout
  - Pseudogout
  - Sarcoidosis
  - Lyme disease
  - Disseminated gonococcemia
  - Rheumatic fever
  - Hepatitis B
  - Subacute bacterial endocarditis
  - Vasculitis
- Noninflammatory joint disease
  - Osteoarthritis
  - Hypertrophic pulmonary osteoarthropathy
  - Myxedema
  - Amyloidosis
  - Sickle cell disease
- Inflammatory periarticular disease
  - Polymyalgia rheumatica
  - Dermatomyositis, polymyositis
  - Eosinophilia-myalgia syndrome
- Noninflammatory periarticular disease
  - Fibromyalgia
  - Reflex sympathetic dystrophy

Adapted from Mainardi CL. Approach to the patient with pain in more than one joint. In: Kelley WN, ed. Textbook of internal medicine, 2nd ed. Philadelphia: JB Lippincott Co, 1993:1002, with permission.

WORKUP

OVERALL STRATEGY

- Focus on these key questions:
  - Is underlying disease process inflammatory or noninflammatory?
  - Is problem systemic or focal?
  - Is it truly articular or periarticular?
  - Is vital organ function or joint integrity endangered?
- Consider synovial fluid analysis if accessible effusion present.
- Avoid routine ordering of "arthritis panel" of blood tests (wasteful, high risk of false-positive results).

HISTORY

- Inquire into joint redness, warmth, soft tissue swelling, and tenderness.
- Identify pain location exactly (joint or extraarticular), what aggravates it (joint movement or not), and what functional loss has occurred; do not mistake tenderness in segment of joint or small effusion as evidence of inflammation.
- Note any response to antiinflammatory agents.
- Inquire into distribution (symmetric or asymmetric, large or small joints, migratory or fixed).
- Perform review of systems for morning stiffness, response to activity, frank feverishness, low-grade fever, rash, concurrent Raynaud's phenomenon, chronic or bloody diarrhea, urethritis, conjunctivitis, chronic fatigue, dry mouth/eyes, nasopharyngeal ulcers, pleuritic chest pain, and mental status changes.
- Take note of gender (e.g., RA, SLE: mostly female; Reiter's syndrome: mostly male) and age (e.g., ankylosing spondylitis onset <age 40).
- Ask about severity [including systemic involvement (fatigue, weight loss, fever)] and effect on daily activity to gauge functional significance; take into account patient's premorbid activity level; check attitudes toward work and pain.
- Note Hx of prior attacks and family Hx of same symptoms (spondyloarthropathies, gout, Heberden's nodes).
- Check travel Hx and any residence in area endemic for Lyme disease in addition to Hx of recent tick bite.

PHYSICAL EXAM

- Document pattern and type of joint involvement and nature of any extraarticular disease.
- Check for dermal clues to underlying illness:
  - Malar rash of SLE
  - Annular erythema chronica migrans (Lyme disease)
  - Papulovesicular lesions with necrotic center (disseminated gonococcemia)
  - Nail pitting and scaling (psoriatic arthritis)
  - Urticaria (hepatitis B)
  - Palpable purpura, ulceration, or livedo reticularis (vasculitis)
  - Red, tender, subcutaneous lesions (erythema nodosum, sarcoidosis, inflammatory bowel disease)
  - Penile ulcers of circinate balanitis and keratoderma blennorrhagicum on heels (Reiter's syndrome)
  - Subcutaneous nodules on elbows, Achilles tendons, pinnae (gout, RA)
  - Clubbing, fingertip atrophy with healed or active ulcers (Raynaud's phenomenon) + calcinosis, subungual telangiectases, and skin tightening (scleroderma)
  - Dry, doughy skin and loss of outer third of eyebrows (hypothyroidism)
- Perform HEENT exam for
  - conjunctivitis and iritis (Reiter's syndrome, other spondyloarthropathies);
  - posterior eye retinopathy: retinal hemorrhages, "cotton-wool" exudates, and ischemic lesions (SLE, vasculitis);
  - oral and mucosal ulcers (painful = SLE; painless = Reiter's syndrome).

- Note on neck, chest, heart, and abdominal exams:
  - Thyroid for goiter
  - Chest for signs of effusion and pleuritis
  - Heart for murmurs (rheumatic fever, SLE, spondyloarthropathies) and rubs (RA and SLE)
  - Abdomen for splenomegaly (RA, SLE)
- Perform musculoskeletal exam for
  - signs of true joint inflammation: entire joint involved, and tenderness, warmth, redness, soft tissue swelling, and effusion;
  - noninflammatory articular disease;
  - any mechanical abnormalities such as limitation of motion, instability, subluxation, or tendon injury;
  - periarticular pathology: bursitis/tendinitis mimicking arthritis, muscle soreness and proximal muscle weakness suggesting myositis, and pressure points in neck and upper back indicating fibromyalgia syndrome;
  - "frozen" joints and tightening of periarticular fibrous tissue from disuse leading to secondary flexion contractures of normal joints;
  - inability to curl fingers while extending MP joints (screening test for disease of finger joints and tendons);
  - loss of lumbar mobility (spondyloarthropathy): place 2 marks on back with patient standing (1 at level of posterior iliac spine level and 1 exactly 10 cm above), then have patient bend forward maximally and measure distance between 2 marks (should be ≥15 cm apart).
- Perform neurologic exam for
  - loss of motor and/or sensory function in extremities (peripheral neuropathy);
  - mental status changes (CNS involvement in suspected SLE and HIV infection).

LAB STUDIES

Approach to Testing

- Test according to clinical evidence; as noted, avoid routine use of panels of tests to "screen" for arthritic conditions (wasteful, erroneous when ordered in absence of clinical evidence).
- To diagnose or rule out "must not miss" conditions, perform Hx and PE, complemented by thoughtfully selected tests that specifically address conditions for which there is at least some clinical evidence.
- Take note that frequency of abnormal test results in absence of disease increases with age, especially with most commonly ordered studies (e.g., ESR, uric acid level, ANA and RF titers).
- Test according to whether clinical evidence suggests inflammatory or noninflammatory disease.

Suspected Inflammatory Articular Disease

- Check ESR to confirm active inflammatory disease.
- Note CBC for hematologic involvement by underlying disease process.
- Consider tests for infectious etiology [blood cultures, Lyme antibody (see Lyme Disease), aminotransferases (viral hepatitis)] if onset acute and duration <6 wks.
- If duration >6 wks and patient has systemic symptoms, test for rheumatoid disease and other systemic conditions; obtain

- RF with cognizance that it neither rules in nor rules out RA but can add to sum of evidence;
- ANA determination (highly sensitive for SLE, but lacking specificity and not necessarily paralleling disease activity).
- If ANA positive (nonspecific) in setting of clinical evidence for inflammatory disease (especially if systemic symptoms present), perform additional tests for antibodies against specific autoantigens; order
  - antibody to native double-stranded DNA (confirms SLE);
  - antibody to Smith antigen (highly specific for SLE, but low sensitivity);
  - antibody to Scl-70 (a nuclear topoisomerase, highly specific for systemic sclerosis, but low sensitivity);
  - anti-Ro and anti-La antibodies (moderate sensitivity, moderate-high specificity for Sjögren's syndrome).
- If Dx remains undetermined, perform joint aspiration if there is effusion, and send synovial fluid for analysis (helps differentiate inflammatory from noninflammatory disease and checks for crystal-induced arthropathy and infection). Note
  - if WBC count >2,000/mm^3 with >75% PMNs (inflammation);
  - if WBC count <1,000/mm^3 (noninflammatory disease).
- Obtain serum uric acid level.
- Consider joint radiography (especially for cases with joint pathology on PE and conditions with early radiologic findings (e.g., sacroiliitis in spondyloarthropathies).
- Avoid routine HLA-B27 testing (positivity in 6–8% of normal persons).
- Check urinalysis to screen for glomerular injury; if positive for RBCs and albumin, obtain BUN and creatinine.

Suspected Noninflammatory Polyarticular Disease

- Order joint radiography to confirm osteoarthritis if necessary.
- Check TSH for suspected hypothyroidism.

Suspected Inflammatory Nonarticular Disease

- Obtain ESR for suspected polymyalgia rheumatica.
- Consider temporal artery biopsy or equivalent test (see Giant Cell Arteritis) for suspected cranial (giant cell) arteritis.
- Check CBC and differential if eosinophilia-myalgia suspected; refer for skin and muscle biopsy if florid peripheral eosinophilia noted.
- Measure serum creatine kinase if polymyositis is concern, and consider muscle biopsy if levels are high.

Suspected Noninflammatory Nonarticular Disease

- No lab tests indicated for Dx of fibromyalgia; Dx is clinical (see Fibromyalgia).
- Similarly, Dx of reflex sympathetic dystrophy is predominantly clinical.

MANAGEMENT

SYMPTOMATIC THERAPY

- Rx should be etiologic, but pending test results and provided that infection has been ruled out, consider high-dose aspirin (up to 12 325-mg tablets/day) or generic NSAID (e.g., 400–800 mg ibuprofen qid) for symptomatic relief of joint inflammation (see specific conditions).

INDICATIONS FOR ADMISSION AND REFERRAL

- If any evidence of bloodstream infection, vasculitis, or involvement of eyes, lungs, heart, kidneys, or nervous system, obtain consultation and consider hospitalization.
- Similarly for persons with severe constitutional symptoms (e.g., disabling fatigue, fever, weight loss), arrange prompt consultation and consider hospitalization.
- Obtain rheumatologic consultation when Dx of less serious illness remains elusive after initial workup completed; timely referral far more productive than exhaustive serologic testing, with its attendant risks of false-positive results.

BIBLIOGRAPHY

- For the current annotated bibliography on polyarticular complaints, see the print edition of *Primary Care Medicine*, 4th edition, Chapter 146, or www.LWWmedicine.com.

Polymyalgia Rheumatica

WORKUP

- Check Hx, PE, and lab studies for diagnostic criteria:
  - Bilateral pain for ≥1 mo in any 2 of these: neck, shoulder girdle, hip girdle, in association with morning stiffness
  - ESR >40 mm/hr by Westergren method
  - Age >50
  - Exclusion of other diagnoses except for giant cell arteritis
  - Marked clinical improvement in response to 1 wk of Rx with <15 mg of prednisone/day
- Also consider patients meeting all criteria except elevated ESR as having polymyalgia rheumatica.

MANAGEMENT

- Begin with low-dose prednisone (10–15 mg/day) provided no evidence of giant cell arteritis.
- For patients with very high ESR and severe symptoms, consider starting prednisone at higher dose (e.g., 20–30 mg/day).
- Taper in decrements of 1–2.5 mg/day q2wk, titrating dose against symptoms and ESR.
- Prescribe lowest dose possible and recommend it be taken qam.
- Continue steady tapering to full cessation of Rx if possible, monitoring symptoms and ESR for 2 yrs for evidence of relapse.
- Restart or increase prednisone by 5–10 mg/day if flare of disease occurs; adjust dose prn and resume tapering as soon as patient achieves remission.
- Instruct patient to report promptly any symptoms suggestive of giant cell arteritis (e.g., vision disturbances, tender cranial artery, headache, fever, jaw claudication).

BIBLIOGRAPHY

- For the current annotated bibliography on polymyalgia rheumatica, see the print edition of *Primary Care Medicine*, 4th edition, Chapter 161, or www.LWWmedicine.com.

Raynaud's Phenomenon

DIFFERENTIAL DIAGNOSIS

- Vasospastic disease
  - Primary
  - Drug-induced (beta blockers, ergot, methysergide)
  - Migraine
- Arterial occlusive disease (± platelet activation)
  - Scleroderma
  - Systemic sclerosis
  - Systemic lupus erythematosus
  - Occupational trauma (e.g., jackhammer operator)
  - Atherosclerotic disease
  - Compression (thoracic outlet, carpal tunnel)
- Hemorheologic disease
  - Paraproteinemia
  - Polycythemia
  - Cryoproteinemia

WORKUP

GENERAL STRATEGY

- Confirm Dx by eliciting characteristic Hx or directly observing characteristic changes in skin color in response to cold or stress.
- If in doubt, immerse patient's hands in ice water and observe for blanching, cyanosis, and reactive hyperemia (≥2 of 3 changes must be present).

HISTORY

- Differentiate primary from secondary disease by inquiring into age at onset, gender, and frequency and severity of attacks, and by examining for distribution of skin changes, ischemic skin changes, manifestations of connective tissue disease, precipitating factors, associated digital swelling, and other vasomotor phenomena, such as migraine and livedo reticularis.
- Consider primary disease if onset in teens, female sex, occurrence of multiple mild daily attacks, symmetric involvement, precipitation of attacks by stress, normal skin except for livedo reticularis, and migraines.
- Consider secondary disease if male patient or in female patient with onset in mid-20s or later, moderate to severe attacks not necessarily daily, asymmetric presentation triggered predominantly by cold, and associated finger swelling, ischemic skin ulcers, or loss of fingertip pulp.
- For patients with presentation suggesting secondary disease, check Hx for skin rash, morning stiffness, arthralgias, joint swelling, fatigue, and fever; note any reports of claudication, angina, and leg ulceration.
- Consider symptoms of thoracic outlet and carpal tunnel syndromes (see Focal Neurologic Complaints) and polycythemia (see Erythrocytosis) if underlying Dx remains unclear.

■ Note occupational Hx for any vibratory injury, and review effects of vasoactive medications (beta blockers, ergotamine, methysergide, or calcium channel blockers) on symptoms.

PHYSICAL EXAM

■ Check for manifestations of connective tissue disease (e.g., malar flush, sclerodactyly, petechial rash, telangiectasia, calcinosis, joint redness, swelling, and effusion).

■ Palpate hand and arm pulses and check capillary filling.

■ Note fingertips for loss of pulp (ischemia) and skin for atrophic changes.

■ Examine nail fold capillary pattern; asymmetry indicates dropout of capillary loops, characteristic and predictive of systemic sclerosis.

LAB STUDIES

■ Omit testing if Hx and PE strongly suggest definite primary disease.

■ Consider ANA test only if evidence of underlying connective tissue disease.

■ For patients who test positive for ANA, obtain anticentromere antibody determination (scleroderma).

■ Obtain noninvasive arterial studies (plethysmography, Doppler ultrasonography) only to confirm anatomic vascular compromise and determine severity.

■ Check CBC and serum globulins to screen for common hematologic problems; reserve immunoelectrophoresis for myeloma candidates (elderly, markedly elevated globulin, anemia).

■ Consider cryoprotein determination for clinical signs of cryoglobulinemia (arthralgias, purpura, proteinuria).

■ Check cold agglutinin test if anemia and splenomegaly present.

MANAGEMENT

PREVENTION

■ Recommend keeping trunk and extremities warm on cold days, with emphasis on truncal warmth.

■ Insist on smoking cessation and elimination of passive smoke exposure.

■ Eliminate or reduce intake of drugs that trigger episodes.

■ Advise elimination or reduction of occupational precipitants (repetitive activity that leads to carpal tunnel syndrome, working on vibrating or rotating tool).

■ Limit exposure to such precipitants to <1 hr/day. Antivibration gloves and coated tool handles have proved insufficient.

SYMPTOMATIC RELIEF

■ Consider calcium channel blocker (e.g., nifedipine, nicardipine, isradipine, felodipine) for patients with primary disease and for many with secondary disease.

■ Avoid short-acting calcium channel blockers; use only with caution in persons with underlying coronary disease (see Stable Angina), and avoid in CHF (see Congestive Heart Failure); watch for side effects (headache, flushing, esophageal dysfunction).

- Consider alpha blockers (e.g., doxazosin); warn of risk of postural light-headedness.
- For patients with vasospastic disease and substantial endothelial injury and platelet activation (e.g., those with systemic sclerosis), add aspirin or dipyridamole to help heal ulcers.
- Consider fish oil supplements rich in omega-3 fatty acids.
- Reserve sympathectomy as measure of last resort; precede by testing response to temporary ganglionic blockade.
- Refer patients who develop ischemic injury.

BIBLIOGRAPHY

- For the current annotated bibliography on Raynaud's phenomenon, see the print edition of *Primary Care Medicine*, 4th edition, Chapter 163, or www.LWWmedicine.com.

Rheumatoid Arthritis

DIFFERENTIAL DIAGNOSIS

- See Polyarticular Complaints.

WORKUP

- See Polyarticular Complaints.

MANAGEMENT

INITIAL MANAGEMENT

Patient Education and Physical Therapy

- Provide comprehensive patient and family ed program that includes psychological support and strategies for maintaining patient's activity, independence, and self-esteem.
- Arrange for physical/occupational Rx consultations to teach exercises, home Rx, and activity programs that help sustain daily activity.

Disease-Modifying Therapy

- At time of initial Dx, consider prompt implementation of disease-modifying Rx (e.g., methotrexate, hydroxychloroquine, sulfasalazine, or any combination); indicated for all patients, but especially those with very active disease or other indicators of poor prognosis (e.g., genotype HLA-DRB1*04/04, high RF titer, extraarticular manifestations, large number of involved joints, age <30, female sex, systemic symptoms).
- Obtain early rheumatologic consultation for selecting disease-modifying regimen.
- Coordinate care with rheumatologist and closely monitor patient for response to Rx and complications of drug program (see below).

Nonsteroidal Antiinflammatory Drug Therapy

- While waiting for disease-modifying Rx to take effect (up to 6 mos), begin antiinflammatory Rx with generic NSAID (e.g., enteric-coated aspirin, 3.6 g/day; ibuprofen, 800 mg tid; or naproxen, 500 mg bid).
- Use NSAIDs with care in patients with impaired renal perfusion; monitor BUN and creatinine.
- Also prescribe cautiously to patients with Hx of peptic ulcer disease or GI bleeding (see Peptic Ulcer Disease).
- Monitor hematocrit and test for fecal occult blood.
- Consider use of selective COX-2 inhibitor only if nonselective NSAIDs are not well tolerated or if patient is at high risk for peptic ulceration and its complications.
- Take into consideration question of cardiovascular risk associated with COX-2 use, especially when contemplating program of daily long-term COX-2 use in persons with known cardiovascular disease or multiple thrombotic cardiovascular risk factors.

Steroid Therapy

- For patients with very active disease whose symptoms are inadequately controlled by initial NSAID Rx, consider adding small dose of corticosteroid Rx (e.g., prednisone, 5 mg/day, in divided doses bid if necessary).
- Reserve qd use of systemic steroids for patients truly incapacitated by symptoms, and use only short-term, low-dose program (e.g., prednisone, 5–7.5 mg/day until disease-modifying Rx takes effect).
- If using steroids, begin program of osteoporosis prevention that includes calcium (1.5 g/day) and vitamin D (400–800 IU/day) + hormone replacement Rx, bisphosphonate (e.g., alendronate, 5–10 mg/day), or both (see Osteoporosis).

SUBSEQUENT MANAGEMENT

- Once disease-modifying Rx takes effect, taper and discontinue NSAIDs and any corticosteroids.
- Continue disease-modifying program indefinitely.
- Prescribe gentle exercise program to maintain range of motion and muscle strength, but avoid stressing severely inflamed joints. Pre-exercise application of heat or cold (either may work) facilitates program.
- Consult with physical therapist to help design program. Morning application of heat is particularly helpful before patient engages in daily activity.
- Selectively rest severely inflamed joints that are too swollen to exercise. Maintain joint in physiologic position by splinting when joint is stressed (e.g., at night) to support weakened joint and prevent flexion contractures.
- Consult rheumatologist if splinting appears necessary.
- Advise daily rest period for patients bothered by generalized fatigue, but outpatients should avoid prolonged bed rest.
- Consult rheumatologist again if patient manifests persistently active disease. It may be necessary to advance or alter disease-modifying regimen. Increasingly, early rheumatologic consultation and aggressive Rx may be necessary to prevent joint destruction, particularly in patients with findings suggesting poor prognosis.
- For patients incapacitated by 1 disproportionately inflamed large, weight-bearing joint, consider single intraarticular injection of long-acting corticosteroid (e.g., triamcinolone acetonide, 2.5–10 mg, depending on joint size, mixed with 1 mL lidocaine). Cleanse knee with iodine and alcohol and perform sterile intraarticular injection. Avoid repeated injections into same joint.

MONITORING

- Monitor disease activity and response to Rx by checking reproducible measures, such as duration of morning stiffness; ESR; number of tender, swollen joints; and grip strength (have patient squeeze blood pressure cuff). Also monitor activities of daily living and psychosocial status.
- For patients on disease-modifying Rx, monitor closely for drug toxicity.
- For those taking hydroxychloroquine, inquire regularly about visual acuity and arrange for ophthalmologic exam q6mos.
- For those taking methotrexate, follow CBC, platelet count, and aminotransferase, alkaline phosphatase, BUN, and creatinine levels.

Inquire regularly about pulmonary symptoms, which might be first manifestation of interstitial pneumonitis and indication for immediate Rx cessation.
- For those taking sulfasalazine, monitor CBC, inquire about GI symptoms, and examine skin for rashes and pruritus.

BIBLIOGRAPHY

- For the current annotated bibliography on rheumatoid arthritis, see the print edition of *Primary Care Medicine*, 4th edition, Chapter 156, or www.LWWmedicine.com.

Shoulder Pain

DIFFERENTIAL DIAGNOSIS

GENERAL CONSIDERATIONS

- Consider causes of shoulder pain in terms of structures that compose shoulder. Vast majority of nontraumatic shoulder complaints are related to tendinitis.

IMPORTANT CAUSES OF SHOULDER PAIN

- Rotator cuff
  - Calcific tendinitis
  - Subacromial impingement
  - Biceps tendinitis
  - Tear
  - Adhesive capsulitis
- Glenohumeral joint
  - Instability
  - Dislocation
  - Arthritis
  - Infection
- Acromioclavicular joint
  - Arthritis
- Referred
  - Cervical spondylosis
  - Myocardial ischemia
  - Shoulder-hand syndrome (reflex sympathetic dystrophy)
  - Diaphragmatic irritation
  - Thoracic outlet syndrome
  - Gallbladder disease

WORKUP

HISTORY

- Inquire about previous trauma or inciting event, location and radiation of pain, specific limitations of movement, associated neurologic deficits, aggravating and alleviating factors, Hx of shoulder problems, and use of Rx.
- Check for symptoms suggesting angina, gallbladder disease, or diaphragmatic irritation.
- Take occupational Hx, especially if patient has engaged in heavy labor or sports (painting, wallpapering, carpentry, throwing, using racquet).
- Note any difficulty sleeping with arm overhead (rotator cuff problems).
- Check medical Hx for shoulder dislocation (glenohumeral instability).

PHYSICAL EXAM

■ Before proceeding to shoulder exam, check neck, chest, heart, and abdomen for sources of referred pain. Note any pain reproduction by neck motion to side of complaint (cervical root compression) or tenderness on deep pressure over neurovascular bundle and scalene muscles of supraclavicular fossa (brachial plexus injury).

■ Examine lungs for effusion, pleural rub, and poor diaphragmatic movement, and heart for signs of ischemia or pericarditis.

■ Check abdomen for tenderness in right or left upper quadrant (subdiaphragmatic disease).

Shoulder Exam

■ Seat patient comfortably and sufficiently disrobed to permit evaluation and comparison of both shoulders.

■ Inspect from front and back for asymmetry or deformity.

■ Instruct patient to place involved shoulder actively through full range of motion, along with similar movements of contralateral limb for comparison, including forward flexion, extension, abduction, and internal and external rotation.

■ Record internal rotation as level at which patient can reach posteriorly, such as buttock or thoracolumbar junction.

■ Observe scapula with forward flexion of shoulder against resistance ("winging" of scapula suggests serratus anterior muscle palsy).

■ Check key etiologic sites for localized tenderness (see Fig. 150-1 in *Primary Care Medicine*, 4th edition), including anterior aspect of acromion, acromioclavicular joint, bicipital groove (best palpated with humerus rotated internally about 10 degrees), greater tuberosity, and cervical spine.

■ With hand on shoulder, put shoulder passively through full range of motion (see Fig. 150-2 in *Primary Care Medicine*, 4th edition), noting any limitations or palpable crepitation.

■ Test muscle strength, including ability to "shrug" shoulder (for trapezius weakness) and forward flexion (for rotator cuff pathology); elicit deep tendon reflexes of upper extremities.

Diagnostic Maneuvers (see also Chapter 150 in *Primary Care Medicine*, 4th edition)

■ Wright's maneuver (for suspected thoracic outlet syndrome): check for reproduction of symptoms and obliteration of radial pulse at wrist when shoulder placed in extreme external rotation and abduction.

■ Neer's test and Hawkins sign (for rotator cuff disease): indicates impingement of greater tuberosity of humerus against undersurface of acromion.

■ Confirm impingement disease of rotator cuff by injecting 5 mL lidocaine (Xylocaine) into subacromial space (relief provided).

■ Consider tests for rotator cuff tear

• Check for external rotation lag (difference between max active and passive external rotation), an indication of infraspinatus tendon tear.

• Perform lift-off test to check for tear in anterior cuff.

• Elicit belly-press sign for tear of subscapularis tendon.

- For supraspinatus tears, note atrophy in supraspinatus fossa of scapula and weakness of resisted abduction with shoulder held in 90-degree abduction.

Tests for Acromioclavicular Joint Disease (see also Chapter 150 in *Primary Care Medicine*, 4th edition)

- Cross-arm adduction test, repeated after injecting acromioclavicular joint with 1 mL lidocaine using 25-ga needle to enter joint.
- Apprehension sign for anterior shoulder instability. Confirmed by performing relocation test.
- Test for laxity of superior glenohumeral ligament by checking for positive sulcus sign.

LAB STUDIES

- Obtain standard A-P views of shoulder to rule out underlying bone tumor, infection, and arthritis of glenohumeral or acromioclavicular joint.
- Obtain A-P views with shoulder in internal and external rotation to best identify calcifications; pay particular attention to diffuse, disorganized pattern of calcification, which suggests acute calcific tendinitis.
- Obtain axillary view if dislocation suspected; note relation of humeral head to glenoid fossa.
- Consider cervical spine films if neck motion reproduces shoulder pain or if root compression symptoms noted.
- Consider MRI for suspected rotator cuff tear; may obviate need for arthrogram; not indicated for initial evaluation of shoulder pain.
- Consider arthrography to identify suspected rotator cuff tear, especially for Dx of full-thickness tears.
- Aspirate joint fluid if infection suspected, and send for Gram's stain, culture, and chemistries (see Monoarticular Arthritis).
- Consider electromyography if PE suggests neuropathy and better characterization is desired.

MANAGEMENT

ROTATOR CUFF TENDINITIS

- Recommend avoidance of exacerbating activities, NSAID Rx (e.g., 375 mg naproxen bid, or 600 mg ibuprofen tid), and exercises to strengthen rotator cuff.
- Refer to physical therapist to teach exercises and provide supervision.
- Teach pendulum exercises and "wall climbing" (see Chapter 150 in *Primary Care Medicine*, 4th edition) if motion is restricted.
- Counsel that some mild discomfort occurs with these exercises.
- Recommend exercising for 5–10 mins, tid–qid.
- Consider subacromial injection of corticosteroid and local anesthetic (see Chapter 150 in *Primary Care Medicine*, 4th edition) when tendon inflammation is so severe that exercises are impossible or when there is severe acute calcific tendinitis; limit to once q6–12mos and to total of 3.
- Consider pulsed ultrasound Rx to help reduce calcification and improve functional status.

- Order orthopedic referral when symptoms are unresponsive or when you suspect large tear.

TORN ROTATOR CUFF

- Institute program of exercise designed to strengthen shoulder rotator muscles.
- Avoid repeated steroid injections.
- Recommend surgical consideration for large tears.

ADHESIVE CAPSULITIS

- Institute active exercise program, preceding each session with 15–20 mins local heat application using heating pad or by taking warm shower.
- Have patient work with physical therapist to learn exercise program.
- Encourage patient to use shoulder as much as possible in activities of daily living.
- Avoid forceful manipulation of shoulder.
- Consider arthroscopic capsulotomy for refractory symptoms.

GLENOHUMERAL ARTHRITIS

- Prescribe exercise and NSAIDs to maintain functional range of motion.
- Recommend same exercises as for adhesive capsulitis qd–bid.
- Refer to physical therapist for exercises directed at maximizing existing muscle strength.
- Consider referral to orthopedic surgeon for cortisone injections into glenohumeral joint (no limit on number of injections permitted).
- Consider total joint arthroplasty in those with marked functional limitation and those refractory to medical management.

ACROMIOCLAVICULAR ARTHRITIS

- Prescribe antiinflammatory medication and activity modification.
- Consider referral to orthopedic specialist for injection of corticosteroid and lidocaine.
- Reserve consideration of surgery for rare cases refractory to all other methods.

INDICATIONS FOR REFERRAL

- Use services of skilled physical therapist to teach and monitor shoulder exercise program.
- Obtain prompt orthopedic consultation for shoulder dislocation or instability, fractures about shoulder, rotator cuff tears, and infection.
- Consider referral for refractory rotator cuff tendinitis refractory to conservative Rx as well as advanced acromioclavicular or glenohumeral joint arthritis.

PATIENT EDUCATION

- Emphasize importance of active participation by patient in Rx program.
- Prepare patient for some pain with exercises, but also note favorable prognosis.

BIBLIOGRAPHY

■ For the current annotated bibliography on shoulder pain, see the print edition of *Primary Care Medicine*, 4th edition, Chapter 150, or www.LWWmedicine.com.

Neurologic Problems

Bell's Palsy

DIFFERENTIAL DIAGNOSIS

CAUSES OF UNILATERAL PERIPHERAL SEVENTH NERVE PALSY

- Bell's palsy (idiopathic, ? herpes)
- Vascular insufficiency
- Bacterial infection (ear)
- Herpes zoster
- Diabetes mellitus
- Sarcoidosis
- Guillain-Barré syndrome
- Tumor (acoustic neuroma, pontine glioma, neurofibroma, cholesteatoma, parotid gland tumor, meningeal carcinomatosis)
- Trauma (fracture, temporal bone)
- Lyme disease

CAUSES OF BILATERAL FACIAL PARALYSIS

- Guillain-Barré syndrome (with or without HIV infection)
- Sarcoidosis
- Lyme disease
- Myasthenia gravis
- Botulism

WORKUP

HISTORY

- Review Hx for elements suggesting other etiologies:
  - Tick bite
  - Rash
  - Generalized or ascending weakness
  - Hearing or other sensory loss
  - Ear pain, tenderness, discharge
  - Localized facial swelling
  - Jaw trauma or pain
  - Enlarged lymph nodes
  - Herpes infection
  - Diabetes mellitus
  - Bilateral involvement

PHYSICAL EXAM

- Look for PE evidence of other causes of facial palsy:
  - Bilateral involvement
  - Other cranial nerve and focal motor deficits
  - Generalized or ascending motor loss

- Otitis media or externa
- Zosteriform lesions (tympanic membrane, external auditory canal, behind ear)
- Erythema migrans and arthritis (see Lyme Disease)
- Cholesteatoma of tympanic membrane
- Jaw tenderness and trauma to temporal bone
- Lymph node enlargement
- Dry rales (sarcoidosis)

LAB STUDIES

- Use lab for further testing only if Hx and/or PE suggest etiology other than Bell's palsy:
  - Consider testing for Lyme disease if patient in area highly endemic for *B. burgdorferi* (see Lyme Disease).
  - Obtain CT or MRI in cases of suspected posterior fossa mass as cause of seventh nerve palsy.
  - In patients with atypical or persistent facial palsy, consider gadolinium-enhanced MRI to help differentiate Bell's palsy from other neurologic causes.
  - Refer for lumbar puncture when CNS inflammation, granuloma, or malignancy is a concern, but note that mild CSF pleocytosis can occur in typical cases of Bell's palsy.
- Consider EMG to help predict recovery, but unneeded for Dx and most informative when ≥3 wks have elapsed after onset of facial paralysis.

MANAGEMENT

- Explain benign nature and good prognosis of condition, but caution about possibility of corneal abrasion.
- Inform patients that they may experience altered taste, decreased tearing and salivation, or altered sensitivity to sound.
- Prescribe methylcellulose eye drops bid and qhs with taping of lid if it cannot close to protect eye.
- If patient seen within 1 wk of onset of facial weakness and if no important contraindications to corticosteroid use (e.g., Lyme disease), begin short course of prednisone (60 mg qam for 5 days).
- If improvement occurs or weakness does not progress during Rx, taper and terminate over 10 more days.
- If improvement does not occur during first 5 days, continue 60 mg prednisone qam for 10 days, then taper over another 10 days.
- If postauricular pain recurs with tapering, reinstitute preceding dose.
- In suspected viral infection or if initial symptoms are severe, consider adding early course of Rx for herpesvirus infection (e.g., acyclovir, 200 mg 5 × day; or valacyclovir 100 mg bid × 7–10 days) to prednisone program (see Herpes Simplex).
- Consider tarsorrhaphy when severe persistent lid weakness exists.
- In 10% of patients who do not achieve acceptable recovery, refer for consideration of autografting with hypoglossal to facial nerve anastomosis; may provide reasonable cosmetic results and afford lasting eye protection.

BIBLIOGRAPHY

■ For the current annotated bibliography on Bell's palsy, see the print edition of *Primary Care Medicine*, 4th edition, Chapter 175, or www.LWWmedicine.com.

DIFFERENTIAL DIAGNOSIS

CAUSES OF INTELLECTUAL IMPAIRMENT

- Neurologic diseases
  - Alzheimer's disease
  - Normal-pressure hydrocephalus
  - Dementia with Lewy bodies (Lewy body disease)
  - Multiinfarct dementia
  - Parkinson's disease
  - Intracranial tumor
  - Neurosyphilis
  - HIV infection
  - Creutzfeldt-Jakob disease
  - Huntington's disease
  - Multiple sclerosis
  - Wilson's disease
  - Progressive supranuclear palsy
- Systemic conditions
  - Infectious
    - Syphilis with CNS involvement
    - HIV infection with CNS involvement
    - Cryptococcal CNS infection
  - Endocrine
    - Hypothyroidism and hyperthyroidism
    - Panhypopituitarism
    - High-dose glucocorticoids
  - Metabolic
    - Vitamin B_{12} deficiency
    - Thiamine deficiency
    - Niacin deficiency (pellagra)
  - Chemical poisons
    - Alcohol
    - Metals (lead, mercury)
    - Aniline dyes
  - Drug intoxications
    - Barbiturates
    - Opiates
    - Anticholinergics
    - Lithium
    - Bromides
    - Haloperidol
    - Antihypertensives

WORKUP

GENERAL STRATEGY

- Differentiate dementia from other causes of mental impairment.

- Identify cause as primarily neurologic or secondarily affecting brain.
- Check for additional manifestations of neurologic impairment to identify diseases that are primarily of brain.
- Check for signs and symptoms of systemic disease to identify conditions that affect brain secondarily.
- Adhere to standard diagnostic criteria for making Dx of Alzheimer's disease (e.g., criteria established by U.S. Department of Health and Human Services):
  - Presence of dementia established by clinical exam and documented by Mini-Mental State Examination . . . or similar exam, with
  - evidence of deficits in ≥2 areas of cognition;
  - progressive worsening of memory and other cognitive function;
  - no disturbance of consciousness; and
  - absence of systemic disorders or other brain disease that alone could account for deficits.

HISTORY

- Explore with patient and family specific cognitive, memory, and behavioral problems and consequences of deficits in patient's daily life, such as difficulties with driving, work, or family relationships.
- Ascertain temporal course of illness and ascertain whether process is chronic and progressive (neurodegenerative), stepwise (multiinfarct), or static (hypotensive, nonprogressive).
- Check risk factors for dementia, including prior severe head trauma, DM, never having been married, and low education level.
- Identify potentially treatable causes by inquiry into risk factors and specific neurologic accompaniments:
  - Cardiovascular risk factors (e.g., smoking, HTN, hyperlipidemia, DM).
  - Gait, incontinence, Hx of meningitis or subarachnoid hemorrhage (increased risk for normal-pressure hydrocephalus).
  - Hx of head trauma, unexplained onset of focal neurologic deficit, and unilateral headache worsening over time (mass lesion).
  - Resting tremor and rigidity (Parkinson's disease).
  - Extrapyramidal symptoms of dysarthria, poor coordination of voluntary movements, or vivid visual hallucinations (Lewy body disease).
  - Hepatocellular dysfunction (Wilson's disease).
  - High-risk sexual behavior (HIV infection, neurosyphilis).
  - Hx of depression (see Depression).
  - Family Hx of dementia, Down syndrome, or psychiatric disorders (hereditary disease).
- Check for causative or exacerbating nonneurologic conditions by reviewing for
  - previous gastric surgery (leading to vitamin B_{12} deficiency);
  - thiamine, niacin, and vitamin B_{12} deficiencies;
  - medications (particularly opiates, sedative-hypnotics, analgesics, anticholinergics, anticonvulsants, corticosteroids, centrally acting antihypertensives, and psychotropics);
  - alcohol abuse and other forms of substance abuse;
  - symptoms of hypothyroidism and pituitary insufficiency;
  - occupational Hx for exposure to toxic substances (e.g., aniline dyes, heavy metals).

PHYSICAL EXAM

- Perform mental status exam to confirm dementia followed by general exam for detection of focal lesions, general brain dysfunction, and contributing factors.

Mental Status Exam

- Consider using Mini-Mental State Exam.
- Include immediate memory testing, with request to remember 3 objects, recite forward and backward numbers given by PCP, and recall short story.
- Check remote memory testing by asking about notable historic events, family milestones, or more recent happenings in newspaper.
- Test language function with naming of parts of objects, following complex commands, and generating word lists.
- Have patient reproduce simple drawings and discern similarities among objects (categorization).
- Ascertain judgment by presenting patient with decision-requiring situations ("finding stamped letter" or "seeing fire in theater").
- Test attention and concentration by having patient reverse sequences, as in naming months of year backward.

General Physical and Neurologic Exams

- Check for signs of cardiovascular risk factors (e.g., elevated BP, xanthomata, atherosclerotic and diabetic retinopathic changes, carotid bruit, LV heave, displaced apical impulse, murmur, S_3, S_4, abdominal aortic enlargement, femoral bruit, loss of distal pulses).
- Check for signs of alcoholism, hepatocellular injury, renal insufficiency, and other systemic illnesses.
- Examine for specific neurologic abnormalities, such as frontal lobe release signs (grasp, suck, snout, root), visual field cut, limitation of extraocular movement, or abnormal pupillary reaction.
- Check for nystagmus (recent drug ingestion, brainstem disease).
- Perform motor exam with particular attention to extrapyramidal features or involuntary movements such as tardive dyskinesias, tremors, asterixis, chorea, or myoclonus.
- Note on sensory exam any evidence of peripheral neuropathy or combined system disease (vitamin B_{12} deficiency).
- Observe gait for small, rigid steps (frontal lobe gait apraxia), wide-based gait (cerebellar disease), and small steps (extrapyramidal disease).
- Consider score on Mini-Mental Status Exam significant only if corroborated by other components of initial evaluation and Hx.
- Repeat testing over time to establish Dx further when in doubt and to identify complicating conditions.

LAB STUDIES

Screening Lab Studies

- Individualize based on patient's Hx, PE, and mental status exams; avoid using "routine battery of tests for dementia."

- Refer to published guidelines more as menu from which to select tests based on patient's clinical presentation than as required series of tests; these include
  - CBC and ESR;
  - chemistry panel (electrolytes, calcium, albumin, BUN, creatinine, transaminase levels);
  - TSH;
  - VDRL or RPR test for syphilis;
  - HIV antibodies;
  - urinalysis;
  - serum vitamin B_{12} and folate levels;
  - CXR;
  - ECG;
  - neuroimaging.
- Consider contrast-enhanced CT or MRI when
  - Hx suggests mass lesion;
  - focal neurologic signs or symptoms present;
  - dementia of abrupt onset;
  - Hx of seizures;
  - Hx of stroke.
- Reserve neuroimaging for patients who meet all of these criteria:
  - Early onset of symptoms
  - Noninsidious course
  - Focal signs or symptoms
  - Early gait disturbance
- Choose MRI with gadolinium contrast over CT for Dx of
  - multiinfarct dementia;
  - posterior fossa disease;
  - tumor.

Other Ancillary Studies

- Consider lumbar puncture in suspected active infection, vasculitis, or normal-pressure hydrocephalus; send CSF for glucose, protein, and gamma globulin levels, cultures, cell count, and serology for syphilis.
- Consider lumbar puncture for Dx of Lyme disease only if strong clinical evidence (see Lyme Disease).
- Watch for recommendations on use of CSF τ-protein determination (highly sensitive and specific for differentiating Alzheimer's from normal aging) and its potential contribution to early Dx.
- Reserve EEG for patients with episodes of altered consciousness or suspected Creutzfeldt-Jakob.
- Consider formal neuropsychological evaluation when Dx in doubt.
- Consider formal psychiatric assessment if depression is complicating clinical picture.

Studies of Limited or Uncertain Utility

- Omit routine use of carotid ultrasonography and transcranial Doppler flow studies unless clinical evidence of cerebrovascular disease or MRI or CT demonstrates infarction.
- Avoid brain biopsy for nonneoplastic and noninfectious diseases unless considering progressive multifocal leukoencephalopathy or Creutzfeldt-Jakob.

- Follow literature for data on utility of cerebral blood flow and metabolism measurements by PET and SPECT for predicting Huntington's and Alzheimer's.

Genetic Testing

- Inform family of issues involved with genetic testing.
- Consider tests for mutations on chromosomes 1, 14, and 21 only when family Hx strongly suggests early-onset Alzheimer's.
- Advise families that *APOE* genotyping, popularized in the press as "the test for Alzheimer's," is too inaccurate to serve as a screening test for Alzheimer's. Test lacks sensitivity to rule out Alzheimer's and is insufficiently predictive of developing dementia to be of prognostic value; potentially useful only when used in combination with full clinical evaluation.
- Discourage taking mail-order "test for Alzheimer's," which is nothing more than *APOE* testing.

MANAGEMENT

ALZHEIMER'S DISEASE AND LEWY BODY DISEASE

Overall Approach

- Offer to serve as main coordinator of patient's care and advisor to family if comfortable handling this responsibility; otherwise refer patient and family for care to those specializing in management of such patients.
- Apprise family members of patient's Dx; provide open discussion of Dx and initial management.
- Suggest that family join a local Alzheimer's disease support group.
- Arrange for social worker to meet early in course of illness with family to help plan care and provide emotional support.
- Advise family on how to establish predictable, well-structured home environment, especially one that limits risk for falls.
- Stop or reduce dosage of all unnecessary medications, especially those that may cause cognitive impairment.
- Consider drug Rx to achieve modest improvement in cognitive function when it will influence overall management (such as ability to maintain patient at home).
- When concomitant psychiatric problem (e.g., depression, anxiety, behavioral disorder, psychosis) develops, consider psychopharmacologic intervention.
- Approach need for nursing home placement carefully and only after home care resources have been used fully.

Use of Psychotropic Agents

- For depression, begin with low dose of SSRI or well-tolerated tricyclic agent (see Depression).
- For anxiety or difficulty sleeping, consider low dose of short-acting benzodiazepine (e.g., 1.0 mg lorazepam; see Anxiety).
- For psychotic behavior or catastrophic reactions, consider low dose of neuroleptic, with atypical neuroleptic preferred for patients with Lewy body disease.

■ If possible, make drug Rx brief (except in depression) and prescribe smallest dose possible in elderly patients.

Use of Psychotropic Agents in the Elderly

■ Antidepressants (mg/day)
- Tricyclics
  - Nortriptyline, 10–150
  - Desipramine, 10–250
- Stimulants
  - Dextroamphetamine, 2.5–40
  - Methylphenidate, 2.5–60
- SSRIs
  - Fluoxetine, 5–60
  - Sertraline, 25–200
  - Paroxetine, 10–40
  - Fluvoxamine, 25–300
  - Citalopram, 10–40
- Others
  - Trazodone, 25–250
  - Nefazodone, 50–600
  - Mirtazapine, 7.5–30.0
  - Venlafaxine (slow-release available), 25–300
  - Bupropion (slow-release available), 75–450

■ Neuroleptics (mg)
- Low potency
  - Thioridazine, 10–50
  - Perphenazine, 0.5–5
- Intermediate potency
  - Haloperidol, 0.25–2.0
- High potency
  - Thiothixene, 0.5–4

■ Atypical neuroleptics
- Clozapine, 6.25–100
- Olanzapine, 2.5–10
- Quetiapine, 12.5–300
- Risperidone, 0.25–3

Side Effects of Atypical Neuroleptics

■ Extrapyramidal effect
- Low: clozapine, olanzapine, quetiapine
- Medium: risperidone

■ Hypotension
- Mild: olanzapine
- Moderate: risperidone
- High: clozapine, quetiapine

■ Sedation
- Mild: risperidone
- Moderate: quetiapine
- High: clozapine, olanzapine

■ Anticholinergic effect
- Mild: risperidone, quetiapine

- Moderate: olanzapine
- High: clozapine

Cognitive Impairment

■ In addition to structuring home environment, prescribe cholinesterase inhibitor (e.g., donepezil, 5–10 mg/day; or rivastigmine, 1.5 mg bid) for Alzheimer's patients with impairment that is compromising daily function at home. Both achieve modest and only temporary improvement in cognitive function and behavioral state, but degree of benefit may be sufficient to permit patient to remain at home rather than be institutionalized.

■ Consider trial of selegiline (5 mg bid) for patients with Lewy body disease.

■ Consider adding vitamin E (2,000 IU/day) to slow functional deterioration

■ Avoid Hydergine, which is ineffective; formerly used for "poor cerebral circulation."

Day Care and Inpatient Programs

■ Consider day care program when demands of home care begin to strain principal caregiver but he or she does not believe that time for inpatient care has arrived.

■ Select day care program that specializes in Alzheimer patients and emphasizes attending to their emotional and physical needs.

■ When disease becomes more advanced and care at home is no longer possible, help family choose specialized inpatient facility.

OTHER CAUSES

■ For vascular dementia, aggressively treat atherosclerotic risk factors; consider need for endarterectomy (see Transient Ischemic Attack) and address risk factors for embolic disease (see Anticoagulant Therapy; Atrial Fibrillation; Valvular Heart Disease).

■ For HIV dementia, treat with intensive antiretroviral Rx (see HIV-1 Infection).

■ For confirmed CNS Lyme disease, begin parenteral antibiotics (see Lyme Disease).

■ For vitamin B_{12} deficiency, provide parenteral replacement (see Anemia).

■ For substance-induced disease, abstaining, avoiding toxins, and discontinuing causative drugs are basic Rx approaches (see Alcohol Abuse; Substance Abuse).

■ For hormonal deficiency, replacement Rx is key (see Diabetes Insipidus; Hypothyroidism).

INDICATIONS FOR REFERRAL AND ADMISSION

■ Consider neurologic consultation for
  - performance of detailed evaluation if beyond resources of PCP;
  - confirmation of Alzheimer's disease Dx when family seeks closure;
  - confirmation of potentially treatable neurologic condition (e.g., Parkinson's disease, normal-pressure hydrocephalus, mass lesion, carotid artery disease);
  - further assessment of suspected hereditary condition and genetic counseling.

■ Admit to hospital for behavioral management or for Rx of intercurrent medical illness, with attention to factors associated with development of delirium and use of lowest possible doses of analgesic and sedative-hypnotic medications.

BIBLIOGRAPHY

■ For the current annotated bibliography on dementia, see the print edition of *Primary Care Medicine*, 4th edition, Chapters 169 and 173, or www.LWWmedicine.com.

Dizziness

DIFFERENTIAL DIAGNOSIS

- Vestibular disease
  - Benign positional vertigo
  - Vestibular neuronitis and ototoxic drugs
  - Meniere's disease
  - Acoustic neuroma and other tumors of cerebellopontine angle
  - Basilar insufficiency
  - Multiple sclerosis
- Cardiac and vascular disease
  - Critical aortic stenosis
  - Carotid sinus hypersensitivity
  - Volume depletion and severe anemia
  - Autonomic insufficiency [drugs, diabetes mellitus (DM)]
  - Diminished vascular reflexes in the elderly
- Multiple sensory deficits
  - DM
  - Cataract surgery
  - Some cases of MS
  - Cervical spondylosis
  - Cerebellar disease
- Psychiatric illness
  - Anxiety
  - Depression
  - Psychosis
- Metabolic disturbances
  - Hypoxia
  - Severe hypoglycemia
  - Hypocapnia and hypercapnia

WORKUP

OVERALL STRATEGY

- Use Hx supplemented by PE to differentiate vestibular from nonvestibular disease.
- If vestibular, determine whether central or peripheral.
- If peripheral, differentiate acoustic neuroma from benign peripheral etiologies.
- If nonvestibular, review psychiatric, metabolic, vascular, and multiple sensory etiologies.

HISTORY

- Obtain best possible description of experience and what patient means by "dizziness"; elicit without leading questions or suggested descriptions.
- Consider vestibular disease when patient reports true vertigo; cardiovascular disorder when postural or paroxysmal faintness reported;

psychogenic cause when ill-defined dizziness or light-headedness unrelated to posture reported; multiple sensory deficits and cerebellar causes when poor balance or disequilibrium noted.

True Vertigo

- Differentiate central from peripheral vestibular disease by inquiring about brainstem symptoms (e.g., diplopia, facial numbness, weakness, hemiplegia, dysphasia).
- If brainstem symptoms present, consider central disease; if absent, consider peripheral disease more likely.
- If suspicious of central disease, check for evidence of and risk factors for MS (see Multiple Sclerosis) and TIA (see Transient Ischemic Attack and Asymptomatic Carotid Bruit).
- If peripheral disease more likely, distinguish among peripheral vestibular causes:
  - Differentiate cochlear from retrocochlear disease (benign from acoustic neuroma) by noting whether clinical course characterized by steadily progressive hearing loss (acoustic neuroma) or episodic or waxing and waning (cochlear etiologies).
  - Note timing and precipitating factors [e.g., symptomatic only on change of position and lasting only moments (benign positional vertigo); single bout of unprovoked persistent symptoms in setting of viral illness (vestibular neuronitis); concurrent inner ear infection (acute labyrinthitis); recurrent paroxysms with tinnitus, pressure, and temporary hearing loss (Meniere's disease)].
  - Review medications and drug Hx (aminoglycoside antibiotics, ethacrynic acid, diuretics, vasodilators, phenothiazines, antihypertensive agents, antidepressants, minor tranquilizers).

Light-Headedness

- Ask about onset with standing or turning.
- If with standing, check for use of antihypertensives, tranquilizers, or antidepressants and for Hx of aortic valve disease.
- If with turning, consider vision problems, multiple sensory deficits, and cerebellar problems.
- If constant and chronic, focus on Hx pertinent to underlying psychiatric disorders (see Anxiety; Depression; Somatization Disorders).

PHYSICAL EXAM

True Vertigo

- Check eyes for nystagmus (a few beats of nystagmus on extreme lateral gaze are normal), and ears for tympanic membrane lesions and hearing acuity.
- Perform neurologic exam, focusing on cranial nerves, sensory modalities, peripheral vision, gait, Romberg's test, and cerebellar maneuvers.
- If peripheral disease suspected, perform Rinne test to differentiate between conductive and sensorineural (cochlear) hearing loss. Also test for speech discrimination (recognizing <20% of words very suggestive of retrocochlear lesion).
- Consider provocative maneuvers:
  - Walking and turning

- Dix-Hallpike or Bárány's maneuver to confirm vestibular disease and to help distinguish peripheral from central vestibular dysfunction.
- Consider alleviating maneuvers (e.g., lying still).

Light-Headedness

- Note general appearance (e.g., overly nervous, hyperventilating, or sighing).
- Take postural signs, noting any postural changes in pulse or BP indicative of postural hypotension.
- Examine skin for pallor.
- Check carotid arteries for bruits and delay in upstroke and left ventricle for signs of hypertrophy and systolic ejection murmur.
- Perform neurologic exam, focusing on sensory modalities, peripheral vision, gait, Romberg's test, and cerebellar maneuvers.
- Consider provocative maneuvers:
  - Hyperventilation
  - Standing up from supine position
- Consider alleviating maneuvers:
  - Rebreathing into paper bag
  - Getting up slowly
  - Touching examiner's hand or walking with cane
  - Withholding suspected drugs

LAB STUDIES

True Vertigo

- Refer for electronystagmography and audiologic testing if clinical and provocative data insufficient to differentiate central and peripheral etiologies.
- Consider brainstem auditory evoked response if acoustic neuroma suspected.
- Follow with MRI of internal auditory canal and cerebellopontine angle only if high clinical suspicion of acoustic neuroma and auditory testing suggestive.
- Consider MRA if basilar TIAs are suggested by transient, isolated vertiginous spells in person with multiple atherosclerotic risk factors.

Light-Headedness

- If volume depletion suspected, check BUN, creatinine, and hematocrit.
- If carotid or cerebrovascular disease suspected clinically, proceed to carotid ultrasound (U/S) and/or transcranial Doppler studies.
- If signs of aortic stenosis presents, check cardiac U/S for critical stenosis.
- If multiple sensory deficits, screen for DM (see Diabetes Mellitus).
- If metabolic etiology suspected, check electrolytes and glucose.

MANAGEMENT

VESTIBULAR DISEASE

Peripheral Cochlear

- Prescribe meclizine (12.5–25 mg q6h prn) or promethazine (25 mg q6h prn) for incapacitating acute vertiginous attack (warn of drowsiness).

- For bothersome benign positional vertigo, refer to ENT specialist for Epley maneuver (relocates free-floating debris) and to trained therapist for balance-vestibular physical Rx.
- Consider Dramamine (50 mg q6h prn) or benzodiazepines for acute vertigo.
- Use salt restriction and diuretics (e.g., acetazolamide, 250 mg bid; or hydrochlorothiazide, 50 mg bid) for Meniere's disease; also limit caffeine and alcohol.

Peripheral Retrocochlear

- Refer to neurosurgery or ENT for consideration of surgical intervention.

Central Vestibular

- Treat etiologically if possible.
- For symptomatic relief pending improvement from etiologic Rx, consider lorazepam (Ativan, 1–2 mg bid). Supplement with gait training and vestibular exercises.

MULTIPLE SENSORY DEFICITS OR CEREBELLAR DYSFUNCTION

- Recommend handrails in home, good lighting, and use of cane or walker.

CARDIOVASCULAR DISEASE

- Treat etiologically (e.g., valve replacement for critical aortic stenosis).
- Supplement with adequate hydration, standing up slowly, and discontinuing or reducing offending drugs.

PSYCHOGENIC LIGHT-HEADEDNESS

- Acutely, apply rebreathing into paper bag for attacks of hyperventilation.
- Follow with rapidly acting anxiolytic agent (e.g., alprazolam, 0.25 mg).
- For chronic anxiety- or depression-related symptoms, consider antidepressant Rx with SSRIs (e.g., see Anxiety; Depression).

BIBLIOGRAPHY

- For the current annotated bibliography on dizziness, see the print edition of *Primary Care Medicine*, 4th edition, Chapter 166, or www.LWWmedicine.com.

DIFFERENTIAL DIAGNOSIS

IMPORTANT PERIPHERAL POLYNEUROPATHIES

- Predominantly motor
  - Acute (days)
    - Guillain-Barré syndrome
    - Diphtheria
    - Porphyria
    - Toxin (organophosphate exposure)
  - Subacute (wks to 1–2 yrs)
    - Toxin exposure (lead poisoning, glue sniffing)
    - Paraproteinemia
  - Chronic
    - Hereditary (Charcot-Marie-Tooth disease)
- Predominantly sensory
  - Acute (days)
    - None
  - Subacute (wks to 1–2 yrs)
    - Amyloidosis
    - Drug toxicity (cisplatin, vitamin B_6 excess)
    - Paraneoplastic syndrome
    - Sjögren's syndrome
  - Chronic (yrs)
    - Hereditary sensory neuropathy
- Sensorimotor
  - Acute (days)
    - Toxin exposure (arsenic)
  - Subacute (wks to 1–2 yrs)
    - Diabetes mellitus
    - Alcohol abuse
    - B vitamin deficiency
    - Renal failure
    - Hypothyroidism
    - Connective tissue disease
    - Paraneoplastic syndrome
    - Drug toxicity (isoniazid, cancer chemotherapeutic agents)
    - AIDS
  - Chronic (yrs)
    - Charcot-Marie-Tooth disease

Adapted from American College of Physicians Medical Knowledge Self-assessment Program IX, 1991, 106, with permission.

WORKUP

OVERALL STRATEGY

- Determine
  - whether problem is peripheral (in nerve root or peripheral nerve) or central (in cord or above).
  - whether peripheral, caused by lesion in peripheral nerve or by nerve root injury.
  - whether cord compression is present, particularly in upper extremity syndromes.
  - whether evidence (in other extremities) of more widespread peripheral neuropathy is present (e.g., diabetic patient with femoral neuropathy who also has diffuse peripheral neuropathy).
  - whether weakness is caused by muscle or nerve lesion.

HISTORY

Peripheral Polyneuropathy

- Inquire into duration (yrs suggests hereditary cause; wks to mos, toxic/metabolic cause or paraproteinemia; days, toxin or Guillain-Barré syndrome).
- Note distribution (helps distinguish polyneuropathy and diabetic mononeuropathy multiplex, which is more multifocal).
- Review medication exposure (e.g., cisplatin, isoniazid, vincristine), habits (alcohol abuse), diet (B vitamin deficiencies), and concurrent medical illnesses (DM, renal failure, liver disease, cancer).

Other Peripheral Nerve Syndromes

- Obtain detailed description of the nature and distribution of symptoms, including any pain radiation and whether there is motor, sensory, or mixed loss of function.
- Be sure to elicit aggravating and alleviating factors and clinical course over time.
- Always check for symptoms of cord and cauda equina compression, including bladder and anal sphincter dysfunction, saddle anesthesia, bilateral deficits, truncal sensory loss.

PHYSICAL EXAM

Peripheral Polyneuropathy

- Clarify distribution and relative sensory and motor components of problem.
- Check for signs of systemic disease.

Other Peripheral Nerve Syndromes

- Perform neurologic exam to address above issues and answer these questions:
  - Is lesion upper motor neuron or lower motor neuron lesion? Check for fasciculations, flaccidity, and lack of reflexes (lower motor neuron lesion originating in anterior horn cell or peripheral nerve); for spasticity and increased reflexes (lesion above anterior horn cell).
  - Is nerve dysfunction focal or more generalized? Check for confinement to 1 root or dermatome or to 1 peripheral nerve (single nerve lesion) and for generalized dysfunction with diffusely decreased deep

tendon reflexes, absent vibration sense at ankles, and stocking-glove pattern of sensory loss (diffuse peripheral neuropathy).
- Is weakness caused by nerve or by muscle disease? Check for weakness in conjunction with altered tendon reflexes and sensory loss (nerve disease) and for normal reflexes and preserved sensation (primary muscle disease). Note involvement of proximal muscle (toxic and metabolic myopathies) or distal musculature (all primary nerve diseases).

LAB STUDIES

Peripheral Polyneuropathy

- Obtain CBC, ESR, and values for blood glucose, serum liver chemistries, BUN, creatinine, and TSH.
- Check CXR and serum immunoelectrophoresis if concerned about malignancy.
- Consider EMG if difficulty differentiating between (1) demyelinating disease and axonal polyneuropathy, (2) root or plexus and more distal nerve trunk involvements, and (3) upper and lower motor neuron weakness.
- Reserve nerve biopsy for hereditary disorders, multifocal mononeuropathy multiplex, or asymmetric clinical syndromes when looking for vasculitis, amyloidosis, or sarcoidosis.
- In monoclonal gammopathy, test for antibody to myelin-associated glycoprotein (anti-MAG antibody) and anti-GM1 antibody to identify candidates for plasmapheresis or immunosuppressive Rx.

Other Peripheral Nerve Syndromes

- Lab studies are usually unnecessary during initial assessment, but sometimes selective testing is informative.
- Check serum for creatine phosphokinase and LDH elevations for suspected primary muscle disease.
- If myotonia present, consider EMG coupled with nerve conduction studies to distinguish primary muscle disease from neuropathic processes.
- Supplement clinical identification of nerve root and peripheral nerve syndromes with selective use of radiologic, nerve conduction, EMG, and serologic studies based on consideration of underlying etiology (see above).

MANAGEMENT

PAINFUL PERIPHERAL NEUROPATHY

- Begin with trial of tricyclic antidepressant (e.g., amitriptyline, nortriptyline).
- If relief insufficient, add or substitute gabapentin (Neurontin).
- Consider mexiletine and topical capsaicin and lidocaine if above measures fail.
- Reserve consideration of plasmapheresis for myasthenia gravis, chronic inflammatory demyelinating polyneuropathy, and monoclonal gammopathy–associated peripheral neuropathy.
- Consider IV immunoglobulin for Guillain-Barré syndrome.

PERIPHERAL POLYNEUROPATHY

- Treat underlying condition.

OTHER PERIPHERAL NEUROPATHY

- Treat etiologically.

INDICATIONS FOR REFERRAL AND ADMISSION

- Admit urgently for suspected acute spinal cord or cauda equina compression; obtain immediate neurosurgical consultation and MRI study of spinal cord.
- Consider neurologic referral for slowly progressive myelopathy to address complex differential (vitamin B_{12} deficiency, MS, and tumor) after mechanical cord compression is excluded by MRI.
- Obtain surgical consultation for root or peripheral nerve compression syndrome if refractory to conservative measures.

BIBLIOGRAPHY

- For the current annotated bibliography on focal neurologic complaints, see the print edition of *Primary Care Medicine*, 4th edition, Chapter 167, or www.LWWmedicine.com.

DIFFERENTIAL DIAGNOSIS

- Acute
  - Meningitis
  - Intracranial hemorrhage (stroke, aneurysm rupture)
  - Stroke
  - Acute increase in intracranial pressure (ICP) (mostly from cerebral edema or hemorrhage, including hypertensive encephalopathy)
  - Acute glaucoma
  - Acute sinusitis
  - Acute metabolic disturbance (carbon monoxide poisoning, hypoglycemia)
  - Acute viral illness
  - Initial presentation of persistent or recurrent headache
- Persistent or recurrent
  - Intracranial mass lesion (neoplasm, abscess, subdural hematoma, large arteriovenous malformation)
  - Tension-type headache
  - Migraine, with and without aura
  - Cluster headache
  - Indomethacin-responsive headache (ice pick, paroxysmal hemicrania)
  - Postconcussion syndrome
  - Cervical spine disease
  - Giant cell arteritis
  - Trigeminal neuralgia
  - HTN
  - Arteriovenous malformation
  - Bruxism/temporomandibular joint (TMJ) dysfunction
  - Medications
  - Substance abuse

WORKUP

OVERALL STRATEGY

- Differentiate primary headache syndromes (migraine ± aura, cluster headache, tension-type headache) from headache secondary to mechanical or systemic process (different Rx).
- Take time to perform Hx and PE; information is often diagnostic, always critical to intelligent test selection, and essential to dealing effectively with patient worries and expectations.
- To distinguish worrisome from harmless headaches, pay special attention to sudden onset, intensity of acute headache, and persistence and worsening over time.

HISTORY

- Obtain full description, particularly clinical course, associated symptoms, precipitants, aggravating and alleviating factors, and patient concerns.

- Review medication Hx for agents that can trigger nonspecific headaches (e.g., indomethacin, nifedipine, cimetidine, captopril, nitrates, atenolol, TMP-SMX, oral contraceptives).
- Note agents associated with drug-related increased ICP (minocycline, isotretinoin, nalidixic acid, tetracycline, TMP-SMX, cimetidine, corticosteroids, and tamoxifen).
- Focus Hx according to whether headache is new or recurrent/chronic.

Headache of New Onset

- Ask about fever, neck stiffness, and neurologic deficits.
- Pay special attention to patient unaccustomed to headaches who presents with sudden onset of "worst headache ever experienced," especially if accompanied by fever, stiff neck (meningitis, meningeal irritation from blood), marked gait ataxia with severe nausea and vomiting (midline cerebellar hemorrhage), alteration in mental status (hypertensive encephalopathy), focal neurologic deficit (migraine, stroke), or visual impairment (acute glaucoma).
- Think about ruptured cerebral aneurysm if there is abrupt onset of severe headache that reaches maximum intensity immediately.
- If headache is throbbing (especially if accompanied by prodromal and aural symptoms), consider migraine; if no prodrome, consider febrile illness, vasodilator use, carbon monoxide exposure, drug withdrawal, and hypoglycemia in addition to migraine.

Recurrent or Persistent Headache

- Differentiate migraine and tension-type headaches (recurrent, waxing and waning course) from brain tumor (increase in severity or frequency with time); intensity of pain is of little value.
- Check for associated symptoms, such as migrainous epiphenomena, new neurologic deficit (tumor), TMJ pain (bruxism), jaw claudication and scalp vessel tenderness (temporal/giant cell arteritis), neck pain (cervical radiculopathy), purulent nasal discharge (sinusitis).
- Note Hx of head trauma (subdural hematoma), parameningeal infection (abscess), depression, situational stress, or substance abuse.
- Review family Hx for headache (migraine, tension-type).
- Note medication Hx for rebound headache caused by overuse of analgesic medication with consequent withdrawal, ergotamine compounds, and serotonergic agonists (triptans).
- Ask about location and quality; tightness or pressure-like quality + whole-head, bandlike, or occipital-nuchal (tension-type, increased ICP); unilateral and throbbing (migraine, tension-type); unilateral and same location with crescendo pattern over time (mass lesion).
- Attend to aggravating and elevating factors [e.g., worsened by straining, coughing, or bending over (mass lesion, sinusitis); brought on by ingesting certain foods or beverages (chocolate, cheese, red wine) or exacerbated by noise, odors, and bright light (migraine); triggered by alcohol (cluster, migraine); induced or exacerbated by cimetidine, ethinyl estradiol, atenolol, indomethacin, danazol, nifedipine, selegiline, and oral contraceptives (drug-induced)].

PHYSICAL EXAM

Acute Headache

- Check BP and temp for elevations, scalp for cranial artery tenderness, sinuses for purulent discharge and tenderness, pupils for loss of reactivity, corneas for clouding (acute glaucoma), disc margins for papilledema, and neck for rigidity on anterior flexion.
- Perform full neurologic exam, especially for ataxia, alteration of mental status, focal deficits, and meningeal signs.

Chronic or Recurrent Headache

- Check detailed neurologic exam, looking for any fixed focal deficit (serious intracranial pathology).
- For facial pain, examine oral cavity for trigger zone (trigeminal neuralgia), teeth for wear (bruxism), TMJ for limitation of motion and crepitus, neck for signs of degenerative disk disease and worsening of headache with neck movement (cervical radiculopathy), and muscles about shoulders, neck, and occiput for excessive tautness (tension-type headache).
- For suspected mass lesion, include consideration of brain abscess and check for source (nasal cavity for purulent discharge, sinuses for tenderness, and ears for signs of chronic otitis media).

LAB STUDIES

Acute Headache

- Hospitalize immediately before testing if acute onset of "worst headache ever" accompanied by meningeal signs, evidence of increased ICP, or persistent new focal neurologic deficit.
- In hospital, obtain emergency head CT to rule out midline cerebellar hemorrhage and CNS mass.
- Follow with lumbar puncture if signs of meningeal irritation but no cerebral mass lesion or increased ICP; send CSF for Gram's stain, culture and sensitivity, CBC and differential, and glucose and protein determinations.
- Check ESR for new onset of headache in elderly patients, especially if accompanied by cranial artery or scalp tenderness; if concern about giant cell arteritis, proceed to temporal artery biopsy (see Giant Cell Arteritis).
- Refer immediately to ophthalmologist for glaucoma testing if there is eye or orbital pain with erythema and blurred vision.

Chronic or Recurrent Headache

- Omit testing in presence of headache Hx characteristic of migraine in conjunction with normal PE and no clinical findings (after detailed Hx and PE) suggesting intracranial disease.
- Avoid ordering neuroimaging studies unless there are worrisome clinical findings (e.g., new neurologic deficit, crescendo pattern to headache).
- Elicit and address patient concerns, and use detailed Hx and PE rather than neuroimaging to provide meaningful reassurance.
- Consider neuroimaging (CT with contrast or MRI) for

- headache of recent onset (<6 mos), especially if unilateral and increasing in frequency or severity (mass lesion).
- presence of seizure-like aural prodrome or loss of consciousness (seizure due to mass lesion).
- persistent personality change (frontal/temporal tumor).
- change in character of long-standing headache or lack of response to Rx directed at initial Dx.

MANAGEMENT

MIGRAINE HEADACHE

Prophylaxis

- Institute if headaches are interfering with work or other activities more than once/wk.
- Educate patients to avoid suspected precipitants (cheese, chocolates, citrus, nuts, red wine, inadequate sleep, and prolonged fasting); headache diary may help identify them.
- Recommend regular exercise and relaxation techniques (see Anxiety), but rest or vacation is of no benefit.
- Investigate family, work, and social circumstances; consider supportive psychotherapy when such stresses are severe.
- Advise that biofeedback is of unproved benefit and probably no better than relaxation exercises and other nonpharmacologic methods.
- Initiate pharmacologic measures when nonpharmacologic measures do not suffice.
- Give particular drug ≥2-mo trial.
- Begin with beta blocker (e.g., atenolol, 25–50 mg qhs) or tricyclic antidepressant (e.g., nortriptyline or amitriptyline, 10–25 mg qhs), especially if there is concurrent depression.
- Consider second-line agents if no response [verapamil, NSAIDs (especially for patients with menstrual migraine when prescribed for several days before, during, and after menstruation)].
- Consider valproate for refractory cases; inform patient of risks of hair loss, weight gain, and teratogenic potential (neural tube defects).
- Advise that there are promising results with high-dose riboflavin (vitamin B_2) when given in doses of 400 mg/day.

Available Agents

- Beta blockers
  - Propranolol, 40–320 mg/day
  - Nadolol, 40–240 mg/day
  - Atenolol, 50–150 mg/day
  - Timolol, 10–30 mg/day
- Tricyclic antidepressants
  - Amitriptyline, 10–300 mg/day
  - Nortriptyline, 10–125 mg/day
  - Doxepin, 10–150 mg/day
- Calcium channel blockers
  - Verapamil, 240–480 mg/day

- NSAIDs
  - Naproxen, 500 mg bid
- Anticonvulsants
  - Valproate: titration to therapeutic level from 250 mg tid
  - Phenytoin: adjustment to therapeutic level, usually 200–400 mg/day
- Serotonin antagonists
  - Methysergide, 2–4 mg in divided doses; usual dose 6–8 mg/day

Abortive Therapy

- Establish effective abortive regimen for patient with only occasional migraines and for those with generally well-controlled but occasional severe breakthroughs.
- For aural symptoms, consider NSAIDs; metoclopramide or prochlorperazine (Compazine) best given 30 mins before analgesic use.
- For abortive Rx choose triptans (selective 5-HT$_{1B/1D}$ agonist) or dihydroergotamine.

Triptan Use

- Consider second-generation agent (longer acting orally) if recurrence of headache problematic after initial dose of sumatriptan.
- Prescribe second dose for pain recurrence, but advise against chronic daily use (risk for rebound phenomenon if used ≥1–2 × wk).
- Avoid in person taking MAOIs or with uncontrolled HTN, CAD, or pregnancy.
- Advise against use during aura phase of migraine and in patients with complicated auras such as hemiparesis or dysphasia.
- Note that chest-related symptoms may occur, but in properly selected patients there is no increased risk of myocardial ischemia or stroke.

Triptan Preparations (Preferred Initial Dose)

- Sumatriptan, (6 mg) SQ
- Imitrex
  - PO: 25 mg, (50 mg), 100 mg
  - Nasal: 5 mg, (20 mg)
- Zolmitriptan (Zomig), (2.5 mg), 5 mg PO
- Naratriptan (Amerge), (2.5 mg) PO
- Rizatriptan (Maxalt), 5 mg, (10 mg) PO
- Maxalt MLT, 5 mg, 10 mg SL
- Eletriptan (Relpax), (40 mg), 80 mg PO

Dihydroergotamine Use

- Recommend nasal administration for home use, preceded if necessary by metoclopramide if nausea is problematic.
- Avoid in patients with coronary disease, peripheral vascular disease, TIA, pregnancy, or sepsis.
- Avoid regular use of analgesics and sedatives [e.g., butalbital, caffeine, and acetaminophen or aspirin (Fioricet and Fiorinal)] and exert marked caution in prescribing them (habituation potential, rebound headache).
- Similarly, avoid regular use of narcotic analgesics.

Reducing Migraine Stroke Risk

- Discourage use of oral contraceptives in premenopausal women with migraine with aura.
- Discourage estrogen use in older women with migraine and other risk factors for stroke.

CLUSTER HEADACHE

Abortive Therapy

- Prescribe
  - inhalation of oxygen (5–8 L/min for 10 mins), or
  - ergotamine suppositories qhs during cluster for patients with night-time symptoms, or
  - dihydroergotamine (SQ), or
  - sumatriptan, or
  - dexamethasone, 8 mg bolus, or prednisone, 20 mg tid tapered over 2 wks.

Prophylaxis

- For severe frequent episodes consider
  - verapamil (360 mg/day), or
  - methysergide (2 mg tid), or
  - lithium (300 mg bid–tid to achieve therapeutic serum level), or
  - sphenopalatine ganglion block, or
  - radio frequency trigeminal rhizotomy (refractory to all medical Rx)

TENSION-TYPE HEADACHE

- Prescribe aspirin, acetaminophen, or nonprescription doses of NSAIDs.
- Attend to any underlying sources of psychological distress.
- Recommend stress reduction measures (see Anxiety) and antidepressant Rx if anxiety or depression concurrent.
- Advise concluding any pending legal proceedings related to trauma-induced headaches.

CHRONIC DAILY HEADACHES

- Check for and eliminate chronic analgesic and ergotamine use (source of rebound headache).
- Attempt total elimination of analgesics and ergotamine compounds.
- Consider hospitalizing for withdrawal of these medications.

OTHER HEADACHE-CAUSING CONDITIONS

- See chapters on specific conditions.

INDICATIONS FOR REFERRAL

- Refer for neurologic consultation if episodes of transient neurologic dysfunction, unilateral headache increasing in frequency and severity, change in personality, or new onset of progressive deficits.
- Consider neurologic consultation for intractable tension-type headache or severe migraine syndrome.
- Obtain dental consultation for TMJ problems refractory to conservative Rx.
- Make surgical referral for temporal artery biopsy when giant cell arteritis is a consideration.

- Arrange ophthalmologic consultation for vision check and assessment of need for refraction if prolonged close work is resulting in headaches.
- Consider psychiatric consultation as diagnostic and learning experience for patients with chronic, intractable, tension-type headache who have completed a full evaluation for other etiologies.

BIBLIOGRAPHY

- For the current annotated bibliography on headache, see the print edition of *Primary Care Medicine*, 4th edition, Chapter 165, or www.LWWmedicine.com.

Multiple Sclerosis

WORKUP

HISTORY

- Consider Dx if multiple (≥2) symptoms of CNS disease develop separated anatomically and in time (>1 mo).

PHYSICAL EXAM

- Check for evidence of multiple lesions (upturned toes bilaterally, subtle internuclear ophthalmoplegia, mild afferent pupillary defect) when symptoms suggest only single lesion.

LAB STUDIES

- Proceed to lab testing if ≥2 separate neurologic lesions are identified clinically.
- Obtain MRI of head and spinal cord to identify characteristic findings (multiple periventricular and spinal cord plaques reported as increased signal intensity on long TR-weighted and proton density-weighted images); found in >90% of MS patients.
- Interpret MRI cautiously and in context of total clinical picture; MRI findings nonspecific (also found in normal elderly, chronic uncontrolled HTN, advanced Lyme disease, and CNS vasculitis).
- For additional confirmation, consider lumbar puncture for CSF exam; send for cell count, protein level, IgG, and electrophoresis for oligoclonal IgG bands.
- Order visual or auditory evoked potentials when MRI results require supporting data.
- Exclude other etiologies by ordering vitamin B_{12} and ANA levels, and consider testing for HIV and Lyme disease antibodies if risk factors or clinical signs present.

MANAGEMENT

OVERALL APPROACH

- Initiate disease-modifying Rx early in course of MS, before irreversible disability has developed.
- Consider disease-modifying Rx for patients with unfavorable prognostic features:
  - Progressive disease from onset
  - Short interval between first 2 relapses
  - Poor recovery from relapse
  - Motor and cerebellar signs at onset
  - Multiple cranial lesions on long TR-weighted MRI.
- Aim to prevent relapses and retard progressive worsening.

ACUTE ATTACK

- Begin high-dose parenteral corticosteroids (e.g., IV methylprednisolone followed by several wks oral prednisone).

- Consider primary prevention with recombinant IFN-β-1a (*Avonex*) after single episode secondary to documented myelination (reduces risk of progression to clinically definite MS).
- Consider recombinant IFN-β-1b (e.g., Betaseron) or glatiramer acetate (Copaxone) as disease-modifying Rx for patients with relapsing-remitting MS; obtain neurological consultation.
- Test serum of patients who continue to have clinical disease activity despite IFN Rx for neutralizing antibodies.

PROGRESSIVE DISEASE

- Offer disease-modifying Rx to patients with secondary progressive disease after thorough patient and family ed regarding proper use and side effects.
- Consider mitoxantrone (Novantrone) for relapsing-progressive or secondary progressive disease.
- Refer for consideration of IV immune globulin if disease progresses despite monthly IFN or copolymer Rx for 2 yrs.
- Refer for consideration of IV cyclophosphamide if rapidly progressive disease ensues unresponsive to other measures; also consider plasmapheresis.

COMPLICATIONS

- Prescribe carbamazepine (200 mg bid) for paroxysmal symptoms (lancinating pain or limb spasms).
- Consider tricyclic antidepressant (e.g., amitriptyline, 25–75 mg/day) to help control emotional lability, relieve neuropathic pain, and counter depression.
- Consider baclofen in low doses (5–10 mg tid) for spasticity, but be aware of side effects (confusion, sedation, increased muscle weakness); diazepam and dantrolene are alternatives.
- Begin anticholinergic Rx (e.g., propantheline, 15 mg bid–qid, prn; or oxybutynin, 5–10 mg bid–tid) for incontinence due to bladder spasm (frequency, urge incontinence).
- Begin cholinergic agent if there is bladder atony (see Incontinence).
- Consider amantadine (Symmetrel; 100 mg bid–tid) for debilitating fatigue.

PATIENT EDUCATION

- Make every effort to eliminate confusion; definitively confirm Dx.
- Review in detail prognosis, Rx options, and their efficacy to enhance patient's sense of control.
- Indicate that progression to disabling disease is not inevitable, that prognosis is highly variable, and that in many cases disease never becomes incapacitating.
- Give detailed advice on handling affairs of everyday life (e.g., avoiding very hot shower, which may transiently exacerbate symptoms).
- Maintain hopeful perspective and establish close, supportive relationship.

INDICATIONS FOR REFERRAL AND ADMISSION

- Obtain neurologic consultation when Dx of MS is suspected on clinical grounds to help determine need for further diagnostic studies (MRI, lumbar puncture with immunoelectrophoresis, evoked potentials) and in selecting Rx modality.

- Refer for consideration of high-dose IV glucocorticoid Rx when there is acute exacerbation of functional significance.
- Obtain neurologic consultation about timing or appropriateness of IFN-β or copolymer Rx.
- Use services of occupational/physical Rx to facilitate maintenance of daily functioning in patients with functionally limiting motor and/or sensory deficits.

BIBLIOGRAPHY

- For the current annotated bibliography on multiple sclerosis, see the print edition of *Primary Care Medicine*, 4th edition, Chapter 172, or www.LWWmedicine.com.

Parkinson's Disease

DIFFERENTIAL DIAGNOSIS

- Idiopathic parkinsonism
  - Parkinson's disease
  - Lewy body disease
- Infectious and postinfectious
  - Postencephalitic parkinsonism (von Economo's disease)
  - Other viral encephalitides
- Toxins
  - Manganese
  - Carbon monoxide
  - Carbon disulfide
  - Cyanide
  - Methanol
  - MPTP
- Drugs
  - Neuroleptics
  - Reserpine
  - Metoclopramide
  - Lithium
  - Amiodarone
  - Methyldopa
- Multisystem degeneration
  - Striatonigral degeneration
  - Progressive supranuclear palsy
  - Olivopontocerebellar degeneration
  - Shy-Drager syndrome
- Primary dementing and other degenerative disorders
  - Alzheimer's disease
  - Creutzfeldt-Jakob disease
- Other CNS disorders
  - Multiple cerebral infarctions (lacunar state, Binswanger's disease)
  - Hydrocephalus (normal-pressure or high-pressure)
  - Posttraumatic encephalopathy (pugilistic parkinsonism)
- Metabolic conditions
  - Hypoparathyroidism
  - Chronic hepatocerebral degeneration
  - Idiopathic basal ganglia calcification
- Hereditary disorders
  - Wilson's disease
  - Juvenile Huntington's disease (rigid variant)

Adapted from Koller WC. How accurately can Parkinson's disease be diagnosed? Neurology 1992;42[Suppl 1]:6, with permission.

WORKUP

HISTORY AND PHYSICAL EXAM

- Base Dx of Parkinson's disease on careful Hx and PE that addresses diagnostic and exclusionary criteria. This necessitates not only checking for resting tremor, bradykinesia, and rigidity but also reviewing medical Hx for medications and toxin exposures; family Hx for hereditary pattern; PE for dementia, cerebellar, and upper and lower motor neuron deficits; and postural signs for autonomic insufficiency.

Criteria for Diagnosis of Parkinson's Disease

- Inclusion criteria
  - Presence for ≥1 yr of 2 of 3 cardinal motor signs
    - Resting or postural tremor
    - Bradykinesia
    - Rigidity
  - Responsiveness to levodopa Rx with moderate to marked improvement lasting ≥1 yr
- Exclusion criteria
  - Abrupt onset of symptoms
  - Remitting or stepwise progression
  - Neurologic Rx within 1 yr
  - Exposure to drugs or toxins associated with parkinsonism
  - Hx of encephalitis
  - Oculogyric crises
  - Supranuclear downward or lateral gaze palsy
  - Cerebellar signs
  - Unexplained upper motor neuron or lower motor neuron signs
  - >1 affected relative
  - Dementia from onset of disease
  - Severe autonomic symptoms

Adapted from Reich SG, DeLong M. Parkinson's disease. In: Johnson R, ed. Current therapy in neurologic disease, 3rd ed. St. Louis: Mosby, 1990, with permission.

- Consider MRI with contrast to exclude significant small vessel vascular disease, which may produce parkinsonian-like state.

MANAGEMENT

INITIAL THERAPY

- After excluding other potential causes of parkinsonism, start selegiline (Deprenyl, 5 mg qam, 5 mg at noon) for Rx of early-stage disease.
- If symptoms progress to impair daily functioning despite selegiline, add dopamine agonist [e.g., pramipexole (Mirapex), 0.125 mg tid].
- Double pramipexole dose at weekly intervals until reaching maintenance dose of about 1 mg tid.

SUBSEQUENT TREATMENT

- If and when symptoms advance despite full initial Rx, add combination preparation levodopa/carbidopa (Sinemet, 25 mg/100 mg tid).
- Adjust dose according to individual response.

- Initiate program of physical Rx and psychological support; watch for and treat any depression that may develop.
- Continue or add selegiline in patients with more advanced disease already taking levodopa/carbidopa (Sinemet) to lower amount of levodopa needed.

ADVANCED DISEASE

- Consider adding anticholinergics, amantadine, and direct dopamine agonists (e.g., bromocriptine, pergolide, ropinirole) to maximize control of symptoms due to advancing disease. Anticholinergics are especially helpful for tremor.

DRUGS FOR PARKINSON'S DISEASE (STARTING AND MAINTENANCE DOSES)

- Anticholinergics (representative examples)
  - Trihexyphenidyl hydrochloride (Artane), 2 mg tid–qid; 2–10 mg tid–qid (you may use timed-release capsule after determining maintenance dose)
  - Benztropine mesylate (Cogentin), 1 mg/day; 0.5–6 mg/day
- Dopamine agonists
  - Carbidopa/levodopa (Sinemet), 50/200 mg in 2 divided doses; 400–500 mg levodopa bid–qid
  - Sinemet CR, 50/200 mg bid; variable
  - Bromocriptine (Parlodel), 1.25 mg/d; 7.5–30 mg bid–tid
  - Pergolide mesylate (Permax), 0.05 mg/day; 1–3 mg tid
  - Deprenyl (Eldepryl, selegiline hydrochloride), 5 mg/day; 10 mg bid
  - Amantadine (Symmetrel), 100 mg/day; 200 mg bid
  - Pramipexole (Mirapex), 0.25 mg tid; variable
  - Ropinirole (Requip), 0.25 mg tid; variable
- COMT inhibitor
  - Tolcapone (Tasmar), 100 mg tid; 100 mg tid

Adapted from Reich SG, DeLong M. Parkinson's disease. In: Johnson R, ed. Current therapy in neurologic disease, 3rd ed. St Louis: Mosby, 1990, and Lang AE, Lozano AM. Medical progress: Parkinson's disease. N Engl J Med 1998;339:1044, 1130, with permission.

PROBLEMS OF LONG-TERM MANAGEMENT

- Watch for loss of efficacy manifested by wearing off of effect at end of dose interval, on-off effect, drug-induced confusion, and loss of dopamine response.
- Consider COMT inhibitor to lessen these problems associated with dopaminergic Rx.
- Obtain neurologic consultation to help design late-stage program.
- Do not neglect important roles of physical Rx, psychological support, and recognition and Rx of depression in day-to-day management.

BIBLIOGRAPHY

- For the current annotated bibliography on Parkinson's disease, see the print edition of *Primary Care Medicine*, 4th edition, Chapter 174, or www.LWWmedicine.com.

Seizures

DIFFERENTIAL DIAGNOSIS

CONDITIONS MIMICKING SEIZURES

With Focal Deficits

- TIA
- Migraine
- Nerve compression

With Episodic Loss of Consciousness

- Transient diminished cerebral perfusion from cardiac source
- TIA
- Panic attack
- Psychotic episode

CONDITIONS CAUSING SEIZURES

In Children

- Primary or idiopathic epilepsy

In Younger Adults

- Drugs (usually alcohol withdrawal)
- Neoplasm
- Trauma

In Older Adults

- Neoplasm
- Trauma
- Cerebrovascular disease

Nonepileptic Convulsions

- Cerebral hypoperfusion
- Hypoglycemia
- Hyperosmolar state
- Hyponatremia

WORKUP

OVERALL STRATEGY

- Attempt to establish etiologic Dx whenever possible. Underlying disorders can be found in >30% of seizures with focal component.
- Consider seizure important manifestation of underlying pathology. After age 30, underlying cause (secondary epilepsy) becomes increasingly likely when patient presents with first seizure.

HISTORY

- Obtain exact description of events from witnesses and patient. Witness reports are especially useful because patient's consciousness and recall were likely compromised.
- Inquire into presence of aura, focal onset, loss of consciousness, and observed injury during convulsion. Such symptoms suggest seizure rather than syncope, although it is impossible to distinguish them absolutely based on any characteristic features.
- Once ascertained that seizure has occurred, check for Hx of focal onset, even in patients with Hx of generalized seizure. Focal onset of witnessed seizure that later became generalized may be important clue to underlying CNS lesion.
- Identify precipitants and underlying disease. Inquire into drugs (e.g., alcohol, cocaine, amphetamines, antidepressants, sedatives, theophylline, insulin, diuretics), cardiac arrhythmias, valvular disease, previous malignancy, stroke, and head trauma.
- Check for symptoms of hyperglycemia and hypoglycemia (see Diabetes Mellitus) in addition to those of meningeal irritation (headache, stiff neck). Seek family Hx of convulsions.

PHYSICAL EXAM

- If possible, perform neurologic exam as quickly as possible after seizure. Focal residual abnormality, such as paralysis of 1 arm (Todd's paralysis), may suggest focal onset even when witnessed event was generalized.
- Check for postural hypotension, abnormalities in heart rate and rhythm, head trauma, carotid disease, cardiac disease, systemic infection, and signs of alcohol and drug abuse (see Alcohol Abuse; Substance Abuse).

LAB STUDIES

Electroencephalogram

- Consider EEG when it is impossible by clinical means to determine whether transient or persistent neurologic event is seizure.
- Interpret EEG result cautiously:
  - Abnormal EEG with epileptiform features (spikes or sharp waves) supports Dx and may provide information about type of seizure disorder, but
  - Abnormal EEG inadequate for Dx of seizures, and normal interictal EEG pattern can be found in up to 20% of patients with purely generalized seizures.
  - EEG concentrates on cortical disturbances; abnormalities of deep temporal lobe or diencephalic structures may not be evident on surface EEG.
  - Obtain sleep EEG to increase sensitivity for detection of partial complex seizures (temporal lobe epilepsy).
  - Consider ambulatory EEG with Digitrace device for up to 72 hrs of monitoring. Patient records clinical events with push button and events are correlated with EEG findings.

Neuroimaging

- Obtain brain MRI with and without gadolinium contrast in patient with first seizure. MRI more sensitive than CT and may be particularly useful in demonstrating abnormalities in medial temporal region.

- Reserve PET and SPECT studies for use by specialists, who might use them to examine cerebral function, confirm organic abnormality, and outline abnormal region for consideration of surgical Rx. Helps differentiate generalized from localization-related seizures and select patients for epilepsy surgery.

Other Testing

- Obtain blood chemistries; measurement of electrolyte, calcium, and alcohol levels; and toxic screen.
- Screen all patients with HIV risk factors for HIV antibody (see HIV-1 Infection).
- Reserve lumbar puncture in patient with first seizure to those with fever, other evidence of infection, or status epilepticus.

MANAGEMENT

OVERALL APPROACH

- Treat etiologically whenever possible, but symptomatic Rx can begin while evaluation is in progress.

ANTICONVULSANT THERAPY

- To prevent further convulsions, begin with loading dose of drug of choice appropriate to seizure type identified. Drug administration can often be on outpatient basis.
- Follow with maintenance dose, and adjust to achieve therapeutic level.
- Check level at interval appropriate for drug half-life.
- If seizures persist, check serum levels of antiepileptic drug and inquire into alcohol and other drug use.
- Add second drug, then taper and discontinue first drug if drug of first choice does not control seizures.
- If seizures are controlled, have patient continue medication for ≥2 yrs.
- If patient remains seizure-free, refer to neurologist to consider cautious attempt to taper medication.
- Teach patient how to recognize warning signals of seizure and how to minimize injury. Instruct patient about role of alcohol in precipitating seizures.
- Educate patient and family about prognosis, activity, and job precautions.

STARTING AND MAINTENANCE ADULT DOSES OF ANTIEPILEPTIC DRUGS (MG/DAY) BY SEIZURE TYPE

Tonic-Clonic Seizures

- Phenytoin (Dilantin), 300; 200–500
- Carbamazepine (Tegretol, Tegretol-XR), 200–400; 600–1,200
- Valproic acid (Depakote), 750; 1,000–4,000
- Phenobarbital, 90; 90–240
- Primidone (Mysoline), 125; 750–1,500
- Gabapentin (Neurontin), 300; 900–4,800
- Topiramate (Topamax), 50; 200–600

- Tiagabine (Gabitril), 4; 32–56
- Gabapentin (Neurontin), 300; 900–4,800
- Tiagabine (Gabitril), 4; 32–56
- Felbamate (Felbatol), 1,200; 1,200–3,600

Complex Partial, Simple Partial Seizures

- Phenytoin (Dilantin), 300; 200–500
- Carbamazepine (Tegretol, Tegretol-XR), 200–400; 600–1,200
- Phenobarbital, 90; 90–240
- Primidone (Mysoline), 125; 750–1,500
- Oxcarbazepine (Trileptal), 150; 600–1,200
- Gabapentin (Neurontin), 300; 900–4,800
- Topiramate (Topamax), 50; 200–600
- Tiagabine (Gabitril), 4; 32–56
- Lamotrigine (Lamictal), 50; 300–500 (not to be used with valproate)
- Felbamate (Felbatol), 1,200; 1,200–3,600

Myoclonic Seizures

- Valproic acid (Depakote), 750; 1,000–4,000
- Clonazepam (Klonopin), 1.5; 1.5–10.0

Absence Seizures

- Valproic acid (Depakote), 750; 1,000–4,000
- Ethosuximide (Zarontin), 500; 500–1,500
- Clonazepam (Klonopin), 1.5; 1.5–10.0
- Lamotrigine (Lamictal), 50; 300–500 (not to be used with valproate)
- Felbamate (Felbatol), 1,200; 1,200–3,600

Atonic Seizures

- Clonazepam (Klonopin), 1.5; 1.5–10.0

Lennox-Gastaut Seizures

- Lamotrigine (Lamictal) with valproate,: 25; 100–400

BIBLIOGRAPHY

- For the current annotated bibliography on seizures, see the print edition of *Primary Care Medicine*, 4th edition, Chapter 170, or www.LWWmedicine.com.

Transient Ischemic Attack and Asymptomatic Carotid Bruit

DIFFERENTIAL DIAGNOSIS

- Carotid or vertebrobasilar occlusive disease
- Small vessel ischemic stroke
- Emboli originating in heart or aortic arch
- Focal seizures
- Focal aura of migraine
- Hyperventilation
- Carpal tunnel syndrome
- Cervical disk or osteophyte

WORKUP

GENERAL STRATEGY

- Evaluate all TIA patients promptly [especially if recent onset (<1 mo)] to assess stroke risk and identify those who require aggressive intervention.

HISTORY

- Confirm that episode was indeed TIA, based on onset and duration (>24 hrs excludes TIA; cessation within 10 mins increases probability of TIA; onset of headache during resolution of neurologic deficit suggests migraine).
- Review symptoms to distinguish vertebrobasilar involvement (binocular vision disturbance, vertigo, paresthesias, diplopia, ataxia, dysarthria, light-headedness, generalized weakness, loss of consciousness, transient global amnesia) from carotid disease (transient monocular blindness; clumsiness, weakness, or numbness of hand; disturbed speech).
- Check frequency of episodes, date of first onset, and presence of underlying heart disease and cardiovascular risk factors.
- Check for subsequent stroke risk factors (HTN, cardiac disease, age >65, carotid symptoms, first few mos after onset of TIAs).
- If carotid bruit found on PE, check Hx for overlooked transient neurologic events (heightened risk for stroke), family Hx of stroke, and stroke risk factors (advanced age, systolic HTN, current smoking, and the presence of DM, AF, or CHD).

PHYSICAL EXAM

- Check for BP elevation, irregularly irregular heart rhythm, and heart murmurs.
- Examine fundus for embolus in retinal artery branch if examining shortly after event.

- Gently palpate and auscultate carotid arteries to note upstroke, volume, and bruits; note pitch and duration of any bruit (correlate with severity of stenosis).
- Palpate facial and superficial temporal pulses with simultaneous assessment of supratrochlear and supraorbital pulses for collateral flow to latter 2 vessels (occlusion of internal carotid artery).

LAB STUDIES

- Check CBC and serum glucose, lipid panel, creatinine, and potassium levels.
- Measure homocysteine, serum folate, and vitamin B_{12}.
- To assess suspected carotid lesions, obtain Doppler and B-mode ultrasonography (U/S) supplemented by transcranial Doppler (flow in ophthalmic system and hemodynamic significance).
- To study posterior circulation, check transcranial Doppler U/S.
- Follow with MRA or standard contrast arteriography to confirm hemodynamically significant disease only if result will affect management (e.g., proceed to endarterectomy or lifelong anticoagulation).
- Consider contrast-enhanced CT or MRI of brain if there is question of silent or prior infarction, unsuspected hemorrhage, or nonvascular disease, such as tumor.
- Obtain transthoracic echocardiography if concerned about embolization to identify predisposing cardiac lesions.
- Strongly consider transesophageal echocardiography when standard echocardiography is unrevealing but clinical suspicion of embolization is strong. Best means of detecting aortic arch sources of embolization.
- Order ambulatory Holter monitoring when AF suspected as source of embolization and results of resting ECG are normal.
- Consider testing for hypercoagulability (anticardiolipin antibodies, protein C and S deficiencies, antithrombin III, factor V Leiden, homocysteine levels) in young patients (age <50) if Hx of unexplained venous thrombosis, family Hx of abnormal clotting, unexplained stroke, or abnormal platelet count, PT, or PTT.

MANAGEMENT

TRANSIENT ISCHEMIC ATTACK

- Attend not only to stroke risk but also to risk factors for CAD [most common cause of death in TIA patients (see Stable Angina)].
- Treat according to degree of symptoms and presence and severity of carotid disease or other sources of embolization.

Symptomatic Transient Ischemic Attack Patients with Tight Carotid Stenosis

- Refer promptly for consideration of carotid endarterectomy if >70% carotid stenosis, especially if recurrent TIAs or TIA within 4 mos of current visit.
- Consider immediate hospital admission, heparinization, and urgent arteriography/MRA in very-high-risk patients.

- Perform preoperative cardiac assessment to gauge overall surgical candidacy.
- Prefer carotid endarterectomy (when performed by skilled surgical team) over medical Rx for patients with recent hemispheric or retinal TIA or nondisabling stroke and ipsilateral high-grade stenosis of internal carotid artery.

Symptomatic Transient Ischemic Attack Patients with Less Severe Carotid Stenosis

- Prefer endarterectomy over medical management for those with recent TIA or stroke and 50–60% carotid stenosis.
- Choose medical Rx if stenosis <50%.
- Emphasize tight control of all cardiovascular risk factors.
- Begin aspirin (60–325 mg/day) as initial Rx.
- Consider dipyridamole/aspirin combination (Aggrenox) and clopidogrel (modestly enhanced efficacy over aspirin alone but at greatly increased cost).
- Prescribe long-term oral anticoagulation with warfarin for presence of AF or if antiplatelet Rx appears ineffective.

Additional Transient Ischemic Attack Candidates for Medical Therapy

- Elect medical Rx for TIA patients who are elderly, cannot tolerate surgery, have single remote TIA, or present in settings in which angiographic and surgical services are unavailable.
- Start aspirin (60–325 mg/day) as initial Rx of choice.

Patients with Transient Ischemic Attack and Normal Carotid Vessels

- Perform thorough cardiac and aortic arch evaluations to rule out an embolic cardiovascular source.
- Place patients with no evident cardiovascular pathology on prophylactic aspirin (325 mg/day).
- Prescribe warfarin for patients with TIA-like episodes caused by cardioembolic disease, including nonrheumatic AF (see Anticoagulant Therapy).

ASYMPTOMATIC CAROTID BRUIT

- Treat aggressively all cardiovascular risk factors.
- Emphasize prompt reporting of any TIA symptoms.
- Refer promptly for consideration of surgical intervention previously asymptomatic patients with high-grade stenosis (70–99%) who subsequently experience TIA.
- Prescribe low-dose aspirin (60–325 mg/day).
- Do not routinely recommend carotid endarterectomy in truly asymptomatic patient with total occlusion or tight stenosis (risk outweighs benefit, especially outside major centers).
- Consider endarterectomy for those who demonstrate rapid progression to hemodynamically and anatomically critical stenosis (e.g., lumen <1 mm), provided that they have no active coronary disease or DM and have anticipated life expectancy >5 yrs.
- Consider surgery only if skilled surgical team with proved record of low perioperative morbidity and mortality (<2%) is available and only after

carrying out careful preoperative cardiac risk assessment (see Stable Angina; Stress Testing).

BIBLIOGRAPHY

■ For the current annotated bibliography on transient ischemic attack and asymptomatic carotid bruit, see the print edition of *Primary Care Medicine*, 4th edition, Chapter 171, or www.LWWmedicine.com.

Tremor

DIFFERENTIAL DIAGNOSIS

COMMON CAUSES OF TREMOR

- Postural
  - Physiologic
- Intention
  - Essential
  - Senile
  - Cerebellar
- Resting
  - Parkinson's disease

OTHER INVOLUNTARY MOVEMENTS

- Dyskinesias
- Tics
- Myoclonus
- Athetosis

WORKUP

HISTORY

- Ascertain circumstances under which tremor occurs (when maintaining posture, during rest, during action).
- Attempt to distinguish resting tremor of early Parkinson's disease from essential tremor, and essential tremor from exaggerated physiologic tremor.

PHYSICAL EXAM

- Observe whether tremor is better or worse with activity by asking patient to hold out hands, write, perform rapid alternating movements, and touch nose with finger repeatedly.
- If resting tremor, check for other signs of parkinsonism (e.g., increased rigidity, cogwheeling, shuffling gait, mask-like facies).
- Observe discretely during Hx and other parts of PE so as not to call excessive attention to tremor (which may worsen or distort with physiologic response of anxiety).

LAB STUDIES

- Request tremor recording by EMG if necessary to differentiate resting from action tremor (or to identify both; may be coexistent).
- Check TSH if hyperthyroidism suspected.

MANAGEMENT

ESSENTIAL TREMOR

- Begin beta blocker (e.g., atenolol, 50 mg/day) and increase prn.
- Alternatively, begin primidone (Mysoline, 50 mg/day) and increase to as much as 250 mg/day in divided doses prn.
- Consider adding alprazolam (Xanax) or another benzodiazepine as intermittent adjunct.

PHYSIOLOGIC TREMOR

- Recommend small pre-performance dose of beta blocker (e.g., propranolol, 20 mg) or short-acting benzodiazepine (e.g., alprazolam, 0.25 mg), but warn of risk of sedation and possibility of hindering performance.

PARKINSON'S DISEASE

- Consider anticholinergic Rx (see Parkinson's Disease).

CEREBELLAR DISEASE

- Advise that drug Rx is usually ineffective.
- Consider wrist weights to dampen amplitude of tremors and make limb more functional.

PATIENT EDUCATION AND INDICATIONS FOR REFERRAL

- Review cause and indicate that often it can be controlled.
- Recommend avoiding agents that worsen symptoms (e.g., alcohol, caffeine).
- Refer patients with intention tremors and cerebellar signs for neurologic consultation, as demyelinating or hereditary degenerative diseases may be responsible.
- Consider referral for disabling tremors refractory to simple Rx for consideration of additional measures.

BIBLIOGRAPHY

- For the current annotated bibliography on tremor, see the print edition of *Primary Care Medicine*, 4th edition, Chapter 168, or www.LWWmedicine.com.

Trigeminal Neuralgia (Tic Douloureux)

DIFFERENTIAL DIAGNOSIS

- Dental disease
- Temporomandibular joint dysfunction
- Giant cell arteritis
- Sphenoid sinusitis
- Cluster headache
- Herpes zoster, pre-eruption
- Postherpetic neuralgia

WORKUP

- See Focal Neurological Complaints.

MANAGEMENT

- Teach patient to avoid repetitive contact with trigger zone.
- Begin drug Rx for disabling and frequent episodes of pain with carbamazepine (100 mg bid, preferably extended-release preparation).
- Increase dosage by 200 mg/day until symptoms are controlled or dosage of 800–1,000 mg/day reached.
- During first 2 mos of carbamazepine Rx, monitor CBC and platelet counts weekly to biweekly; monthly thereafter.
- Stop carbamazepine immediately if WBC count falls <3,000/mm^3 or if skin rash, easy bruising, fever, mouth sores, or petechiae develop.
- Consider baclofen (10 mg bid) as alternative to carbamazepine. Increase dosage by 10 mg/d q3d until patient responds or maximum of 60 mg/day reached. Discontinue medication gradually; do not withdraw it abruptly.
- If carbamazepine or baclofen alone is insufficient to control symptoms, add phenytoin, 300 mg/day.
- If above medicines are unsuccessful, start gabapentin (Neurontin), 300 mg qhs, and increase by 300 mg q4d until reaching 1,800 mg/day divided into 3 doses. Sedation may be limiting side effect.
- Avoid narcotics because they are unlikely to help long-term pain control and may lead to drug dependency.
- Refer patient unresponsive to pharmacologic measures to neurosurgeon skilled in selective radio frequency rhizotomy or microvascular decompression.

BIBLIOGRAPHY

- For the current annotated bibliography on trigeminal neuralgia (tic douloureux), see the print edition of *Primary Care Medicine*, 4th edition, Chapter 176, or www.LWWmedicine.com.

Dermatologic Problems

Acne

MANAGEMENT

- Patient ed is essential in acne Rx to enlist patient understanding and cooperation.
- Eliminate acnegenic drugs, such as steroids or androgens, exposure to oils, and habits such as face rubbing.
- For obstructive acne, use retinoic acid (tretinoin) cream or gel, 0.025% or 0.05% qhs.
- Recommend sunscreen use with tretinoin, which causes increased sun sensitivity.
- If papules or pustules are present, prescribe topical erythromycin or clindamycin (as lotion, solution, or gel) or topical benzoyl peroxide.
- If partial but insufficient response to single topical agent, consider combination topical Rx with erythromycin or clindamycin + benzoyl peroxide [e.g., combination preparation erythromycin/benzoyl peroxide (Benzamycin)].
- In more severe inflammatory acne, prescribe systemic antibiotic (e.g., tetracycline, doxycycline, minocycline, or erythromycin).
- Start with full dose and reduce to maintenance after acne is under control. Advise patient to take doxycycline with adequate amount of liquid because it can cause esophagitis if taken with only small sips.
- For severe nodulocystic acne resistant to conventional Rx, consider systemic 13-*cis*-retinoic acid, with full awareness of its risks, especially teratogenesis, and requirement for appropriate monitoring.

BIBLIOGRAPHY

- For the current annotated bibliography on acne, see the print edition of *Primary Care Medicine*, 4th edition, Chapter 185, or www.LWWmedicine.com.

Aphthous Stomatitis

DIFFERENTIAL DIAGNOSIS

- Pemphigus
- Herpes simplex
- Behçet's syndrome
- Hand-foot-and-mouth disease

MANAGEMENT

- Reassure patient that lesions will heal spontaneously and do not represent more serious pathology.
- For patients with large lesions and those bothered by discomfort, consider additional measures.
- For extremely painful lesions, use topical anesthetic agent (e.g., viscous lidocaine, ac) to allow eating.
- Recommend avoiding abrasive foods.
- Consider tetracycline liquid used as mouthwash (250 mg qid, held in mouth for several mins).
- Consider topical Rx: topical corticosteroid paste (e.g., Orabase) applied to mucous membrane, carbamide peroxide gel, or topical use of sucralfate liquid.
- For women with definite premenstrual flare, consider estrogen-dominated oral contraceptive.
- Identify and correct any existing folate, vitamin B_{12}, or iron deficiencies.
- For lesions precipitated by emotional stress, attend to underlying stress (see Anxiety).
- Reserve chemical cauterization with silver nitrate sticks for exceptional situations (risk of destroying normal tissue).
- Recommend avoiding mucosal trauma (foods with sharp surfaces, salt, and talking while chewing) and maintaining good nutrition and oral hygiene (soft-bristled toothbrush).
- Prescribe vitamin supplement for patients with dietary vitamin or mineral deficiency.

BIBLIOGRAPHY

- For the current annotated bibliography on aphthous stomatitis, see the print edition of *Primary Care Medicine*, 4th edition, Chapter 224, or www.LWWmedicine.com.

Bites (Animal and Human)

MANAGEMENT

OVERALL APPROACH

- Clean wounds vigorously with soap and water.
- Copiously irrigate with normal saline solution. Use syringe with needle to generate high-pressure jet to cleanse puncture wounds.
- Immunize with 0.5 mL IM tetanus toxoid if previously immunized but no booster in past 5–10 yrs.

ANIMAL BITES

- Clean thoroughly and follow expectantly if puncture wound trivial and clean, without crush injury, and not involving hand.
- Treat moderate or severe fresh, uninfected animal tear wounds with cleansing, débridement, and phenoxymethyl penicillin (250 mg qid), followed by secondary closure in 24–48 hrs if no signs of infection.
- Treat infected animal bite wounds with débridement, drainage, and cleansing. Culture wound, delay wound closure until infection subsides, and begin penicillin (500 mg qid).
- Add penicillinase-resistant penicillin (e.g., 500 mg dicloxacillin qid) if erythema appears to be spreading or if *S. aureus* suspected.
- For infected cat bites, use amoxicillin/clavulanic acid (875/125 mg bid) as single agent, or cefuroxime (500 mg bid).
- If patient is allergic to penicillin, use doxycycline (100 mg bid) for initial antibiotic Rx.
- Treat for 7–10 days for uncomplicated cellulitis.

HUMAN BITES

- Treat initially with penicillin and penicillinase-resistant agent (e.g., dicloxacillin). Delay wound closure.
- Elevate affected limb until swelling declines, usually after 3–5 days.
- Immobilize clenched-fist injuries and obtain hand surgery consultation promptly.
- Instruct patient to watch for signs of infection, such as pain, redness, warmth, swelling, or purulent exudate.

BIBLIOGRAPHY

- For the current annotated bibliography on animal and human bites, see the print edition of *Primary Care Medicine*, 4th edition, Chapter 196, or www.LWWmedicine.com.

Cellulitis

WORKUP

OVERALL STRATEGY

- First rule out other causes of focal erythema, swelling, and tenderness (superficial thrombophlebitis, arterial insufficiency, and erythema nodosum).
- Then examine for precipitating factors.
- Remember also that cellulitis can also exist concurrently with any one of these conditions.

HISTORY

- Note any Hx of phlebitis, varicose veins, claudication, or pretibial nodularity.
- Review Hx for predisposing factors for cellulitis (e.g., DM, heart failure, recent trauma, leg edema, vascular insufficiency, leg ulcers, previous infection, tinea pedis, and loss of sensation).
- Also ask about IV drug use, occupational exposure, and any recent bites and stings.
- Note any report of fever with rigors, suggesting bacteremia.

PHYSICAL EXAM

- Check for superficial thrombophlebitis by examining for inflammatory response centered about a superficial vein, causing it to be enlarged and focally tender.
- Examine for dependent rubor of arterial insufficiency, which is generalized, nontender, and associated with diminished or absent pulses and cold extremity.
- Look for characteristic findings of erythema nodosum (multiple, exquisitely tender nodules often located pretibially).
- Once cellulitis confirmed, check for signs of predisposing factors (e.g., skin atrophy or ulceration, leg edema, poor pulses, trauma, tinea pedis, and loss of sensation.
- Note temp, area(s) of skin involved, lymphangitic streaking, proximal lymphadenopathy, and any skin breaks, ulceration, or atrophy.
- Mark borders of lesion with indelible pen to allow objective and rapid assessment of progression and resolution.
- Check for crepitus and foul odor suggesting anaerobic infection.
- Palpate for fluctuance and inspect viability of surrounding tissue.

LAB STUDIES

- Obtain CBC and differential to help gauge severity of infection and hematologic response.
- Omit routine culturing of area, because most cases of cellulitis are caused by streptococci or staphylococci.

- Do culture skin in setting of open weeping wounds or infection in unusual areas, such as perineum.
- Order material from such areas to be cultured anaerobically and aerobically.
- When rigors, fever, heart murmur, or lymphangitic spread present or patient is immunocompromised, obtain 2 separate sets of blood cultures before administering antibiotics.
- If crepitus, fluctuance, or devitalization present, obtain x-ray to look for gas production in soft tissue, indicative of gangrene. In diabetic or immunocompromised patients, or in situations of previous injury, radiography is important check for osteomyelitis beneath cellulitis.

MANAGEMENT

- Promptly hospitalize any patient unable to be cared for at home and also anyone with high fever, rigors, lymphangitis, rapid progression, compromised host defenses, or involvement of face, orbit, or perineum.
- Treat patient with mild, uncomplicated illness on ambulatory basis, beginning with phenoxymethyl penicillin (500 mg PO qid, 1 hr ac and qhs).
- Monitor closely during next 48 hrs.
- If inflammation and fever do not begin to resolve after 48 hrs or if close monitoring is impossible, prescribe penicillinase-resistant penicillin (e.g., dicloxacillin, 500 mg PO qid).
- For patients markedly allergic to penicillin (type I hypersensitivity), prescribe erythromycin (500 mg qid).
- If allergy to penicillin is not well documented and was not anaphylactoid, consider first-generation cephalosporin, such as cephalexin, 500 mg tid. First-generation agents have good antistaph coverage.
- Reserve fluoroquinolones, such as ciprofloxacin, for gram-negative cellulitis. They have only moderate antistrep and antistaph activity in vitro; use with caution in cellulitis.
- If anaerobes suspected, use fluoroquinolone + clindamycin or metronidazole.
- Give 0.5 mL tetanus toxoid IM to patients with open wound but without tetanus booster in past 10 yrs.

BIBLIOGRAPHY

- For the current annotated bibliography on cellulitis, see the print edition of *Primary Care Medicine*, 4th edition, Chapter 190, or www.LWWmedicine.com.

Corns and Calluses

MANAGEMENT

- Advise patient to avoid tight shoes with pointed toes, to wear shoes that fit properly, and to change them frequently. Socks should cushion sensitive area.
- Patient may treat corns and calluses with proprietary plasters. PCP or patient can apply keratolytic agent to lesion in form of 40% salicylic acid plaster for several days. After lesion has improved, use of circular pads may prevent recurrence.
- Consider paring down large lesion. Patients can perform procedure themselves, but instruct them never to pull loose skin. Protect tender area with moleskin after paring.
- After lesions have been removed or pared down, ensure that foot is not subjected to same pressures that produced problem.
- Refer patients with refractory lesions and lesions caused by underlying orthopedic disease to podiatrist or orthopedist for definitive Rx of structural problem. Molded shoe insert device may be prescribed. Patients with DM and others with insufficient vascular supply to foot should receive regular foot care from podiatrist.

BIBLIOGRAPHY

- For the current annotated bibliography on corns and calluses, see the print edition of *Primary Care Medicine*, 4th edition, Chapter 189, or www.LWWmedicine.com.

Dermatitis (Atopic or Contact)

MANAGEMENT

- Identify and remove potential contacts, allergens, and irritants. Treat any skin dryness (see Dry Skin). Using rubber gloves with cotton linings may be beneficial.
- Dry oozing lesions with Burow's solution compresses bid–qid for 10–30 mins, depending on degree of vesiculation; colloidal oatmeal baths indicated for more generalized lesions.
- Suppress pruritus if possible with topical antipruritic (e.g., Pramosone ointment) or systemic antihistamine (see Pruritus).
- For acute dermatitis, begin with fluorinated corticosteroid cream. Start with highest potency necessary and reduce as soon as acute inflammation is controlled.
- If acute process is extensive and severe, begin oral prednisone, 1 mg/kg/day, and taper rapidly to full cessation within 10–14 days. Alternatively, give IM corticosteroid injections as triamcinolone acetonide (40 mg/mL).
- For chronic lichenified eruptions, treat for prolonged periods with ointment formulations or, if unresponsive, steroid cream under occlusion. In refractory cases, intralesional injection of diluted triamcinolone solution (2–3 mg/mL) by experienced physician may be effective.
- Refer patients with refractory hand dermatitis to dermatologist.

BIBLIOGRAPHY

- For the current annotated bibliography on atopic or contact dermatitis, see the print edition of *Primary Care Medicine*, 4th edition, Chapter 184, or www.LWWmedicine.com.

Dermatitis (Seborrheic)

MANAGEMENT

- Provide patient with list of OTC shampoos and suggest selecting one that meets personal preferences.
- For oily hair, advise daily shampooing for first wk; patient can sometimes decrease to 2–3 times/wk for maintenance.
- For resistant cases, prescribe use of ketoconazole shampoo qod.
- For mild to moderate facial or chest involvement, consider 2% ketoconazole cream applied to affected areas bid until clearing.
- Recommend maintenance Rx 1–2 times/wk indefinitely if necessary.
- If erythema present, prescribe topical nonfluorinated corticosteroid preparation (e.g., 1% or 2.5% hydrocortisone cream) for face; fluorinated lotion is appropriate for scalp (e.g., 0.1% betamethasone valerate lotion).
- Remove heavy crusts by softening with keratolytic lotions or oil-based agents before shampooing.
- Treat exudative intertriginous lesions with drying and nonfluorinated topical steroid lotion.
- Treat blepharitis hygienically by gentle rubbing of eyelashes with washcloth and No More Tears shampoo. Occasionally, patient can use steroid-containing eye ointment, such as Metimyd or Blephamide solution, taking care to avoid prolonged use.

BIBLIOGRAPHY

- For the current annotated bibliography on seborrheic dermatitis, see the print edition of *Primary Care Medicine*, 4th edition, Chapter 184, or www.LWWmedicine.com.

MANAGEMENT

- Instruct patient about environmental modifications to increase ambient humidity. Keep room temperature as low as is comfortable.
- Caution patients to avoid dehydrating soaps, solvents, or disinfectants. They should not scrub skin.
- Encourage use of bath oils and well-oiled soaps. Patient should soak in tub for 1–10 mins before adding bath oil. Warn patient that bath oil may make tub slippery.
- Use emollients after showering or bathing. Try several agents, beginning with cheapest, to find acceptable one. Newer emollients with esterified alcohols or emulsifiers are most cosmetically acceptable but also most costly.
- Lotions or creams that contain 2–20% urea or 5–12% ammonium lactate help hold water in stratum corneum and may increase skin plasticity.
- In presence of eczematous change or for patient who insists on rapid resolution, use topical corticosteroid ointments ± occlusion.
- Most important aspect of management is patient ed. Reinforce use of measures that prevent dryness.

BIBLIOGRAPHY

- For the current annotated bibliography on dry skin, see the print edition of *Primary Care Medicine*, 4th edition, Chapter 183, or www.LWWmedicine.com.

Excessive Sweating

DIFFERENTIAL DIAGNOSIS

- Normal physiologic response
  - Menopause
  - Fever
  - Infectious disease
  - Malignancy (night sweats)
  - Central neurologic injury
  - Peripheral autonomic neuropathy
  - Thyrotoxicosis
  - Pheochromocytoma (rare)
  - Parkinson's disease
  - Drugs
    - Antipyretics
    - Insulin
    - Meperidine
    - Emetics
    - Alcohol
    - Pilocarpine
- Gustatory
  - Diabetic neuropathy
  - Damage to seventh cranial nerve
  - Frey's syndrome (rare)
  - Injury to sympathetic trunk after surgery

WORKUP

HISTORY

- Determine whether excess sweating is restricted to axillae, palms, and soles (indicative of normal response to everyday events) or more generalized (underlying medical condition).
- Ask whether excess sweating began recently and can be correlated with stress.
- If sweating occurs primarily at night, inquire about fever, fatigue, adenopathy, cough, sputum production, and other symptoms of infection and malignancy (see Fever).
- If generalized sweating, ask about hyperthyroidism (see Hyperthyroidism) and menopause (see Menopause). Paroxysms of sweating suggest panic disorder (see Anxiety) and pheochromocytoma (see Hypertension).
- Obtain drug Hx, checking for use of antipyretics, insulin, meperidine, emetics, alcohol, and pilocarpine.

PHYSICAL EXAM

- Note degree and location of sweating. If Hx of fever or generalized night sweats, examine for underlying infection and cancer (see Fever). Examine for signs of hyperthyroidism (see Hyperthyroidism).

- Note any increases in BP because elevated BP in setting of paroxysmal flushing and sweating suggests pheochromocytoma.
- Perform neurologic exam in patients with suspected CNS disease or peripheral autonomic neuropathy.

LAB STUDIES

- No lab studies are mandatory. Base test selection on Hx and PE findings. Screening "panscan" is of little use and likely to generate false-positive results.

MANAGEMENT

- Reassure patient that excess sweating is not consequence of pathologic condition once you have ruled out medical causes.
- For axillary sweating, recommend frequent washing and changes of clothing.
- For excess sweating of palms or axillae, recommend 20% alcoholic solution of aluminum chloride hexahydrate (Drysol). Effective alternative is 6.25% aluminum tetrachloride (Xerac AC) applied qhs and covered with plastic food wrap; patient can wear polyethylene or vinyl gloves if palms are affected.
- Recommend patient wash treated areas qam with soap and water.
- Prescribe 1–3 consecutive treatments/wk. Once dryness occurs, maintenance with 1 Rx/wk should suffice.
- Consider electrical current to block sweat glands temporarily. Use of device (Drionic) daily for 1 wk may relieve sweating for up to 1 mo.
- Consider intradermal injection of botulinum toxin, which is gaining in popularity and is relatively noninvasive.
- Consider as extreme measure liposuction techniques if all else fails in obese patient and problem is compromising health.
- If topical Rx, reassurance, and less invasive approaches fail, consider sympathectomy performed via thoracoscope, but only if hyperhidrosis is truly incapacitating. Refer to neurosurgeon or vascular surgeon for evaluation.

BIBLIOGRAPHY

- For the current annotated bibliography on excessive sweating, see the print edition of *Primary Care Medicine*, 4th edition, Chapter 183, or www.LWWmedicine.com.

Fungal Infections

DIFFERENTIAL DIAGNOSIS

- Intertrigo
- Erythrasma

WORKUP

- Check for scaly, erythematous lesions with defined margins in damp, dark areas (groin, axilla, inframammary region).
- In intertriginous areas, differentiate from intertrigo (slight maceration and erythema) and erythrasma (asymptomatic, slightly erythematous to light brown, finely scaling patches with little or no central clearing).
- When dermatophyte infection suspected, obtain scraping from involved area and perform microscopic exam.
- To prep specimen for microscopic exam, scrape lesion border lightly with No. 15 scalpel blade or edge of microscope slide.
- Collect scale onto clean microscope slide and push all scale into small mound.
- Place 1 or, at most, 2 drops of 20% potassium hydroxide ± DMSO in center of mound and lay coverslip over it.
- Heat slide gently if solution does not contain DMSO.
- Under 40× magnification, examine for threadlike hyphae and any budding spores and pseudohyphae (*Candida*).
- Confirm by using higher power (100×) to ensure that artifacts are not mistaken for hyphae.
- Consider culturing scraping by planting on Sabouraud's dextrose agar.
- If candidal infection is identified or topical fungal infection is recurrent or extensive, check for underlying HIV infection, DM, cirrhosis, lymphoma, steroid use, and chemotherapy.

MANAGEMENT

- Prescribe topical antifungal preparation approved for qd use (e.g., clotrimazole). This is cost-effective and likely to improve patient compliance.
- For intertriginous areas, prescribe lotion or solution preparation; creams can increase risk of skin maceration.
- If clearing is incomplete after 2–3 wks, consider short-term systemic antifungal use, but only after weighing benefits against risk of adverse drug effects.
- Similarly, for patients with onychomycosis, weigh expense of systemic agents and potential for serious adverse effects (especially hepatic) against cosmetic consequences of living with untreated condition.

BIBLIOGRAPHY

■ For the current annotated bibliography on fungal infections, see the print edition of *Primary Care Medicine*, 4th edition, Chapter 191, or www.LWWmedicine.com.

Hair Loss

DIFFERENTIAL DIAGNOSIS

- Nonscarring alopecia
  - Androgenic
    - Male pattern
    - Female pattern
  - Alopecia areata
  - Post febrile infection
  - Folliculitis (mild)
  - Tinea capitis (ectothrix)
  - Hypothyroidism
  - Iron deficiency
  - Systemic lupus erythematosus (SLE)
  - Syphilis
  - Medications
    - Antineoplastics
    - Antimetabolites
    - Antidepressants
    - Anticonvulsants
    - Anticoagulants
    - Allopurinol, probenecid
    - Beta blockers
    - Quinine
    - High-dose vitamin A, isotretinoin
    - Oral contraceptives
  - Discontinuation of corticosteroids
  - Trichotillomania
  - Telogen effluvium
  - Crash diets
  - Post pregnancy
- Scarring alopecia
  - Physical trauma
    - Burns
    - Radiation
    - Chronic traction
  - Infection
  - Bacterial folliculitis (severe)
  - Fungal (endothrix)
  - Discoid lupus erythematosus
  - Morphea
  - Lichen planopilaris
  - Pseudopelade
  - Neoplasms
  - Granulomatous disease
  - Factitial

WORKUP

HISTORY

- Identify nature of problem: is it specific area of hair loss or generalized hair loss?
- Inquire into symptoms of precipitating illness, such as hypothyroidism, SLE, granulomatous disease, iron deficiency, or febrile infection.
- Note any Hx of physical trauma (e.g., pulling hair or use of curlers, bleaches, permanent wave lotions, straightening lotions, hot combs).
- Review family Hx for male or female pattern baldness.
- Check medication Hx for antimetabolites, anticonvulsants, anticoagulants, beta blockers, colchicine, antithyroid drugs, androgens, oral contraceptives, lithium, and excessive amounts of isotretinoin (Accutane) and vitamin A.
- Note recent pregnancy, strenuous dieting, and presence of skin conditions such as folliculitis and tinea.
- Quantify and confirm hair loss by having patient collect hairs lost each day in separate envelopes and count total (<100 hairs/day WNL).

PHYSICAL EXAM

- Check pattern of hair loss (localized or diffuse) and androgenetic pattern.
- Examine scalp for areas of reduced hair growth, hair loss, and scarring; differentiate scarring from nonscarring alopecia.
- If necessary, differentiate perceived from actual loss by performing "pluck" or "pull" test (25–30 hairs grasped and extracted from scalp by hand or with instrument such as hemostat); finding <5 telogen hairs (has terminal club on hair shaft) is normal.
- Note presence of short, broken hairs (pulling).
- Observe surrounding areas for evidence of inflammation, cellulitis, folliculitis, and fungal infection.
- If available, use Wood's light to demonstrate fungal infection.
- Scrape any inflamed area for microscopic exam (see Fungal Infections) and culture.
- If circular areas characteristic of alopecia areata noted, apply light traction to hairs at edge of bald area; if hairs come out with ease, extension of alopecic area is likely.
- Check for signs of systemic illness (hypothyroidism, SLE, iron deficiency, sarcoidosis).
- In woman with male pattern hair loss, examine for hirsutism and virilization.
- Examine nails for Beau's lines (suggestive of systemic process affecting nail and hair growth).

LAB STUDIES

- Consider skin biopsy, particularly in cases of scarring alopecia with suspected inflammation.
- If systemic disease suspected clinically, test accordingly (e.g., CBC; serum iron, ferritin, TIBC, TSH, T4, ANA, testosterone, and other androgenic hormone levels).

MANAGEMENT

OVERALL APPROACH

- Reassure patient with harmless etiology (e.g., women with hair loss after pregnancy) or unsubstantiated loss.
- Discontinue if possible any drugs associated with hair loss and seek alternatives.
- Treat etiologically [e.g., scalp infection (see Cellulitis; Fungal Infections; Pyoderma), underlying systemic conditions].
- Advise that hair loss associated with chemotherapy is usually self-limited and best managed by wearing wig or scarf [see Cancer (General)].

SYMPTOMATIC MEASURES

Alopecia Areata

- Reassure that condition is likely self-limited and that watchful waiting is safest and most cost-effective approach.
- If severe and psychologically troubling, refer to dermatologist for consideration of
  - phenol or UV light Rx (irritant stimulus);
  - superpotent topical fluorinated corticosteroid under occlusion;
  - scalp injection of triamcinolone acetonide, if topical Rx fails; prepared as dilute solution for injection (5 mg/mL) to minimize risk of dermal atrophy; small volumes used; multiple injections necessary;
  - systemic corticosteroids, but only after weighing cosmetic benefits against long-term risks;
  - anthralin, applied qhs and removed qam;
  - psoralen + UVA light Rx.

Male Pattern Baldness

- Consider finasteride (Propecia) if patient prepared for small risk of side effects (loss of libido, erectile dysfunction, or decrease in ejaculatory volume occurring in about 2%) in return for 50% likelihood of noticeable improvement.
- Consider full-strength (5%) topical minoxidil (Rogaine) for younger men (aged <40) who have been bald for <10 yrs and have balding area on vertex, diameter <4 in.; note that 6 mos daily minoxidil Rx may be necessary before hair growth becomes apparent, and new hair persists only as long as bid applications continue; relapse occurs in 2–6 mos.
- Suggest use of finasteride and topical minoxidil for enhanced results in those willing to bear cost, inconvenience, and possible side effects.
- Consider spironolactone and dexamethasone for symptomatic Rx of male pattern hair loss in women with associated hirsutism due to androgen excess (see Hirsutism); begin spironolactone (75–200 mg/day × 6 mos); if unsuccessful consider dexamethasone (0.125–0.250 mg qhs × 6 mos); treat underlying condition etiologically.

Female Pattern Hair Loss

- Reassure that male pattern hair loss will not ensue.
- Consider low-strength (2%) minoxidil; warn that there may be short-term increased hair loss, but new hair growth expected within 12 mos.

- Advise women not to use 5% minoxidil because facial hirsutism may develop.
- Warn women of childbearing age not to take finasteride, and pregnant women not even to handle crushed or broken tablets (risk of congenital genitourinary abnormalities in male offspring).

PATIENT EDUCATION

- Review prognosis and reassure when Dx is self-limited or harmless condition.
- Help patient come to terms with hair loss.
- Provide advice on hair care; recommend:
  - avoiding alkaline pH shampoos and excessive toweling after hair washing;
  - using conditioner and combing instead of brushing;
  - disentangling hair from brush gently and use of brush with natural bristles or nylon brush with rounded edges;
  - avoiding bleaching, permanent waving, straightening, hot combs, and excessive sun exposure.
- Advise that weaving is relatively safe and successful procedure, but must be repeated periodically (expensive and a nuisance).
- Advise that hair transplants are painful, expensive, and have varying rate of success; best candidates have coarse, dark hair.
- Discourage implants of artificial hair (elicit chronic foreign body reaction).

INDICATIONS FOR REFERRAL

- Consider dermatologic referral for further evaluation when Dx unclear and for performance of clip test and telogen counts when perceived hair loss cannot be confirmed clinically.
- Refer for symptomatic Rx of psychologically disabling alopecia areata.
- Obtain endocrinologic consultation when there is concern about hirsutism due to androgen excess.

BIBLIOGRAPHY

- For the current annotated bibliography on hair loss, see the print edition of *Primary Care Medicine*, 4th edition, Chapter 182, or www.LWWmedicine.com.

Herpes Simplex

DIFFERENTIAL DIAGNOSIS

- Genital ulcer (+ adenopathy)
  - Genital herpes simplex virus (HSV-II)
  - Syphilis
  - Chancroid
- Genital ulcer (− adenopathy)
  - Causes of genital ulceration with adenopathy
  - Behçet's syndrome
  - Inflammatory bowel disease
  - Excoriation
  - Secondary bacterial infection

WORKUP

OVERALL STRATEGY

- Attempt to make initial Dx of HSV infection on basis of Hx and characteristic lesions on PE.
- Reserve lab testing for atypical disease, and include testing for syphilis when considering genital lesions.

HISTORY

- Obtain detailed sexual Hx including inquiry about oral-genital sexual activity.
- Review Hx for genital redness, spotting, fissures, pain, and paresthesias, even in absence of skin lesions (raises suspicion of genital herpes).
- Note any Hx of fever blisters or cold sores, because it indicates prior HSV infection and helps identify patients with first episode of nonprimary disease.

PHYSICAL EXAM

- Look for characteristic "dew-drop-on-a-rose-petal" lesions of HSV infection.
- Differentiate lesions of HSV infection (very tender with clean base and tender, nonfluctuant inguinal adenopathy) from other causes of genital ulcer with adenopathy:
  - Primary syphilis: nontender ulcer (chancre); indurated and painless or minimally uncomfortable; clean base and nonfluctuant inguinal adenopathy.
  - Chancroid: very tender, soft, purulent ulcerations in conjunction with sore, fluctuant lymph nodes and erythema of overlying skin.

LAB STUDIES

- If lesion is atypical, unroof vesicle and perform Tzanck prep (see Herpes Zoster); useful for quick Dx (multinucleated giant cells), but less specific than viral culture (most sensitive of commonly available tests).

- Culture for HSV within 48 hrs of onset of symptoms; highest-yielding lesions are intact vesicles, pustules, and early moist ulcers.
- Consider PCR testing for HSV identification; identifies viral genetic material; most sensitive and specific means to Dx active disease; cost is high; far better than testing for HSV antigen by direct fluorescent antibody testing (limited sensitivity; false-negative rates high when used in populations with low prevalence of HSV infection).
- Consider use of HSV serology to confirm prior infection, but in most instances such testing less useful to evaluate ongoing episode because titers often rise insufficiently, and cross-reactivity between HSV-1 and HSV-2 occurs. HSV serology by Western blot assay promises sensitive and type-specific antibody testing but is not yet widely available.
- Reserve antibody testing for persons at increased risk for primary infection (i.e., pregnant women with no prior exposure or prior antibody titers).
- Be aware that most commercial labs are presently unable to provide reliable type-specific antibody testing. Also, serology has disadvantage of not producing data while patient is clinically affected, and once exposed, patients carry titers forever, whether or not infection becomes reactivated.
- Differentiate benign inflammatory cervical abnormality of HSV infection from real metaplastic or anaplastic disease when performing PAP smear (see Cervical Cancer). Genital herpes is major cause of types II and III abnormalities on Pap smear.

MANAGEMENT

PRIMARY INFECTION AND NONPRIMARY INITIAL GENITAL DISEASE

- Begin 7- to 10-day course of oral acyclovir (200 mg 5 times/day), valacyclovir (1,000 mg bid), or famciclovir (250 mg tid).
- Then decide on need for continued Rx and titrate doses according to Rx response.
- Continue Rx until lesions have healed.
- Reduce dose for patients with renal failure.
- Provide supply for use during recurrences, which are likely in first yr after initial infection.

RECURRENT DISEASE

- Begin Rx at first sign of illness, preferably during prodromal phase before skin lesions emerge.
- Treat symptomatic recurrences for 5 days with acyclovir (200 mg 5 times/day, or 400 mg tid), famciclovir (125 mg bid), or valacyclovir (500 mg bid).
- Consider long-term suppressive Rx for patients with >6–8 recurrences/yr, those who want to minimize risk for asymptomatic viral transmission, and immunocompromised patients.
- Prescribe for suppression acyclovir (400 mg bid), famciclovir (250 mg bid), or valacyclovir (500–1,000 mg/day).

- Titrate prophylactic dose to lowest level possible without reactivation, and continue for up to 12 mos.
- After 12 mos, halt suppressive Rx and reassess need for continuation.

ADDITIONAL MEASURES FOR ALL PATIENTS

- Teach about transmissibility of genital herpes, including risk for genital infection associated with oral-genital sexual activity and with asymptomatic viral shedding.
- Recommend condoms when 1 partner is antibody-negative.
- Help patient keep problem in perspective and address common misconceptions regarding meaning of infection.
- Watch for secondary bacterial infection and disseminated HSV disease. In immunosuppressed patients, dissemination may present as gangrenous ulcers or deep-seated eschars.
- Follow genital infections closely during pregnancy; consider monitoring antibody status in latter part of pregnancy to determine susceptibility to primary infection and need for extra precautions or use of suppressive Rx in infected male partner.

BIBLIOGRAPHY

- For the current annotated bibliography on herpes simplex, see the print edition of *Primary Care Medicine*, 4th edition, Chapter 192, or www.LWWmedicine.com.

Herpes Zoster

WORKUP

HISTORY

- Check Hx for characteristic herpetic rash ("dew drop on rose petal") in dermatomal distribution and any pain in similar distribution.
- Note any report of fever, malaise, or adenopathy.
- Consider Dx in absence of rash during prodromal phase, when patients present with periorbital headache, unexplained back pain, or chest wall pain in dermatomal distribution; expect characteristic eruption in 2–5 days.
- Review medical Hx for immunocompromising illnesses (e.g., HIV infection) or their risk factors.
- If immunocompromise suspected, check Hx for disseminated Zoster (>10 lesions outside single dermatome).

PHYSICAL EXAM

- Identify characteristic dermatomal "dew-drop-on-rose-petal" rash and accompanying pain.
- Note any spread beyond dermatomal distribution, eye or otic involvement, and meningeal signs.

LAB STUDIES

- Support clinical Dx by performing Tzanck prep; sample taken from unroofed vesicle demonstrates multinucleated giant cells; superior to viral isolation in Dx of early lesions.
- If necessary, confirm Dx by sending material for viral culture or PCR assay (detects viral genetic material); serology is least useful for Dx because it requires 2 separate determinations and demonstration of rising antibody titers.

MANAGEMENT

INITIAL SYMPTOMATIC MEASURES

- Dry vesicles, relieve pain, and treat secondary infection.
- Keep lesions clean and dry by applying wet-to-dry compress soaked with Burow's solution tid–qid.
- Use antibiotics only if purulence and worsening erythema suggests secondary infection.
- Relieve discomfort by prescribing mild analgesic such as aspirin or acetaminophen; consider narcotic analgesia (e.g., codeine or oxycodone) if pain incapacitating.
- Start antiviral Rx as soon as Dx made (preferably ≤72 hrs after rash onset).
- Prescribe nucleoside antiviral agent (e.g., acyclovir, famciclovir, valacyclovir), especially to those who present early with severe pain or ophthalmic involvement, are aged >50, or have ophthalmic involvement.

- Use high doses (e.g., acyclovir, 800 mg 5 times/day × 10 days; famciclovir, 500–750 mg tid × 7 days; or valacyclovir, 1 g tid × 7 days).
- Preferentially prescribe newer cyclovirs (more convenient, lower cost, fewer CNS side effects in the elderly compared to acyclovir).
- For painful thoracic or truncal involvement, consider wrapping affected area, first with nonadherent dressing then with elastic bandage.
- Recommend rest if there is generalized malaise and fatigue.
- Consider intralesional injections of triamcinolone (2 mg/mL) in lidocaine for severe local pain (no evidence that systemic steroids lessen acute pain).
- Treat pruritus with oral antihistamines or calamine lotion (both reduce itching and dry rash).
- Consider topical capsaicin (not very effective).

SHORTENING CLINICAL COURSE AND REDUCING RISK FOR POSTHERPETIC NEURALGIA

- Start antiviral Rx within 72 hrs of rash onset.
- Make sure that patients at high risk for postherpetic neuralgia receive early Rx (present early with severe pain, aged >50, ophthalmic involvement).
- Consider prophylactic use of systemic glucocorticosteroids with antiviral Rx, particularly in patients aged >50 with severe pain and many herpetic lesions.
- Start high-dose prednisone (60 mg qam) at same time as antiviral Rx.
- Taper over next 2–4 wks, then discontinue.
- Watch for availability of varicella vaccine (under development).
- Refer immunosuppressed patients with generalized zoster for IV Rx.

TREATMENT OF POSTHERPETIC NEURALGIA

- Begin tricyclic antidepressant (e.g., amitriptyline, start at 25 mg qhs).
- Add, or use instead, gabapentin (Neurontin, start at 300 mg tid and titrate to 3,600 mg/day).
- Consider second-line agent carbamazepine.
- Add brief course of narcotics if first-line drug insufficient.
- Consider topical capsaicin (efficacy modest; burning sensation with prolonged use).

INDICATIONS FOR REFERRAL

- Refer immediately to ophthalmology if any suggestion of visual compromise or other ocular involvement.
- Refer to ENT for any otic involvement.
- Hospitalize and promptly obtain infectious disease consultation if patient with herpetic skin lesions shows any signs of meningeal irritation or generalization of infection, especially in suspected immunocompromise.

BIBLIOGRAPHY

- For the current annotated bibliography on herpes zoster, see the print edition of *Primary Care Medicine*, 4th edition, Chapter 193, or www.LWWmedicine.com.

Intertrigo and Intertriginous Dermatoses

DIFFERENTIAL DIAGNOSIS

- Intertrigo in groin
  - Tinea cruris
  - Candidiasis
  - Condyloma
  - Herpes
  - Scabies
  - Pediculosis
  - Lichen sclerosus et atrophicus
  - Lichen simplex chronicus
- Intertrigo in axilla
  - Candidiasis
  - Tinea
  - Erythrasma
  - Contact dermatitis
  - Fox-Fordyce disease
  - Hidradenitis suppurativa
- Intertrigo of inframammary region
  - Candidal infection

MANAGEMENT

- Give priority to eliminating precipitating conditions, especially moisture and friction.
- Carefully dry skin fold areas with absorbent material: dust with drying powders and recommend loose, absorbent clothing.
- For exudative lesions, use compresses of drying agent such as Burow's solution.
- Advise avoiding irritant contactants (e.g., irritant deodorants) in axillary eruptions.
- Treat areas of mild to moderate inflammation with topical hydrocortisone (1–2.5%). For more severe cases, use medium-potency fluorinated topical corticosteroid, but limit to short periods to minimize risk of dermal atrophy.
- Treat any intertriginous bacterial or fungal infection etiologically (steroid Rx alone may worsen symptoms; see Cellulitis; Fungal Infections; Pyoderma).

BIBLIOGRAPHY

- For the current annotated bibliography on intertrigo and intertriginous dermatoses, see the print edition of *Primary Care Medicine*, 4th edition, Chapter 188, or www.LWWmedicine.com.

Minor Burns

MANAGEMENT

- For first-degree burns, immediately apply cold; continue application until area remains pain-free even when cold is withdrawn.
- If skin is broken, cleanse with mild soap and water before applying cold water or ice.
- No dressing or antibiotic indicated for first-degree burns. Use emollients such as petrolatum (Eucerin) or aloe vera if blistering does not occur after several days.
- For severe sunburn, prescribe gentle topical corticosteroid lotion for symptomatic relief. Aspirin or ibuprofen provides analgesia and limits inflammation.
- Consider brief course of systemic steroids for extensive sunburn.
- For second-degree burns, spread silver sulfadiazine (Silvadene) over involved area in thickness sufficient to prevent burn from showing through. Refrigerating sulfadiazine minimizes pain.
- Wrap area with 6–7 gauze layers for protection.
- Prescribe systemic antibiotics, usually dicloxacillin, for any secondary cellulitis. Do not use prophylactic oral antibiotics for fear of selecting out resistant gram-negative organisms.

BIBLIOGRAPHY

- For the current annotated bibliography on minor burns, see the print edition of *Primary Care Medicine*, 4th edition, Chapter 196, or www.LWWmedicine.com.

DIFFERENTIAL DIAGNOSIS

CAUSES OF PIGMENTATION DISTURBANCES

Hyperpigmentation

- Circumscribed
  - Freckle
  - Lentigines
  - Melasma (pregnancy, estrogen, oral contraceptives)
  - Postinflammatory
  - Physical trauma
- Diffuse
  - Addison's disease
  - Systemic conditions (Wilson's disease, hemochromatosis, hepatic insufficiency, biliary cirrhosis, porphyria cutanea tarda, rheumatoid arthritis, scleroderma)
  - Drugs (arsenic, antimalarials, chlorpromazine, busulfan, cyclophos-phamide, clofazimine, gold, silver, zidovudine)
  - Nutritional (pellagra, malabsorption syndromes, starvation, folic acid deficiency)
  - Malignancy (lymphomas)

Hypopigmentation

- Hereditary conditions
  - Partial albinism
  - Phenylketonuria
  - Homocysteinuria
- Vitiligo (± concurrent autoimmune disease, including pernicious anemia, Hashimoto's thyroiditis, male hypogonadism, DM)
- Dermatoses
  - Tinea versicolor
  - Pityriasis alba
  - Eczema
- Chemical exposure
  - Rubber
  - Antioxidants
  - Germicides
  - Phenols

WORKUP

LOCALIZED HYPERPIGMENTATION

- Inspect lesions and inquire about previous dermatoses, inflammatory lesions, and oral contraceptive use (melasma).
- Check for signs of dysplastic pigmented lesion (see Skin Cancer).

DIFFUSE HYPERPIGMENTATION

- Inquire into onset and possible sun exposure.
- Review Hx for exposure to agents known to produce pigmentary changes (see differential diagnosis).
- Check review of systems for weakness and postural hypotension (Addison's disease) and pruritus (hepatic dysfunction).
- Inquire into any period of severe vitamin deficiency or malnutrition.
- Examine for hyperpigmentation in palmar creases and scars (Addison's disease) and signs of malignancy, hepatic insufficiency, or malabsorption.
- Test for underlying disease if suggested clinically, and consider skin biopsy in suspected deposition of heavy metal or hemosiderosis.

HYPOPIGMENTATION

- Ascertain onset and possible exposure to bleaching agents (phenol-containing industrial cleaners such as those used in janitorial work).
- If vitiligo suspected, inquire into symptoms of related autoimmune diseases (pernicious anemia, Hashimoto's thyroiditis, DM, connective tissue disease).
- Differentiate total depigmentation of vitiligo from partial postinflammatory hypopigmentation.
- Order ophthalmoscopic exam to detect any retinal pigmentary changes.
- Examine person with suspected vitiligo for manifestations of pernicious anemia, thyroid disease, DM, and collagen vascular disease.
- Scrape hypopigmented areas and perform potassium hydroxide wet mount of scrapings for characteristic hyphae of tinea versicolor.
- Consider testing for manifestations of concurrent autoimmune disease (serum vitamin B_{12}, TSH), antithyroid antibodies, glucose, and ANA.

MANAGEMENT

HYPERPIGMENTATION

- Advise strict avoidance of sunlight.
- Consider topical bleaching with hydroquinone cream, potent corticosteroids, and retinoic acid (e.g., bleaching solution of 0.1% retinoic acid, 5% hydroquinone, and 0.1% dexamethasone in hydrophilic ointment or alcohol).
- For melasma, prescribe hydroquinone/sunscreen combination (e.g., Solaquin, Solaquin Forte) or alcoholic solution of hydroquinone (Melanex).
- Explain that pigment lightening may require months of Rx and can be undone in ≤1 day of unprotected sun exposure.

HYPOPIGMENTATION

- Review Rx options: masking with application of appropriate cosmetic, bleaching of normal skin, or repigmentation with psoralen and UVA radiation (PUVA); note that hundreds of PUVA treatments may be required.
- Refer to dermatologist experienced in using psoralen and PUVA to achieve optimal cosmetic results; titration is very important (blistering can occur).
- Provide psychological support and counseling.

BIBLIOGRAPHY

■ For the current annotated bibliography on pigmentation disturbances, see the print edition of *Primary Care Medicine*, 4th edition, Chapter 180, or www.LWWmedicine.com.

Pruritus

DIFFERENTIAL DIAGNOSIS

- Dermatologic
  - Arthropod bites and stings
  - Bullous pemphigoid
  - Dermatitis
    - Atopic dermatitis
    - Contact dermatitis (allergic and irritant)
    - Dermatitis herpetiformis
  - Dermatophytosis
  - Infestation
    - Scabies
    - Pediculosis
  - Lichen planus
  - Lichen simplex chronicus
  - Pityriasis rosea
  - Psoriasis
  - Urticaria and dermatographism
    - Varicella
    - Xerosis
- Psychological
  - Neurotic excoriations
  - Depression
  - Delusions of parasitosis
- Systemic
  - HIV infection
  - Hyperthyroidism
  - Renal failure, chronic
  - Drug reaction
  - Hematologic disease
    - Iron deficiency anemia
    - Mycosis fungoides
    - Polycythemia vera
    - Paraproteinemia
  - Systemic mastocytosis
  - Hepatobiliary problems
    - Intrahepatic cholestasis
    - Extrahepatic obstruction
    - Third trimester of pregnancy
  - Malignancy
    - Malignant carcinoid
    - Lymphoma, leukemia
    - Multiple myeloma
  - Parasitosis
    - Ascariasis
    - Hookworm
    - Onchocerciasis
    - Trichinosis

WORKUP

OVERALL APPROACH

- Search first for primary dermatologic disease or scabies infestation.
- When no evidence for these, perform more detailed Hx and PE supplemented by selected lab studies.

HISTORY

- Elicit location, associated symptoms, precipitants, clinical course, and severity (including effect on sleep and daily activity).
- Include detailed description of any skin changes or rashes.
- Check for Hx of atopy, asthma, or urticaria.
- Note any concurrent pruritus in household members (scabies) and worsening in winter (dry skin).
- Review environmental factors such as sunburn, prickly heat, cats in household, exposure to fiberglass, and excessive drying.
- Review all medications (subclinical allergic reaction), including those that can intrinsically cause itching (e.g., opiates, amphetamines, quinidine, aspirin, B vitamins, and niacin).
- In setting of generalized pruritus, check for symptoms, risk factors, and Hx of hyperthyroidism, renal failure, lymphoma, polycythemia, cholestatic liver disease, and HIV infection.
- Suspect pregnancy as cause if patient is woman in third trimester.
- If cause is not evident from medical Hx, explore relation between psychological or situational stresses and onset of pruritus; note any depression.

PHYSICAL EXAM

- Carefully inspect skin, noting presence and distribution of any rash, excoriations, lichenification, inflammatory changes, and xerosis (scaling and dryness, especially evident on legs and revealed best by tangential lighting).
- If localized, check area in more detail:
  - Scalp: psoriasis and seborrhea
  - Trunk: urticaria, scabies, contact dermatitis
  - Inguinal area: *Candida* infection, pediculosis, tinea, scabies
  - Hands: eczema, contact dermatitis, scabies
  - Legs: neurotic excoriations, stasis dermatitis, atopic dermatitis (popliteal fossa), lichen simplex (lateral malleoli), dermatitis herpetiformis (knees)
  - Feet: tinea, contact dermatitis
- If generalized and no evidence of primary dermatologic disease, check for jaundice, rash of HIV infection (see HIV-1 Infection), scleral icterus, lymphadenopathy, goiter, and organomegaly.

LAB STUDIES

- Test selectively and avoid "panscan" (wasteful, false-positives).
- Perform skin scraping to confirm clinical Dx of scabies or dermatophytosis (see Fungal Infections; Scabies and Pediculosis).
- Order serum bilirubin, alkaline phosphatase, and transaminase levels + abdominal ultrasound of biliary tree in suspected cholestasis.
- Proceed to CXR and CT if concerned about lymphoma or carcinoid.

- Obtain HIV antibody testing if Hx suggestive.
- If Dx remains elusive, check CBC, BUN, TSH, calcium, albumin, and globulin levels.
- Pruritus *per se* is not predictor of malignancy; do not initiate workup for occult malignancy in absence of other clinical evidence for cancer.
- Obtain dermatologic referral and consideration of skin biopsy if pruritus defies Dx; skin biopsy exam should include special stains or direct immunofluorescence for mastocytosis, mycosis fungoides, or autoimmune bullous disease.

MANAGEMENT

OVERALL APPROACH

- Treat etiologically for greatest efficacy.
- Treat symptomatically when etiology is irreversible or not yet established, especially if itching is disturbing sleep and interfering with daily life.
- Teach avoidance of provocative factors and how to overcome itch-scratch-itch cycle.
- Provide advice regarding nonspecific behavioral, topical, and systemic measures.

NONSPECIFIC BEHAVIORAL AND TOPICAL MEASURES

- Trim fingernails and keep them clean; rub with palms rather than scratching.
- Minimize use of coffee, spices, or alcohol if they precipitate itching.
- Change 1 sheet at a time (reduces static electricity).
- Avoid rough clothing, particularly wool; prefer cotton clothing that has been doubly rinsed of detergents.
- Humidify indoor environment.
- Avoid frequent or prolonged showering; do not use hot water (increases cutaneous blood flow).
- Use mild soaps (Dove, Basis, Neutrogena, Purpose, Aveeno Bar) rather than drying antiperspirant products.
- Sponge skin with cool water and use moisturizers before bedtime.
- Encourage use of simple emollient preparations (Moisturel, Eucerin, Lubriderm, Aveeno lotion), especially after bathing; add Alpha Keri or other lubricating agents to rinse cycle when sheets are washed.
- Consider preparations containing menthol, phenol, and camphor (e.g., Sarna lotion) applied several times daily to provide symptomatic relief.
- Reserve calamine lotion for weeping lesions (can be drying).
- Consider pramoxine-containing products (PrameGel, Prax, Pramosone), but avoid other topical anesthetics and antihistamines (potent sensitizers).
- Consider hydrocortisone cream, lotion, or ointment, but restrict use of higher-potency corticosteroids to specific steroid-responsive dermatoses (dermal atrophy).

NONSPECIFIC SYSTEMIC MEASURES

- Consider H_1 blocker for allergen-mediated itch; especially useful at nighttime (e.g., hydroxyzine, 25 mg tid or 50 mg qhs); of little benefit for nonallergen itch except for sedation.

- If sedation undesirable, prescribe cetirizine (Zyrtec, 5–10 mg/day).
- Consider antiinflammatory Rx with *aspirin* if suspected mechanism is kinin- or prostaglandin-mediated; avoid systemic steroids unless treating etiologically.

SPECIFIC SYMPTOMATIC MEASURES

Hepatobiliary Disease

- Identify and relieve any extrahepatic obstruction.
- For intrahepatic cholestasis, including pruritus of pregnancy, prescribe cholestyramine and colestipol.
- Consider ursodeoxycholic acid in persons with primary biliary cirrhosis for intense and refractory pruritus.
- Refer for consideration of UV Rx [UVB, psoralen with UVA (PUVA)] if all else fails.

Psychiatric Illness

- Begin benzodiazepine for acute anxiety-related pruritus (e.g., diazepam, 2–5 mg qhs × 2–5 days), especially if accompanied by difficulty sleeping, but avoid long-term use.
- Begin antidepressant Rx if concurrent depression; consider starting with qhs dose of doxepin (sedating and antihistaminic; see Depression).
- For psychotic delusions of parasitosis, consider neuroleptic such as pimozide.
- Consider mental health referral when pruritus represents somatic response to psychological distress.

Human Immunodeficiency Virus Infection

- Treat with antiretroviral Rx (see HIV-1 Infection).
- Also treat etiologically if complicated by scabies (see Scabies and Pediculosis), dry skin (see above), psoriasis flare (see Psoriasis), sulfa allergy associated with TMP-SMX prophylaxis, staphylococcal folliculitis, or liver failure (see HIV infection).

Renal Failure

- Treat etiologically if possible.
- Give trials of topical capsaicin and PO cimetidine.
- Consider opiate antagonist naloxone (see Renal Failure).
- For recalcitrant uremic pruritus, refer for consideration of UV photochemotherapy, IV xylocaine, activated charcoal, IV erythropoietin, exchange transfusion, and parathyroidectomy.

BIBLIOGRAPHY

- For the current annotated bibliography on pruritus, see the print edition of *Primary Care Medicine*, 4th edition, Chapter 178, or www.LWWmedicine.com.

Psoriasis

MANAGEMENT

- Treat localized, mild to moderate disease topically.
- Emphasize importance of keeping skin well hydrated and avoiding sunburn and other skin injuries.
- Allow cautious sun exposure, but advise avoiding sunburn, and do not recommend sun exposure for those with increased skin cancer risk (fair skin, easily burned, Hx of skin irradiation).
- Review medications for potential exacerbating drugs (lithium, beta blockers, NSAIDs); reduce dose or substitute if possible.
- Consider topical steroid program for control of visible lesions.
- Begin with "superpotent" preparation [e.g., betamethasone (Diprolene), diflorasone (Psorcon), clobetasol (Temovate), halobetasol (Ultravate)].
- Prescribe ointment preparation for lesions with considerable scale, although cream may be more acceptable for daytime use and suffice for plaques with minimal scale.
- Use twice-daily regimen of steroid application to achieve best results.
- Switch to less potent preparation for maintenance Rx.
- Consider the effective nonsteroidal preparations calcipotriene (Dovonex) or tazarotene as alternatives to topical steroids.
- Use only milder steroids on face and skin folds.
- For patients with excessive scale, recommend gentle removal by warm bathing.
- For mild scalp involvement, prescribe nightly use of tar shampoo. Instruct patient to rub in gently, leave on for 10 mins, and then rinse gently.
- For more severe scalp disease, follow tar shampoo with gentle application of topical steroid lotion [e.g., fluocinolone (Synalar)].
- If scalp involvement marked, recommend covering head with shower cap after steroid application and use of superpotent topical steroid lotion [e.g., betamethasone (Diprolene)].
- As alternatives to superpotent topical steroid lotion application, consider nonsteroidal topicals such as anthralin scalp preparation, calcipotriene (Dovonex) scalp lotion, or tazarotene (Tazorac) gel.
- Refer patients who do not respond and those with extensive disease (>20% of skin area involved) to dermatologist for consideration of methotrexate or other systemic Rx.
- Promptly admit to hospital if generalized pustular or erythrodermal disease develops.
- Refer patients with more extensive or refractory disease to dermatologist.

BIBLIOGRAPHY

- For the current annotated bibliography on psoriasis, see the print edition of *Primary Care Medicine*, 4th edition, Chapter 187, or www.LWWmedicine.com.

DIFFERENTIAL DIAGNOSIS

CAUSES OF PURPURA

- Thrombocytopenic
- Thrombocytopathic
- Clotting factor deficiency
- Vascular
- Connective tissue disease
- Idiopathic (see Bleeding Problems)

PALPABLE PURPURA: IMPORTANT CAUSES OF LEUKOCYTOCLASTIC SMALL VESSEL VASCULITIS

- ANCA-associated
  - Drug-induced
  - Wegener's granulomatosis
  - Microscopic polyangiitis
  - Churg-Strauss syndrome
- Immune complex
  - Rheumatoid disease
    - SLE
    - RA
    - Sjögren's syndrome
  - Cryoglobulinemia (mixed type)
  - Drug-induced immune complex (penicillins, thiazides, aspirin, amphetamines)
  - Schönlein-Henoch purpura
  - Serum sickness
  - Goodpasture's syndrome
  - Inflammatory bowel disease
  - Ulcerative colitis
  - Primary biliary cirrhosis
  - Chronic active hepatitis
- Paraneoplastic
  - Lymphoproliferative disease
  - Myeloproliferative disease
  - Carcinoma

Adapted from Jennette JC, Falk RJ, Andrassey K, et al. Nomenclature of systemic vasculitides: proposal of an international consensus conference. Arthritis Rheum 1994;37:187, with permission.

WORKUP

OVERALL STRATEGY

- Differentiate benign processes (e.g., ecchymoses diameter <6 cm, localized areas of trauma) from more serious hematologic, vasculitic, or infectious pathologies (e.g., palpable purpura, petechial macules in dependent areas).

HISTORY

- Obtain careful description of location, size, and clinical course of purpuric lesions, along with associated symptoms and precipitants.
- Screen for bleeding diathesis by inquiring about blood loss from other sites; easy bruising; bleeding into joint; abnormally heavy bleeding with menstruation, surgery, or dental work; and family Hx of bleeding problems.
- Review all medications, especially aspirin, NSAIDs, dipyridamole, ticlopidine, sulfinpyrazone, and those associated with hypersensitivity reactions that affect platelets (e.g., antibiotics, quinidine, phenothiazines).
- Check for Hx of renal or hepatocellular failure.
- If vasculitis suspected,
  - inquire into symptoms of vasculitic disease and its etiologies (e.g., fever, pruritus, joint pain, urticaria, dry mouth/eyes, morning stiffness, pleuritic pain, abdominal pain, melena, hematuria, lymphadenopathy, jaundice, symptoms of inflammatory bowel disease, chronic leg edema, paresthesias) in patients with early petechial rash or palpable purpura;
  - note any recent streptococcal or staphylococcal infection (hypersensitivity vasculitis);
  - check for medications that might contribute (penicillins, thiazides, aspirin, amphetamines);
  - inquire into sources and sites of recent infection (purulent penile or vaginal discharge, pelvic pain, other recent infection, IV drug abuse, HIV infection, recent dental work).

PHYSICAL EXAM

- Inspect skin lesions; if they appear petechial, press glass slide over them to see if they blanch (nonpurpuric) or do not blanch (purpuric).
- Also check for blanching vascular lesions (telangiectasias, spider angiomata).
- Shine light tangentially to skin to detect elevated lesions, and confirm by careful palpation.
- Note size, number, and location of purpuric lesions and whether they are palpable or macular, petechial or ecchymotic.
- Circle any ecchymosis to follow extension or regression objectively.
- If Hx suggests bleeding problem or if PE reveals petechiae in dependent areas or large ecchymoses, direct PE toward hematologic causes (see Bleeding Problems).
- If palpable purpura is present, check for splinter hemorrhages, rheumatoid nodules, separate malar rash, dry mucous membranes, jaundice, lymphadenopathy, pleural effusion, heart murmur, pericardial rub, hepatic abnormalities, purulent vaginal or urethral discharge, joint inflammation, and changes of stasis dermatitis.
- If Hx reveals only easy bruising and no evidence for hematologic or vasculitic pathology, consider connective tissue and idiopathic causes

and check for cushingoid appearance, signs of everyday trauma, and tender ecchymoses in absence of trauma.

LAB STUDIES

- There is no standard battery of lab tests. Select studies based on clinical findings.

Flat Petechial Rash/Suspected Hematologic Disorder

- Platelet count
- Bleeding time
- PT
- PTT
- Other hematologic testing as determined by initial test results
- See also Bleeding Problems

Palpable Purpura/Suspected Vasculitis

- Blood cultures (rule out bacteremia)
- ANA and RF
- ANCA
- Urinalysis
- Skin biopsy for histologic processing + culture and Gram's stain
- If leukocytoclastic vasculitis confirmed by skin biopsy, then
  - no further testing if otherwise healthy patient with resolving skin lesions and nothing more than Hx of using potentially offending drug;
  - serum immunoelectrophoresis if elderly and if lesions persist;
  - cryoprotein and serum complement if young woman with leukocytoclastic histology or if Hx of hepatitis C;
  - ANCA if small vessel vasculitis present on biopsy and test not already obtained;
  - obtain rheumatologic consultation to optimize test selection and interpretation, particularly in ANCA-positive persons.

MANAGEMENT

OVERALL APPROACH

- Reassure patient with no hematologic or systemic abnormality, but only after completing thorough evaluation (e.g., elderly with senile purpura, or young woman with syndrome of easy bruising).
- Advise against taking large doses of vitamins C and vitamin K, but do recommend avoiding aspirin and NSAIDs.
- Advise, if possible, dose reductions or elimination of drugs that impair platelet function or compromise connective tissue integrity.

INDICATIONS FOR ADMISSION

- Admit any patient with fever and purpura (possible bloodstream infection or systemic vasculitis).
- Admit if evidence of bleeding from multiple sites, severe thrombocytopenia, or marked prolongation of PT or PTT (see Bleeding Problems).

BIBLIOGRAPHY

■ For the current annotated bibliography on purpura, see the print edition of *Primary Care Medicine*, 4th edition, Chapter 179, or www.LWWmedicine.com.

Pyoderma

MANAGEMENT

IMPETIGO

- Apply compresses soaked in Burow's solution for 20 mins bid–qid, then débride gently with washcloth and cleanse with chlorhexidine-containing agent.
- Lightly apply mupirocin to area after drying. Nighttime application also advised.
- Advise patient to keep lesions uncovered, and family should avoid using same towel or washcloth; keep children away from patient with impetigo.

FOLLICULITIS

- Treat with débridement and topical antibiotics, as for impetigo.

FURUNCLES AND CARBUNCLES

- Treat with hot compresses until lesions are fluctuant and drain spontaneously. Larger lesions may require removal of core with 4-mm biopsy punch to facilitate drainage.
- Treat furuncles or carbuncles associated with cellulitis or fever or located on face with oral antistaphylococcal antibiotics, either erythromycin (333 mg tid × 10 days) or dicloxacillin (250 mg qid × 10 days).
- Treat recurrent infection with 10- to 14-day course of systemic antibiotic, and remove bacteria from potential sources, such as skin, nares, nails, and razors and other fomites.

ERYSIPELAS

- Treat with cool compresses and phenoxymethyl penicillin (500 mg qid) × 7–10 days.

RECURRENT PYODERMA

- Eradicate staph nasal carrier state. Prescribe oral dicloxacillin (500 mg qid × 10–14 days) + with topical mupirocin applied bid for ≥5 days.

BIBLIOGRAPHY

- For the current annotated bibliography on pyoderma, see the print edition of *Primary Care Medicine*, 4th edition, Chapter 190, or www.LWWmedicine.com.

Rosacea and Other Acneiform Dermatoses

MANAGEMENT

ROSACEA

- Begin oral tetracycline (500 mg bid) and continue for several wks to mos.
- Gradually reduce dosage to 250 mg qod before considering cessation. Prolonged low-dose Rx may be necessary.
- Alternatively, use doxycycline (100 mg bid) or minocycline (50 mg bid).
- Add topical metronidazole gel (0.75% bid or 1% qd) to systemic antibiotic program, and maintain topical Rx even after discontinuing systemic Rx.
- If patient cannot tolerate topical metronidazole, use topical sulfur and sodium sulfacetamide lotions bid.
- Have patient avoid sunlight and fluorinated steroids and limit systemic medications and foods known to exacerbate condition.
- Consider short-term course of low-potency, nonfluorinated topical corticosteroid (e.g., 1% or 2.5% hydrocortisone cream bid) if erythema is refractory.
- Refer patient for consideration of surgical management if rhinophyma or telangiectases are prominent.

PERIORAL DERMATITIS

- Begin with tetracycline (500 mg bid) and gradually taper dose over several wks after resolution occurs.
- Avoid use of heavy cosmetics, creams, and fluoride toothpastes.
- Consider short course of hydrocortisone cream (1% or 2.5% bid).

PERIORBITAL COMEDONES

- Refer for comedo extraction prn.
- Initiate topical tretinoin (0.025% cream, 0.1% microsphere gel qhs) to affected areas. Warn patients that tretinoin may cause irritation and to avoid sunlight during use.
- For patients who cannot tolerate tretinoin, prescribe topical adapalene (0.1% solution or gel qhs).
- Prescribe sun protection with noncomedogenic sunscreen.
- Consider referral for surgical approaches in severe cases.

BIBLIOGRAPHY

- For the current annotated bibliography on rosacea and other acneiform dermatoses, see the print edition of *Primary Care Medicine*, 4th edition, Chapter 186, or www.LWWmedicine.com.

Scabies and Pediculosis

WORKUP

SCABIES

- Review Hx for intense pruritus, most severe at night or when over-heated or taking off clothes.
- Check for characteristic burrows, most commonly found on fingers, interdigital areas, and wrists, and almost always below neck unless elderly or immunocompromised; lesions typically linear, several mm in length, with dark dot at 1 end.
- Scrape open roof of burrow, remove contents, and microscopically examine material suspended in drop of light mineral oil under low power. Look for adult organism.

PEDICULOSIS

- Review for risk factors such as exposure to school-age population (head lice), poor personal hygiene (body lice), and sexual contacts (pubic lice).
- Check base of hair shaft for diagnostic finding of nits (egg cases). Use gloves to avoid infestation.
- Note any vertical excoriations on trunk (cardinal sign of body lice).
- Suspect head lice if pyoderma of nape of neck or occiput found.

MANAGEMENT

SCABIES

- Prescribe 5% permethrin cream, applied from neck down (including all body folds and creases) and left on overnight for 8–12 hrs. About 30 g suffices for average adult; 1 Rx usually adequate.
- Consider application to scalp. Application beneath nails may prevent reinfestation.
- Advise changing and cleaning underwear and bed linen.
- Treat all household members.
- Only if reinfestation occurs should second Rx course be necessary.
- Prescribe topical corticosteroids and oral antihistamines for bothersome rash and pruritus; if severe, consider oral steroids.
- For crusted scabies, use keratolytic agent (10% salicylic acid or 20% urea) to hasten shedding of affected horny skin layer. Have patient carefully coat subungual areas with permethrin cream.

PEDICULOSIS CAPITIS

- Have patient routinely shampoo without medication and thoroughly dry hair because excess water slows neural activity of insect and protects it from neurotoxic effects of permethrin.
- Apply sufficient permethrin 1% cream rinse to wet hair thoroughly; leave on for 10 mins, then rinse.

- Alternatively, recommend synergized pyrethrins shampoo, applied undiluted until infested areas are entirely wet. After 10 mins, wash areas thoroughly with warm water, then dry. Because Rx is less effective as ovicide, repeat in 7–10 days to kill newly hatched lice.
- Advise drying hair with clean towel after Rx with pediculicide and removing any remaining nits with fine-toothed comb. Nit removal is believed to reduce chance of reinfestation.
- Recommend washing combs, clothing, and bed linens.

PEDICULOSIS CORPORIS AND PEDICULOSIS PUBIS

- Treat in manner similar to pediculosis capitis.
- Recommend application of permethrin 1% cream rinse or 1% cream to body for 10 mins before washing off.
- Treat sexual partners of patients with pediculosis pubis.
- Treat eyelash involvement by advising application of petrolatum jelly up to 5 times/day × 5–7 days. Alternately, recommend 0.25% physostigmine ophthalmic ointment, applied to lashes qid for 3 consecutive days.
- Advise washing clothing and bed linens.

BIBLIOGRAPHY

- For the current annotated bibliography on scabies and pediculosis, see the print edition of *Primary Care Medicine*, 4th edition, Chapter 195, or www.LWWmedicine.com.

Skin Ulceration

MANAGEMENT

VENOUS INSUFFICIENCY AND STASIS DERMATITIS

- In all patients with stasis changes, control edema with rest, elevation, diuretics, avoidance of dependency, and external compression with stockings or bandages.
- Treat any concurrent nutritional deficiency, HTN, DM, or CHF.
- Treat pruritus with intermediate-potency topical corticosteroids (e.g., 0.1% triamcinolone acetonide).
- Use ointment preparation if area is dry and scaly; use cream if area is moist. Avoid application near or on ulcers because corticosteroids may delay wound healing.
- Treat acute exudative dermatitis with cool Burow's compresses (1:40 dilution) bid–tid × 30–60 mins.
- Discourage scratching and using OTC medicaments.

CUTANEOUS ULCERATION

- Prescribe application of wet-to-wet dressings, followed by cleaning and gentle débridement with gauze sponges several times/day.
- Use dilute hydrogen peroxide to clean ulcerated area.
- Try occlusive dressings because they may ease pain, débride ulcers, and lead to healing without surgical intervention.
- For secondary infection, culture for aerobic and anaerobic bacteria, and treat accordingly with PO or IV antibiotics.
- For mild skin infection, consider topical antibiotic creams such as mupirocin for short-term use (<2 wks), but avoid preparations that contain neomycin.
- For persistent deep ulcers, consider underlying osteomyelitis. Radiographs may be useful.
- Refer for surgical consultation patients with ulcers refractory to proper conservative management. Pinch grafting is relatively simple in-office approach. Culture-derived human skin-equivalent grafts (Apligraf) have been successful but are very expensive. Becaplermin (recombinant human platelet-derived growth factor, Regranex Gel) has been shown clinically effective in healing ulcers but is also very expensive.
- Surgical débridement and split-thickness or full-thickness skin grafting may be necessary.

BIBLIOGRAPHY

- For the current annotated bibliography on skin ulceration, see the print edition of *Primary Care Medicine*, 4th edition, Chapter 197, or www.LWWmedicine.com.

Urticaria and Angioedema

DIFFERENTIAL DIAGNOSIS

COMMON CAUSES OF URTICARIA AND ANGIOEDEMA

- Acute disease (episodes for <6 wks)
  - Infection
    - Viral
    - Bacterial
    - Fungal
    - Parasitic
  - Foods (eggs, shellfish, nuts)
  - Food additives (sodium benzoate, azo dyes such as tartrazine and yellow dye No. 5)
  - Drugs
    - Immunologic release of mediators (penicillins, sulfa-containing agents)
    - Direct mediator release (IV iodinated contrast agents, opiates, amphetamines)
    - Prostaglandin inhibition (aspirin, other NSAIDs)
  - Other sensitizing antigens (e.g., latex, blood transfusion)
  - Insect sting
  - All causes of chronic urticaria
- Chronic disease (episodes for >6 wks)
  - Idiopathic
  - Physical
    - Cold
    - Pressure
    - Dermatographism
    - Cholinergic (exercise, hot shower, emotional stress)
    - Solar
    - Vibratory
  - Hereditary C1 inhibitor deficiency
  - Acquired angioedema (lymphoma, adenocarcinoma, chronic lympho-cytic leukemia)
  - Causes of acute urticaria

WORKUP

HISTORY

- Obtain description of urticarial response and its precipitants; Hx is key to Dx.
- Note whether predominant reaction is angioedema (suggesting possible C1 INH deficiency) or urticaria.
- Ascertain whether individual wheals persist for >24 hrs (suggesting urticarial vasculitis, especially if accompanied by purpura and pigmentation) or clear quickly.

- Inquire into illnesses, medications, foods, activities, and exposures associated with urticaria or angioedema (see above); include review of nonprescription drugs (NSAIDs and aspirin).
- Consider latex allergy in health care workers with urticaria.
- Encourage keeping food diary when food allergy suspected.
- Do not overlook agents that may be entering through conjunctivae, nasal mucosa, rectum, or vaginal area.
- Keep in mind that penicillin antigen may be present in dairy products, and yeast antigen in beer.
- Note whether exposure to pressure, cold, light, heat, or exercise precipitates lesions.
- Check travel Hx for possible parasitic infestation.
- Inquire into agents and factors that might modulate intensity of urticarial reaction (e.g., alcohol, NSAIDs, heat, humidity, occlusive clothing, psychological stress).
- Review family Hx for angioedema, but negative family Hx does not rule out C1 INH deficiency.
- Perform systems review for symptoms of systemic illness, infection, and malignancy, including night sweats, fatigue, weight loss, lymphadenopathy, recurrent peptic ulcer disease (*Helicobacter* infection), jaundice, easy bruising, cold intolerance, dry skin, thyroid enlargement, dysuria, vaginal or sinus discharge, and pain in teeth, joints, or sinuses.

PHYSICAL EXAM

- Observe lesions and their distribution: linear wheals (dermatographism), small lesions with erythematous flares (cholinergic urticaria), periorbital or perioral swelling (angioedema), lesions persisting >24 hrs with purpura and hyperpigmentation (urticarial vasculitis).
- Examine ears, pharynx, sinuses, and teeth for focal infection.
- Check nodes for enlargement and abdomen for hepatosplenomegaly (lymphoma, hepatocellular disease).
- Note any joint inflammation (active rheumatoid disease).

LAB STUDIES

- Avoid attempting Dx using extensive panel of lab tests in absence of suggestive Hx and PE.
- Limit initial studies to CBC and differential (for infection and myeloproliferative disease) and ESR (for active connective tissue disease).
- Consider skin biopsy only in suspected vasculitis (see Purpura); take sample from margin of lesion to include normal and involved skin.
- Measure serum C4 if evidence for C1 INH deficiency.
- Check for antithyroid antibodies and TSH when autoimmune pathophysiology suggested.
- Order ANA determination and urinalysis if ESR is high and urticarial vasculitis is concern.
- Obtain serology for *H. pylori* exposure if there is recurrent peptic ulcer disease with urticaria.
- Omit skin testing, IgE radioallergosorbent test, and serum IgE levels.
- Reserve radiologic exams for suspected focal infection or malignancy.

- Check stool for O&P only if recent diarrheal illness, travel to endemic area, or peripheral eosinophilia.
- Avoid "cytotoxic food allergy" testing (no scientific validity).
- Consider provocative tests:
  - Ice cube on skin (cold urticaria)
  - Stroking skin (dermatographism)
  - Intradermal injection of methacholine using 0.1 mL of 1:500 dilution (cholinergic urticaria)
  - Pressing at right angle to skin with redness and swelling at site after latent period of 0.5–4.0 hrs (pressure urticaria)
  - Placebo-controlled challenge testing for reactivity to food additives (food allergy); avoid in persons with Hx of asthma or airway involvement
- Therapeutic trials
  - Consider elimination diet that consists of lamb, rice, string beans, fresh peas, tea, and rye crackers (excludes most common food allergens) or more limited approach eliminating dairy products, beer, nuts, shellfish, berries, and food additives.
  - Stop all drugs or change preparations or brands, including toothpastes and cosmetics, to eliminate tartrazine dyes and potentially offending additives.

MANAGEMENT

OVERALL APPROACH

- Treat etiologically whenever possible.
- Recommend avoiding substances that may aggravate symptoms (e.g., aspirin, NSAIDs, alcohol, ACE inhibitors).
- Reassure that 50% with urticaria alone and 25% with associated angioedema become symptom-free within 1 yr even if etiologic Dx is not made.
- If symptoms are problematic, consider these for symptomatic relief:
  - Antihistamines
    - H_1 blockers (e.g., hydroxyzine, 10–25 mg qhs; or nonprescription preparations diphenhydramine, 25–50 mg qhs; or chlorpheniramine 4–8 mg qhs).
    - Nonsedating H_1 blocker (e.g., fexofenadine, 60 mg qam) for daytime use.
    - In refractory cases, add H_2 blocker (e.g., cimetidine, 400 mg tid) or doxepin, a tricyclic antidepressant with H_1 blocker activity (e.g., 25 mg bid or qhs; avoid concurrent use of nonsedating H_1 blocker terfenadine).
  - Steroids and other drugs (for severe refractory cases)
    - Course of oral glucocorticosteroids (e.g., prednisone, 20–40 mg qam × 7–10 days with rapid taper after 10–14 days and switch to qod Rx with elimination by 3–4 wks).
    - Trial of β_2 agonist terbutaline in fairly high doses (1.25 mg tid).
    - Trial of nifedipine (extended-release formulation, 30 mg qam).
    - Trial of anabolic steroids (e.g., danazol, stanozolol) for hereditary angioedema.
- Avoid Rx of unproved efficacy, including empiric trials of broad-spectrum antibiotics and antifungal agents.

■ Advise against topical preparations of corticosteroids, antihistamines, and local anesthetics (expensive, no benefit in chronic urticaria).

ACUTE ATTACKS

■ Mild to moderate attacks: full program of oral antihistamines.
■ Severe attacks complicated by angioedema: prompt administration of SQ aqueous epinephrine (0.3 mL of 1:1,000 dilution).
■ For severe acute urticaria uncomplicated by angioedema: short course of systemic steroids (e.g., prednisone, started at 40 mg/day and rapidly tapered to full cessation by 1 wk).
■ For physical urticaria of aquagenic, cold-induced, or dermatographic origin: H_1 blocker cyproheptadine.
■ For cold-induced and localized heat-induced urticaria: topical capsaicin (results variable).
■ For vibratory physical urticaria: antihistamines.
■ For exercise-induced urticaria: minimize vigorous exercise, especially after eating or when taking aspirin or NSAIDs.

CHRONIC AND REFRACTORY URTICARIA

■ Begin with nonsedating H_1 blocker.
■ Add H_2 blocker, such as cimetidine, if necessary.
■ Substitute doxepin if control inadequate.
■ Consider brief course of systemic corticosteroids (as described above); use only if symptoms intolerable. Avoid longer-term systemic steroid Rx.
■ Prescribe trial of exogenous thyroid hormone replacement if TSH elevated and antithyroid antibodies present.
■ Consider course of antibiotic Rx for patient with idiopathic urticaria and positive *Helicobacter* serology (see Peptic Ulcer Disease).

HEREDITARY ANGIOEDEMA

■ Treat with SQ epinephrine (0.3 mL of 1:1,000 dilution) for acute attack that threatens airway obstruction.
■ Advise carrying epinephrine self-administration kit.
■ Consider anabolic steroids (e.g., danazol, stanozolol) for prophylaxis when attacks frequent or severe; monitor C1 esterase inhibitor level and liver function periodically.

INDICATIONS FOR REFERRAL AND ADMISSION

■ Consider referral to allergist for (1) confirmatory placebo-controlled testing for patients with repeated episodes believed caused by food allergies; (2) penicillin skin testing, particularly with minor determinants if antibiotic sensitivity suspected; or (3) comfort and reassurance.
■ Refer patient with suspected urticarial vasculitis to rheumatologist or dermatologist for skin biopsy and immunohistologic staining of sample.
■ Admit patients with acute angioedema complicated by airway obstruction or GI symptoms for respiratory support and observation.

PATIENT EDUCATION

■ Prepare patient for likelihood that cause is usually not found.

- Reassure patient that medical workup will exclude serious and treatable diseases and that many options are available to shorten process and alleviate symptoms.
- Emphasize variable natural Hx of urticaria and high probability that lesions will disappear spontaneously.
- Prepare patient for likelihood that urticaria will recur.
- Instruct patients to avoid exacerbating factors (e.g., aspirin, NSAIDs, heat, exertion, alcoholic beverages).
- Provide specific advice, such as avoiding swimming in cold water for patients with cold urticaria.

BIBLIOGRAPHY

- For the current annotated bibliography on urticaria and angioedema, see the print edition of *Primary Care Medicine*, 4th edition, Chapter 181, or www.LWWmedicine.com.

Warts

MANAGEMENT

- Use liquid nitrogen for initial Rx of common warts. Apply with cotton swab to area that includes small rim of surrounding skin.
- Treat plantar warts by paring down with scalpel and applying 40% salicylic acid plaster cut in shape of, but slightly smaller than, wart. Cover with occlusive adhesive tape and leave in place for 24–72 hrs.
- Continue Rx at home, with gentle paring and reapplication of salicylic acid plaster prn. Check progress regularly.
- Treat flat warts with topical 5-FU, retinoic acid, or Keralyt (6% salicylic acid gel).
- Treat moist anogenital warts with topical podophyllum; remind patient to remove medication after 4–6 hrs.
- Consider topical podofilox for patient administration at home if repeated Rx needed.
- Consider imiquimod for anogenital lesions that do not respond to less-expensive Rx.
- If topical Rx proves ineffective or if patient has extensive anal or genital involvement, refer for consultation and consideration of more aggressive Rx, such as carbon dioxide laser.

BIBLIOGRAPHY

- For the current annotated bibliography on warts, see the print edition of *Primary Care Medicine*, 4th edition, Chapter 194, or www.LWWmedicine.com.

Age-Related Macular Degeneration

SCREENING AND/OR PREVENTION

- Insist on full smoking cessation.
- Instruct patient in daily use of Amsler's grid and emphasize importance of promptly reporting any vision distortion.
- Inform patient that no definitive evidence supports prophylactic use of high-dose zinc or antioxidant vitamins (e.g., C, E, and beta carotene); use is unwarranted.

WORKUP

- Inquire into gradual or sudden loss of central visual acuity in elderly persons.
- Ask about distorted vision (metamorphopsia, indicative of serous retinal detachment due to neovascularization).
- Examine macula for drusen, irregularities in pigmentation, hemorrhage, and discoid scarring.
- Use Amsler's grid to check for defects in central visual acuity; test each eye separately with any prescribed corrective lenses worn and grid held at comfortable reading distance.
- If macular degeneration suspected, obtain prompt ophthalmologic consultation to confirm and to determine whether disease is exudative or nonexudative and whether patient is candidate for prophylactic Rx.

MANAGEMENT

EXUDATIVE DISEASE WITH NEOVASCULARIZATION

- Arrange urgent ophthalmologic referral for patients reporting new distortion of vision with Amsler's grid use.
- Have patient considered for immediate argon laser photocoagulation Rx to preserve central vision if neovascularization not unacceptably close to fovea.
- For patients with central vision loss due to neovascularization disease, arrange for use of low-vision aids.

NONEXUDATIVE DISEASE WITHOUT NEOVASCULARIZATION

- Inform patient that there is no definitive prophylactic Rx, but prognosis is good.

PATIENT EDUCATION

- Reassure that regardless of severity of macular degeneration, blindness will not ensue because peripheral vision is largely unaffected.

- Reemphasize importance of early detection of neovascularization and its consequences through daily use of Amsler's grid and prompt reporting of distorted vision.
- Make complete smoking cessation top priority.

INDICATIONS FOR REFERRAL

- Refer to ophthalmologist any elderly patient suspected on basis of Hx or PE to have macular degeneration; promptness is critical if there is distorted vision (early serous retinal detachment, neovascularization).

BIBLIOGRAPHY

- For the current annotated bibliography on age-related macular degeneration, see the print edition of *Primary Care Medicine*, 4th edition, Chapter 206, or www.LWWmedicine.com.

Cataracts

SCREENING AND/OR PREVENTION

- Recommend protective eyewear (treated to block all UV transmission) as best means of reducing cortical cataract risk due to solar UVB radiation.
- Also suggest wearing brimmed hat.
- Advise that sunglasses with plastic untreated lenses do not reduce exposure, and darkness of lens's tint is not necessarily measure of protective capacity.
- Inform that dark, unprotective sunglasses may actually exacerbate exposure by blocking visible light transmission, causing pupillary dilation and thus increasing penetration of UV radiation.
- Advise outdoor workers to wear close-fitting protective sunglasses.
- Insist on smoking cessation.
- Limit steroid use to lowest dose and minimum strength necessary (particularly in the elderly).
- Inform that nutritional supplements such as antioxidants have not been shown to slow rate of cataract progression.

WORKUP

- Check visual acuity near and at distance.
- Identify lenticular opacity with direct ophthalmoscope while attempting to visualize fundus:
  - Set lens at 0 D, stand about 12 in. from patient, and check for disruption of red reflex.
  - Reset ophthalmoscope to +15 or +20 D and come close to patient to visualize lens and check for retinal abnormalities, particularly macular degeneration (manifested by hemorrhage, scarring, and drusen), which can cause vision loss symptomatically similar to that from cataract.
- As in all cases of visual impairment, obtain ophthalmic consultation.

MANAGEMENT

CONSERVATIVE MEASURES

- Before considering surgery, initiate conservative measures, especially during early disease when eyeglasses prescription (early nuclear sclerosis) or pupillary dilator Rx (posterior subcapsular cataract) may suffice.
- Suggest conservative approach when vision is good in 1 eye and there are no important functional limitations.
- Review with elderly patients with age-related nuclear cataracts that condition is not a "growth" and poses no harm to vision.

SURGERY

- Refer for consideration of surgery when conservative measures no longer suffice and patient believes visual dysfunction is impairing quality of life.

■ Consider surgery if visual impairment marked [interferes with daily living (e.g., causes falls, prohibits reading or watching TV, or interferes with driving)].

■ Note that although surgical correction is highly successful in up to 99% of patients, it is not risk-free.

■ To ensure safety and quality of result, note whether age, mental status, or medical condition necessitates or prohibits use of general anesthesia to minimize risk of movement during surgery.

■ For patients who want to know more about surgery, review most common approach: phacoemulsification [uses ultrasound to break up hard nucleus, followed by aspiration through small (3-mm) opening that is often self-sealing and requires no sutures].

■ Note that visual rehabilitation requires contact lenses or permanent lens implantation (the latter usually preferred for the elderly).

■ Inform patient that phacoemulsification allows rapid return to full physical activity but that transient use of topical medications may be necessary after surgery, and it may be several wks after surgery before fully corrected vision is realized.

BIBLIOGRAPHY

■ For the current annotated bibliography on cataracts, see the print edition of *Primary Care Medicine*, 4th edition, Chapter 208, or www.LWWmedicine.com.

Contact Lenses

MANAGEMENT

HARD AND RIGID CONTACT LENSES

- Advise patient that gas-permeable lenses are preferred form of rigid lens, replacing original hard design.
- Review advantages and disadvantages:
  - Improved comfort and longer wearing times.
  - Longer initial adaptation and may dislodge more frequently than soft contact lenses.
  - Excellent results, especially with astigmatic patients.
  - Relatively easy to clean and can last several yrs if cared for properly.
  - Good long-term tolerance; low risk of corneal ulcerations, corneal neovascularization, and infection.
  - Advanced skill and knowledge required by practitioner in fitting and designing lenses.

SOFT LENSES

- Note that soft lenses are another option; very popular due to their comfort.
- Review advantages and disadvantages:
  - Good initial comfort and tolerance.
  - Can be worn for longer periods, do not dislodge easily, and allow switching easily between contacts and glasses (less molding effect on cornea).
  - Less effective for astigmatic correction compared with rigid lenses.
  - Require more frequent thorough cleaning and disinfection.
  - Require more frequent replacement.
  - Pose low risk of infection and ulcerative keratitis if removed before bed and properly cleaned and disinfected before insertion.

DISPOSABLE SOFT LENSES

- Note that disposables have become very popular due to enhanced convenience and comfort.
- Review advantages and disadvantages:
  - Available for single use, weekly, bimonthly, monthly, and quarterly.
  - Must be removed for sleep if designed for daily wear and cleaned and disinfected before reinsertion the following day.
  - Pose low risk of infection.
  - Extended-wear lenses allow occasional sleeping with lenses, but continuous use restricted to ≤7 days.
  - Prolonged use associated with changes in ocular tissues and markedly increased risk of infection and resultant ulcerative keratitis (can result in permanent vision loss; destroys corneal stroma).
- Refer promptly to ophthalmologist for antibiotic Rx in suspected ulcerative keratitis.

BIBLIOGRAPHY

■ For the current annotated bibliography on contact lenses, see the print edition of *Primary Care Medicine*, 4th edition, Chapter 210, or www.LWWmedicine.com.

Diabetic Retinopathy

SCREENING AND/OR PREVENTION

SCREENING

- Arrange yearly dilated ophthalmoscopy to detect proliferative retinopathy (handheld ophthalmoscope inadequate for screening, especially when performed by nonophthalmologic physician).
- Consider stereophotography if it becomes available at reduced cost (allows evaluation of macular edema).
- Implement current consensus screening guidelines:
  - For type I DM, screen annually beginning 5 yrs after onset, generally not before puberty.
  - For type II DM, screen initially at time of Dx and then annually.
  - If initial exam uses stereo fundus photography and is normal, next exam need not occur for 4 yrs. After that, annual screening is required, regardless of method used.
  - For pregnant diabetics, have dilated ophthalmoscopy performed during first trimester and provide close follow-up throughout pregnancy; counsel on risk of developing or worsening retinopathy during pregnancy; no screening needed for gestational DM.
- Supplement formal ophthalmologic screening with handheld ophthalmoscopic exam during regular medical visits.

PREVENTION

- Aim for tight control of serum glucose in all diabetics (HBA1C <7.0; see Diabetes Mellitus).
- Achieve tight control of any concurrent systemic HTN or hypercholesterolemia.
- Insist on smoking cessation.

MANAGEMENT

- Refer patient with proliferative retinopathy to retinal specialist for consideration of panretinal laser photocoagulation.
- Refer patient with nonproliferative retinopathy complicated by clinically significant macular edema to retinal specialist for consideration of focal laser Rx.
- Consider surgical vitrectomy if vitreous hemorrhage will not spontaneously clear or when dense fibrovascular proliferation affects macula and causes severe vision loss (also allows more aggressive laser photocoagulation).
- Reestablish tight glycemic control (see Diabetes Mellitus) if visual blurring occurs from hyperglycemia-induced osmotic swelling.
- Restore and maintain tight glycemic control (see Diabetes Mellitus) if diplopia develops from localized demyelination of third, fourth, or sixth cranial nerves; usually recovers within 1–3 mos.
- Treat any cataracts that form (see Cataracts).

PATIENT EDUCATION

- Review importance of and approaches to tight glycemic control (see Diabetes Mellitus).
- Stress benefits of smoking cessation, HTN control, and regular ophthalmologic exams.
- Teach immediate reporting of eye symptoms.
- Provide good news that vision loss can be prevented.

INDICATIONS FOR REFERRAL

- Arrange prompt ophthalmologic referral for change in vision, new appearance of floaters, eye pain, discovery of retinopathy (particularly neovascularization due to proliferative retinopathy), any symptoms or signs of macular edema (distorted vision, moderate to severe nonproliferative retinopathy), or loss of ability to visualize fundus.

BIBLIOGRAPHY

- For the current annotated bibliography on diabetic retinopathy, see the print edition of *Primary Care Medicine*, 4th edition, Chapter 209, or www.LWWmedicine.com.

Dry Eyes

DIFFERENTIAL DIAGNOSIS

- Lacrimal gland dysfunction
  - Age
  - Systemic disease (Sjögren's syndrome, sarcoidosis, Hodgkin's disease)
  - Anticholinergic drugs (atropine, antihistamines, tricyclics)
- Compromised eyelid function
  - Fifth or seventh nerve palsy
  - Exophthalmos
  - Scar formation
- Mucin deficiency
  - Chemical burns
  - Hypovitaminosis A
  - Isotretinoin (Accutane)
  - Benign ocular pemphigoid
  - Trachoma
- Environmental factors
  - Excessive dryness
  - Excessive exposure (e.g., exophthalmos, Bell's palsy)
- Lipid abnormalities
  - Chronic blepharitis
  - Meibomitis

WORKUP

HISTORY

- Note duration and frequency of symptoms and particularly if onset is related to dry environmental conditions.
- Check for suggestive symptoms (more pronounced as day progresses, exacerbated by tobacco smoke, lack of tears with crying, strands of mucus from inner canthi on awakening).
- Inquire into any associated dry mouth, joint pains, prior ocular disease, infection, or surgery.
- Review medications, especially in elderly (e.g., tricyclics, anxiolytics, antihypertensives).
- Note any Hx of rheumatoid disease or its symptoms.

PHYSICAL EXAM

- Observe frequency and completeness of blinking.
- Note any lid pathology (lid margin crusting, engorgement of meibomian glands).
- Check for thick yellow mucous strands in lower fornix, hyperemic and edematous bulbar conjunctiva, and corneal dullness.
- Observe completeness of lid closure and position of eyelashes.

- Test corneal reflex if concerned about neuroparalytic keratitis or facial nerve palsy.
- Examine skin and joints for signs of rheumatoid disease.

LAB STUDIES

- Perform Schirmer's test to document aqueous deficiency (measures wetting of filter paper strip).
- If Sjögren's syndrome suspected, obtain ANA determination (95% sensitive in Sjögren's; specificity low) and RF (75% sensitive; specificity low).
- If positive, follow up with more specific anti-Ro and anti-La antibodies (>90% specificity).
- Reserve lip biopsy for cases in which clinical findings strongly suggestive but lab studies negative.

MANAGEMENT

- If no signs of ocular disease, consider symptomatic measures.
- Stop or reduce unnecessary medications that may be contributing.
- Eliminate environmental dryness.
- Suggest 2-wk trial of artificial tear substitutes such as methylcellulose (Visulose, 0.5% or 1%), polyvinyl alcohol (Liquifilm Tears, 1.4%; or Liquifilm Forte, 3%), or hydroxypropyl methylcellulose 1% (Ultra Tears, Tears Naturale, and Adsorbotear).
- Advise patients that they may instill drops prn, starting with 1–2 drops qid and increasing to as frequently as hourly to achieve comfort.
- Refer for further evaluation and consideration of punctal plugs if simple measures do not suffice.
- Avoid prescribing steroids and antibiotics for uncomplicated disease.
- Arrange immediate ophthalmologic referral if red eye, visual disturbance, or eye pain develops.

PATIENT EDUCATION

- Teach proper instillation of eyedrops:
  - Apply drop into lower fornix without contact occurring between dropper and eye.
  - Apply digital pressure in punctal or inner region of lower lid to reduce drainage and prolong contact.
  - Avoid instilling >1 drop at a time.

BIBLIOGRAPHY

- For the current annotated bibliography on dry eyes, see the print edition of *Primary Care Medicine*, 4th edition, Chapter 202, or www.LWWmedicine.com.

Excessive Tearing

DIFFERENTIAL DIAGNOSIS

- Excessive tear production
  - Keratitis
  - Blepharitis
  - Conjunctivitis
  - Atopy
  - Sinusitis
  - Facial palsies
  - Reflex tearing of dry eyes
- Impaired tear drainage
  - Dacryocystitis
  - Punctal obstruction (tumor, burn, senile atresia, infection)
  - Ectropion
  - Sagging of lower lid
  - Obstruction of lacrimal sac and nasolacrimal duct (idiopathic, congenital, neoplasms, ethmoiditis, and turbinate disease)

WORKUP

HISTORY

- Confirm excessive tearing (do tears actually run down cheeks?).
- Determine frequency and whether unilateral (more likely to be structural eye pathology) or bilateral (less likely to be localized eye pathology).
- Inquire into overflowing tears in absence of environmental irritants (structural pathology).
- Check for watery eyes noted on exposure to cold, air conditioning, or dry environment (exaggerated physiologic tearing).
- Ask about sinus disease, facial fractures, infections, prior surgery, and symptoms suggesting Sjögren's syndrome (paradoxical tearing).

PHYSICAL EXAM

- Observe lid structure and motion, and examine patency of puncta under low magnification.
- Exert gentle pressure over lacrimal sac on side of nose and over canaliculi to attempt to express purulent material for exam and culture.
- Examine for signs of dry eye to rule out paradoxical tearing.

LAB STUDIES

- Arrange ophthalmologic referral for testing of lacrimal drainage (fluorescein dye, saline irrigation, and/or probing).
- If positive, consider dacryocystography (radiocontrast dye injection) to outline obstruction and proximal lacrimal system, and dacryoscintigraphy to demonstrate functional impairment (pump failure).

MANAGEMENT

- Eliminate environmental irritants.
- Treat any underlying dry eye or sicca syndrome with appropriate lubricants (see Dry Eyes).
- Treat any contributing dacryocystitis with hot compresses ≥qid and oral antistaphylococcal antibiotics (e.g., erythromycin, 250 mg qid; or dicloxacillin, 250 mg qid).
- Reassure patients without infection that condition is harmless.
- Refer patients unresponsive to simple measures to ophthalmologist for formal testing and consideration of surgical Rx (including lid surgery to correct malposition or dacryocystorhinostomy to relieve nasolacrimal obstruction).

BIBLIOGRAPHY

- For the current annotated bibliography on excessive tearing, see the print edition of *Primary Care Medicine*, 4th edition, Chapter 205, or www.LWWmedicine.com.

Exophthalmos

DIFFERENTIAL DIAGNOSIS

- Bilateral exophthalmos
  - Graves' disease
  - Cushing's syndrome
  - Acromegaly
  - Lithium ingestion
  - Metastatic tumor
  - Orbital lymphoma
- Unilateral exophthalmos
  - Tumor
    - Orbital: hemangioma, meningioma, optic nerve glioma
    - Extending into orbit: tumors of eye, lid, paranasal sinus
  - Inflammatory: orbital pseudotumor, sarcoidosis, foreign body, orbital thrombophlebitis, periorbital infection, ruptured dermoid cyst
  - Vascular: hemangioma, aneurysm, varices, carotid cavernous fistula, and cavernous sinus thrombosis
  - Skeletal: Paget's disease
  - Other, mimicking exophthalmos: asymmetry of orbits, severe unilateral myopia, facial nerve paresis, eyelid retraction, congenital glaucoma, ptosis or enophthalmos of opposite eye

WORKUP

OVERALL STRATEGY

- First establish whether condition is unilateral or bilateral; then proceed accordingly.

HISTORY

- Inquire into time course (old photographs helpful).
- Check relevant medical Hx and review of systems (e.g., trauma to orbit, hyperthyroidism, cancer, periorbital tumor, lithium ingestion, severe sinus infection, worsening headache, and change in skin, facial features, or hands).
- Note any consequences of exophthalmos (visual acuity changes, diplopia, pain, excessive lacrimation, photophobia, foreign body sensation).

PHYSICAL EXAM

- Document degree of exophthalmos by measuring distance from lateral orbital rim to apex of cornea with patient looking straight ahead (ULN = 21–22 mm with difference between both eyes <2 mm).
- Examine for signs of orbital infection/inflammation (orbital cellulitis) and compromised eye function.
- Check or have measured visual acuity, IOP, and extraocular muscle function.

- Assess color vision, pupillary reactivity, and visual fields for signs of optic nerve compression, and note any pallor or swelling of optic nerve head on ophthalmoscopic exam.
- Auscultate globe and orbit for bruits and pulsation.
- Check sinuses for tenderness and purulent discharge.
- Note any conjunctival or corneal drying.
- In setting of bilateral disease, examine neck for goiter and bruit, pretibial region for myxedematous changes, and remainder of exam for other signs of thyroid hormone excess (see Hyperthyroidism).
- Note any cushingoid or acromegalic features.

LAB STUDIES

- If bilateral disease (even in absence of clinical hyperthyroidism), screen for Grave's disease with TSH determination, supplemented by testing for antibodies to thyrotropin receptors and peroxidase; also order total T_3 and free T_4 index if TSH low or undetectable.
- If unilateral disease, proceed to orbital imaging with axial and coronal CT if suspected mass lesion or bony pathology; screen with ultrasound if more evidence of a mass needed before CT scan.
- Consider orbital MRI for better definition of suspected vascular or neoplastic lesion.
- If patient appears cushingoid or acromegalic, proceed with appropriate workup.

MANAGEMENT

GENERAL APPROACH

- Recommend elevating head of bed.
- Suggest using artificial tear lubricants and taping eyelids closed qhs if patient reports foreign body sensation (exposure keratopathy).
- Instruct patient to immediately report any vision change, ocular pain, redness, or diplopia.

GRAVES' OPHTHALMOPATHY

- Insist on complete smoking cessation.
- Treat underlying Graves' disease carefully, because ophthalmopathy can worsen with use of modalities that cause gland destruction (see Hyperthyroidism).
- Consider antithyroid drugs in preference to radioiodine Rx, or consider adding high-dose corticosteroids (e.g., prednisone, 0.5 mg/kg × 1 mo, beginning several days after radioiodine administration; see Hyperthyroidism).
- Refer to thyroid specialist for design of specific Rx program.

INDICATIONS FOR REFERRAL AND ADMISSION

- Obtain prompt consultation early in unilateral, severe, or unexplained exophthalmos, especially when infection, inflammation, mass, or vascular lesion is suspected.

- Order endocrinologic consultation for managing ophthalmopathy of Graves' disease.
- Arrange emergency admission if orbital cellulitis is encountered.

BIBLIOGRAPHY

- For the current annotated bibliography on exophthalmos, see the print edition of *Primary Care Medicine*, 4th edition, Chapter 204, or www.LWWmedicine.com.

Eye Pain

DIFFERENTIAL DIAGNOSIS

- Extraocular causes
  - Lid
    - Hordeolum (a small abscess of the lid)
    - Acute dacryocystitis
    - Cellulitis
    - Chalazion
  - Conjunctival
    - Irritant exposure (prolonged sun exposure, pollution, occupational irritants, aerosol propellants, wind, dust)
    - Infection (viral or bacterial)
    - Lack of sleep
  - Corneal
    - Incipient zoster
    - Abrasions
    - Foreign bodies
    - Ulcers
    - Ingrown lashes
    - Contact lens abuse
    - Excessive exposure to sun or other forms of ultraviolet radiation
    - Infection (bacterial or viral)
  - Scleral
    - Episcleritis
    - Scleritis (connective tissue disease)
- Intraocular conditions
  - Anterior eye
    - Acute angle-closure glaucoma
    - Acute anterior uveitis (idiopathic, connective tissue disease, sarcoidosis, inflammatory bowel disease)
    - Refractive error (mild pain only)
  - Posterior eye
    - Posterior uveitis
- Orbital disease
  - Tumor
  - Inflammatory disease
  - Retrobulbar optic neuritis
- Referred pain from extraocular sources
  - Sinusitis
  - Tooth abscess
  - Tension headache
  - Giant cell arteritis
  - Prodrome of herpes zoster
  - Ocular muscle imbalance

WORKUP

OVERALL STRATEGY

- First check to ensure no threat to vision. Most intraocular conditions that cause eye pain may compromise vision and should be carefully checked for, as should corneal injuries.
- Arrange prompt referral if corneal or intraocular problem suspected

HISTORY

- Review Hx for important clues:
  - Deep pain: intraocular problem
  - Foreign body sensation: problem is on eye surface or extraocular
  - Any change in visual acuity or color vision: retinal problem
  - Diplopia and displacement of eye: orbital problem
- Note aggravating and alleviating factors:
  - Pain exacerbated by lid movement and relieved by cessation of lid motion: foreign body or corneal lesion.
  - Pain worsened by eye motion: retrobulbar optic neuritis, especially if accompanied by loss of central vision and normal-appearing optic disc.
- Note important associated symptoms:
  - Photophobia: acute anterior uveitis; migraine
  - Headache: migraine, sinusitis
  - Purulent nasal discharge: sinusitis
- Check for sources of conjunctival irritation:
  - Occupational exposures
  - Trauma
  - Sun, sun lamp, and other forms of UV radiation (e.g., arc welding)
  - Foreign body contact

PHYSICAL EXAM

- First test and record visual acuity, color vision, and extraocular movements.
- Inspect eye, lid, and conjunctiva for masses and redness, pupil for reactivity, cornea for clarity, and fundus for any disc abnormalities. Note:
  - Cloudy cornea in conjunction with a fixed midposition pupil: acute glaucoma; eye may be red.
  - Constricted pupil with excessive tearing: anterior uveitis; in severe cases, eye also may be red and anterior chamber hazy.
  - Central scotoma with normal appearing disc: retrobulbar neuritis.
- Invert lid with cotton-tipped applicator to check for foreign body and chalazion.
- Inspect cornea with penlight and small hand lens for gross injury.
- Examine iris for dilated vessels around limbus (ciliary flush): intraocular inflammation of anterior uveitis.

Fluorescein Staining

- If corneal lesion is a concern, consider obtaining fluorescein stain exam using cobalt blue filtered light.
- Be sure fluorescein instilled by means of single-dose container or sterile fluorescein strips wetted with sterile saline to avoid using infected solution.

- Touch strip to inferior cul de sac while patient looks upward; then ask patient to blink once.
- Observe any fluorescein staining of denuded areas of corneal epithelium (bright green color when viewed by normal light, intensity enhanced by cobalt blue light).
- Check for dendritic ulcers of herpes keratitis, abrasions, small foreign bodies, and punctate defects caused by irradiation.

Intraocular Pressure

- Have IOP measured to rule out glaucoma if pain not clearly related to external eye or adnexa and no infection, foreign bodies, or globe puncture.

MANAGEMENT

OVERALL APPROACH

- Most serious causes of eye pain require prompt ophthalmologic referral, but consider managing minor foreign bodies and abrasions in office.

FOREIGN BODIES

- Irrigate with normal saline from squirt bottle, syringe without needle, or IV tubing to flush out foreign material.
- If irrigation fails, do not make any further attempt to remove foreign body if it is firmly embedded in cornea.

ABRASIONS

- Apply topical antibiotic (e.g., erythromycin ointment) and tight pressure patch for 24–48 hrs.
- Never apply antibiotic ointment if possibility of perforation. Under such circumstances, patch eye with protective metal or plastic shield and arrange referral; do not place any pressure on globe.

CONJUNCTIVITIS

- See Red Eye.

GLAUCOMA

- See Glaucoma.

INDICATIONS FOR REFERRAL

- Obtain prompt ophthalmologic consultation for vision loss or impairment.
- Also obtain consultation for progressive pain, redness, or discharge unresponsive to conservative Rx.
- Refer if pupil eccentric or anterior chamber shallow, suggesting loss of aqueous humor.

BIBLIOGRAPHY

- For the current annotated bibliography on eye pain, see the print edition of *Primary Care Medicine*, 4th edition, Chapter 201, or www.LWWmedicine.com.

Glaucoma

SCREENING AND/OR PREVENTION

GENERAL APPROACH

- Have all persons aged >40 screened for increased intraocular pressure (IOP).
- Note any optic nerve cupping during routine ophthalmoscopy.
- Refer promptly for Rx persons with ocular HTN or suspected optic nerve cupping.
- Refer urgently persons with suspected acute angle-closure glaucoma (e.g., painful red eye, decreased visual acuity, markedly elevated IOP, redness, fixed and nonreactive pupil in mid-dilation, and corneal haziness).

OPEN-ANGLE GLAUCOMA

- Determine onset and frequency of screening according to patient's risk factors:
  - Asymptomatic African-Americans: q3–5yrs between age 20–39, q2–4yrs between age 40–64, and q1–2yrs at age ≥65.
  - Other asymptomatic patients: <q3–5yrs between age 20–39, q2–4yrs between age 40–64, and q1–2yrs at age ≥65.
- As part of routine health maintenance exam, perform funduscopic exam, checking for notching, increased depth and width of physiologic cup, and progressive pallor; note any disc hemorrhages.
- Refer to eye specialist for direct measurement of IOP. Use of Schiøtz tonometer by PCP has not been demonstrated to have adequate specificity or sensitivity in detecting glaucoma to be valuable.
- Automated perimetry or nerve fiber layer analysis may be valuable future screening adjunct, but cost is too great, false-positives too frequent, and equipment too immobile to recommend at present.

MANAGEMENT

- Begin with a topical beta blocker, an agonist, topical carbonic anhydrase inhibitor, and/or prostaglandin analogue singly or in combination to reach target pressure.
- If medical Rx proves inadequate or intolerable, consider laser trabeculoplasty or surgery.
- Instruct patients taking drops on how to occlude nasal lacrimal ducts to minimize risk of systemic absorption through nasal mucosa.
- Have IOP, optic nerve appearance, visual field, and nerve fiber layer monitored by ophthalmologist to watch for disease progression.
- Know patient's ocular medications and their systemic side effects.
- Monitor IOP carefully in persons (especially elderly) taking high-dose nasal or inhaled steroids.

BIBLIOGRAPHY

■ For the current annotated bibliography on open-angle glaucoma, see the print edition of *Primary Care Medicine*, 4th edition, Chapters 198 and 207, or www.LWWmedicine.com.

Impaired Vision

SCREENING AND/OR PREVENTION

- Perform visual screening on all adults, especially hypertensives, diabetics, and the elderly.
- Refer for more detailed ophthalmologic evaluation if age >65, Hx of DM, glaucoma, eye trauma, eye infection, other eye problem, vision worse than 20/40 by Snellen's testing, or difference of >2 Snellen's lines between eyes.
- Arrange early and regular ophthalmologic screening of all diabetics (see Diabetic Retinopathy).

DIFFERENTIAL DIAGNOSIS

CAUSES OF IMPAIRED VISION

- Eyelids
  - Edema
  - Blepharospasm
- Cornea
  - Abrasion
  - Infection
  - Edema
  - Degeneration
- Anterior chamber
  - Inflammatory cells (from iritis)
  - Hyphema
- Lens
  - Cataract
  - Swelling [e.g., poorly controlled diabetes mellitus (DM)]
- Vitreous
  - Hemorrhage
  - Floaters
- Retina
  - Age-related macular degeneration
  - Central serous retinopathy
  - Inflammation
  - Trauma
  - Detachment
  - DM
  - Hypertension
- Vasculature
  - Central retinal artery occlusion
  - Giant cell (cranial or temporal) arteritis
  - Anterior ischemic optic neuropathy
  - Retinal vein occlusion

- Optic nerve
  - Compression (glaucoma, tumor)
- Psychiatric
  - Hysteria
  - Malingering
- Refractive error

WORKUP

HISTORY

- Establish onset, duration, clinical course, and pattern of vision loss (acute loss suggests vascular event, retinal detachment).
- Note any associated visual phenomena and pain.
- Inquire into telltale premonitory and associated symptoms:
  - Amaurosis fugax: central retinal artery occlusion, giant cell arteritis.
  - Sudden flurry of light flashes and vitreous floaters: retinal detachment.
  - Scintillating scotomata: migraine.
  - Progressive vision loss: cataract, macular degeneration, glaucoma.
  - Previous episodes of decreased visual acuity with halos around lights and pain: angle-closure glaucoma.
  - Foreign body sensation: corneal abrasion, foreign body, or herpes simplex keratitis.
- Check for contributing conditions (DM, HTN, heart disease, HIV infection, polymyalgia rheumatica, sickle cell anemia).
- Note any Hx of trauma or smoking.

PHYSICAL EXAM

- Check visual acuity, 1 eye at a time.
- If patient complains of associated pain, refer immediately for ophthalmologic evaluation.
- If lids tightly swollen, pry apart to test vision.
- Test with patient wearing distance glasses.
- For convenience, use Snellen's eye chart. If patient cannot read letters, note distance at which patient can accurately count fingers or identify hand motions.
- If patient cannot see targets, determine whether eye can perceive light.
- Recheck with patient looking through pinhole to eliminate any residual refractive error.
- Examine pupils carefully, noting size, direct and consensual light reactions, and presence of any afferent pupillary defect:
  - Afferent pupillary defect: optic neuritis, central retinal artery occlusion, giant cell arteritis, and extensive retinal diseases.
  - Fixed pupil with red eye: acute angle-closure glaucoma.
- Examine conjunctivae for signs of inflammation (trauma, acute glaucoma, and infection).
- Note cornea for clarity and crisp light reflex.

- If tonometer available, measure IOP.
- Perform ophthalmoscopy and note
  - whether you can visualize fundus or dense cataract or vitreous opacity is present;
  - optic disc for papilledema and atrophy;
  - macula for cherry-red spot, hemorrhages, and scars;
  - retinal vessels for caliber and any emboli.
- Check cranial arteries for enlargement, tenderness, and loss of pulsations in patients aged >50 with sudden vision loss (giant cell arteritis).
- Check opticokinetic responses (pass front page of newspaper before eyes) if malingering or hysteria suspected.

LAB STUDIES

- Obtain ESR if giant cell arteritis suspected, and consider need for temporal artery biopsy (see Giant Cell Arteritis).
- If retinal vein thrombosis noted, check for hypercoagulable state (see Deep Vein Thrombophlebitis).
- If diabetic retinopathy noted, check for glycemic control (see Diabetes Mellitus).
- If central retinal artery occlusion encountered, check for source of emboli.

MANAGEMENT

OVERALL APPROACH

- Obtain immediate ophthalmologic consultation if sudden vision loss.
- If ophthalmologist is not immediately available, initiate appropriate first aid emergency measures.

CENTRAL RETINAL ARTERY OCCLUSION (<24 HRS)

- Gently massage globe with fingers (to dislodge embolus).
- Have patient breathe mixture of 5% carbon dioxide and 95% oxygen (dilates retinal vessels, allows delivery of high PO_2 to any viable retinal cells) or have patient breathe into paper bag.
- Give 500 mg IV acetazolamide [decrease aqueous humor production, lower intraocular pressure (IOP)].

GIANT CELL ARTERITIS

- See also Giant Cell Arteritis.
- Start high-dose systemic glucocorticosteroids (e.g., prednisone, 60 mg/day; or IV Rx if vision loss marked and very recent).
- Refer for consideration of temporal artery biopsy.

ACUTE ANGLE-CLOSURE GLAUCOMA

- See also Glaucoma.
- Begin immediately topical pilocarpine 2% in both eyes and acetazolamide 500 mg IV.
- Consider other topical medications to help lower intraocular pressure [topical beta blockers (e.g., timolol, betaxolol, levobunolol), α-agonists

(brimonidine, apraclonidine), and carbonic anhydrase inhibitors (dorzolamide, brinzolamide)].

- Consider analgesics and antiemetics.
- If available, administer osmotic agents (IV mannitol or PO glycerol).
- Refer for laser iridotomy or peripheral iridectomy to prevent further attacks.

INDICATIONS FOR REFERRAL

- Refer all patients with acute vision loss immediately for ophthalmologic exam, especially if glaucoma, macular degeneration, retinal vein occlusion, retinal artery occlusion, or infectious etiology suspected or cause unclear.
- Refer all type 1 diabetics for annual ophthalmologic exam starting 5 yrs after onset of disease, and all type 2 diabetics at time of Dx.
- Refer patients with refractive error to eye specialist for proper refraction and consideration of refractive surgery if difficulty with glasses and/or contact lenses.

BIBLIOGRAPHY

- For the current annotated bibliography on impaired vision, see the print edition of *Primary Care Medicine*, 4th edition, Chapter 200, or www.LWWmedicine.com.

DIFFERENTIAL DIAGNOSIS

SOME IMPORTANT CAUSES OF RED EYE

- Conjunctival disease
  - Infection (bacterial, viral, chlamydial)
  - Allergy
  - Foreign body
  - Subconjunctival hemorrhage
  - Pinguecula
  - Pterygium
  - Episcleritis
  - Scleritis
  - Abrasion
- Corneal disease
  - HSV
  - Adenovirus
  - Herpes zoster
  - Keratoconjunctivitis sicca
  - Exposure keratopathy
  - Chemical trauma
  - Corneal ulceration (± concomitant infection)
- Uveal tract disease
  - Primary iritis and choroiditis
  - Secondary iritis (infection, trauma)
  - Systemic diseases (collagen vascular)
- Diseases of eyelid and orbit
  - Blepharitis
  - Chalazion
  - Hordeolum
  - Dacryocystitis
  - Cellulitis
  - Hemorrhage
- Intraocular disease
  - Acute glaucoma

CAUSES OF EYELID INFLAMMATION

- Bacterial infection
  - Impetigo
  - Erysipelas
- Viral infection
  - Herpes simplex virus
  - Molluscum contagiosum
  - Varicella zoster
  - Human papillomavirus
- Parasitic infection
  - *P. pubis*

602

■ Immunologic skin condition
  • Atopic dermatitis
  • Contact dermatitis
  • Erythema multiforme
  • Pemphigus foliaceus
  • Connective tissue disorders
  • SLE
  • Dermatomyositis
■ Dermatoses
  • Psoriasis
  • Ichthyosis
  • Exfoliative
  • Erythroderma
■ Benign eyelid tumors
  • Pseudoepitheliomatous hyperplasia
  • Actinic keratosis
  • Squamous cell papilloma
  • Sebaceous gland hyperplasia
  • Hemangioma
  • Pyogenic granuloma
■ Malignant eyelid tumors
  • Basal cell carcinoma
  • Squamous cell carcinoma
  • Sebaceous cell carcinoma
  • Melanoma
  • Kaposi's sarcoma
■ Other
  • Neurofibromatosis
  • Sarcoidosis
  • Down syndrome

WORKUP

OVERALL STRATEGY

■ Use clinical presentation and reference to characteristic findings to quickly assess underlying etiology:
  • Bacterial conjunctivitis: itching, tearing, mucopurulent discharge, diffuse conjunctival hyperemia, clear cornea, normal intraocular pressure (IOP).
  • Viral conjunctivitis: photophobia, foreign body sensation, itching, tearing, mucoid discharge, preauricular adenopathy, diffuse conjunctival hyperemia, cornea sometimes with faint punctate staining or infiltrates, normal IOP.
  • Allergic conjunctivitis: foreign body sensation, itching, tearing, diffuse conjunctival hyperemia, clear cornea, normal IOP.
  • Corneal injury or infection: decreased vision, pain, photophobia, foreign body sensation, tearing, preauricular adenopathy (in herpes keratitis), pupil normal or small (indicates secondary iritis), diffuse conjunctival hyperemia and ciliary flush, IOP normal or very low (in perforating trauma).
  • Iritis: decreased vision, pain, photophobia, tearing, small pupils, ciliary flush, clear or lightly cloudy cornea, IOP increased, normal, or decreased.

- Acute glaucoma: pain, pupils mid-dilated and fixed, diffuse conjuncti-val hyperemia and ciliary flush, cloudy cornea, increased IOP.

HISTORY

- Ascertain duration of redness, rapidity of onset, activity at onset, and degree and quality of symptoms.
- Inquire about any vision changes, pain, itching, morning crusting, tearing, mucoid or purulent discharge, photophobia, and foreign body sensation.
- Remember that viral conjunctivitis may cause foreign body sensation and herpes simplex keratitis may feel like "chemical" in eye.

PHYSICAL EXAM

- Accurately measure visual acuity, preferably at distance; if abnormal, check for uncorrected optical abnormality by use of pinhole.
- Immediately refer to ophthalmologist any patient with reduced vision accompanying red eye that is not readily explained by preexisting or obviously harmless condition (e.g., mucus or tearing may reduce vision by 1 or 2 lines at most; corneal lesions further reduce vision, with only partial improvement on pinhole testing; central epithelial abrasion typ-ically maintains vision at about 20/100 or better).
- Palpate preauricular nodes for enlargement (viral infection).
- Inspect lid margins for crusting, ulceration, inspissations, and masses, and conjunctiva for distribution of redness, ciliary flush, and foreign bodies (including lid eversion).
- Note any corneal clarity with flashlight supplemented by direct ophthal-moscope set at about +15 D to magnify corneal details.
- Refer immediately for slit lamp exam if corneal injury suspected.
- If glaucoma suspected, have the IOP measured.
- Note depth of anterior chamber by aiming flashlight parallel to iris (coronal plane) from temporal side (shallow anterior chamber will cast shadow on nasal iris).

LAB STUDIES

- Obtain CBC and differential and blood cultures in suspected cellulitis.
- Consider clotting studies for subconjunctival hemorrhage, but only if other evidence of coagulopathy is present or patient is on anticoagulant Rx.
- If bacterial or serious viral eye infection suspected, refer to ophthal-mologist for sampling of discharge, smear preparation, and culturing.
- Ensure that purulent discharges are Gram's stained and then cultured on blood agar and, if *Neisseria* suspected, on chocolate agar.

MANAGEMENT

GENERAL APPROACH

- Refer immediately any patient with red eye problem associated with eye pain, visual disturbance, or corneal damage; also refer if acute glaucoma suspected.
- Never prescribe topical steroid or steroid-antibiotic combination drops without ophthalmologic consultation (infection may worsen, corneal ulcer may rapidly form and cause perforation).

CONJUNCTIVAL DISEASE

- Immediately refer if severe photophobia, eye pain, or change in visual acuity, otherwise begin initial management.

Viral Conjunctivitis

- Instruct patient to refrain from eye rubbing and transmitting infection to other eye or other persons (live virus shed in tears up to 2 wks).
- Treat expectantly (self-limited, clearing within 2–3 wks).
- Refer if failure to clear spontaneously.

Bacterial Conjunctivitis

- Prescribe erythromycin ophthalmic ointment (qid) or polymyxin/trimethoprim (Polytrim) drops (qid); alternatives include bacitracin ophthalmic ointment and sodium sulfacetamide.
- Avoid neomycin (allergic keratitis in 5%) and more potent topical antibiotics (aminoglycosides, fluoroquinolones; reserved for use by ophthalmologists).

Allergic Conjunctivitis

- Recommend in seasonal allergies cool compresses and decongestant-antihistamine drops [naphazoline (Vasocon-A, Naphcon-A, Albalon-A)], antihistamine [levocabastine (Livostin)], or topical mast cell stabilizers [cromolyn (Opticrom), olopatadine (Patanol), and others] up to qid.
- Avoid long-term use of decongestant drops (marked rebound vasodilation).
- Consider ocular (ketorolac) ophthalmic drops (NSAID).
- Alternatively, prescribe oral antihistamines.
- If unresponsive, refer for consideration of topical steroid Rx.

Subconjunctival Hemorrhage

- Provide reassurance (harmless and self-limited).
- If marked swelling, recommend compresses (initially cool, then warm) and erythromycin ophthalmic ointment or lubricating ointment.

Conjunctival Foreign Bodies

- Remove with cotton swab and apply erythromycin ointment (tid × 2 days).

EYELID AND ORBITAL DISEASE

Blepharitis

- Recommend lid hygiene measures and topical antibiotics.
- Instruct patient to dilute Johnson's baby shampoo with water (50:50) and use cotton ball to scrub lids well with eyes closed.
- Follow with water rinse and application of hot compress to closed lids for 5–10 mins.
- Have patient then apply erythromycin or bacitracin ophthalmic ointment tid–qid into inferior fornix, rubbing excess into eyelash base; continue until improved.
- Recommend maintaining nightly lid hygiene and warm compresses.

Chronic Blepharitis and Meibomian Gland Inflammatory Disease

- Consider oral Rx for acne rosacea (usual cause) in addition to topical Rx.

- Prescribe low-dose tetracycline antibiotic (e.g., tetracycline, 250 mg/day; doxycycline, 50 or 100 mg/day; or minocycline 50 mg/day) or 7- to 14-day course of double- or triple-antibiotic Rx for *H. pylori* infection (e.g., amoxicillin, metronidazole, bismuth subsalicylate; see Peptic Ulcer Disease).

Hordeolum

- For mild cellulitis of lid margin (preseptal cellulitis), prescribe topical lid Rx (as above) + oral antibiotics (e.g., dicloxacillin, 250 mg qid; or erythromycin, 250–500 mg tid if penicillin allergic).
- For orbital cellulitis and orbital cellulitis complicated by cavernous sinus thrombosis, admit urgently.

Acute Dacryocystitis

- Recommend warm compresses and oral antibiotics, but refer if local abscess (requires incision and drainage).

Mild Hypersensitivity Reactions

- Advise discontinuing offending agent and applying cool compresses.
- Consider systemic antihistamines in moderately severe reactions and systemic steroids in severe reactions causing lids to swell shut.

Traumatic Lid Ecchymoses

- Apply cool compresses and ice packs early; then switch to warm compresses.

CORNEAL DISEASE

Corneal Ulcers

- Refer for intensive emergency evaluation and Rx by ophthalmologist.
- If ophthalmologist not immediately available and patient presents with typical herpes simplex dendritic keratitis, consider starting trifluridine (Viroptic) drops (up to 9 times/day) or vidarabine (Vira-A) ointment (5 times/day), + erythromycin ointment bid.

Corneal Abrasions

- Prescribe erythromycin ointment and tight sterile patch that prevents lid motion for 24–48 hrs.
- If initial abrasion was sizable (≥25% of cornea), check after patch removal; consider cycloplegia for painful secondary iritis.
- After reepithelialization, advise ointment application tid × 4 days.

Foreign Bodies

- Treat first with vigorous irrigation.
- Manage rust rings as abrasions after washing away foreign body.
- Consider using cotton swab for foreign bodies that do not wash away (do not use sharp instruments unless trained in technique).
- Débride rust on surface carefully; avoid scraping (damage to Bowman's membrane, permanent scarring). If rust cannot be removed, leave it (untreated, it will surface and slough in 1–2 wks, although may be irritating transiently).

Contact Lens Overwear and Ultraviolet Keratitis

- Prescribe brief cycloplegia, erythromycin ointment, and sterile pressure patching for 24 hrs.
- Consider analgesics for severe associated pain.

Suspected Corneal Laceration and Perforation

- Refer emergently; place protective metal shield ("Fox shield") over eye; do not instill medication.

UVEAL TRACT DISEASE

- Refer to ophthalmologist for initial evaluation and management.
- If ophthalmologist not immediately available, consider cycloplegia.
- If secondary to corneal abrasion, prescribe tropicamide 1% qid or cyclopentolate 1% qid, or in eye that will be patched for 1–2 days, several drops scopolamine 0.25% for longer cycloplegia (avoid atropine; effects persist for 1–2 wks).

INTRAOCULAR DISEASE

Acute Glaucoma

- Treat immediately with acetazolamide, 500 mg IV, and glycerol, 120 mL PO in orange juice.
- Instill pilocarpine 2% q15min to break attack.
- Refer immediately for definitive Rx (laser or surgical iridotomy).

BIBLIOGRAPHY

- For the current annotated bibliography on red eye, see the print edition of *Primary Care Medicine*, 4th edition, Chapter 199, or www.LWWmedicine.com.

Refractive Surgery

MANAGEMENT

OVERALL APPROACH

- Provide overview and basic information by reviewing with patient advantages and disadvantages of available procedures.
- Refer to ophthalmologist skilled in performing these procedures for further consultation if surgery makes good medical sense.

LASER PROCEDURES

- Refractive surgery offers way of reducing or eliminating dependence on glasses and/or contact lenses to obtain clear vision.
- Ophthalmic lasers correct myopia, hyperopia, and astigmatism by reshaping cornea.
- LASIK is currently most advanced and predictable refractive procedure available.
- PRK is an earlier laser application, but more risk of corneal scarring.
- Postoperatively, epithelium heals across recontoured anterior corneal stromal surface.
- In LASIK, surgeon first creates flap of anterior corneal tissue; much less of corneal surface is disrupted than in PRK, and return of vision is faster, with minimal pain, and elimination of risk of anterior corneal scarring.
- LASIK requires higher surgical skills than PRK (flap creation with microkeratome).
- About two-thirds of patients see 20/20 or better with no glasses, and 95% see 20/40 or better.
- Surgeon can perform retreatments within several mos after LASIK and ≥6 mos after PRK if refractive error not acceptably corrected.
- Laser procedures can treat hyperopia and astigmatism but not eliminate need for reading glasses in presbyopia.
- Anterior corneal scarring is risk with PRK; virtually eliminated with LASIK.
- Flap complications in LASIK are function of surgeon's experience, but rarely lead to decrease in visual acuity.
- LASIK patients may experience transient glare, halos, monocular diplopia, and/or dry eyes, which decrease with time.
- Patient selection is important and includes
  - age >21;
  - relatively stable refractive error;
  - LASIK relatively contraindicated in ocular Hx of herpes simplex keratitis, irregular astigmatism, keratoconus, corneal scars, exposure keratitis, and autoimmune disease that could alter wound healing;
  - PRK absolutely contraindicated with RA and SLE, in immunocompromised patients, and those with other systemic illness that affect wound healing, and in keloid formers.

INTRASTROMAL CORNEAL RING SEGMENTS

- Review advantages (preservation of central corneal visual zone and removability) and disadvantages (deposits around implants and corneal instability with diurnal variation causing myopic shift at end of day).

INTRAOCULAR LENSES

- Investigational; correction of myopia with intraocular lens implantation.
- Provides predictable, high-quality, higher-range approach to vision correction.
- Serious potential complications: corneal edema, iritis, cataract development, and glaucoma.
- Long-term follow-up in controlled studies needed.
- Reserved for levels of myopia and hyperopia untreatable by other corrective surgeries.

THERMOKERATOPLASTY

- Investigational; reshaping cornea by precision heat from infrared holmium laser.
- May prove useful for low to moderate hyperopia, offering technical simplicity and nearly immediate useful vision.

BIBLIOGRAPHY

- For the current annotated bibliography on refractive surgery, see the print edition of *Primary Care Medicine*, 4th edition, Chapter 210, or www.LWWmedicine.com.

Visual Disturbances

DIFFERENTIAL DIAGNOSIS

CAUSES OF FLOATERS AND FLASHING LIGHTS

- Floaters
  - Myopia
  - Aging
  - Vitreous detachment
  - Retinal tear
  - Retinal detachment
  - Intraocular inflammation (uveitis, retinitis)
  - Vitreous hemorrhage
- Flashing lights
  - Vitreoretinal traction
  - Retinal detachment
  - Mechanical stimulation (cough, rubbing eyes, head trauma)
  - Classic migraine
  - Seizure activity in visual cortex (static light, colored flashes)

WORKUP

HISTORY

- Obtain complete, detailed description of visual disturbance with no leading questions.
- Note onset, course, and any associated symptoms (e.g., headache, decreased visual acuity).
- Check for sudden onset of flashing lights and/or floaters (vitreoretinal traction due to vitreous detachment, retinal tear, or retinal detachment), new onset in immunocompromised patient (CMV retinitis), flashes of light on waking and rubbing eyes (harmless), and floaters present for extended time without marked increase in number (harmless).
- If halos reported, check for glaucoma (see Glaucoma).
- If reports of lightning flashes, yellow discoloration, or frost over objects, review medications and clinical Hx for digitalis toxicity.
- If vision distortion, consider subretinal fluid accumulation and macular degeneration.
- Check for Hx of migraine or family Hx of headaches.

PHYSICAL EXAM

- Test visual acuity and visual fields, and have IOP measured (see Glaucoma).
- Examine fundus for vitreous hemorrhage, ballooning white area suggesting retinal detachment, areas of retinal inflammation, and macular abnormalities.

■ In immunocompromised patients, look for signs of CMV retinitis (e.g., focal, granular, perivascular yellow-white lesions ± hemorrhage in "brushfire" pattern).

LAB STUDIES

■ Refer promptly to ophthalmologist for indirect ophthalmoscopy and scleral depression if patient reports new flashes and/or floaters.
■ Refer patients with metamorphopsia for fluorescein angiography.
■ Arrange measurement of IOP in patient with halos.
■ Check serum levels of digoxin, potassium, BUN, and creatinine in suspected digitalis toxicity (see Congestive Heart Failure).
■ Arrange EEG and MRI scanning of head if patient reports visual hallucinations.

MANAGEMENT

■ Arrange urgent referral for new onset of unexplained flashes or floaters (retinal tear, retinal detachment, or inflammatory/infectious process— e.g., CMV retinitis), especially if field loss detected.
■ Also refer urgently for vision distortion (age-related macular degeneration) and consideration of need for macular photocoagulation.
■ Make prompt referral for report of halos indicating glaucoma.
■ Encourage complete eye exam for patients with chronic flashes and floaters.
■ Advise all patients with flashes and floaters of need to immediately report onset of new floaters or flashes or appearance of peripheral visual field defects.
■ Reassure patient with chronic floaters in absence of ocular disease and person with migraine that ophthalmologic prognosis is excellent.
■ Reassure patients with flashes that occur with minor mechanical stimulation (cough, rubbing of eyes) as long as there is no evidence of more serious pathology.

BIBLIOGRAPHY

■ For the current annotated bibliography on visual disturbances, see the print edition of *Primary Care Medicine*, 4th edition, Chapter 203, or www.LWWmedicine.com.

Ear, Nose, and Throat Problems

Epistaxis

SCREENING AND/OR PREVENTION

- Instruct patient on avoiding trauma to mucosa. Specifically, warn against habitual nose picking, constant rubbing with handkerchief, and excessively forceful blowing. Trim fingernails of children short.
- Have patient keep septum well coated with petrolatum-based ointment, such as zinc oxide, A and D ointment, or antibiotic ointment, until healed, usually in 3–5 days.
- Teach control of minor recurrent bleeding by use of cotton pledgets soaked in vasoconstricting solution (e.g., 1:1,000 epinephrine) or vasoconstricting nosedrop (e.g., Neo-Synephrine or Afrin) and pressed against bleeding site.
- Explain importance of humidifying home environment; have patient keep several windows partially open, place containers of water near radiators or stoves, or install humidifier.
- Consider patient application of water-based lubricant to rims of nostrils to maintain mucosal moisture.

DIFFERENTIAL DIAGNOSIS

MAJOR CAUSES OF EPISTAXIS

- Local disease
  - Dry indoor environment
  - URI
  - Chronic sinusitis
  - Trauma (nose picking, forceful blowing)
  - Occupational irritant exposure
  - Cocaine abuse
  - Angiomas
  - Allergies
  - Lack of humidification
  - Malignancy
- Systemic disease
  - Granulomatous disease (Wegener's, sarcoidosis)
  - Hereditary hemorrhagic telangiectasia
  - Infection (chickenpox, influenza)
  - Bleeding diathesis
  - Malignant HTN

WORKUP

HISTORY

- Inquire into amount of bleeding, duration, and frequency.
- Review for risk factors and Hx of bleeding diathesis (easy bruising, hematuria, melena, heavy menstrual periods, family Hx of bleeding disorders, use of oral anticoagulants, antiplatelet agents).

- Check for environmental and traumatic factors (occupational exposure to irritating chemicals or dust, dry home, chronic cocaine use, and repeated nose blowing or picking).

PHYSICAL EXAM

- Have patient sit up and lean forward so that any blood flows from nose (allowing assessment of rate and site of bleeding and preventing emesis from swallowing blood).
- Check pulse and BP for any postural hypotension.
- Note skin, mucous membranes, and conjunctiva for pallor, purpura, petechiae, telangiectasias, and rash.
- Examine lymph nodes for enlargement (sarcoidosis, tuberculosis, malignancy).
- Percuss sinuses for evidence of sinusitis (suggesting Wegener's, midline granuloma, and nasal tumor).

LAB STUDIES

- Use findings from Hx and PE to guide testing.
- Obtain PT, PTT, bleeding time, blood smear, and platelet count if bleeding diathesis suspected (see Bleeding Problems).
- Check sinus films if there are recurrent bouts of sinus pain, tenderness, and bleeding.

MANAGEMENT

FIRST AID

- Teach patient-administered first aid:
  - Instruct patient to sit up and remain calm, lean forward, and pinch against septum nostril that is bleeding to tamponade flow.
  - Then have patient spray nose with phenylephrine-containing OTC nasal spray (e.g., Neo-Synephrine or Afrin).
  - Follow with use of small pledget of cotton lightly soaked with spray and pressed against bleeding portion of septum. After 10 mins, most nosebleeds stop.
  - Have patient apply petrolatum-based ointment such as zinc oxide or bacitracin to septum to prevent further drying and abrasion. Keep in for several days.
  - Instruct patient to limit heavy lifting, other forms of straining, bending over, intake of spicy or hot foods, hot showers, and medications that might impair hemostasis (see Bleeding Disorders).
  - Reassure patient when nosebleed is purely local phenomenon; many people attribute nosebleeds to HTN and fear cerebral hemorrhage.

ANTERIOR SEPTAL BLEEDING

- Have patient sit up (reduces venous pressure) and lean forward (prevents swallowing blood).
- Soak small piece of cotton or cotton ball in 1:1,000 epinephrine or vasoconstricting nosedrop such as phenylephrine (Neo-Synephrine) or oxymetazoline (Afrin) and place it in nasal vestibule, pressed against bleeding site for 10–15 mins.
- Remove to observe for rebleeding.

- Prescribe humidification and lubricant such as petrolatum ointment to promote healing.
- If these remedies fail, anesthetize mucous membrane by applying cotton soaked with 4% lidocaine (or 4% cocaine, if available) for 5 mins and apply silver nitrate stick to bleeding site and any prominent vessels.
- If small artery in septal mucous membrane continues bleeding or rebleeds short time later, repeat silver nitrate cautery procedure.
- Follow by placing small amount of oxidized regenerated cellulose (Surgicel) against bleeding artery or small packing of petroleum gauze strip and leave in nasal vestibule for 24 hrs.
- Avoid abrading mucous membrane, especially if bleeding disorder present.
- Recommend humidification, copious lubricants, and soft cotton tamponades wetted with long-acting vasoconstricting drops [oxymetazoline 0.05% (Afrin nasal solution)].
- Avoid packing if possible; if unavoidable, use piece of oxidized cellulose (does not require removal).
- Treat any underlying bleeding disorder.

POSTERIOR EPISTAXIS

- If postural hypotension present, arrange for immediate ER care by ENT specialist.
- Meanwhile, instruct patient to sit up and lean forward.
- If bleeding stops temporarily, spray nose with topical anesthetic and vasoconstricting substance (e.g., oxymetazoline 0.05%, or cocaine 4%, if available).
- Do not have patient blow nose in absence of means of dealing with brisk bleeding that might ensue.
- If blood pressure permits, administer parenteral analgesic [e.g., meperidine (Demerol), 50 or 100 mg IM] in preparation for surgical electrocautery of posterior nose or placement of compressing balloons, packs, or tampons.

INDICATIONS FOR REFERRAL AND ADMISSION

- Refer for prompt emergency ENT care (including endoscopic cautery) if active posterior bleeding.
- Admit for observation, IV hydration, pain control, and possibly antibiotics any patient who undergoes extensive posterior nasal packing (airway obstruction, painful difficult swallowing, infection); elderly at greatest risk.

BIBLIOGRAPHY

- For the current annotated bibliography on epistaxis, see the print edition of *Primary Care Medicine*, 4th edition, Chapter 213, or www.LWWmedicine.com.

Facial Pain and Swelling

SCREENING AND/OR PREVENTION

- Inquire into time of last dental exam.
- Examine teeth and gums for plaque and gingival disease.
- Urge regular brushing with fluoride-containing dentifrice and flossing.
- Recommend yearly dental exam and plaque removal.
- Know fluoridation status of local public water supply before prescribing fluoride-containing vitamins to pediatric patients.

DIFFERENTIAL DIAGNOSIS

IMPORTANT CAUSES OF FACIAL PAIN OR SWELLING

- Odontogenic pain
  - Caries
  - Pulpitis
  - Periapical abscess
  - Alveolar abscess
- Nonodontogenic pain
  - Trigeminal neuralgia
  - Temporomandibular joint dysfunction
  - Myocardial ischemia (referred jaw pain)
  - Giant cell arteritis (masseter claudication)
- Salivary pain and swelling
  - Viral infection (mumps)
  - Bacterial infection
  - Ductal obstruction
  - Sjögren's syndrome
  - Lymphoproliferative disease
  - Tumor
  - Chemical irritant

WORKUP

HISTORY

- Elicit onset, severity, quality, location, radiation, aggravating and ameliorating factors, and duration of pain.
- Note if brought on by contact with hot, cold, or sweet substances (dental caries) or if aggravated by heat and relieved by cold (periapical abscess).
- Check for fever and swelling (alveolar abscess).
- Inquire into any lancinating pain precipitated by contact with trigger zone (trigeminal neuralgia); distinguish from abscess by lack of effect of temperature on pain and absence of swelling.

617

- In patient who complains of salivary gland enlargement, inquire into site(s) of involvement, presence of fever or tenderness, Hx of chronic illness, malignancy, toxin or drug exposure, and symptoms of rheumatologic disease or sicca syndrome (dry eyes/mouth).
- Note any report of acute unilateral salivary gland swelling and pain, especially in elderly, debilitated, or postoperative patient (sialadenitis).
- Check for any painless progressive parotid enlargement, be it unilateral (tumor) or bilateral (lymphoma, sarcoidosis, Sjögren's syndrome).
- Consider coronary ischemia whenever jaw pain reported, especially if exertional.

PHYSICAL EXAM

- Examine in semi-sitting position.
- Use lighting fixture that can illuminate oral cavity while leaving hands free.
- Inspect mouth for fractured, decayed, or heavily restored teeth and for heavy deposits of debris and calculus (tartar) on teeth and gingivae (odontogenic disease).
- If available, use dental mirror or short-handled laryngoscopy mirror to retract tongue; otherwise use wooden tongue blade.
- Palpate teeth to determine any tenderness and mobility, and soft tissues for indurated or fluctuant swelling adjacent to suspicious tooth (abscess).
- Percuss teeth for tenderness (diagnostic of abscessed tooth).
- Palpate salivary glands bimanually (intraorally and extraorally).
- Observe salivary duct orifices for salivary flow and any purulent drainage.
- Palpate all lymph nodes for enlargement and tenderness.

LAB STUDIES

- Confirm suspected dental caries or abscess by dental referral for x-ray.
- Check WBC count if acute sialadenitis suspected clinically, and glucose in diabetics with facial pain.
- If Sjögren's syndrome suspected, screen for connective tissue disease with serum ANA testing and, if positive, follow with anti-Ro and anti-La antibody determinations (see Dry Eyes).
- Send any purulent salivary gland drainage for Gram's stain, culture, and sensitivity testing.

MANAGEMENT

TOOTH OR PERIODONTAL ABSCESS

- While awaiting dental evaluation, provide patient with sufficient analgesia (e.g., ibuprofen, 800 mg q8h; or codeine sulfate, 30 mg q4–6h).
- Begin penicillin V potassium (250–500 mg PO q6h) if clinical evidence of infection.
- If underlying valvular heart disease, consider endocarditis prophylaxis before dental procedure (e.g., amoxicillin, single 2-g dose PO 1 hr before; or, if penicillin allergic, clindamycin, 600 mg; cephalexin, 2 g; or azithromycin, 500 PO 1 hr before procedure; see Bacterial Endocarditis).

■ Promptly refer to oral surgeon for definitive drainage of infection at earliest opportunity; do not rely on antibiotics to clear infection.

SIALADENITIS

■ Stimulate salivary flow with sour candies and warm compresses.

■ For submandibular sialadenitis, begin penicillin (as above).

■ For acute bacterial parotitis, start with antistaphylococcal Rx (e.g., dicloxacillin, 500 mg qid).

■ Culture any purulent discharge to guide further antibiotic Rx.

INDICATIONS FOR REFERRAL

■ Make early dental referral for any signs of dental decay or gingival inflammation, especially in patients with compromised oral hygiene due to bulimia, Sjögren's syndrome, HIV infection, or upcoming cancer Rx (e.g., head and neck irradiation, chemotherapy).

■ Recommend regular periodic full dental evaluation for patient with valvular heart disease, especially before consideration of valvular prosthesis; provide endocarditis prophylaxis before each visit (see Bacterial Endocarditis).

■ Arrange dental/oral surgical consultation when PE suggests oral cavity source of facial pain.

■ Promptly refer patient with abscess for definitive drainage procedure.

■ If deep facial pathology suspected as source of pain (fever, trismus, elevation of tongue, or ophthalmoplegia), refer emergently to oral surgeon and arrange for prompt admission to hospital for parenteral antibiotics.

■ For acute salivary swelling, set up oral surgery visit quickly for exam and radiographic study to detect and relieve any obstructing sialoliths (sialography is contraindicated in acute period of infection; CT or MRI usually suffices).

■ Consider biopsy of minor salivary gland of lip if Sjögren's syndrome, sarcoidosis, or lymphoma is a consideration (obviating parotid biopsy).

BIBLIOGRAPHY

■ For the current annotated bibliography on facial pain and swelling, see the print edition of *Primary Care Medicine*, 4th edition, Chapter 214, or www.LWWmedicine.com.

Halitosis

DIFFERENTIAL DIAGNOSIS

- Oral cavity: poorly fitting dental work, periodontal disease, sialadenitis, abscess
- Posterior pharynx: tonsillitis, diverticulum, tumor
- Sinus: sinusitis, tumor, necrotic disease
- Esophagus: reflux, diverticulum, motor dysfunction
- Lungs: abscess
- Metabolic: renal or hepatic failure; ketoacidosis
- Psychiatric: psychosis (self-perception only)

WORKUP

- Concentrate on detecting oral cavity and nasal pathology.
- Directly confirm reported odor.
- Differentiate oral source from nasal one by pinching nares closed while patient exhales and by having patient exhale through nose with mouth closed.
- Check for poorly fitting dental work, periodontal disease, glossitis, tooth abscess, and tonsillar disease.
- Assess salivary glands for purulent discharge and obstruction of saliva flow.
- When oral cavity and sinus tracts appear normal, consider gastroesophageal reflux, pulmonary disease, and metabolic dysfunction.
- Order psychiatric consultation when there are no objective findings but psychotic behavior is evident in addition to olfactory hallucinations.

MANAGEMENT

- Treat etiologically for best results.
- Emphasize good oral hygiene, especially in the elderly; encourage regular flossing and brushing; arrange regular dental checkups; mouthwashes are poor substitute for good oral hygiene.
- Refer to endodontist if gum disease prevalent.
- Consider empirical course of acid suppression for suspected reflux-induced disease.

BIBLIOGRAPHY

- For the current annotated bibliography on halitosis, see the print edition of *Primary Care Medicine*, 4th edition, Chapter 215, or www.LWWmedicine.com.

Hearing Loss

SCREENING AND/OR PREVENTION

- Perform periodic hearing assessment of all elderly persons.
- Consider self-administered questionnaire for screening and determining who requires testing.
- Hold off screening for hearing-loss gene mutations (in *GJB2*) until benefits are clearer.

DIFFERENTIAL DIAGNOSIS

COMMON AND IMPORTANT CAUSES OF HEARING LOSS

- Conductive
  - Impacted cerumen
  - Foreign body
  - Occlusive edema of auditory canal
  - Perforation of tympanic membrane
  - Chronic otitis media
  - Serous otitis media
  - External otitis
  - Otosclerosis
  - Exostoses
  - Developmental defects
  - Glomus tumors
- Sensorineural
  - Presbycusis
  - Noise-induced deafness
  - Drugs (aminoglycosides, loop diuretics, quinidine, aspirin)
  - Meniere's disease
  - Acoustic neuroma
  - Hypothyroidism (mild loss)
  - Idiopathic sudden deafness
  - Congenital syphilis
  - Diabetes mellitus
  - Perilymph leak
  - Multiple sclerosis

WORKUP

HISTORY

- Focus on detecting site of lesion, aided by identifying whether impairment is conductive or sensorineural.
- Ascertain sounds or situations in which patient has most trouble hearing (difficulty understanding spoken words suggests sensorineural hearing loss).

- Inquire into drug use, focusing on aminoglycosides, quinine derivatives, salicylates, chemotherapeutics, and loop diuretics (furosemide, ethacrynic acid).
- Note any Hx of otitis, noise trauma (both recreational and work related), or head trauma.
- Check family Hx [gene mutations, otosclerosis, acoustic neuromas (associated with von Recklinghausen's disease)].

PHYSICAL EXAM

- Inspect external auditory canal for obstruction (impacted cerumen, foreign body, external otitis, exostoses).
- Examine tympanic membranes for inflammation, perforation, and scarring.
- Check for fluid in middle ear and for reddish mass visible through intact tympanic membrane (high-riding jugular bulb, aberrant internal carotid artery, or glomus tumor).
- Perform pneumatic otoscopy to assess tympanic membrane mobility.
- Conduct nasopharyngeal exam in patients with persisting serous otitis media, particularly if unilateral.
- If vertigo or suspected glomus or acoustic tumor, conduct complete cranial nerve exam.

Hearing Testing

- Use old-fashioned mechanical watch ticking as crude screen for high-frequency impairment.
- Otherwise, perform whispering, gradually increasing its intensity, asking patient to repeat words whispered into tested ear while masking contralateral ear with some background noise.
- Use familiar disyllabic words in which both syllables are equally accented (e.g., pancake, hot dog).
- With these measures, roughly estimate patient's hearing thresholds.
- Use high-frequency (512-Hz) tuning fork to detect hearing loss; assess threshold of perception by striking tuning fork against heel of hand, withdrawing it at 1 ft/sec, starting 1 in. from ear, until it becomes imperceptible, and noting distance.

Differentiating Conductive from Sensorineural Hearing Loss

- Perform Weber's test [placing vibrating tuning fork midline on skull and noting any difference in perceived loudness (conductive loss = sound clearer in involved ear; sensorineural loss = sound clearer in better ear)].
- Perform Rinne test (vibrating fork placed on mastoid process until sound gone, then rapidly repositioned without reactivation in front of external auditory canal to see if, and how long, sound is heard again). Normally sound by air conduction twice as long as by bone conduction; reduced in conductive loss.
- Alternatively, place vibrating tuning fork on mastoid process for several seconds and then in front of external auditory canal to determine which produces "louder" sound (in conductive loss, bone conduction > air conduction; in sensorineural and normal, air conduction > bone conduction).
- Compare examiner's bone conduction hearing (if normal) with patient's (Schwabach test; sensorineural loss = patient perceives sound for less time than examiner; conductive loss = patient perceives sound for longer time than examiner).

LAB STUDIES

- Obtain audiogram to help classify hearing loss as conductive or sensorineural and to subclassify according to pattern detected (see appendix to Chapter 212 in *Primary Care Medicine*, 4th edition).
- Order additional studies only as suggested by initial testing and usually only after expert consultation.
- Consider CT scanning only if there is concern about specific middle ear or mastoid disorders (e.g., chronic infection, glomus tumors).
- Reserve MRI with gadolinium enhancement for strong clinical/audiologic suspicion of retrocochlear disease (e.g., acoustic neuroma, MS).
- Similarly, consider auditory brainstem response testing and electronystagmography only with expert consultation to determine site of lesion.
- In patients who are difficult to test, consider evaluation of otoacoustic emissions.

MANAGEMENT

- Recommend that elderly patients cup hand behind ear if having trouble hearing.
- Suggest supplementary speech reading (interpreting what is being said by extrapolating from words heard and facial expressions).
- Advise household members to clearly enunciate, rather than just speak louder, and to directly face patient with presbycusis while speaking.
- Remove any impacted cerumen or other obstruction.
- Cease use of ototoxic drugs.
- Treat any concurrent otitis media.
- Advise limiting exposure to occupational and recreational noise and to use ear protection when exposure unavoidable.

INDICATIONS FOR REFERRAL

- Obtain otoneurologic referral when conductive etiology or acoustic neuroma suggested by clinical findings.
- Arrange otologic assessment when simple symptomatic measures insufficient and quality of life being seriously compromised by hearing loss. Similarly, refer when clinical findings suggest conduction disease and when there is sensorineural hearing loss that may benefit from hearing aid (e.g., flat hearing threshold and good discrimination).
- Initiate immediate otolaryngologic referral when there is true sudden hearing loss.

BIBLIOGRAPHY

- For the current annotated bibliography on hearing loss, see the print edition of *Primary Care Medicine*, 4th edition, Chapter 212, or www.LWWmedicine.com.

Hiccups

DIFFERENTIAL DIAGNOSIS

CONDITIONS ASSOCIATED WITH PERSISTENT HICCUP (UNPROVED ETIOLOGIES)

- Structural pathology
  - Pericarditis
  - Tumor
  - Pneumonia
  - Pleuritis
  - Myocardial infarction
  - Hiatal hernia
  - Peritonitis
  - Gastric dilatation
  - Pancreatitis
  - Biliary tract disease
  - Tympanic membrane irritation
  - Aortic aneurysm
- Metabolic disturbances
  - Uremia
  - Diabetes mellitus
  - Alcoholism
- CNS disease
  - Tumor
  - Infection
  - Surgery
- Psychogenic disease
  - Hysteria
  - Anorexia nervosa
  - Anxiety

WORKUP

HISTORY

- Inquire into recent abdominal, thoracic, or neurologic surgery, abdominal pain (especially radiating to tip of shoulder or worsened by respiration), prior renal disease, excess alcohol consumption, fever, cough, DM, and emotional problems.
- Review methods patient has tried for symptom relief.
- Note any neurologic complaints.

PHYSICAL EXAM

- Check temp and tympanic membranes; percuss lungs for evidence of reduced diaphragmatic excursion; and auscultate for signs of infiltrate, effusion, or pleuritis.

- Examine abdomen for distention, organomegaly, upper abdominal tenderness, and signs of peritonitis.
- Conduct neurologic exam if there is Hx of neurologic difficulties.

LAB STUDIES

- Test only if hiccups persist for days.
- Begin with CXR.
- Obtain serum determinations of sodium, creatinine, and BUN.
- Consider abdominal CT, concentrating on subdiaphragmatic region.
- If CNS disease suspected, consider neuroimaging (CT or MRI).

MANAGEMENT

- For patients with no serious underlying disease, recommend home remedies that interrupt reflex arc:
  - Holding breath and breathing into paper bag
  - Swallowing tsp granulated sugar
  - Placing finger into back of pharynx and stimulating gag reflex
  - Drinking from wrong side of glass
  - Rubbing nasopharynx with cotton swab
  - Passing nasogastric tube, if other methods fail
- For persistent symptoms when cause remains undiagnosed or untreatable, consider
  - chlorpromazine, 25–50 mg IV, then oral maintenance Rx of 25 mg qid;
  - metoclopramide IV, followed by oral Rx (10 mg tid);
  - phenytoin and carbamazepine in patients with CNS etiology.
- When all other measures fail and hiccups remain disabling, consider surgical infiltration of phrenic nerve on involved side.

BIBLIOGRAPHY

- For the current annotated bibliography on hiccups, see the print edition of *Primary Care Medicine*, 4th edition, Chapter 221, or www.LWWmedicine.com.

DIFFERENTIAL DIAGNOSIS

- Acute hoarseness
  - Acute laryngitis
    - Viral infection
    - Vocal abuse
    - Toxic fumes
    - Allergy (seasonal)
  - Acute laryngeal edema
    - Angioneurotic edema
    - Infection
    - Direct injury
    - Nephritis
  - Acute epiglottitis
- Chronic hoarseness
  - Chronic laryngitis
    - Chronic or recurrent vocal abuse
    - Smoking
    - Allergy
    - Persistent irritant exposure
  - Carcinoma of larynx
    - Intrinsic to vocal cords
    - Extrinsic to vocal cords
  - Vocal cord lesions
    - Polyps
    - Leukoplakia
    - Contact ulcer and granuloma
    - Vocal nodule
    - Benign tumors
  - Vocal cord paralysis
    - Laryngeal nerve injury (tumor, neck surgery, aortic aneurysm)
    - Brainstem lesion
  - Vocal cord trauma
    - Chronic intubation
  - Systemic disorders
    - Hypothyroidism
    - Rheumatoid arthritis
    - Virilization
- Psychogenic

WORKUP

HISTORY

- Determine whether onset was sudden or gradual, and course self-limited or progressive.
- Note any difficulty breathing or stridor (obstruction); if present, admit to hospital emergently.

- Check for hoarseness exacerbated by talking; ask whether voice completely disappeared, and, if so, for how long.
- Inquire into any recent excessive voice use, URI, sore throat, fever, chills, sputum, and myalgias.
- Document irritant exposures (cigarette smoking, dust, fire, smoke, or irritant fumes).
- Note alcohol intake.
- Ask about Hx of neck mass, neck surgery, intubation, and lung tumor.
- Check for symptoms of hypothyroidism.

PHYSICAL EXAM

- Note voice quality:
  - Breathy voice suggests poor cord apposition (tumor, polyp, nodule).
  - Raspy voice indicates cord thickening due to edema or inflammation (chemical irritation, vocal abuse, infection).
  - High, shaky or very soft voice indicates trouble mounting adequate respiratory force.
- Examine oropharynx and carefully palpate thyroid and cervical lymph nodes.
- If there is unexplained neck mass or lymph node, check nose, paranasal sinuses, and nasopharynx.
- Proceed to indirect laryngoscopy if hoarseness duration >2–3 wks. Note any unilateral paresis, thickening, nodularity, or signs of inflammation.
- Premedicate readily gagging patient using diazepam, 10 mg PO, + analgesic throat spray [benzocaine (Cetacaine) or lidocaine (Xylocaine) spray].
- Refer for fiberoptic laryngoscopy patients with uncontrollable gag reflexes.
- Refer for emergency laryngoscopy by airway specialist if there is dyspnea (see below).

LAB STUDIES

- Obtain CXR, and if negative, films of skull base and neck for patient with unilateral paresis of left vocal cord (recurrent laryngeal nerve syndrome).
- Check TSH if cords appear chronically edematous and there is clinical suspicion of hypothyroidism.
- Consider small-needle biopsy for patient with suspected carcinoma of larynx or unexplained enlarged neck node and hoarseness.
- Check C1 esterase inhibitor level when there are recurrent soft tissue edematous episodes and positive family Hx (angioneurotic edema).
- Obtain lateral soft tissue films in acutely dyspneic patients.

MANAGEMENT

OVERALL APPROACH

- Advise all patients with hoarseness to quit smoking immediately (see Smoking Cessation).

ACUTE LARYNGITIS

- Recommend voice rest and, when necessary to speak, use moderate voice, not whisper.

- Advise professional singers and speakers to rest voice when they become hoarse (especially during URIs) to prevent permanent vocal cord injury.
- Suggest warm sialogogues, such as hot tea with sugar and lemon.
- Avoid antibiotics unless definite bacterial infection evident.
- Prescribe cough suppressant, particularly with mucolytic agent.
- Recommend humidification of home environment; for immediate relief, inhalation of steam in hot shower or breathing through moist hot towel.
- Prescribe topical steroid spray (e.g., dexamethasone or flunisolide) when cause is hay fever; avoid steroids if there is no allergic etiology.
- Consider vasoconstricting spray and analgesics when voice use by professional is absolutely necessary. Occasionally, you may give professional singers short course of topical or oral steroids to get through singing commitment, but further cord injury may ensue.

ACUTE LARYNGEAL EDEMA

- Hospitalize immediately.
- Assess degree of swelling and airway compromise.
- Consider emergency airway.
- Administer 0.3 mL adrenaline 1:1,000 SQ, and dexamethasone (Decadron, 12 mg IV).

VOCAL CORD NODULES

- Treat early with voice rest and vocal Rx.
- Refer for consideration of excision any nodule that does not promptly respond to conservative Rx; use of atraumatic technique (microlaryngeal surgery, carbon dioxide laser) is mandatory.

ANGIONEUROTIC EDEMA

- In acute situation with airway narrowing that does not respond to epinephrine or glucocorticosteroids, arrange emergency intubation or tracheotomy.
- If available, infuse C1 esterase inhibitor.
- Consider prophylactic Rx using anabolic steroids with attenuated androgenic effect (e.g., danazol or stanozolol) to stimulate synthesis of C1 esterase inhibitor; may be given for several days before any planned surgery.

TEMPORARY AND PERMANENT UNILATERAL VOCAL CORD PARALYSIS

- Refer to otolaryngologist for consideration of collagen paste injection into musculature of paralyzed cord, moving it to midline for 3–6 mos.
- Refer for consideration of thyroplasty and arytenoid adduction procedure patients with permanent vocal cord paralysis.

CARCINOMA OF LARYNX

- Obtain early consultation to choose among surgery, laser, and radiation Rx for early stage (T1N0) disease (highly curable); better voice results usually with irradiation.
- Consider induction chemotherapy and radiation with surgery for salvage in larger lesions.

- Emphasize importance of smoking cessation as best form of prevention.
- Treat leukoplakia by ordering vocal cord stripping under microscopic control; arrange for regular follow-up exams and repeated vocal cord stripping, particularly if patient does not limit irritant use.
- Have dependent polyps removed by microsurgery.

INDICATIONS FOR REFERRAL AND ADMISSION

- Refer if
  - unable to visualize vocal cords;
  - Hx of unexplained hoarseness lasting >3 wks, particularly in patient at-risk for cancer (smoker, drinker) in absence of acute infectious process;
  - there is cord nodule, thickening, or paralysis on indirect laryngoscopy;
  - voice Rx needed for professional speaker/singer who experiences repeated vocal trauma and for person with organic disease in need of voice rehabilitation.
- Admit any patient with concurrent acute dyspnea.

BIBLIOGRAPHY

- For the current annotated bibliography on hoarseness, see the print edition of *Primary Care Medicine*, 4th edition, Chapter 216, or www.LWWmedicine.com.

Nasal Congestion and Discharge

DIFFERENTIAL DIAGNOSIS

- Allergic
  - Seasonal allergic rhinitis (pollens)
  - Perennial allergic rhinitis (dusts, molds)
- Vasomotor
  - Idiopathic (vasomotor rhinitis)
  - Abuse of nosedrops
  - Drugs (reserpine, guanethidine, prazosin, cocaine abuse)
  - Psychologic stimulation (anger, sexual arousal)
- Mechanical
  - Polyps
  - Tumor
  - Deviated septum
  - Crusting (as in atrophic rhinitis)
  - Hypertrophied turbinates (chronic vasomotor rhinitis)
  - Foreign body (usually in children)
- Chronic inflammatory
  - Sarcoidosis
  - Wegener's granulomatosis
  - Midline granuloma
- Infectious
  - Atrophic rhinitis (secondary infection)
- Hormonal
  - Pregnancy
  - Hypothyroidism

WORKUP

OVERALL STRATEGY

- Distinguish allergic from vasomotor disease and identify any mechanical obstruction, chronic inflammatory disease, or drug-induced illness.

HISTORY

- Check timing of symptoms, particularly concurrence with pollination periods (seasonal allergic rhinitis), continuous waxing and waning throughout yr with exacerbations during hay fever season (combination perennial and seasonal allergic disease), chronic without respect to seasons (vasomotor rhinitis, perennial allergy, mechanical obstruction, or chronic inflammatory condition), frequent "colds" (perennial rhinitis).
- Inquire into aggravating and alleviating factors, especially if bothered by dusts (atopy) or aggravated by quick changes in temperature, emotion, or drugs (vasomotor disease).
- Review medications, substance abuses, and environmental exposures for antihypertensive agents; nasal decongestant overuse; cocaine

abuse; exposure to fur-bearing animals, feathers, and other animal danders; and chemical irritants and pollutants.

- Note associated symptoms, such as acute fever and purulent nasal discharge (sinusitis); chronic fetid, foul-smelling discharge accompanied by crusting (secondary infection in atrophic rhinitis, Wegener's granulomatosis, and midline granuloma); bloody discharge and unilateral obstruction (tumor); asthma or aspirin sensitivity (nasal polyps); and itching of eyes, tearing, and conjunctival redness (allergic mechanism).
- Consider epidemiologic data, including onset in childhood (allergic disease), or chronic progressive nasal congestion in middle-aged woman (atrophic rhinitis or necrotizing inflammatory disease).
- Review medical Hx for hypothyroidism, sarcoidosis, and pregnancy.
- Ask about family Hx of similar symptoms (allergic disease).

PHYSICAL EXAM

- Examine nasal mucous membranes for erythema, pallor, atrophy, edema, crusting, and discharge, but realize that although pale, boggy appearance to mucosa is allegedly classic sign of allergic disease, erythema does not rule it out.
- Using nasal speculum, note any polyps, erosions, or septal perforations and deviations.
- Check eyes for conjunctival erythema, tearing, photophobia, and papillary edema of lids (allergic mechanism).
- Transilluminate and palpate sinuses, examine pharynx for erythema and discharge, and check ears for otitis.
- Palpate cervical nodes for enlargement and auscultate chest for wheezes.

LAB STUDIES

- Consider antigen challenge to help differentiate allergic and nonallergic disease and to provide basis for immunotherapy, but unnecessary when Hx provides ready allergen(s) identification.
- Use skin testing as procedure of choice for detection of allergen-specific IgE, including that due to inhaled allergens:
  - For environmental allergens, order epicutaneous (needle prick) test; avoid intradermal injection (false-positives, severe systemic reactions).
  - Consider test "positive" when wheal and flare occur within 20 mins; proves sensitization only; correlate with Hx and PE to establish causation.
  - Omit antihistamines for 12–24 hrs before testing.
  - Use saline control to rule out dermatographism as cause of wheal and flare.
  - Note any eczema and concurrent antipsychotic drug use (interferes with interpretation).
- Consider total serum IgE and total eosinophil count when skin prick testing is unavailable; sensitivity low, diagnostically helpful only if markedly elevated; absence of elevation does not rule out allergic disease.
- Consider *in vitro* radioallergoabsorbent testing to identify and quantitate allergen-specific IgE; expensive, modest sensitivity (<skin testing), but specific. Reserve for use when skin tests equivocal.

- Consider *in vitro* IgE immunoassays as alternative *in vitro* test for specific IgE antibodies; positive test that correlates with symptoms on natural exposure often sufficient for initiating environmental Rx.
- Consider smears of nasal secretions for eosinophils; limited specificity (eosinophils present in vasomotor and allergic rhinitis), but abundance more suggestive of allergy; also informative for infection (large numbers of neutrophils).
- Obtain sinus films to confirm sinusitis, but clinical Dx usually suffices (see Sinusitis).

MANAGEMENT

ALLERGIC DISEASE

Overall Approach

- Implement avoidance and environmental measures.
- Start with trial of first-generation antihistamine, beginning with qhs dose of long-acting preparation (e.g., sustained-release chlorpheniramine, 8–12 mg).
- Add small daytime dose of shorter-acting preparation (e.g., chlorpheniramine, 4 mg) if needed and continue if well tolerated, but exert caution in persons whose work requires unimpaired psychomotor performance (e.g., those operating machinery, heavy equipment, or motor vehicle).
- If sedation problematic and short-term Rx sufficient, consider short-term addition of sympathomimetic (e.g., pseudoephedrine, 60 mg); avoid if there is HTN or underlying heart disease.
- If sedation problematic and longer-term Rx needed for mild to moderate disease, begin least costly bid nonsedating antihistamine (e.g., fexofenadine, 60 mg qam only); recommend OTC first-generation antihistamine qhs.
- If control inadequate, switch to qd sustained use of topically active, nonabsorbable, nasal steroid preparation (e.g., beclomethasone, 1–2 puffs bid) or cromolyn.
- Consider immunotherapy only for those who do not respond within 1 yr of above measures and for those who expect chronic unavoidable exposure to offending allergen(s).

Allergen Avoidance

Seasonal Allergic Rhinitis

- Advise avoiding long walks in woods during pollination period and staying indoors with windows closed when symptoms are severe and pollen count high (e.g., hot, windy, sunny days).
- Inform that although air conditioners make indoor living more comfortable on hot days, filters do not remove pollen from air; keep air intake on air conditioner closed.
- Advise keeping daisies, dahlias, and chrysanthemums outdoors if ragweed problematic.
- Recommend keeping bedroom free of excess dust and avoiding tobacco smoke, chemical vapors, and strong perfumes.

Perennial Allergic Rhinitis

- Recommend cleaning house, especially bedroom, with damp mop 2–3 times/wk, replacing feather pillows with Dacron or polyester ones, and covering mattress with elastic fabric casing.
- Advise using dehumidifier in damp basement and removing any old newspapers or furniture there.
- Suggest humidifying household bedroom air in winter and purchasing only furnishings with synthetic fabrics to minimize dust collection.
- Avoid African violets and geraniums at home if allergic to molds.
- Recommend no new fur-bearing pets and removing current pets if symptoms disabling (keeping pet out of bedroom insufficient).

Pharmacotherapy

Classes

ANTIHISTAMINES

- Begin with first-generation H_1 blocker (e.g., chlorpheniramine, diphenhydramine, clemastine).
- If sedation or psychomotor retardation bothersome, consider second-generation H_1 blocker (e.g., loratadine, fexofenadine) for daytime use; also less dry mouth and constipation; extremely expensive; continue first-generation preparation qhs.
- Advise taking on empty stomach (better absorption).

SYMPATHOMIMETICS

- Add sympathomimetic (e.g., pseudoephedrine, 60 mg q4–6h) to antihistamine program if marked nasal congestion persists despite antihistamine use.
- Avoid in patients with HTN, CAD, or heart failure.
- Avoid fixed combinations as initial Rx.
- Avoid sustained use of topical sympathomimetic decongestant sprays [e.g., phenylephrine (Neo-Synephrine) or oxymetazoline (Afrin)] because of tachyphylaxis and rebound nasal congestion if used >3 consecutive days.

TOPICAL CORTICOSTEROIDS

- Begin intranasal corticosteroid if symptoms of seasonal or perennial allergic rhinitis persist despite antihistamine Rx; halt antihistamines.
- Prescribe nonabsorbable topically active preparation used qd–bid (e.g., flunisolide, budesonide, beclomethasone, fluticasone, triamcinolone, mometasone).
- Prefer liquid to powdered formulation in patients with dryness and crusting.
- Watch for mucosal irritation, friability, and nosebleeds.

CROMOLYN SODIUM

- Consider as alternative to inhaled steroids in persons with less severe disease; most effective when used prophylactically before anticipated allergen exposure.
- Prescribe as inhaled powder or as dissolved liquid up to 6 times/day.
- Patients with very high IgE levels are most responsive; many others are not.

NEDOCROMIL

■ Consider in same fashion as cromolyn; also possesses antiinflammatory activity; clinical efficacy in allergic rhinitis similar, but only bid administration required.

Dosing

FIRST-GENERATION ANTIHISTAMINES

■ Chlorpheniramine (generic), 4 mg qid; long-acting, 12 mg bid
■ Brompheniramine (generic), 4 mg qid
■ Diphenhydramine (generic), 25 mg qid
■ Clemastine (Tavist), 1 mg bid

SECOND-GENERATION ANTIHISTAMINES

■ Fexofenadine (Allegra), 60 mg bid
■ Loratadine (Claritin), 10 mg qd–bid
■ Cetirizine (Zyrtec), 5–10 mg qd

INHALED ANTIHISTAMINES

■ Azelastine (Astelin spray), 137 mg bid

COMBINATION PREPARATIONS

■ Chlorpheniramine/pseudoephedrine, 8/120 mg bid
■ Loratadine/pseudoephedrine, 5/60 mg bid

TOPICAL CORTICOSTEROIDS

■ Beclomethasone
  • Beconase (also AQ), 42 µg, 1 spray bid
  • Vancenase, 42 µg, 1 spray bid
  • Vancenase AQ, 84 µg, 1 spray qd
  • Budesonide (Rhinocort), 32 µg, 2 sprays bid
  • Flunisolide (Nasalide), 25 µg, 2 sprays bid
  • Fluticasone (Flonase), 50 µg, 2 sprays bid
  • Mometasone (Nasonex), 50 µg, 2 sprays qd
  • Triamcinolone (Nasacort AQ), 55 µg, 2 sprays qd
■ Mast cell stabilizers
  • Cromolyn, 5.2 mg, 1 spray tid

Immunotherapy (Hyposensitization)

■ Consider as last resort in patients facing prolonged (>6 wks) exposure to known allergen and who remain incapacitated despite 1-yr trial of full program of pharmacotherapy and environmental measures.
■ Use as complement to medical Rx because most responses not dramatic.
■ Unless Hx definitive, perform skin testing for definitive identification of causative allergen(s) before prescribing.
■ Assess response to immunotherapy (improvement in symptoms, reduction in medication requirements) q6mos; discontinue immunotherapy if substantial benefit not evident after 12–18 mos.

VASOMOTOR RHINITIS

Overall Approach

■ Recommend avoiding tobacco smoke, rapid temperature and humidity changes, and irritant chemical vapors.

- Advise humidification of home in winter.
- Cease all nasal sprays.
- Consider change in antihypertensive medication if hypertensive.
- Prescribe trial of mild adrenergic agent with some α activity (e.g., pseudoephedrine).
- Add antihistamine for nonspecific drying effect.
- Treat any concurrent reactive depression; consider using antidepressant having some anticholinergic activity (e.g., amitriptyline).
- Avoid immunotherapy and steroids.
- Reserve consideration of surgical approaches (e.g., cryosurgery of inferior and middle turbinates or sectioning parasympathetic nerve supply to nose) only for patients seriously impaired by symptoms, because chances of success limited and risk of complications substantial.

INDICATIONS FOR REFERRAL

- Refer to allergist for skin testing and consideration of immunotherapy if allergic rhinitis inadequately controlled despite 1 yr of well-designed medical Rx.
- Consider allergy referral when allergic etiology cannot be distinguished from vasomotor rhinitis and when antigen(s) must be identified for management purposes.
- Refer to ENT specialist if polyp, foreign body, or deviated septum is obstructing and requires removal or if there is suspected tumor, necrotizing inflammatory condition, or atrophic rhinitis.
- Referral might also be worthwhile for patients with incapacitating vasomotor rhinitis.

BIBLIOGRAPHY

- For the current annotated bibliography on nasal congestion and discharge, see the print edition of *Primary Care Medicine*, 4th edition, Chapter 222, or www.LWWmedicine.com.

Otitis

WORKUP

ACUTE OTITIS MEDIA

- Note any fever or chills.
- Check tympanic membrane for mobility and presence of bony landmarks.
- Check for middle ear effusion and note its appearance (translucent or cloudy).
- Avoid cultures of nasopharynx (not helpful).
- Reserve needle aspiration of middle ear for cases unresponsive to appropriate antibiotic Rx and cases involving immunocompromised individuals.

CHRONIC OTITIS MEDIA

- Check for presence of perforated drum and discharge (chronic otitis media).
- Differentiate seemingly recurrent external otitis from unrecognized tympanic membrane perforation and chronic otitis media by careful otoscopic exam after resolution of acute external infection.

EXTERNAL OTITIS

- Review Hx for DM or HIV infection.
- Examine pinna for erythema and pain on movement in conjunction with any discharge in external canal.
- Check for expending erythema and pain suggesting signs of cellulitis.

MANAGEMENT

ACUTE PURULENT OTITIS MEDIA

- Begin amoxicillin or, for penicillin-allergic persons, trimethoprim-sulfa or erythromycin.
- If inadequate response to 7- to 10-day course, switch to amoxicillin-clavulanate (Augmentin) to cover resistant strains of *H. influenzae* and *M. catarrhalis.*
- Add sympathomimetic decongestant (e.g., pseudoephedrine).
- Avoid antihistamines (may lead to inspissated secretions).
- Refer to otolaryngologist if intractable pain, progressive hearing loss, persistent fever, headache, or no response to medical Rx; patient may require consideration of myringotomy.

ACUTE SEROUS OTITIS MEDIA

- Begin sympathomimetic decongestant (see Nasal Congestion and Discharge).
- When allergy clearly evident, consider adding antihistamine (see Nasal Congestion and Discharge).

- Advise patients who must travel by air without delay to use oral and intranasal decongestants (see Nasal Congestion and Discharge), especially in anticipation of descent for landing when risk of barotrauma is greatest.
- Consider teaching self-inflation of eustachian tubes for symptomatic relief; instruct patient to pinch nose closed, inhale deeply, close mouth, and try to blow nose while keeping it pinched.

CHRONIC OTITIS MEDIA

- Instruct avoiding swimming and other sources of water in canal; suggest using cotton plug to help keep ear canal dry when showering.
- Prescribe careful aural toilet with 1.5% acetic acid irrigation and topical ophthalmic antibiotic drops.
- Consider surgery if response insufficient.
- Monitor closely for complications (e.g., intracranial suppuration, facial paralysis, sensorineural hearing loss, and vertigo).
- Refer promptly to otolaryngologist if persistent fever and headache ensue.

OTITIS EXTERNA

- Prevent water contamination by using cotton ball coated with petrolatum ointment.
- Treat with topical antibiotics (e.g., polymyxin/hydrocortisone/neomycin eardrops 4 drops qid × 1 wk) and analgesic. Avoid neomycin-containing eardrops, such as Cortisporin (allergic skin reaction).
- Refer to otolaryngologist for suction aspiration of debris and insertion of wick to promote antibiotic penetration when canal is obstructed by edema or purulent material.

CELLULITIS/MALIGNANT EXTERNAL OTITIS

- Admit promptly for parenteral antibiotics, with coverage against *P. aeruginosa*; especially urgent if DM or HIV infection present.
- Refer to otolaryngologist for consideration of débridement.

BIBLIOGRAPHY

- For the current annotated bibliography on otitis, see the print edition of *Primary Care Medicine*, 4th edition, Chapter 218, or www.LWWmedicine.com.

Pharyngitis

DIFFERENTIAL DIAGNOSIS

- *S. pyrogenes*
- Chlamydia
- Viruses
- Fusobacteria
- Gonococcus
- Meningococcus
- Diphtheria
- Candida
- Acid reflux

WORKUP

HISTORY

- Estimate risk of *S. pyogenes* by telephone triage.
- Check for triaging clusters, such as fever, difficulty swallowing, and absence of cough.
- Consider using scoring system to enhance estimation of risk (fever and difficulty swallowing scored from 0–3, based on severity; final score derived by subtracting score for cough; score of ≥2 "positive" for Dx of *S. pyogenes* infection).
- Although far from perfect, consider this scheme to help decide who should come in for further evaluation.
- Inquire into exposure to family members with current documented streptococcal pharyngitis and any Hx of rheumatic fever.
- Inquire into positive throat culture in preceding yr, tender anterior cervical adenopathy, temp >101° F, and absence of rhinorrhea and itchy eyes.
- Regarding other sore throat etiologies and complications, ask about orogenital sexual contact, concurrent steroid or immunosuppressive Rx, and any dyspnea (epiglottitis).

PHYSICAL EXAM

- Check for marked tonsillar exudate, anterior cervical adenopathy, and temp >101° F (positive predictive value 30% when prevalence of strep infection 10%; absence of these features + presence of cough reduces probability to 3%).
- Examine pharynx for signs of other etiologies (e.g., white cheesy exudate of thrush), gingivitis, and necrotic tonsillar ulcers of fusobacteria and spirochetes).
- Note any viral exanthem, conjunctivitis, petechiae, generalized lymphadenopathy, splenomegaly, or hepatic tenderness.
- Check for "sandpaper" erythematous rash with accentuation in groin and axillae (scarlet fever).

- If severe dysphagia or dyspnea, urgently evaluate to exclude airway obstruction; if epiglottitis suspected, do not instrument airway.

LAB STUDIES

For Suspected Strep Pharyngitis

- Take swab of posterior pharynx and subject specimen to rapid strep antigen testing; swab tonsils and posterior pharynx.
- Omit testing and treat directly pharyngitis patients at high risk for rheumatic fever (e.g., Hx of rheumatic fever) and those with high probability of strep infection (closed population experiencing strep epidemic).
- Send retropharyngeal swab for culture when rapid antigen testing is negative yet clinical suspicion remains high.
- Omit culturing any patient with typical symptoms and signs of viral URI and no Hx or PE evidence of strep infection.
- Omit repeat culture after antibiotic Rx; most positive cultures after Rx represent strep carriers and not true infection.
- Limit repeat culturing to patients with Hx of rheumatic fever and during outbreaks of strep throat, especially when reinfection by close contacts suspected.

For Other Etiologies

- Obtain heterophile antibody if clinical suspicion is high and there is no Hx of infectious mononucleosis; repeat test in several wks if initially negative or check serology for antibodies to EBV.
- Plate throat swab onto Thayer-Martin media if Hx of orogenital contact and possible gonococcal infection.
- Confirm suspected candidal infection by scraping exudate and examining potassium hydroxide prep for yeast forms.

MANAGEMENT

SUSPECTED *S. PYOGENES* INFECTION

- Treat according to probability of strep infection, likelihood of patient compliance, chance of adverse reaction to antibiotics, and benefits of treating immediately vs waiting for culture results.
- Treat immediately without testing when Hx of rheumatic fever and when household member has documented group A β-strep infection.
- Consider empiric antibiotic Rx for patients with high clinical probability of strep infection (e.g., exudative pharyngitis, temp >101° F, tender bilateral anterior cervical adenopathy, and no rhinorrhea or cough), especially if no Hx of allergic reactions to antibiotics.
- Prescribe antibiotics only after confirmation by rapid strep testing or culture in pharyngitis patients with low-intermediate probability of strep infection (≥2 predictive factors).

Antibiotic Program

- Administer single IM injection of 1.2 million U benzathine penicillin or prescribe 10-day course of oral phenoxymethyl penicillin (250 mg tid–qid); 5- to 10-fold increase in risk of allergic reaction with IM penicillin.
- In penicillin-allergic patient, prescribe oral erythromycin (250 mg qid × 10 days).

- Limit antibiotic Rx to penicillin or erythromycin due to their proven efficacy, narrow spectrum, and low cost.

RECURRENT STREP INFECTION

- For recurrent pharyngitis and positive strep culture, check for noncompliance with oral antibiotics; if so, administer benzathine penicillin.
- If positive culture, consider carrier state for group A strep and concurrent noninfectious etiology for sore throat.
- Avoid routine tonsillectomy as means of reducing recurrent infections (unproved); obtain ENT consultation.
- Obtain otolaryngology consult for recalcitrant cases.

OTHER TYPES OF PHARYNGITIS

Meningococcal Carrier State

- Treat carriers with rifampin when evidence of active meningococcal disease in household or dormitory contacts.

Gonococcal Pharyngitis

- Begin with ceftriaxone, 250 mg IM.
- Alternatively, use ciprofloxacin or azithromycin (see Gonorrhea).

Diphtheria

- Administer antitoxin to prevent myocarditis and peripheral neuritis.
- Prescribe erythromycin or penicillin to eliminate organism from upper respiratory tract.
- Hospitalize for Rx of epiglottitis.

Necrotizing Pharyngitis (Fusobacteria)

- Prescribe penicillin and good nutrition.

Chlamydia, Mycoplasma

- No Rx necessary.

Pharyngeal Candidiasis

- In immunocompromised patients, prescribe gargling with 15 mL oral nystatin suspension (100,000 U/mL, swish-and-swallow 6 times/day) or using 10-mg clotrimazole troche held in mouth (15–30 mins tid).

Viral Sore Throat

- Treat symptomatically with voice rest, humidification, and lozenges or hard candy + saline gargling and aspirin or acetaminophen.

PATIENT EDUCATION

- Maximize patient satisfaction by addressing patient concerns and communicating Dx and rationale for Rx.
- When probability of strep infection is deemed too low to warrant testing or Rx (see above), reassure patient that risk is nil and that antibiotics are unlikely to provide any benefit.
- For insistent person or one with intermediate risk by triage Hx, recommend coming in for rapid antigen testing.
- Be sure to instruct patient with proven *S. pyogenes* infection to complete full 10-day course of antibiotics to reduce risk of rheumatic fever fully.
- Review risks and benefits of tonsillectomy over medical Rx in patients with recurrent strep infections and intact tonsils.

BIBLIOGRAPHY

■ For the current annotated bibliography on pharyngitis, see the print edition of *Primary Care Medicine*, 4th edition, Chapter 220, or www.LWWmedicine.com.

DIFFERENTIAL DIAGNOSIS

- Common cold
- Allergic rhinitis
- Vasomotor rhinitis
- Polyps
- Tumors
- Cysts
- Foreign bodies
- Vasculitis (Wegener's granulomatosis)
- See also Nasal Congestion and Discharge.

WORKUP

HISTORY

- Consider sinusitis in patients with symptoms of nasal congestion and discharge that persist >7–10 days.
- Note Hx of purulent rhinorrhea, maxillary toothache, and poor response to decongestants (useful predictors of sinusitis).
- Check for symptom of "double sickening" (URI symptoms with initial improvement followed by increasing nasal symptoms; also suggestive of sinusitis).
- Inquire about risk factors such as nasal polyps, deviated nasal septum, trauma, foreign bodies, and rapid altitude changes.
- Pay attention to toxic symptoms of high fever and rigors associated with complaints suggesting extended infection, such as eyelid edema and diplopia.

PHYSICAL EXAM

- Examine nasal cavity for purulent discharge draining from turbinate, and transilluminate maxillary sinuses for impaired light transmission.
- If dental abscess suspected as source of maxillary sinus infection, tap maxillary teeth for focal tenderness (sign of abscessed tooth).
- Palpate maxillary and frontal sinuses to elicit sinus tenderness, but absence does not reliably rule out sinusitis.

LAB STUDIES

- Although Dx usually clinical, consider testing in confusing cases and in patients who do not improve or have suspected complication or frequent recurrences.

Sinus Films

- Sinusitis confirmed by finding mucosal thickening, sinus opacification, or air-fluid levels on conventional sinus x-rays.

- Normal sinus x-rays in person with suspected sinusitis rules out maxillary and frontal disease; ethmoidal involvement harder to exclude.
- For maxillary sinusitis, single occipitomental (Waters') view acceptable to examine sinuses. Bone erosion can be present in chronic sinusitis.

Computed Tomography and Magnetic Resonance Imaging

- CT best reserved for complicated disease and search for occult ethmoidal disease in patients with refractory symptoms and negative conventional x-rays. Also useful to delineate anatomy before endoscopic surgery.
- MRI useful for differentiating mucosal inflammation from tumor.
- Neither study appropriate for patients with routine sinus infection.

Ultrasound

- Sensitivity of ultrasound lower than that for sinus x-rays, but specificity higher. Expertise not widely available.

Sinus and Nasal Cultures

- Although used as gold standard for research purposes, culture of aspirate from maxillary sinus negative in up to 40% of patients with suspected sinusitis.
- Cultures obtained from nasal swabs and even protected endoscopes invariably contaminated with nasal flora and unreliable; false-positive isolates of staphylococcal species common.

MANAGEMENT

ACUTE SINUSITIS

- Attend to any underlying etiologies, such as allergic rhinitis (see Nasal Discharge and Congestion).
- Begin antibiotic Rx with amoxicillin (500 mg PO tid) or TMP-SMX (TMS-DS, 160/800 mg bid) unless patient is immunocompromised or there is known highly clinically resistant organism prevalent in community. If patient is penicillin and sulfa allergic, consider doxycycline.
- Consider concurrent use of sympathomimetic decongestant (e.g., sustained-release pseudoephedrine, 120 mg bid). Avoid routine use of decongestants that contain antihistamines because of drying effect, which thickens secretions and risks aggravating obstruction.
- Treat with antibiotics for 7–14 days, supplemented by decongestants and systemic and topical hydration (e.g., humidification, isotonic saline nasal spray). Continue program for additional 5–7 days if response is incomplete.
- Consider broad-spectrum penicillinase-resistant antibiotic agent (e.g., amoxicillin-clavulanate, 500/125 mg tid; cefuroxime, 250–500 mg bid; loracarbef, 200–400 mg bid; azithromycin, 500 mg on first day, then 250 mg/day on days 2–5; clarithromycin, 500 mg bid; levofloxacin, 500 mg/day) only if there is known highly clinically resistant organism prevalent in community or if patient unresponsive to initial 2-wk course of first-line antibiotic Rx with amoxicillin or TMP-SMX.
- Consider referral to otolaryngologist when patient does not respond to 2 courses of antibiotics, has suspected anatomic abnormality that predisposes to sinusitis, or has frequent recurrences (>3/yr).

■ Obtain dental referral in suspected eroding tooth abscess and add anaerobic antibiotic coverage (e.g., clindamycin or metronidazole).

CHRONIC SINUSITIS

■ Refer to ENT specialist for identification and definitive correction of causative pathology.
■ Meanwhile, treat with broad-spectrum penicillinase-resistant antibiotic (e.g., amoxicillin/clavulanate 875/125 mg bid).

BIBLIOGRAPHY

■ For the current annotated bibliography on sinusitis, see the print edition of *Primary Care Medicine*, 4th edition, Chapter 219, or www.LWWmedicine.com.

Smell Disturbances

DIFFERENTIAL DIAGNOSIS

- Nasal
  - URI
  - Polyps
  - Ozena
  - Chronic sinusitis
  - Allergic rhinitis
  - Influenza and other virus
  - Chemical injury (e.g., tar, formaldehyde)
- Cranial nerve
  - Trauma
  - Meningioma
  - Cerebral aneurysm
- Cerebral cortex
  - Seizure disorder
  - Meningioma
  - Aneurysm
  - Schizophrenia
- Metabolic-endocrine
  - Hypothyroidism
  - Hypogonadism
  - Liver disease

WORKUP

HISTORY

- Distinguish local nasal pathology from central or cranial nerve lesions.
- Check Hx for head trauma, worsening headaches, olfactory hallucinations, personality change, unexplained forgetfulness, visual disturbances, gradual onset, or steady progression of symptoms (disease beyond nasal cavity).
- Note any Hx of head congestion, nasal discharge, allergies, sinus problems, influenza, chemical exposure, or recent cold (nasal source).
- Inquire into symptoms of hepatocellular failure and hypothyroidism (metabolic-endocrine etiology).
- Take psychiatric Hx when abnormal smells reported in absence of overt evidence of pathology.

PHYSICAL EXAM

- Document disorder by challenging each nostril with representative sample of each primary odor: pungent, floral, mint, and putrid (most accurately assessed using chemicals, such as pyridine, garlic-like odor, nitrobenzene, bitter almond, thiophene, and burnt rubber odor; kits are available).

- Examine head for trauma, and nares for polyps, deviated septum, mucosal inflammation, and discharge.
- Transilluminate sinuses for opacity (sinusitis).
- Check fundi for blurring of disc margins and visual fields for field cuts suggestive of optic chiasm compression (see Diabetes Insipidus; Galactorrhea and Hyperprolactinemia; Headache).
- Note skin, thyroid, and ankle jerks for signs of hypothyroidism, and hair, voice, muscles, and testes for evidence of hypogonadism.
- Note any jaundice, hepatomegaly, ascites, or asterixis.

LAB STUDIES

- Reserve sinus films for patients with clinical evidence of sinusitis (see Sinusitis) and neuroimaging studies (CT or MRI) if there is Hx of recent head trauma or symptoms and signs suggestive of mass lesion (see Diabetes Insipidus; Galactorrhea and Hyperprolactinemia; Headache).
- Similarly, obtain appropriate liver, thyroid, and/or gonadotropin studies (see Cirrhosis and Chronic Liver Failure; Hypothyroidism; Infertility) in patients with clinical suspicion of any one of these conditions.

MANAGEMENT

- Treat any local nasal pathology that is not self-limited (e.g., chronic sinusitis or persistent allergic rhinitis; see Nasal Congestion and Discharge; Sinusitis).
- Consider local or even systemic antibiotic Rx for ozena; prescribe saline irrigations to remove obstructing crusts (see Nasal Congestion and Discharge).
- Correct any underlying hypothyroidism.
- Recommend avoiding toxic fumes (e.g., formaldehyde).
- Consider removing symptomatic nasal polyps.
- Advise that influenza-induced, sudden, complete loss of smell may not be fully recoverable, but often some smell may return.
- Watch literature for data on zinc salts in restoring normal olfaction and taste.

BIBLIOGRAPHY

- For the current annotated bibliography on smell disturbances, see the print edition of *Primary Care Medicine*, 4th edition, Chapter 215, or www.LWWmedicine.com.

Snoring

WORKUP

- Check for symptoms of sleep apnea (e.g., habitual snoring, daytime sleepiness, Hx of motor vehicle accidents caused by falling asleep at wheel, or witnessed apneas).
- Inquire in women about atypical symptoms and signs of sleep apnea (chronic fatigue without associated obesity or daytime sleepiness, overbite).
- Examine mouth and upper airway for obstructing anatomy.
- Refer for formal ENT evaluation if obstructing lesion suspected.
- Consider nocturnal oxygen saturation monitoring and formal sleep study if sleep apnea suspected (see Sleep Apnea).

MANAGEMENT

- Advise losing excess weight and avoiding alcohol and sedatives.
- Recommend sleeping on one's side rather than on back and avoiding excessive neck flexion that comes from sleeping supine on several pillows; consider elevating head of bed.
- Treat any nasal obstruction from chronic rhinitis (see Nasal Congestion and Discharge).
- Consider trial of external nasal dilator (e.g., Breathe Right nasal strip).
- For patients with disturbingly refractory snoring, consider qhs use of CPAP (see Sleep Apnea); device usually reserved for sleep apnea but may be worth trying in households in which excessive nonapneic snoring threatens marital harmony and restful sleep.
- Consider dental orthosis if severe overbite or other obstructing maxillomandibular pathology.
- Obtain pulmonary consultation when concerned about sleep apnea (daytime sleepiness, nocturnal apnea; see Sleep Apnea).
- Obtain ENT consultation if snoring intractable and associated with anatomic oropharyngeal pathology.

BIBLIOGRAPHY

- For the current annotated bibliography on snoring, see the print edition of *Primary Care Medicine*, 4th edition, Chapter 223, or www.LWWmedicine.com.

Taste Disturbances

DIFFERENTIAL DIAGNOSIS

- Disturbances in smell
- Injury to taste buds
  - Age
  - Smoking
  - Hot liquids
  - Dental disease
  - Sjögren's syndrome
  - Idiopathic conditions
- Cranial nerve lesions (seventh or ninth, partial loss only)
  - Ear surgery
  - Bell's palsy
  - Ramsay Hunt syndrome (herpes zoster infection of geniculate ganglion)
  - Cholesteatoma
  - Cerebellopontine angle tumors (advanced disease)
- Central lesions
  - Head trauma
  - Tumors (rare)
- Psychiatric disorders
  - Depression
  - Drugs
  - Captopril
  - Imipramine (and other tricyclic agents)
  - Clofibrate
  - Lithium
  - L-dopa
  - Acetazolamide
  - Metronidazole
  - Glipizide
  - Iron
  - Tetracycline
  - Allopurinol
- Metabolic-endocrine conditions
  - Hypogonadism
  - Uremia
  - Hypothyroidism
  - Hepatitis
  - Pregnancy

WORKUP

HISTORY

- Use Hx to localize underlying pathophysiology; because intracranial disease is distinctly rare, concentrate on disease in mouth and in distribution of chorda tympani and seventh nerve.

- Check for Hx of alcohol abuse, smoking, dental disease, and severe mouth dryness (buccal cavity source).
- Ask about facial palsy, herpes zoster rash about ears, recent ear surgery, hearing problems, vertigo, and tinnitus (injury to seventh nerve).
- Review drug use and inquire into concurrent metabolic or endocrinologic problems (see above).
- Inquire into smell impairment, concurrent depression, and dry eyes/mouth, especially if RA is present (Sjögren's syndrome).

PHYSICAL EXAM

- Examine nose, ears, oral cavity, tongue, teeth, and gums.
- Assess taste by challenging withdrawn tongue with sweet, salty, bitter, and sour stimuli on each side; ask what it tastes like.
- Note any lateralization (seventh nerve lesion).
- Check other cranial nerves, concentrating on olfaction, hearing, and facial motor functions.

LAB STUDIES

- Check TSH if Hx or PE suggests hypothyroidism.
- Obtain renal function studies (BUN, creatinine) if renal disease suspected.
- Order ANA in suspected rheumatoid disease and Sjögren's syndrome. If the latter strongly suspected clinically, confirm with anti-Ro and anti-La antibody determinations (moderate sensitivity, moderate-high specificity for Sjögren's syndrome).
- Consider MRI if cerebellopontine angle tumor is a concern.

MANAGEMENT

- Advise complete smoking cessation and reduction in alcohol consumption.
- If possible, curtail or stop medications that may impair taste.
- Correct any dental disease of consequence.
- Treat any underlying hypothyroidism (see Hypothyroidism).
- Address depression (see Depression).

INDICATIONS FOR REFERRAL

- Obtain neurological consultation if olfactory hallucinations, changes in personality, visual field defects, or memory impairment uncovered in conjunction with disordered smell.
- Arrange neurological consultation if multiple cranial nerve defects, vertigo, or tinnitus in conjunction with altered taste.
- Consider psychiatric consultation when olfactory hallucinations are accompanied by other evidence of thought disorder.
- Refer to otolaryngologist patients with ozena, nasal polyps, deviated nasal septum, refractory sinusitis, or chorda tympani lesion.

BIBLIOGRAPHY

- For the current annotated bibliography on taste disturbances, see the print edition of *Primary Care Medicine*, 4th edition, Chapter 215, or www.LWWmedicine.com.

Temporomandibular Joint Dysfunction

DIFFERENTIAL DIAGNOSIS

- Acute otitis media
- Parotitis
- Giant cell arteritis
- Chronic pain syndrome

WORKUP

HISTORY

- Inquire into chronic unilateral jaw or facial pain exacerbated by jaw movement or chewing; note any radiation behind eyes and ears and down neck into shoulders.
- Ask about clicking sounds, jaw locking, and difficulty opening mouth widely, especially in the morning.
- Check for Hx of nocturnal bruxism, include questioning of spouse or family members.
- Note any pain complaints that extend far beyond temporomandibular joints (TMJs) and globally affect daily activity, suggesting chronic pain syndrome (see Nonmalignant Pain); if present, gently explore Hx for refractory pain complaints, multiple doctors, and psychosocial stresses, but avoid initial suggestion of "psychological" cause and instead continue assessment with full exploration of all etiologies.
- Distinguish from acute otitis media and parotitis by chronicity and absence of associated inflammatory symptoms.
- Rule out giant cell arteritis by reviewing Hx for focal scalp tenderness, shoulder and hip girdle arthralgias/myalgias, and transient visual difficulties (see Giant Cell Arteritis).

PHYSICAL EXAM

- Check for presence of markedly limited jaw movement with mandibular hypomotility, jaw deviation on opening mouth, masticatory muscle tenderness, and crepitus and clicking on jaw movement.
- Inspect molar prominences for flattening from chronic grinding.
- Palpate scalp for enlarged and tender cranial arteries (giant cell arteritis) and parotids for tenderness and swelling; check tympanic membranes for bulging, erythema, and middle ear effusion (otitis).

LAB STUDIES

- Check WBC count and ESR to rule out concurrent inflammatory disease.
- Confirm internal TMJ derangement using MRI of TMJ; minimize test expense by imaging only TMJ, and limit test to patients who do not respond to conservative measures and are being considered for more aggressive Rx.

MANAGEMENT

NONSURGICAL

- Recommend dietary measures, including cutting food into small pieces and using diet that minimizes hard repetitive chewing (e.g., no chewing gum or biting into big submarine sandwiches).
- Suggest local heat and massage to muscles of mastication; consider ultrasound, but probably no better than application of warm pack or even cold pack.
- Prescribe aspirin or low-dose NSAIDs for prominent pain.
- Refer to dentist for consideration of custom-made splint or bite guard for qhs use if there is severe grinding.
- If major psychosocial stresses identified, address them when symptomatic measures prescribed; begin with supportive counseling and consider cognitive/behavioral Rx (see Anxiety) if symptoms are incapacitating.
- Restrict minor tranquilizer use to short-term Rx qhs for severe nocturnal muscle spasm (e.g., diazepam, 2 mg qhs × 3–5 days); avoid long-term tranquilizer use; no additional benefit from so-called muscle relaxants [e.g., methocarbamol (Robaxin), carisoprodol (Soma)].
- Consider 2-mo trial of sedating tricyclic antidepressant (e.g., nortriptyline, 25 mg qhs) if pain refractory.
- Arrange referral for patients who report refractory pain; they may have suffered joint damage and require consideration for regrinding or surgical intervention.
- When clinical presentation is one of refractory pain accompanied by more global musculoskeletal dysfunction and disproportionately little evidence of TMJ destruction, approach condition as chronic pain syndrome (see Nonmalignant Pain).

REGRINDING AND SURGERY

- Consider only if patient has severe malocclusion leading to marked joint trauma.
- Refer only after full conservative measures have provided no relief and there is clinical and MRI evidence of internal joint derangement and secondary degenerative arthritis.
- Make referral to oral surgeon experienced in treating TMJ disease (no large-scale, prospective, randomized studies to guide choice of surgery); consider arthroscopic approaches.

BIBLIOGRAPHY

- For the current annotated bibliography on temporomandibular joint dysfunction, see the print edition of *Primary Care Medicine*, 4th edition, Chapter 225, or www.LWWmedicine.com.

Tinnitus

DIFFERENTIAL DIAGNOSIS

- Consider same otologic etiologies as for hearing loss (see Hearing Loss).
- When encountering subjective complaints of ear or head noise in absence of otologic pathology, consider psychogenic disease and causes of objective tinnitus (cerebrovascular pathology, palatal myoclonus, and patulous eustachian tube).

WORKUP

- Start with same pattern of diagnostic assessment as for hearing loss (see Hearing Loss).
- Add the following workup specific to tinnitus.

HISTORY

- Inquire into whether tinnitus is pulsatile or nonpulsatile (i.e., vascular or not) and subjective or objective; do not spend much time defining pitch of tinnitus (limited diagnostic value).
- Check for associated hearing loss and any association with drug use, vertigo, noise trauma, ear infection, or respiration.
- Inquire into any Hx of head trauma (development of arteriovenous fistula or aneurysm of intrapetrous portion of internal carotid artery).
- Note if present only at night (increased awareness of normal head sounds).

PHYSICAL EXAM

- Inspect external ear and tympanic membrane for cerumen impaction, foreign bodies, perforation, signs of otitis media, and abnormal middle ear masses.
- Perform Weber's and Rinne testing to determine sensorineural or conductive hearing loss (see Hearing Loss).
- Examine cranial nerves for evidence of neuropathy and signs of acoustic neuroma or glomus tumor.
- Check for nystagmus (see Dizziness) if vertigo reported.
- Auscultate skull for bruit if origin of problem remains obscure.
- Compress ipsilateral jugular vein to see if it abolishes objective tinnitus (jugular megabulb anomaly).

LAB STUDIES

- Obtain audiogram to help identify and localize site of underlying otologic disease.
- Consider neuroimaging studies (e.g., CT or MRI), but only in conjunction with otolaryngology consultation; usually best reserved for evaluation of unilateral or asymmetric tinnitus with or without hearing loss.

MANAGEMENT

OVERALL APPROACH

- Inform patient that no medication has proved effective for tinnitus relief.
- Suggest qhs use of clock radio playing background music that shuts off after 30 mins.
- Recommend keeping radio on during day when patient has to work in quiet room.
- Advise that hearing aid-like devices promoted as tinnitus maskers are of questionable value.
- Consider biofeedback in cases of stress-related disease.

INDICATIONS FOR REFERRAL

- Refer when conductive hearing loss is discovered or when there is clinical suspicion of acoustic neuroma, glomus tumor, or cerebrovascular abnormality, especially before embarking on expensive workup.
- Consider referral to satisfy anxious patient that everything has been explored and that there is no serious or correctable underlying condition.

BIBLIOGRAPHY

- For the current annotated bibliography on tinnitus, see the print edition of *Primary Care Medicine*, 4th edition, Chapter 217, or www.LWWmedicine.com.

Psychiatric and Behavioral Problems

Alcohol Abuse

SCREENING AND/OR PREVENTION

- Screen asymptomatic persons for alcohol abuse by asking CAGE questions:
  - Have you ever felt the need to **C**ut down on drinking?
  - Have you ever felt **A**nnoyed by criticism of your drinking?
  - Have you ever had **G**uilty feelings about drinking?
  - Have you ever taken a morning **E**ye opener?
- Also consider use of self-administered alcohol dependence scale for screening.

WORKUP

OVERALL STRATEGY

- On completion of workup, refer to consensus criteria for substance abuse and dependence for Dx (DSM-IV Criteria for Substance Abuse and Dependence; see Substance Abuse).

HISTORY

- Take detailed alcohol Hx in all patients identified by screening or suspected clinically to have alcohol abuse problem.
- Elicit drinking profile:
  - Setting for drinking
  - Social network for drinking
  - Amount, rate, and frequency of consumption
  - Pressures to drink
  - Other activities related to drinking
- Inquire into attempts at cessation; withdrawal symptoms; effects on work, family, and social interactions; and any associated medical, legal, or social consequences or complications.
- Check for abuse of other substances (e.g., tobacco, drugs).
- Perform thorough review of systems as it pertains to hepatic and neurologic symptoms.

PHYSICAL EXAM

- Check for signs of hepatocellular dysfunction (see Cirrhosis and Chronic Liver Failure) and substance abuse (see Substance Abuse).

LAB STUDIES

- Check CBC, liver function tests, and vitamin B_{12} and folate levels.

MANAGEMENT

OVERALL APPROACH

- Establish rapport. Let patients know you accept and understand them by approaching problem in respectful and comfortable manner.

- Offer appropriate and sufficient instruction and explanation as you go along, always engaging patient in establishing realistic goals and not pushing beyond limits.
- Maintain proper balance of support, caring, and limit-setting; remain flexible and adaptable to patient's needs.
- Think of Rx as series of short-term programs to develop and increase patient's sense of mastery.
- Never insist on immediate abstinence. This goal is to be negotiated and accomplished in context of harm reduction when patient resists abstinence. Only if all else fails should you confront and control in this area.
- If serious health problems may result from any alcohol intake and you must ask patient to abstain, do it in context of supportive educational-advice session to ensure patient's return.
- If patient comes to session drunk, kindly and calmly explain why session is pointless, and reschedule appointment. If behavior continues, renegotiate Rx agreement to include rules about it.
- Keep motivation high by using patient's fear of losing his or her health, or something or someone very important, and by getting him or her to seek and define reinforcers.
- Help patient to identify, objectify, and deal with anger and other emotions to enhance emotional control.
- When patient is ready, help pinpoint actual behaviors to change and work on them progressively. One may need to provide information, modeling, practice, feedback, and homework as patient learns to handle feelings and develop new social skills, tools necessary to assess and modify behavior.
- Encourage self-monitoring of drinking behavior via logs, teaching patient to detect causes, consequences, and maintaining factors and thus helping to learn alternate ways of coping with people, places, situations, and feelings associated with heavy drinking.
- Select components of available specialized Rx programs that match patient's needs, wants, and coping ability. Standard formula of detoxification—disulfiram and Alcoholics Anonymous—is no longer most acceptable or recommended Rx for alcoholism.
- For spree- and binge-drinking patients whose interpersonal and psychologic problems are likely to predominate, consider outpatient psychotherapy if they are socially intact, intellectually curious, and psychologically minded.
- For patients strongly motivated to attain total abstinence and specifically requesting disulfiram Rx, begin 250 mg qhs and renew monthly, reevaluating need for continued drug Rx while working on psychosocial interventions that sustain long-term abstinence. Rx contraindicated in those with underlying psychiatric illness or cardiovascular disease.
- Consider naltrexone, 50 mg/day, for those who relapse because of intense craving for alcohol.
- Use drug Rx only as complement to and means of participating effectively in comprehensive program of care.
- For patients who are rigid, repressed, and resistant to open-ended Rx, consider behavioral-cognitive methods. Brief physician intervention that is personalized can be effective.

- For patients willing to dedicate themselves to lifelong sobriety or who will benefit from peer counseling, consider Alcoholics Anonymous, especially if there is religious interest.
- For patients who are homeless, jobless, or have other serious social problems, refer to community social service agency for direct aid.
- For patients unresponsive to outpatient Rx who can afford time and need to leave their environment to cease drinking, consider inpatient alcohol program.

WITHDRAWAL

- Consider outpatient management if patient is reliable, has no or only mild symptoms, has no active underlying medical illnesses, has no Hx of severe withdrawal, and has supportive family that can supervise.
- Prescribe long-acting benzodiazepine (e.g., fixed-schedule program of diazepam, 10 mg q6h for 4 doses, then 5 mg q6h for 8 doses); achieve tapering by normal drug metabolism.
- Admit promptly for inpatient Rx unstable patients and those with other medical conditions or with symptoms suggesting potentially severe withdrawal (e.g., tachycardia, tremor, hallucinations, increased irritability).

BIBLIOGRAPHY

- For the current annotated bibliography on alcohol abuse, see the print edition of *Primary Care Medicine*, 4th edition, Chapter 228, or www.LWWmedicine.com.

Angry Patient

WORKUP

- Note verbal and nonverbal manifestations [demands, annoyance, resentment, Hx of temper outbursts and undirected violence (slamming doors), cynicism, sarcasm, negativism, and obstructive (i.e., passive-aggressive) behavior].
- Check for self-destructive behaviors, such as not adhering to medical regimen, canceling appointments, or continuing harmful habits.
- Observe clenched fists and jaws, frowning, narrowed palpebral fissures, compressed lips, widened nostrils, abrupt gestures, and jerky gait.
- Be aware of one's own subjective emotional response to patient during interview; note any feelings of irritation or boredom with patient (? unconscious response to anger and hostility).
- Learn what patient is angry about by noting subject matter that brings out irritation, annoyance, or hostility.
- Identify borderline patient by checking for interpersonal relationships that are superficial or very dependent and manipulative; intense labile emotions; extreme emptiness and anger; life story marked by lack of fulfillment and frequent failures; and impulsive, manipulative, and self-destructive behavior.

MANAGEMENT

OVERALL APPROACH

- Acknowledge patient's feelings by explicitly presenting patient with observations and reasons for concluding that patient is angry.
- Reassure that anger will not destroy therapeutic relationship.
- Convey neither fear nor rejection of patient's feelings but rather interest in trying to understand them to be helpful; no need to agree with patient's feelings.
- Set limits on patient's behavior while making it clear that there will be no counterattack in retribution; point out in noncondemnatory and nonjudgmental fashion when patient's hostility interferes with communication, therapeutic regimen, or coping with illness.
- Indicate that although you recognize and acknowledge patient's anger, it is problematic because it is self-destructive and interferes with patient's care or recovery.
- Explore causes of anger and respond appropriately:
  - If angry about being ill, investigate exact fears and sources of despair.
  - If angry about being thrust into patient role, try to structure relationship to minimize aspects that most threaten patient.
  - If anger is displaced from another situation or relationship, point this out without encouraging patient to vent hostility on actual source.
- Avoid retaliation; do not react with hostility; maintain clinical distance on situation; view patient's anger not as criticism but rather as response to patient's own fears, threats, and frustrated wishes.

659

INDICATIONS FOR REFERRAL

- Consider psychiatric referral for patient with suspected borderline personality disorder to confirm Dx and suggest management approach.
- Before suggesting referral to patient, obtain "curbside" psychiatric consult with colleague to help formulate strategy for raising issue of consultation with patient and successfully arranging referral.

BIBLIOGRAPHY

- For the current annotated bibliography on anger, see the print edition of *Primary Care Medicine*, 4th edition, Chapter 231, or www.LWWmedicine.com.

Anxiety

DIFFERENTIAL DIAGNOSIS

ANXIETY DISORDERS

- Generalized anxiety disorder
- Panic disorder
- Specific phobia
- Adjustment disorder with anxious mood
- Obsessive-compulsive disorder
- Posttraumatic stress disorder

MEDICAL CAUSES OF ANXIOUSNESS

- Cardiovascular
  - Angina pectoris
  - Arrhythmias
  - Congestive Heart Failure
  - Hypertension
  - Hypovolemia
  - Myocardial infarction
  - Syncope (of multiple causes)
  - Valvular disease
  - Vascular collapse (shock)
- Dietary
  - Caffeinism
  - Monosodium glutamate (Chinese restaurant syndrome)
  - Vitamin deficiency diseases
- Drug-related
  - Akathisia (secondary to antipsychotic drugs)
  - Anticholinergic toxicity
  - Digitalis toxicity
  - Hallucinogens
  - Hypotensive agents
  - Stimulants (amphetamines, cocaine, and related drugs)
  - Withdrawal syndromes (alcohol or sedative-hypnotics)
- Hematologic
  - Anemias
- Immunologic
  - Anaphylaxis
  - Systemic lupus erythematosus
- Hormonal/metabolic
  - Cushing's disease
  - Hyperkalemia
  - Hyperthermia
  - Hyperthyroidism
  - Hypocalcemia
  - Hypoglycemia

- Hyponatremia
- Hypothyroidism
- Menopause
- Porphyria (acute intermittent)

■ Neurologic
- Encephalopathies (infectious, metabolic, and toxic)
- Essential tremor
- Intracranial mass lesions
- Postconcussion syndrome
- Seizure disorders (especially of temporal lobe)
- Vertigo

■ Respiratory
- Asthma
- COPD
- Pneumonia
- Pneumothorax
- Pulmonary edema
- Pulmonary embolism

■ Secreting tumors
- Carcinoid
- Insulinoma
- Pheochromocytoma

WORKUP

HISTORY

■ Take psychiatric and medical Hx.

■ Check for symptoms of generalized anxiety disorder:
- Chronic anxiety lasting ≥6 mos
- Concern over ≥2 different issues (usually many)
- Panic attacks

■ Review for manifestations of panic disorder:
- Episodic extreme anxiety
- ≥1 attack being followed by ≥1 mo of 1 of these:
  - Persistent concern about having additional attacks;
  - Worry about implications of attack or its consequences (e.g., losing control, having heart attack); or
  - Significant change in behavior related to attacks.

■ Note any specific phobias, characterized by irrational fear associated with particular stimulus or presence of social phobia, with anxiety associated with scrutiny by others.

■ Inquire into symptoms of obsessive-compulsive disorder:
- Obsessions (intrusive unwanted bizarre thoughts), compulsions (repetitive behaviors performed in ritualistic or stereotypical fashion), or both.

■ Check for posttraumatic stress disorder, noting
- Hx of severe traumatic exposure;
- subsequent anxiety symptoms lasting ≥1 mo;
- reexperiencing trauma (e.g., flashbacks), avoiding stimuli associated with trauma, and increased arousal;
- possible delayed onset (>6 mos after original trauma).

- Search for features of adjustment disorder with anxious mood, such as
  - anxiety developing as maladaptive response to identifiable stressor;
  - symptoms lasting <6 mos.
- Conduct careful and thorough medical Hx (including use of medications and substances) and review of systems to check for medical etiologies (see above).

PHYSICAL EXAM

- Perform complete PE to rule out important medical etiologies, emphasizing check for signs of cardiac, pulmonary, hormonal, metabolic, and neurologic diseases (see above).

LAB STUDIES

- Test accordingly for any medical conditions suggested by Hx and PE.
- Also screen for occult hyperthyroidism with TSH determination.
- Consider testing for pheochromocytoma, but only when there is clinical evidence suggestive of Dx (see Hypertension).
- Test for hypoglycemia only when symptoms occur in fasting state or in context of insulin use.

MANAGEMENT

OVERALL APPROACH

- Begin with supportive psychotherapy that includes explanation, empathic listening, meaningful reassurance, guidance, and encouragement.
- Teach relaxation techniques for patients willing to use them (see below).
- Consider referral for insight-oriented Rx if emotional upheaval or disabling symptoms.
- Supplement psychotherapeutic measures with anxiolytic drug Rx to improve patient's ability to perform daily activities previously impaired by anxiety.
- For short-term or acute Rx, consider a benzodiazepine, but in most instances, use only in adjunctive role for limited duration.
- If selecting benzodiazepine Rx, pay attention to onset and duration of action (see below).
- Warn about risk of physical dependence with chronic benzodiazepine use.
- Inform patient that drug Rx is likely to reduce but not eradicate symptoms.
- Consider use of antidepressant with anxiolytic effects (e.g. SSRI) if chronic pharmacologic Rx needed.
- Refer if there is evidence of substance abuse, either as etiologic factor or as mode of self-Rx.

SITUATIONAL ANXIETY AND ADJUSTMENT DISORDER

- Initiate supportive psychotherapy and behavioral measures (see below), including identification of specific provocative stressors and their association with symptom onset.

- If distress from anxiety impairs daily functioning, begin short course (up to 5 days) of benzodiazepine Rx (e.g., clonazepam, 0.5 mg bid).
- If distress represents 1 of many such episodes in pattern of emotional upheaval, refer for insight-oriented Rx. Also refer if symptoms endure beyond stressful period or worsen despite Rx.

GENERALIZED ANXIETY DISORDER

- Initiate supportive psychotherapy and consider insight-oriented Rx to help diminish role of psychosocial stressors.
- Consider short course of benzodiazepine Rx for periods of exacerbation (e.g., alprazolam, 0.5 mg tid for up to 5 days).
- Avoid chronic benzodiazepine Rx due to risk of dependency. If patient is discontinuing long-term Rx, taper over several wks according to patient's ability to tolerate decreases. Monitor for withdrawal symptoms (e.g., tinnitus, perceptual changes, involuntary movements).
- Prescribe SSRI if chronic anxiolysis needed, especially if there is Hx of associated panic attacks or depression.
- Begin with low-dose SSRI program (e.g., paroxetine, 10 mg/day) and advance dose as tolerated (e.g., to 40 mg/day).
- If SSRI Rx does not suffice, consider atypical antidepressant [e.g., venlafaxine, extended release (e.g., Effexor XR), 37.5 mg bid, and advance dose as tolerated to 150 mg bid].
- Alternatively, consider trial of buspirone for chronic anxiolysis. Begin with 5 mg tid and gradually advance to max of 60 mg/d. Risks of physiologic dependence and withdrawal are nil, but potency is low and it may take wks to notice any effect.
- Refer patients with disabling chronic anxiety for psychiatric care.

PANIC DISORDER

- Use pharmacologic Rx to achieve control and minimize phobic avoidance and depression.
- Screen for suicidality (see Depression), especially if patient is despondent; refer urgently if there is concern. Otherwise, begin Rx with low-dose SSRI (e.g., paroxetine, 10 mg/day).
- If agitation is not increased, proceed gradually to full antidepressant doses (e.g., paroxetine, 40 mg/day; sertraline, 150 mg/day).
- In situations in which cost benefits of generic tricyclic antidepressant override better tolerability of SSRI, start with small "test" dose (e.g., imipramine, 10 mg qhs, and proceed gradually as tolerated to 100–200 mg qhs). Factor into cost-benefit equation added costs of cardiac monitoring and blood levels of tricyclic antidepressants.
- Alternatively, consider an MAOI antidepressant, but this requires dietary restriction and expertise in its use (see Depression).
- If patient seeks rapid relief from disabling phobic behavior, start with potent benzodiazepine (e.g., alprazolam, 0.25–0.5 mg qid; or clonazepam, 0.5 mg qhs or bid) pending onset of benefit from antidepressant Rx.
- After period of well-being, taper benzodiazepine to lowest possible maintenance dose or proceed to discontinuation.
- Weigh continued benzodiazepine use against risk of dependence. Use of potent benzodiazepines poses risks of dependence and severe withdrawal.

- Taper slowly over several wks when discontinuing Rx that has continued >6 wks.
- Refer patients with prominent phobic behavior and those with suicidal ideation.
- For patients requiring longer-term maintenance Rx, it is important to continue antidepressant medication at full acute-phase dose.

SOCIAL PHOBIA

- Refer for behavioral Rx.
- Prescribe benzodiazepine on prn, single-dose basis to help attenuate anxiety, decrease avoidance, and facilitate daily functioning and behavioral Rx.
- Prescribe low-dose SSRI (e.g., paroxetine, 10 mg qhs) and proceed gradually to full antidepressant doses (paroxetine, 40 mg qhs; or fluoxetine, 20–40 mg qam).
- For patients whose performances are compromised by ordinary "stage fright," consider trial of beta blocker prn (e.g., propranolol, 10 mg, up to 20 mg qid). Give pre-performance trial dose to be sure performance is not compromised by medication.

SPECIFIC PHOBIAS

- Refer for behavioral Rx.
- Consider rapidly acting single-dose benzodiazepine Rx prn (e.g., alprazolam, 0.25–0.50 mg; or diazepam, 10 mg) to provide symptomatic control in anxiety-provoking situations and to facilitate behavioral Rx.
- Refer for more specific behavioral and pharmacologic Rx.

OBSESSIVE-COMPULSIVE DISORDER

- Refer for behavioral Rx.
- Initiate pharmacologic Rx with SSRI.
- Refer to experienced psychopharmacologist for further management of drug Rx program.

POSTTRAUMATIC STRESS DISORDER

- Refer to psychiatrist specializing in Rx of such persons. Most programs begin with SSRI. Mood stabilizers may help prominent irritability or anger. Benzodiazepines may sometimes help in short term, but use with caution because of risk of substance abuse in this vulnerable patient population.
- Refer to experienced psychotherapist. Three psychotherapy techniques—exposure Rx, cognitive Rx, and anxiety management—are considered most useful in Rx of posttraumatic stress disorder. Expert therapists make distinctions among techniques depending on which specific type of symptom presentation is most prominent. Insight-oriented psychotherapy helps overcome emotional memories of traumatic event; behavioral techniques may also be of benefit.

TREATMENT OF THE ELDERLY

- Reduce starting doses of medications by half of usual adult dose.
- When using benzodiazepines as short-term anxiolytic, prescribe lorazepam or oxazepam. For chronic anxiety, use longer half-life agents with caution and at reduced doses and dose intervals.

- If antidepressants are indicated, consider SSRI (e.g., fluoxetine) or MAOI (see Depression).
- If agitation, sundowning, or psychotic features accompany anxiety, prescribe small doses of atypical neuroleptic (e.g., risperidone, 0.5 mg qd–bid).

BENZODIAZEPINE DOSING AND HALF-LIFE

- Alprazolam (Xanax), 0.5 mg (12–15 hrs)
- Chlordiazepoxide (Librium), 10 mg (5–30 hrs)
- Clonazepam (Klonopin), 0.25 mg (15–50 hrs)
- Clorazepate (Tranxene), 7.5 mg (30–200 hrs)
- Diazepam (Valium), 5 mg (20–100 hrs)
- Lorazepam (Ativan), 1 mg (10–20 hrs)
- Oxazepam (Serax), 15 mg (5–15 hrs)

BEHAVIORAL STRATEGIES FOR STRESS MANAGEMENT

- Before proceeding to train patient in relaxation as self-control procedure, advise reduction or elimination of caffeine.

Diaphragmatic Breathing

- Effective means of coping with and reducing stress; quickest and simplest method of relaxation.
- Involves breathing slowly and deeply from abdomen.
- Prevents possibility of hyperventilation and, after 50–60 s of such breathing, brings feeling of quiescence to body and reduction in bodily symptoms of stress.
- Have patient conduct exercise either sitting or lying down, with pillow placed at small of back to force abdomen out.
- Instruct breathing to begin by pushing stomach out as inhalation takes place slowly and deeply.
- Advise taking care to minimize chest movement during each inhalation.
- Suggest saying "relax" silently before exhaling, and stomach should fall with exhalation.
- While breathing in, abdomen should be pushed out; while breathing out, stomach should come in.

Progressive Deep Muscle Relaxation

- Based on finding that anxiety is not experienced when muscles are relaxed.
- Recommend progressive deep muscle relaxation as simple procedure alternating tension with relaxation.
- Ask patient first to tense set of muscles as hard as possible until tension is felt in muscles.
- Then have patient relax muscles and become aware of ("to feel internally") difference between tension and relaxation.
- Have patient focus attention on specific muscle groups, actively tensing each muscle group for 10–15 s, then letting go of tension in muscles and observing difference.
- Teach patient to apply approach systematically to host of muscle groups starting at head and ending at toes.

Autogenic Training

- Relaxation technique composed of set of exercises intended to induce heaviness and warmth in muscles through mental imagery.
- With patient sitting comfortably in armchair in quiet room with eyes closed, introduce verbal formulas (e.g., "my arm is heavy") and instruct visualizing and then feeling relaxation of focused muscle while silently repeating and passively concentrating on that formula.
- Use formulas (verbal somatic suggestions) to facilitate concentration and "mental contact" with selected body parts.
- Consider classic training program with psychophysiologic exercises performed several times/day:
  - Theme of heaviness (e.g., "my arm feels heavy and relaxed")
  - Theme of warmth (e.g., "my arm feels warm and relaxed")
  - Passive concentration on cardiac activity (e.g., "my heartbeat feels calm and regular")
  - Breathing and respiration
  - Warmth in chest and abdomen
  - Passive concentration on cooling of forehead
- If time and convenience are concerns, condense exercises so that whole round can be practiced in 5–10 mins.
- In condensed version, focus primarily on physiologic aspects, interspersed with general suggestions for relaxation.

BIBLIOGRAPHY

- For the current annotated bibliography on anxiety, see the print edition of *Primary Care Medicine*, 4th edition, Chapter 226, or www.LWWmedicine.com.

Depression

DIFFERENTIAL DIAGNOSIS

CLASSIFICATION OF DEPRESSIVE SYNDROMES

- Major affective disorders
  - Major depression (unipolar depression)
  - Bipolar disorder (manic-depressive illness)
- Chronic affective disorders
  - Dysthymic disorder
  - Cyclothymic disorder
- Other conditions
  - Adjustment disorder with depressed mood
- Organic brain syndrome
  - Organic affective disorder

ORGANIC ETIOLOGIES OF DEPRESSION

- Drug induced (alpha-methyldopa, antiarrhythmics, benzodiazepines, barbiturates and other CNS depressants, beta blockers, cholinergic drugs, corticosteroids, digoxin, H_2 blockers, and reserpine).
- Substance abuse related (alcohol abuse, sedative-hypnotic abuse, cocaine and other psychostimulant withdrawal).
- Toxic/metabolic disorders (hypothyroidism, hyperthyroidism of the elderly, Cushing's syndrome, hypercalcemia, hyponatremia, DM).
- Neurologic disorders (stroke, subdural hematoma, MS, brain tumor, Parkinson's disease, Huntington's disease, epilepsy, dementia).
- Infectious disorders (viral, especially mononucleosis and influenza; HIV ± AIDS; and syphilis).
- Nutritional disorders (vitamin B_{12} deficiency and pellagra).
- Other (carcinomas, especially pancreatic carcinoma, and postsurgical, especially cardiac surgery).

CONDITIONS MIMICKING DEPRESSION

- Fibromyalgia
- Vasculitis/connective tissue disease
- Lyme disease
- Endocrinopathies
- CFS

WORKUP

HISTORY

- When depression is suspected, inquire specifically into its psychological and neurovegetative manifestations.
- Ask about depressed mood, including its clinical course and associated symptoms. Note any reports of mania or hypomania.

- Screen for cardinal symptoms of major depression, designated by the acronym SIGECAPS:
  - Sleep disturbance, including early morning awakening
  - Interest or libido loss
  - Guilt or self-deprecatory feelings
  - Energy level decrease
  - Concentration difficulties
  - Appetite disturbance or weight change
  - Psychomotor disturbance
  - Suicidal thoughts
- Take note of any atypical presentations such as chronic pain, hypochondriasis, or cognitive difficulties.
- Check for manifestations of bipolar disorder, including attacks of mania or hypomania interspersed with episodes of severe depression.
- Inquire into any psychotic episodes and symptoms.
- Consider cyclothymic disorder when symptoms are less severe, accompanied by chronic mood swings.
- Consider dysthymic disorder when symptoms are chronic, less severe, with fewer neurovegetative symptoms and concurrent personality disorder.
- Consider adjustment disorder when there is depressed mood that is time limited, without neurovegetative symptoms, and in response to identifiable precipitant.
- Rule out "organic" etiologies by checking for symptoms associated with medical causes (see above and see also Chronic Fatigue).
- When there are multiple bodily symptoms and chronic fatigue, check for symptoms of connective tissue disease, vasculitis, fibromyalgia, CFS, Lyme disease, and endocrinopathies (see Chronic Fatigue).
- Include thorough review of medications and inquire into substance abuse.
- Conduct complete review of systems.
- If depression suspected, check for suicidality by specifically asking about suicidal thoughts and intentions. If patient appears suicidal, especially if plans are reported, refer immediately for emergency psychiatric care.

PHYSICAL EXAM

- Conduct complete PE and formal mental status exam to address patient concerns about organic illness and to rule out medical causes of depression, fatigue, and multiple bodily complaints (see above and see also Chronic Fatigue).
- If antidepressant medication is likely to be used, check for preexisting postural hypotension, especially in the elderly.

LAB STUDIES

- Choose lab studies carefully and only when Hx and PE provide sufficient evidence of organicity to warrant testing.
- Order only those tests suggested by clinical findings. Avoid routine batteries of tests or "panscans" because of very high risk of generating false-positive results with indiscriminate testing.
- If patient is likely to need antidepressant medication, obtain baseline resting ECG to check for cardiac rhythm disturbances and conduction system disease, especially if tricyclic agents are to be used.

MANAGEMENT

OVERALL APPROACH

- Recheck suicide risk before proceeding with primary care management.
- If patient appears suicidal, psychotic, or severely depressed with no social supports or ability to care for self, arrange prompt psychiatric consultation with view toward possible hospitalization.
- For other patients, begin supportive psychotherapy and make any social and environmental interventions that may help. Especially with elderly or severely depressed patients, involve family in Rx plan.
- Consider antidepressant medication for those with major depression or with subtype associated with marked neurovegetative symptoms.
- Begin pharmacotherapy with an SSRI, the antidepressant class of first choice based on safety and tolerability.
- Advise patients that it may take 4–6 wks for benefit to become evident and that benefit requires taking antidepressant regularly.
- Advise patient of common SSRI side effects (nausea, headache, insomnia, sedation, lack of appetite, sexual dysfunction), but also reassure that side effects are usually mild, often transient, and not basis for discontinuing Rx.
- Base choice of SSRI on cost (generic fluoxetine now available) when minor differences in side-effect profiles are not clinically important.
- Start with modest dose and titrate upward as tolerated to full dose (see below).
- In the elderly, reduce starting dose to one-half to one-third standard starting dose (see below).
- If patient responds to antidepressant Rx, continue for at least 6–9 mos and then slowly taper.
- If patient unresponsive to 4- to 8-wk trial of full-dose SSRI Rx, consider switching to tricyclic antidepressant. (If severely depressed and unresponsive, proceed directly to psychiatric consultation for design of antidepressant program.)
- If considering tricyclic antidepressant Rx, check cardiac status first (see above), then select specific agent based on degree of sedation desired and amount of anticholinergic effect tolerable. Prescribe generic tricyclic antidepressant preparation for lowest cost.
- If there is any possible suicide risk, do not prescribe ≥1 week's tricyclic antidepressant supply or >1 g.

ANTIDEPRESSANT AGENTS

Selective Serotonin Reuptake Inhibitors

- Citalopram (Celexa), 20 mg/day, titrate to 20–40 mg/day
- Fluoxetine (Prozac), 20 mg/day, titrate to 20–40 mg/day
- Fluvoxamine (Luvox), 50 mg/day, titrate to 100–250 mg/day
- Paroxetine (Paxil), 20 mg/day, titrate to 20–60 mg/day
- Sertraline (Zoloft), 50 mg/day, titrate to 100–250 mg/day

Atypical Antidepressants

- Bupropion sustained release (Wellbutrin SR), 150 mg qam, titrate to 150–200 mg bid

- Mirtazapine (Remeron), 15 mg qhs, titrate to 30-45 mg qhs
- Nefazodone (Serzone), 50 mg bid, titrate to 150–300 mg bid
- Trazodone (Desyrel), 50–100 mg qhs, titrate to 200–600 mg/day
- Venlafaxine extended release (Effexor XR), 37.5 mg bid, titrate to 75–150 mg bid

Tricyclic Antidepressants

- Amitriptyline (Elavil), 25 mg qhs, titrate to 150–300 mg qhs
- Clomipramine (Anafranil), 25 mg qhs, titrate to 150–200 mg qhs
- Desipramine (Norpramin), 25 mg qam, titrate to 150–300 mg qam
- Doxepin (Adapin), 25 mg qhs, titrate to 150–300 gm qhs
- Imipramine (Tofranil), 25 mg qhs, titrate to 150–300 mg qhs
- Nortriptyline (Pamelor), 10 mg qhs, titrate to 50–150 mg qhs
- Protriptyline (Vivactil), 10 mg qam, titrate to 30–60 mg qam
- Trimipramine (Surmontil), 25 mg qhs, titrate to 150–250 mg qhs

Monoamine Oxidase Inhibitors

- Phenelzine (Nardil), 15 mg bid, titrate to 45–90 mg/day
- Tranylcypromine (Parnate), 10 mg bid, titrate to 40–80 mg/day
- L-deprenyl (Eldepryl), 10 mg bid, titrate to 30–40 mg/day

BIBLIOGRAPHY

- For the current annotated bibliography on depression, see the print edition of *Primary Care Medicine*, 4th edition, Chapter 227, or www.LWWmedicine.com.

Eating Disorders

DIFFERENTIAL DIAGNOSIS

- Malignancy
- Chronic infection
- Intestinal disorders
  - Malabsorption
  - Inflammatory bowel disease
  - Hepatitis
- Endocrinopathies
  - Hyperthyroidism
  - Panhypopituitarism
  - Adrenal insufficiency
  - Diabetes mellitus
- Psychiatric illnesses
  - Depression
  - Schizophrenia
  - Obsessive-compulsive neurosis
- Organic brain syndrome
- Tumors of CNS (in rare cases mimic anorexia nervosa)

WORKUP

OVERALL STRATEGY

American Psychiatric Association Diagnostic Criteria for Eating Disorders

- Anorexia nervosa
  - Low body weight (<85% of expected or BMI <17.5 kg/m^2)
  - Inaccurate perception of own body size, weight, or shape
  - Intense fear of weight gain
  - Amenorrhea (if female)
- Bulimia nervosa
  - Excessive concern about body weight or shape
  - Recurrent binge eating (≥2 times/wk for 3 mos)
  - Recurrent purging, excessive exercise, or fasting (≥2 times/wk for 3 mos)
  - Absence of anorexia nervosa
- Binge-eating disorder
  - Recurrent binge eating (≥2 times/wk for 6 mos)
  - Marked distress with ≥3 of these:
    - Eating very rapidly
    - Eating until uncomfortably full
    - Eating when not hungry
    - Eating alone
  - No recurrent purging, excessive exercise, or fasting
  - Absence of anorexia nervosa

HISTORY

Anorexia Nervosa

- Explore patient's attitudes toward weight loss, desired weight, and eating habits; 24-hr dietary recall is more revealing than answers to general questions about diet.
- Obtain detailed weight and menstrual Hx, including date and circumstances at onset of weight loss, minimum and maximum weights, recent weight changes, and last normal menstrual period.
- Ask about bingeing, vomiting, and use of laxatives, diuretics, diet pills, and emetics; ask patient to quantify daily exercise (excessive exercise may be variant of anorexia).
- Inquire into symptoms of malnutrition (fatigue, skin or hair changes), dehydration (light-headedness, syncope, thirst), hypokalemia (cramps, weakness, paresthesias, polyuria, palpitations), and other problems common to purgers (e.g., heartburn, abdominal pain, rectal bleeding).
- Screen for suicidality during initial visit (see Depression), because risk is increased among those with eating disorders.
- Likewise, explore psychosocial Hx and check for depression, anxiety, and personality disorders (see Anxiety; Depression; Somatization Disorders).

Bulimia

- Maintain high index of suspicion because bingeing and purging may be concealed and no physical signs are characteristic.
- Check for preoccupation with weight and food, Hx of frequent weight fluctuations, and problems common to patients who purge and become dehydrated (dizziness, thirst, syncope) or hypokalemic (muscle cramps or weakness, paresthesias, polyuria).
- Also inquire into hematemesis and heartburn (suggests excessive vomiting) and constipation, rectal bleeding, and fluid retention (laxative abuse).
- When Dx suspected, ask directly about bingeing and purging. Direct inquiry may elicit Hx from patient seeking help but ashamed to volunteer information. Some patients who vomit deny that it is voluntary. Exclude organic causes of chronic vomiting in these cases (see Nausea and Vomiting).

Binge-Eating Disorder

- Focus on Hx because PE and lab findings are almost always normal.
- Explore patient's experiences with eating, because distress is characteristic, as are feelings of disgust and guilt after binge.

PHYSICAL EXAM

Anorexia Nervosa

- Check for signs of malnutrition and dehydration by measuring height and weight (without street clothing) and checking postural signs by noting BP and pulse response to postural change.
- Take temp, looking for hypothermia.
- Examine skin for pallor, hair changes of lanugo, chest for rales, and extremities for edema and signs of peripheral vasoconstriction.
- Auscultate apical pulse for arrhythmias.

- Perform anorectal exam for blood (laxative abuse).
- Elicit the deep tendon reflexes for delayed relaxation (secondary hypothyroidism).
- Also use exam to rule out other causes of weight loss (see Weight Loss).

Bulimia

- Check postural signs for evidence of volume depletion.
- Note any salivary gland enlargement or scars on dorsum of hand, suggesting chronic self-induced vomiting. Also examine teeth for erosion and discoloration.
- Perform neurologic exam to rule out any focal abnormalities indicative of CNS tumor or seizure disorder, which can mimic bulimia (rare).

LAB STUDIES

Anorexia Nervosa

- Obtain full set of serum electrolytes + BUN, creatinine, and ECG with rhythm strip.
- If hyponatremia found, consider excess water intake or inappropriate ADH secretion.
- Obtain serum calcium (+ albumin) and magnesium levels if dysrhythmia noted or laxative abuse suspected.
- Test for complications of starvation, such as anemia, leukopenia, secondary hypothyroidism, hypoglycemia, fatty liver, and hypothalamic amenorrhea with ordering of CBC, TSH, glucose, alkaline phosphatase, gonadotropins, and serum estrogens.
- If amenorrhea persistent, weight loss marked, and nutrition poor, obtain DEXA bone scan for detection of osteoporosis (see Osteoporosis).
- Consider additional lab and imaging studies if worried about other etiologies of unexplained weight loss (see Weight Loss).

Bulimia

- Check serum and urine electrolytes, BUN, creatinine, and ECG. Measure calcium and magnesium in laxative abusers.
- Take note of serum and urine electrolyte findings to help determine mode of purging. Hypokalemic alkalosis suggests frequent vomiting or diuretic use. Nonanion gap acidosis suggests laxative abuse.

MANAGEMENT

OVERALL APPROACH

- At first visit, decide whether care should proceed on inpatient or outpatient basis by assessing degree of malnutrition, dehydration, and electrolyte disturbance.
- Before starting management, be sure other causes of weight loss and its complications have been ruled out (see Hyperthyroidism; Nausea and Vomiting; Palpitations; Secondary Amenorrhea; Weight Loss).
- Organize and coordinate multidisciplinary team approach. Obtain expert psychiatric and nutritional consultations.

■ Educate patient about medical complications of eating disorders and bingeing and purging.
■ Set and review with patient guidelines for outpatient management:
  • Minimum acceptable weight
  • Weight goal
  • Weight gain of 1–2 lbs/wk for underweight patients
  • Maintenance of normal electrolytes
■ Monitor weight, postural signs, cardiac rhythm, and electrolytes.
■ Treat any hypokalemia with potassium chloride.
■ Address and treat any endocrinologic complications (see Hypothyroidism; Secondary Amenorrhea).

INDICATIONS FOR ADMISSION

■ Weight loss >40% of normal (or >30% if within 3 mos).
■ Weight loss rapidly progressive.
■ Cardiac arrhythmia (urgent).
■ Persistent hypokalemia unresponsive to outpatient Rx.
■ Syncope, severe dizziness, or listlessness (urgent).
■ Severe depression (urgent if patient becomes suicidal).

BIBLIOGRAPHY

■ For the current annotated bibliography on eating disorders, see the print edition of *Primary Care Medicine*, 4th edition, Chapter 234, or www.LWWmedicine.com.

DIFFERENTIAL DIAGNOSIS

- Psychiatric disorders
  - Depression (major depression, dysthymia, bipolar disorder)
  - Stimulating antidepressants (desipramine, imipramine, bupropion, fluoxetine, sertraline)
  - Substance abuse (sedative abuse and withdrawal: alcohol, narcotics, benzodiazepines)
  - Stimulant abuse and withdrawal (amphetamines, cocaine, phencyclidine)
  - Cigarette and nicotine dependence and withdrawal
  - Character disorders
  - Psychosis
  - Antipsychotic agent production of periodic leg movements of sleep
- Medical/surgical problems
  - Musculoskeletal: arthritic pain
  - Cardiovascular: nocturnal angina, orthopnea, paroxysmal nocturnal dyspnea; medications: quinidine, propranolol, atenolol, pindolol, clonidine, methyldopa
  - Respiratory: COPD, asthma; medications (terbutaline, albuterol, salmeterol, metaproterenol, phenylpropanolamine, pseudoephedrine, phenylephrine)
  - Endocrine: hyperthyroidism; medications (oral contraceptives, cortisone); dysthymia, bipolar disorder
  - Neuropsychiatric: delirium
- Primary sleep problems
  - Sleep apnea
  - Circadian rhythm disturbance
    - Jet lag
    - Shift work
    - Delayed sleep phase syndrome
  - Periodic leg movements of sleep
    - Nocturnal myoclonus
    - Restless leg syndrome
- Miscellaneous
  - Caffeine
  - OTC medications
  - "Diet pills"
  - Environmental factors: noise, temperature

WORKUP

OVERALL STRATEGY

- Search for underlying etiology when complaint is persistent, sleep latency (time between lights out and falling asleep) is consistently >60 mins, or insomnia is associated with compromised daytime functioning.

HISTORY

- Obtain full description of problem, facilitated by patient's keeping sleep log or diary, which includes time in bed, estimate of time asleep, any awakenings, time of morning arousal, estimate of sleep quality, and comments on unusual events and any associated symptoms (e.g., orthopnea, urinary frequency, pain, palpitations). Patient should record entries directly on getting up qam.
- Pay attention to use of sedatives, hypnotics (including OTC preparations), and stimulants.
- Screen for alcohol and other substance abuse (see Alcohol Abuse; Substance Abuse).
- Listen carefully for and inquire directly about symptoms of depression, bipolar disease, anxiety disorder, and psychosis (see Anxiety; Depression).
- Note occupational and travel patterns.
- Whenever possible, interview spouse, bed partner, or family member, particularly for symptoms suggesting sleep apnea (e.g., excessive snoring, apneic episodes, disturbed sleep; see Sleep Apnea).
- Review medical and psychiatric Hx of patient and family.

PHYSICAL EXAM

- Customize according to findings on Hx. Check for upper airway soft tissue obstruction in patient with suspected sleep apnea; for jugular venous distention, rales, wheezes, heaves, and gallops when concerned about cardiopulmonary etiology; for moist skin, tachycardia, proptosis, goiter, and tremor when hyperthyroidism is possibility; and for prostatic enlargement in elderly man with sleep-disturbing nocturia.
- Evaluate and confirm any reported sources of pain.
- Perform mental status exam to help detect psychiatric disease (see Anxiety; Depression).

LAB STUDIES

- Testing should be limited, selective, and based on evidence from Hx and PE (e.g., TSH for suspected hyperthyroidism, CXR for cardiopulmonary disease, toxic screen for substance abuse).
- Refer selectively to sleep lab, predominantly when obstructive sleep apnea or primary sleep disorder suspected, such as central sleep apnea or nocturnal myoclonus (see Sleep Apnea).
- Consider psychiatric evaluation only when character problems interfere with Dx or management or if nature of suspected mental or emotional problem is obscure.

MANAGEMENT

INSOMNIA DUE TO DEPRESSION

- If insomnia is related to underlying affective disorder, begin sedating tricyclic antidepressant, such as nortriptyline (10 mg) or an SSRI (e.g., paroxetine, 20 mg; or mirtazapine, 20 mg, taken 1 hr before bedtime for 2 wks).

- See patient frequently until symptoms resolve, and increase dose prn to treat depression fully.
- Offer patient ed and arrange social support to elderly patients who have normal daytime functioning but who are lonely or upset and who may awaken in early morning as consequence of their psychological state or from normal age-related changes in their sleep pattern.

INSOMNIA DUE TO ANXIETY

- If insomnia is related to anxiety disorder, prescribe a short course of triazolam (starting at 0.125 mg qhs) when problem is staying asleep, and zolpidem (5–10 mg qhs) when main problem is falling asleep.
- Consider clonazepam (0.5 mg) or flurazepam (15 mg) qhs if daytime anxiety is present.
- If symptoms recur after 2 wks of Rx for anxiety-related insomnia, institute behavioral and relaxation Rx (see Anxiety) and consider psychiatric consultation.

INSOMNIA DUE TO CHARACTER DISORDER

- If insomnia is related to character disorder, seek psychiatric consultation, require close adherence to good sleep hygiene, and use benzodiazepines only with caution.

INSOMNIA DUE TO SUBSTANCE ABUSE

- Make sure to obtain from all patients complete Hx of alcohol and substance use, including cigarettes, caffeine, nonprescription drugs, and stimulants.
- Interview family members and obtain toxic screens of urine or blood when there is doubt.
- Do not prescribe benzodiazepines for patients with current or past alcohol or substance abuse.
- Supervise withdrawal and abstinence, and seek psychiatric consultation when withdrawal symptoms or abstinence are problematic.

INSOMNIA DUE TO PAIN OR MEDICAL CONDITION

- Treat pain and underlying medical problems aggressively.
- Consider a short course of benzodiazepines (e.g., zolpidem, 5–10 mg qhs) to help reestablish normal sleep pattern.

BIBLIOGRAPHY

- For the current annotated bibliography on insomnia, see the print edition of *Primary Care Medicine*, 4th edition, Chapter 232, or www.LWWmedicine.com.

Nonmalignant Pain

DIFFERENTIAL DIAGNOSIS

CAUSES OF CHRONIC PAIN BY LOCATION

- Head and face
  - Tension headache
  - Sinusitis
  - Glaucoma
  - Migraine
  - Chronic otitis
  - Medication
  - Cluster
  - Trigeminal neuralgia
  - Giant cell arteritis
  - Abscess
  - Postconcussive
  - Large arteriovenous malformation
  - Subdural hematoma
  - Hypertension
  - Tumor
  - Bruxism
  - Dentalgia
  - Temporomandibular joint disorder
  - Sialadenitis
- Musculoskeletal system
  - Fibromyalgia
  - RA
  - Paget's disease
  - Polymyalgia rheumatica
  - Osteoarthritis
  - Tumor
  - Myositis
  - Gout/pseudogout
  - Cramps
  - Systemic lupus erythematosus
  - Bursitis/tendinitis
  - Osteomyelitis
  - Reflex sympathetic dystrophy
  - Hypothyroidism
  - Trichinosis
  - Sickle cell disease
  - Trauma
  - Lyme disease
  - Secondary syphilis
- Low back
  - Chronic disk disease
  - Osteoporotic fracture
  - Tumor (bone/retroperitoneum)
  - Sciatica

- Spinal stenosis
- Seronegative spondyloarthropathy
- Epidural abscess
- Abdomen/pelvis
  - Irritable bowel syndrome
  - Inflammatory bowel disease
  - Kidney stones
  - Biliary colic
  - Diverticulitis
  - Chronic pyelonephritis
  - Esophagitis
  - Gastritis/peptic ulcer disease
  - Polycystic kidney
  - Pancreatitis
  - Hepatitis
  - Endometriosis
  - Parasitosis
  - Malignancy
  - Ovarian cyst
  - Aortic aneurysm
  - Abdominal angina
  - PID/tubo-ovarian abscess
  - Sickle cell
  - Poisoning (e.g., lead)
  - Familial Mediterranean fever
  - Medication
  - Hernia
  - Porphyria
  - PMS
- Peripheral nerve
  - Diabetic neuropathy
  - Vitamin B_{12} deficiency
  - Charcot-Marie-Tooth disease
  - HIV neuropathy
  - Connective tissue disease
  - Hypothyroidism
  - Paraneoplastic syndrome
  - Renal failure
  - Poisoning (ethanol, platinum, isoniazid)

PSYCHOLOGICAL AND SOCIAL FACTORS CONTRIBUTING TO CHRONIC PAIN

- Psychological factors
  - Major depression
  - Anxiety disorders
  - Somatoform disorders
  - Personality disorders
  - Substance abuse
  - Malingering
- Social factors
  - Domestic violence
  - Daily activities causing pain
  - Activities hindered by pain

- Work hindered by pain
- Work contributing to pain
- Secondary gain

WORKUP

OVERALL STRATEGY

- Explore biologic and psychosocial dimensions of problem.
- Define patient's psychosocial context.
- Classify pain process as precisely as possible.
- Determine likelihood of serious underlying biologic pathology.

DEFINING PSYCHOSOCIAL CONTEXT

- Screen all patients with chronic pain for depression, anxiety, somatization, personality disorder, substance use/abuse, and malingering.
- Note important clues suggesting primary psychological or social cause:
  - Depressed or anxious affect
  - Hx of substance abuse
  - Multiple unrelated pain sites
  - Onset in adolescence
  - Hx of difficult social interactions
  - Absence of clear pathophysiologic mechanism
  - Evidence of physical, sexual, or emotional abuse
  - Potential for or Hx of pursuing secondary gains litigation reward or worker's compensation
  - Review home, work, and leisure activities in depth for possible precipitating and aggravating social factors.
- Screen for domestic violence by asking a few basic questions:
  - Do you feel unsafe at home?
  - Has anyone at home hit you or tried to injure you?
  - Have you ever been afraid of your partner?
  - Has anyone ever threatened you or tried to control you?

CLASSIFYING PAIN PROCESS

- Document classic cardinal features of pain (i.e., onset, duration, quality/severity, location/radiation, alleviating/aggravating factors, associated symptoms, circumstances surrounding onset).
- Determine from presentation whether pain is acute or chronic, localized or diffuse, somatic or visceral, and nociceptive (due to tissue/organ damage) or neuropathic (due to direct nerve stimulation).
- Assess whether presentation makes anatomic/biologic sense or is best explained by psychological or psychosocial mechanisms.
- Take into account cultural influences on pain presentation and description.
- Assess pain severity using standard severity scales, most of which are cross-culturally reproducible (e.g., visual analogue pain scale or 1–10 rating scales).

DETERMINING LIKELIHOOD OF SERIOUS UNDERLYING BIOLOGIC PATHOLOGY

- Note important clues for predominantly biologic etiology:

- Pain of recent onset
- Little associated psychiatric symptomatology
- Presence of constitutional symptoms
- Objective findings prominent

MANAGEMENT

OVERALL APPROACH

- Identify and address focal treatable pathology, but be prepared to approach chronic pain as chronic disease that may not have "cure."
- Use mechanistic classification of pain (nociceptive vs neuropathic) to determine pharmacologic approach to pain control.
- If pain incurable, focus on improving daily functioning and quality of life rather than on eliminating pain.
- Take into account and address psychosocial factors in design of Rx program.
- Identify and address any primary psychiatric processes, and treat secondary processes along with pain.
- Organize multidisciplinary approach to Rx of difficult cases:
  - Arrange psychiatric referral when there is primary psychiatric disorder or when behavioral training might be useful.
  - Consider referral to pain center/pain specialist for help in design of comprehensive program and for consideration of invasive techniques.

NOCICEPTIVE PAIN

- Treat nociceptive pain stepwise, starting with non-opiate analgesics and progressing to opiates as necessary.
- Use acetaminophen as non-opiate of choice. Avoid depending on long-term NSAID use if possible due to adverse effects from chronic use (peptic ulcer, renal impairment, bleeding).
- If chronic NSAID use unavoidable, consider concomitant PPI (e.g., omeprazole) or misoprostol; also consider COX-2 inhibitor.
- Do not hesitate to prescribe opiates on long-term basis if following criteria are met:
  - Pain inhibits daily functioning and quality of life.
  - Patient consistently reports subjective chronic pain on more than one occasion.
  - More conservative measures have failed.
  - Patient does not meet formal criteria for substance abuse (see Substance Abuse) or other primary psychiatric disorder (see Anxiety; Depression; Somatization Disorders).
- Start with short-acting opiate to determine necessary daily dose, then switch to long-acting opiate preparation for chronic use, supplemented by short-acting agent for breakthrough pain (see below).
- Treat proactively in preference to reactively.
- Consider use of opiate contract in patients with potential for narcotic abuse.

NEUROPATHIC PAIN

- In addition to analgesics, consider use of antidepressants, anticonvulsants, and topical anesthetics (see below).

INITIAL AND MAXIMUM DOSES (MG) OF MEDICATIONS FOR PAIN

Non-Narcotic Analgesics

- Acetaminophen (Tylenol), 500–1,000 q4–6h, max 1,000 qd
- Tramadol (Ultram), 50–100 q6h, max 400 qd
- Aspirin (Ecotrin, Bayer), 325–650 q4–6h, max 650 q4h
- Ibuprofen (Advil, Motrin, Nuprin), 200–800 q6h, max 800 q6h
- Naproxen (Naprosyn, Aleve), 250–500 q12h, max 500 q12h
- Etodolac (Lodine), 200 q8h, max 400 q8h
- Indomethacin (Indocin), 25–50 q8h, max 50 q8h
- Ketorolac (Toradol), 10 q6h, max 10 q4h
- Salsalate (Disalcid), 500 bid, max 1,000 tid
- Celecoxib (Celebrex), 100 bid, max 200 bid

Opioids

- Codeine (in Tylenol nos. 2–4), 15 q4h, max 60 q4h
- Oxycodone (in Percocet), 5 q6h, max 10 q4h
- Oxycodone sustained release (OxyContin), 10 q12h, max 30 q8h
- Morphine (Roxanol elixir), 10 q6h, max 30 q4h
- Morphine sustained release (MS Contin), 60 q12h, max 180 q8h
- Hydromorphone (Dilaudid), 2 q6h, max 2 q4h
- Methadone (Dolophine), 20 q8h, max 20 q4h
- Meperidine (Demerol), 50 q4h, max 150 q3h
- Fentanyl patch (Duragesic), 25 µg/hr q72h, max 200 µg/hr q72h

Anticonvulsants

- Gabapentin (Neurontin), 100 qhs, max 1,200 tid
- Baclofen (Lioresal), 5 q8h, max 20 q6h
- Phenytoin (Dilantin), 150 qd, max 300 qd (level)
- Carbamazepine (Tegretol), 200 q8h, max 400 q8h (level)
- Clonazepam (Klonopin), 0.5 q6h, max 1–5 q6h

Antidepressants

- Doxepin (Sinequan), 25 bid, max 100 q8h
- Amitriptyline (Elavil), 25 qhs, max 75 bid
- Imipramine (Tofranil), 75 qhs, max 75 bid
- Nortriptyline (Pamelor), 25 qhs, max 25 q6h
- Desipramine (Norpramin), 25 qhs, max 150 bid
- Paroxetine (Paxil), 20 qd, max 50 qd
- Fluoxetine (Prozac), 20 qd, max 80 qd

BIBLIOGRAPHY

- For the current annotated bibliography on nonmalignant pain, see the print edition of *Primary Care Medicine*, 4th edition, Chapter 236, or www.LWWmedicine.com.

Sexual Dysfunction

SCREENING AND/OR PREVENTION

- Screen for sexual dysfunction by asking a few simple questions during genitourinary review of systems:
  - Does your present sexual functioning meet your expectations?
  - Has there been a change in your sexual functioning?
  - Would you like to change anything in your sexual functioning?

DIFFERENTIAL DIAGNOSIS

DISORDERS IN WOMEN

General Considerations

- Sexual pain syndromes include dyspareunia with pain on insertion or deep penetration, and vaginismus.
- More common than pain syndromes are problems related to women's interest in and desire for sex, physiologic and subjective response to stimuli, or frequency of orgasm.

Causes of Dyspareunia

- Pain greatest on insertion
  - Inadequate lubrication
  - Vaginitis
  - Incompletely ruptured hymen
  - Bartholin's gland cyst
  - Stricture
  - Inadequate episiotomy
  - Vulvovaginal atrophy
  - Vulvar vestibulitis
  - Pudendal neuralgia
  - Vaginismus
- Pain greatest on deep penetration
  - PID
  - Ovarian cyst
  - Endometriosis
  - Pelvic adhesions
  - Relaxation of pelvic support
  - Uterine fibroids

Secondary Causes of Sexual Dysfunction

- Medical
  - Cushing's disease
  - Addison's disease
  - Diabetes mellitus (DM)
  - Hypopituitarism
  - Hyperprolactinemia
  - Degenerative joint disease
  - Hypothyroidism

684

- Multiple sclerosis
- Temporal lobe lesions
- Coronary heart disease
- Psychiatric
  - Bipolar disorder
  - Anxiety disorder
  - Major depression
  - Panic disorder
  - Somatization disorder
  - Somatoform pain disorder

DISORDERS IN MEN

General Considerations

- It is normal to have occasional episodes of erectile failure at times of stress, fatigue, or distraction. Rate of failure that approaches 25% of attempts to achieve or sustain erection sufficient for intercourse defines Dx of impotence or erectile dysfunction.
- Condition affects up to 10% of men; prevalence increases among older men.

Important Organic Causes of Secondary Sexual Dysfunction

- Decreased libido
  - Drugs
    - Alcohol
    - Guanethidine
    - H_2 blockers (cimetidine)
    - Phenothiazines
  - Cord lesions (sensation abolished)
  - Endocrine-metabolic disease
    - Addison's disease
    - Cushing's syndrome
    - Hypothyroidism
    - Hypogonadism
- Impotence
  - Drugs
    - Alcohol
    - Amphetamines
    - Antidepressants
    - Antihypertensive agents (methyldopa, clonidine, beta blockers, diuretics, reserpine)
    - Barbiturates
    - Cocaine (priapism with chronic abuse)
    - H_2 blockers
    - Methadone
    - Phenothiazines
  - Cord lesions
    - Below T-11
  - Peripheral autonomic neuropathy
    - DM
  - Surgical procedure
    - Simple prostatectomy (occasional; all approaches)
    - Perineal prostatectomy
    - Open perineal biopsy

- Radical prostatectomy, bladder or rectal surgery
- Prostatic disease
  - Prostate cancer
  - Vesiculoprostatitis
- Penile and urethral lesions
  - Pelvic fractures
  - Phimosis, herpes, balanitis (painful intromission)
  - Peyronie's disease (painful intromission)
  - Hernia or hydrocele (interferes with coitus)
- Endocrine-metabolic disease
  - Addison's disease
  - Cushing's syndrome
  - Hypothyroidism
  - Acromegaly
  - Hypogonadism
  - Hyperprolactinemia
  - Zinc deficiency (severe, in dialysis patients)
- Vascular disease
  - Aortoiliac insufficiency
  - Venous disease
- Ejaculatory failure
  - Drugs
    - Alcohol
    - Guanethidine (retrograde)
    - Phenothiazines
  - Cord lesions
  - Peripheral autonomic neuropathy
    - DM (retrograde)
  - Surgical procedure
    - Simple prostatectomy (retrograde; all approaches)
    - Radical retroperitoneal node dissection
    - Bilateral sympathectomy
  - Prostatic disease
    - Prostatitis (painful)
  - Penile and urethral lesions
    - Pelvic fractures
    - Hypospadias
    - Priapism

WORKUP

OVERALL STRATEGY

- Thoroughly and nonjudgmentally explore problem in detail as elicited by screening or direct complaint.
- Ask patient to describe problem in own words, noting duration, circumstances, precipitating and alleviating factors, and severity.
- Elicit Rx patient thinks might be helpful.
- Check medical Hx for medications, substances, and illnesses that might affect sexual function.
- Conduct thorough psychological, endocrinologic, vascular, and genitourinary reviews of systems.

- In men, establish that erectile function is significantly compromised before undertaking extensive workup. Once confirmed, evaluation shifts to differentiating psychogenic from organic disease. Sudden onset and preservation of erections on awakening or masturbation suggest psychogenic causes.

HISTORY

In Women

- Determine whether patient noticed dyspareunia with first experience of sexual intercourse or whether it has developed recently, secondary to organic change or situational problem.
- Ask patient whether pain occurs before penetration, on penetration, or only after deep penetration. Establish whether patient can insert tampons without pain; if she can, mechanical obstruction is unlikely.
- Hx of recent infection, previous surgery, or pelvic pathology may suggest etiology.
- Take complete Hx, including current and previous sexual experiences. Recent studies underscore new awareness of prevalence of sexual abuse, including incest, rape (including date rape), and domestic violence. Patients may not be forthcoming with these experiences.
- Explore any Hx of sexual fears. Sensitively obtain understanding of patient's current sexual experience (circumstances, time spent on foreplay, etc.) and feelings toward partner. Interviewing husband or sexual partner is part of complete evaluation and is appropriate in many cases.

In Men

- In exploring medical etiologies, check for signs and symptoms of DM (see Diabetes Mellitus), alcohol abuse (see Alcohol Abuse), and aortoiliac disease (see Arterial Insufficiency).
- Note atherosclerotic risk factors (HTN, smoking, DM, hyperlipidemia).
- Review medications, especially antihypertensives, major tranquilizers, antidepressants, other drugs with anticholinergic activity, and H_2 blockers with antiandrogenic effects (e.g., cimetidine).
- If patient reports reduced libido, check for symptoms of thyroid disease (see Hyperthyroidism; Hypothyroidism), hyperprolactinemia (see Galactorrhea and Hyperprolactinemia), hypogonadism (see Infertility), and adrenal disease.
- Review medical Hx for radical prostate or pelvic surgery, pelvic irradiation, spinal cord injury, MS, cancer, and pelvic fracture.

PHYSICAL EXAM

In Women

- Perform thorough PE, concentrating on vascular, endocrinologic, and neurologic aspects. Also perform mental status exam, checking for depression and other psychological problems.
- Pelvic exam is most important part of workup. Inspect for signs of vulvovaginitis, atrophic vaginitis, narrowed introitus, cervicitis, and congenital abnormalities. Palpation may identify uterine mass, retroverted uterus, or tenderness.
- Determine whether manipulation of cervix produces pain. Examine for loss of pelvic support, rectocele, or cystocele.

■ Obtain smear for cervical cytology to detect underlying malignancy.

In Men

■ Perform thorough PE, concentrating on vascular, endocrinologic, and neurologic aspects. Also perform mental status exam, checking for depression and other psychological problems.

■ Check vital signs for postural fall in BP (indicative of autonomic or adrenal insufficiency), general appearance for loss of secondary sexual characteristics, and skin for spider angiomata, palmar erythema, excessive dryness, hyperpigmentation, and other dermatologic signs of endocrinopathy. Note neck for goiter.

■ Inspect flaccid penis for tumor, inflammation, discharge, phimosis of foreskin, and hard plaques of Peyronie's disease along dorsolateral aspect of shaft.

■ If possible, assess erect penis, especially if you suspect disease of shaft, so that you can obtain precise information on degree of chordee or erectile weakness.

■ Check testicles and prostate for size, masses, nodules, and tenderness. Small, soft testes suggest hypogonadism. Intrascrotal pathology such as varicocele, hydrocele, or inguinal hernia may mechanically interfere with performance and you can detect them with exam (see Scrotal Masses, Pain, and Swelling).

■ Palpate and auscultate aorta and femoral arteries for bruits and other signs of occlusive disease, especially if patient has Hx of claudication (see Arterial Insufficiency). Note any femoral bruits.

■ Check spine for focal tenderness and evidence of cord compression (see Back Pain). Neurologic assessment includes testing for pain sensation in genital and perianal areas and checking the bulbocavernosus reflex to determine integrity of second, third, and fourth sacral segments of spinal cord. Positive response indicates that S2, S3, and S4 are intact.

■ Other aspects of neurologic function also deserve thorough testing. Evidence of cortical, brainstem, spinal cord, or peripheral deficit may be important etiologic clue.

LAB STUDIES

In Women

■ Obtain CBC, ESR, and cervical culture if PE suggests PID (see Menstrual or Pelvic Pain). Pelvic ultrasound may be indicated to help define suspected pelvic mass. Referral to gynecologist for laparoscopy is indicated if endometriosis, adhesions, or adnexal mass is a consideration.

In Men

■ Ordering routine battery of tests is not recommended. Best approach is to tailor lab workup to match patient's clinical presentation. For example, 2-hr postprandial serum glucose determination is indicated when you suspect DM (see Diabetes Mellitus). Elevated TSH level confirms hypothyroidism. Measure serum total testosterone and LH when reduced libido accompanies erectile dysfunction.

■ Absence of nocturnal penile tumescence indicates advanced organic disease and remains gold standard for detecting organic erectile dysfunction. The "postage stamp test" (wrapping snug ring of postage stamps around flaccid penis at bedtime) is simple, inexpensive method of screening for nocturnal tumescence.

- Order most other studies only on basis of consultation with specialist in male erectile dysfunction.

MANAGEMENT

FOR WOMEN

Overall Approach

- When Hx and pelvic exam do not reveal cause, and simple measures (e.g., advice about prolonging foreplay, sexual positions, use of lubricants) do not help, refer to gynecologist experienced in and sensitive about Rx of sexual dysfunction.
- Treat underlying vaginal or pelvic infection, and advise patient to refrain temporarily from intercourse (see Menstrual or Pelvic Pain; Vaginal Discharge).
- Cyst of Bartholin's gland duct may spontaneously drain after frequent warm soaks in bathtub and sometimes relieves obstruction; patient may require marsupialization by gynecologist to provide adequate drainage if cyst is inflamed and infected.
- Patients with pain from herpes simplex infection can obtain relief with acyclovir (see Herpes Zoster).
- Retained suture material in episiotomy scars, vulvar islands of adenosis (ectopic columnar epithelium), or nerve endings previously damaged by herpetic infection may require local excision for relief of pain.
- Rx of vaginismus, which may involve education, relaxation, and exercises, is best instituted by experienced therapist.
- Medications, especially antihypertensives and antidepressants, may cause problems with desire, excitement, or orgasm. Changes in regimen, including addition of buspirone to an SSRI that may cause problem but is required can be curative.
- Most problems involving desire, excitement, or orgasm are related to interplay of psychological and relationship issues; referral to experienced therapist is prudent course.
- Complement psychological counseling with small doses of testosterone in postmenopausal women. Sildenafil, ephedrine, and oral phentolamine have also been used but should be prescribed by those with expertise in this area.

Female Sexual Arousal Disorder (Excitement Phase Disorder)

- Arrange referral because this condition often results from more severe psychopathology and usually requires expert attention.
- Pending etiologic Rx, suggest supplemental lubrication such as saliva or K-Y Jelly.

Orgasmic Dysfunction

- Help change goal of sexual activity away from orgasm and toward enjoyment of experience.
- Give permission to woman to express sexual feelings.
- Begin sensate focus exercises, nongenital massage to genital massage. Use back-protected position (man in seated position with woman

between his legs with her back against his chest) with female in control to alleviate self-consciousness or spectatoring.

- Instruct man in stimulative technique: he should not force responsivity but rather seek to accommodate desires; he should not approach clitoris directly because of sensitivity.
- After success in manual genital stimulation, suggest controlled intercourse in female-superior position with man making no demands comes next, followed by lateral position that allows for mutual freedom of pelvic movement.
- For women who have never experienced orgasm, suggest self-stimulation supplemented by fantasy material.
- For women who have orgasms with masturbation but not intercourse, consider teaching "bridge technique":
  • After insertion of penis, man stimulates woman (clitorally) manually or with vibrator. This pairing can be helpful in achieving orgasm, and often after woman experiences orgasm in this way, need for supplementary stimulation disappears.

Vaginismus

- Explain to patient and her partner that condition is involuntary and not willful.
- Consider giving physical demonstration of involuntary vaginal spasm by inserting gloved finger into vaginal entrance.
- Ask couple to refrain from intercourse during early Rx.
- Encourage woman to accept larger and larger objects into vagina in stepwise gradual fashion, accomplished using graduated Hegar dilators in office and at home, or by using her fingers, first 1 and then several, approximately size of penis. She may use her partner's fingers. Syringe containers of different sizes make good dilators.
- Next, in female-superior position, woman gradually inserts penis.

FOR MEN

Erectile Dysfunction

- Erectile dysfunction necessitates empathic, understanding, and thorough approach that recognizes emotional impact it can have on men. Education is essential to help patient comprehend and cope with condition.

Behavioral Therapy

- Before rushing directly to medical Rx, consider behavioral methods.
- Educate patient about his ability to satisfy his partner without intercourse.
- Begin "sensate focus" exercises, which start with nongenital massage and progress to genital massage. Prohibit intercourse, even if erections occur.
- After patient obtains erection by genital massage, have him progress to attempting intercourse. In female-superior position, woman may manually stimulate penis, and if erection occurs, she may insert it into her vagina in slow, undemanding fashion, relieving partner of any responsibility for insertion. She may also do this with partial erections. Gradual movement is begun. There is an emphasis on pleasures of vaginal containment.
- If behavioral methods fail, then proceed to consideration of medical Rx.

Medical Therapy

- When you implicate medications, dose reduction or change in drug can resolve erectile dysfunction. For example, changes to ACE inhibitors, to ranitidine from cimetidine, and to tricyclic antidepressant with less anticholinergic activity (e.g., nortriptyline, desipramine) might help patients with HTN, GERD, and depression, respectively.
- Sildenafil (Viagra) is effective for most men with erectile dysfunction. Exceptions include marked vascular insufficiency, cavernosal fibrosis, and radical prostatectomy-induced problems when bilateral sparing of neurovascular bundles was not achieved. Do not prescribe sildenafil to men taking nitrates for ischemic heart disease. Dose ranges from 25–100 mg no more than once/day and should begin at lower doses. Sildenafil is expensive, averaging >$10/dose.
- Local intracavernosal injection of papaverine, phentolamine or alprostadil has been effective in patients with DM, neurologic injury, psychogenic erectile dysfunction, and vascular insufficiency.
- Consider prosthesis for patient with refractory erectile dysfunction who expresses serious need to regain capacity to engage in coitus. Of 3 prostheses available, simpler ones (semirigid and adjustable malleable types) have proved most satisfactory.
- Alternative is vacuum suction device placed over flaccid penis and connected to hand-operated vacuum pump. Negative pressure in cylinder facilitates passive blood flow into penis. Device works best in patients who respond to penile injection Rx and is alternative to such Rx.
- Correction of aortoiliac disease often meets with disappointing results because of high frequency of coexisting disease in distal vessels; it is not advised. Microsurgical techniques have been used to correct vascular disease within penis. Success rates range from 20–80%. Best results occur in young men with traumatic vascular injury; worst results are in older men with diffuse atherosclerotic involvement of cavernosal artery.
- Reserve testosterone Rx for patients with hypogonadism, manifested by low serum testosterone level. Do not use testosterone as all-purpose sexual stimulant. It has little effect in impotent patients with normal testosterone concentrations (although it may add to frustration by increasing libido).

Premature Ejaculation

- Educate patient that condition has little to do with sensitivity of penis but is usually result of previous conditioning and anxiety.
- Suggest increase in frequency of sexual activity.
- Teach the Masters and Johnson "squeeze" technique:
  - Woman manually stimulates penis. When ejaculation is approaching point of inevitability, as indicated by the man, the woman squeezes penis with her thumb on frenulum, her index finger placed above, and her middle finger below coronal ridge on dorsal side of penis.
  - Pressure is applied until man no longer feels urgency to ejaculate (15–60 s).
- Repeat squeeze technique 2–3 times before allowing ejaculation.

- Once there are good results with squeeze technique, encourage couple to try intercourse in this manner:
  - In female-superior position, woman remains motionless to accustom man to vaginal containment. Gradual thrusting begins, using squeeze technique as excitement intensifies.
  - Alternative to squeeze technique is "stop-start" method. Woman stimulates man to point of ejaculation, then stops stimulation. Erection may or may not subside. She then resumes stimulating penis. After several stop-start procedures, man may ejaculate.

Retarded Ejaculation (During Intercourse)

- Suggest behavioral approach:
  - Woman stimulates penis, asking for directions (verbal and physical) to enhance feeling.
  - Extravaginal ejaculation is obtained by continued stimulation. In man's mind, the woman should become associated with ejaculatory release.
  - The woman stimulates penis manually until orgasm becomes inevitable. Penis is then inserted and female thrusts demandingly. Manual stimulation is repeated if there is no successful ejaculation.

BIBLIOGRAPHY

- For the current annotated bibliography on sexual dysfunction, see the print edition of *Primary Care Medicine*, 4th edition, Chapters 115, 132, and 229, or www.LWWmedicine.com.

Somatization Disorders

DIFFERENTIAL DIAGNOSIS

- Anxiety
- Depression
- Conversion reaction
- Hypochondriasis
- Schizophrenia
- Malingering
- Medical conditions causing multiple bodily complaints:
  - Multiple sclerosis
  - Connective tissue disease
  - Vasculitis
  - Fibromyalgia
  - Lyme disease
  - Chronic fatigue syndrome
  - Thyroid disease

WORKUP

HISTORY

- Differentiate somatization from organic disease by noting the following:
  - Quality of symptoms
    - Complaints with characteristics inconsistent with known pathophysiology are likely psychogenic.
    - Psychogenic sensory complaints often involve combinations of sensory modalities that are neurologically impossible [e.g., patient reports loss of position and vibratory sense but walks normally (see Focal Neurologic Complaints)].
    - Psychogenic symptoms are more likely to resemble symptoms that have afflicted someone important to patient (so-called figure of identity) or to be excessively vague or overly detailed.
    - Diffuse inconsistent descriptions and vivid, elaborate, highly personalized, or idiosyncratic complaints are very suggestive. Patient may reveal psychological factors in choice of words (e.g., "pain in the neck" or "not having a leg to stand on").
  - Timing and precipitants
    - Psychogenic pain is typically unaffected by activity or passage of time, and patient often seems more concerned with PCP accepting authenticity of pain than with relieving it.
    - Although stress can precipitate physical and psychological illness, onset of psychogenic complaints is often closely associated with significant emotional stress, such as loss of loved one or onset of major interpersonal conflict or sexual problem.
    - Functional complaints are also prone to occur on anniversary of psychologically meaningful event.

- Attitude toward symptoms
  - When patient is unconcerned, inappropriately calm, or more concerned with establishing authenticity than with obtaining relief, suspect strong emotional component. Remember that stoic and stolid patients may remain very unemotional when afflicted with serious organic disease.
  - Patients with psychogenic complaints who unconsciously derive considerable gain from their illness are often reluctant to consider emotional cause for symptoms.
- Define the underlying psychopathology by inquiry into the following:
  - Precipitants and response to illness
    - Ongoing psychological stress, pending litigation or disability proceedings, prior medical complaints without demonstrable physical cause, depression, or anxiety disorder.
    - Previous medical care experiences, Hx of consulting many physicians for same complaints, immediate replacement of treated symptom with new one.
  - Personality
    - Illness, discomfort, and disability become way of life, extent patient uses them to deal with emotional discomfort, interpersonal difficulties, and environmental stress.
    - Patient sees himself or herself as suffering and unfortunate person whose life is filled with disappointment, "bad luck," defeat, and illness.
    - Patient may express anger and hostility indirectly, as in cynicism, sarcasm, and uncooperativeness.
    - Individual feels deprived and imposed on, and reproaches, accuses, and blames others.
    - Excessive dependence on others; overpowering desire for care, attention, sympathy, and human contact.
    - Attitude toward physician may have clinging and hungry quality.
  - Personal significance and secondary gain
    - Personal significance attached to symptoms or to suspected illness.
    - Possible secondary gains, such as receiving sympathy, attention, and support (including financial support) from family and friends; being excused from duties, challenges, and responsibilities; and acquiring power to influence and manipulate others by virtue of being sick.

PHYSICAL EXAM

- Conduct thorough PE and mental status exam looking for evidence of organicity (see Fatigue) and for psychopathology (see Anxiety; Depression). Unexpected evidence of organic illness may turn up, and normal exam is prerequisite for effective reassurance and avoiding unnecessary lab testing.

LAB STUDIES

- Unless there is strongly suggestive evidence of organic pathology, avoid testing, especially elaborate or invasive studies. High risk of false-positive results in absence of suggestive clinical evidence.
- Omit performing tests to reassure patient because such action is usually futile. Patients who are highly anxious about their health often find new concerns when result is negative, and likelihood of false-positive result is higher when pretest probability of organic pathology is low.

MANAGEMENT

- Explain results of medical workup without denying reality of patient's discomfort.
- Encourage discussion of psychosocial problems and set up regular schedule of appointments for further elaboration and supportive Rx.
- Make it clear to patient that physical symptoms need not be present to see doctor. Avoid prn appointments when possible.
- Treat underlying psychological problem specifically; do not attempt nonspecific suppression of symptoms with tranquilizers.
- Do not try to remove or cure symptoms in patient with somatizing personality disorder. Acknowledge suffering and provide support. Avoid use of medication and extensive workup of vague symptoms. Goal of care should be adaptation to chronic discomfort.

BIBLIOGRAPHY

- For the current annotated bibliography on somatization disorders, see the print edition of *Primary Care Medicine*, 4th edition, Chapter 230, or www.LWWmedicine.com.

SCREENING AND/OR PREVENTION

GENERAL CONSIDERATIONS

- Ask about substance use and abuse in straightforward fashion as part of standard review of habits.
- During screening Hx and PE, observe for characteristic findings suggesting substance abuse.
- Consider obtaining toxic screen of blood and urine if suspicion is high and confirmation unavailable by Hx.

HISTORY AND PHYSICAL EXAM FINDINGS SUGGESTING SUBSTANCE ABUSE

- Opiates
  - Hx: fever, HIV infection, hepatitis B, pneumonia, TB
  - PE: needle tracks, petechiae, murmur, lymphadenopathy, rash, jaundice, hepatomegaly/tenderness, pulmonary consolidation
- Sedatives
  - Hx: depression, seizures, lethargy, amnesia
  - PE: psychomotor retardation, sadness, observed convulsion, cognitive impairment
- Stimulants
  - Hx: agitation, nasal congestion: stroke, focal neurologic deficits, chest pain, infarction, syncope, palpitations
  - PE: delirium, perforated septum, mucosal edema, new neurologic deficits, new S_4 gallop, single S_2, arrhythmia, enlarged heart, S_3
- Hallucinogens
  - Hx: psychosis, hallucinations, enlarged breasts (males)
  - PE: disordered thinking; gynecomastia
- Alcohol (see Alcohol Abuse)
- Any substance
  - Hx: withdrawal syndrome
  - PE: tremor, tachycardia, agitation, fever

Adapted from Shine RD. The diagnosis of drug dependence by primary care providers. J Gen Intern Med 1991;6(Suppl):S32, with permission.

WORKUP

OVERALL STRATEGY

DSM-IV Criteria for Substance Abuse and Dependence

Substance Abuse

- Maladaptive pattern of substance use leading to clinically significant impairment or distress, as manifested by ≥1 of these occurring within 12 mos:

- Recurrent substance use resulting in failure to fulfill major role obligations at work, school, or home.
- Recurrent substance use in situations in which it is physically hazardous.
- Recurrent substance-related legal problems.
- Continued substance use despite persistent or recurrent social or interpersonal problems caused or exacerbated by effects of substance.

■ Symptoms have never met criteria for substance dependence for this class of drugs.

Substance Dependence

■ Maladaptive pattern of substance use, leading to clinically significant impairment or distress, as manifested by ≥3 of these occurring within 12 mos:
- Tolerance, as defined by 1 of these:
  - Need for markedly increased amounts of substance to achieve intoxication or desired effect.
  - Markedly diminished effect with continued use of same amount of substance.
- Withdrawal as manifested by 1 of these:
  - Characteristic withdrawal syndrome for substance.
  - Same (or closely related) substance taken to relieve or avoid withdrawal symptoms.
- Substance is often taken in larger amounts or over longer period than intended.
- Persistent desire or unsuccessful efforts to reduce or control substance use.
- Great deal of time spent to obtain and use substance or recover from its effects.
- Important social, occupational, or recreational activities given up or reduced because of substance use.
- Substance use continues despite knowledge of persistent or recurrent physical or psychological problem caused or exacerbated by substance use.

HISTORY

■ If screening raises suspicion of substance abuse, proceed directly to more formal evaluation.

■ As with screening, ask about substance abuse in straightforward fashion after establishing some rapport; neither apologize nor suggest blame.

■ Perform evaluation with reference to consensus criteria for Dx of substance abuse and dependence (DSM-IV criteria for substance abuse and dependence, above).

■ Check Hx first for key elements that define substance abuse (see criteria above); examine impact on daily functioning and note any continued use despite adverse consequences.

■ Then review Hx for elements that indicate substance dependence (see criteria above), focusing on symptoms of tolerance and withdrawal and substance-seeking behavior.

■ Also check for risk factors and characteristic findings suggesting substance abuse potential (see Screening in this topic).

PHYSICAL EXAM

- Check for signs associated with abuse of specific substances (see Screening in this topic) as well as signs of withdrawal (fever, tachycardia, HTN, anxiety, cognitive impairment).

LAB STUDIES

- Obtain toxic screen when substance abuse is strongly suspected but unconfirmed by Hx.
- If febrile, begin with blood cultures and proceed according to clinical findings (see Fever).

MANAGEMENT

GETTING PATIENT INTO CARE

- Match Rx strategy with patient's stage of change:
  - Precontemplative: take empathetic stance that encourages patient to seek help later; point out problems (liver disease, employment loss) that may result from substance abuse.
  - Contemplative: use patient's ambivalence and review downside of substance use.
  - Planning: help patient and family plan concrete steps to implement change.
  - Active: support behavioral changes that result in abstinence.
  - Maintenance: focus on prevention of relapse.
- Honor confidentiality, but include family in matching Rx with stage of change.
- Have referral numbers available so that patient's moment of motivation is not lost.

COMPREHENSIVE SUBSTANCE ABUSE TREATMENT

- Refer to specialists and specialized organizations for implementation of comprehensive substance abuse Rx.
- Be sure program has these critical components:
  - Evaluation for comorbid psychiatric or medical disorders (presence of comorbid psychiatric disorder worsens prognosis).
  - Education about effects of drug and nature of addiction.
  - Use of mutual support groups such as Alcoholics Anonymous or similarly organized Narcotics Anonymous.
  - Individual psychotherapy.
  - Family involvement and promotion of sense of belonging, and use of other supportive measures such as exercise, meditation, and discussion of spirituality that may include organized religion.
  - Emphasis on complete abstinence and rehabilitation.

MEDICATION

- Consider drugs that produce aversive reactions (disulfiram for alcohol) or block pleasure (naltrexone for opiates) for short-term use in very motivated patients receiving intensive support.

- Consider methadone maintenance for opiate addicts not ready for detoxification; refer patient to specially licensed Rx center.
- Prescribe nicotine patches or bupropion as part of program for smoking cessation (see Smoking Cessation).

TREATMENT OF ACUTE OVERDOSES AND TOXIC REACTIONS

- Arrange ER admission.
- In decision making and triage, consider the following:
  - Cocaine: no specific antagonist. Rx aimed at relieving symptoms and providing cardiovascular support.
  - Opiates: cardiovascular and airway supportive care. Opiate antagonist naloxone (Narcan) administered IV; usual dose is 0.01 mg/kg; average person will take approximately 2 ampules (0.8 mg). Half-life of naloxone is shorter than that of heroin, so continuous observation and possibly repeated dosing are necessary. Subsequently consider opiate detoxification protocols based on
    - substitution of long-acting oral opiate, methadone, for short-acting injected opiates such as heroin, with taper during 4 days–2 wks depending on setting; or
    - use of opiate buprenorphine (agonist/antagonist), IM or SL during 4- to 5-day course.
  - Sedative-hypnotics: airway and cardiovascular support. Benzodiazepine antagonist flumazenil is available, but clinical experience limited.
  - Marijuana: for panic reaction, reassurance that feeling will pass and ensuring that patient is safe.
  - Hallucinogens: for "bad trip," reassure and maintain safety; rarely, 1–2 mg lorazepam PO (or equivalent) for agitation; for extreme agitation or delirium, physical restraint and 2 mg lorazepam q2h (or equivalent) prn. Obtain toxic screen to search for adulterants and additional drugs. For flashbacks, reassurance is best.

INDICATIONS FOR ADMISSION AND REFERRAL

- Refer for inpatient Rx
  - patients physically dependent on sedative-hypnotics;
  - alcoholic patients with Hx of severe withdrawal symptoms;
  - persons with serious complicating medical or psychiatric conditions;
  - those who have previously failed to improve with outpatient Rx.
- Consider referral for outpatient detoxification if comprehensive specialized program is available and patient has no indications for admission.
- Be sure detoxification program is accompanied by strong psychological and social support, education, and planning for long-term Rx, including the continued support and involvement of PCP.

BIBLIOGRAPHY

- For the current annotated bibliography on substance abuse, see the print edition of *Primary Care Medicine*, 4th edition, Chapter 235, or www.LWWmedicine.com.

Allied Fields

WORKUP

OVERALL APPROACH

■ Consent
  • Review state laws regarding specific services that minors may obtain without parental consent [e.g., related to pregnancy, birth control, abortion, and evaluation and Rx of STDs (including HIV infection), substance abuse, and sexual assault].
  • Note rights of "emancipated" minors (married, have children, serve in military, live apart from parents, or are homeless) and "mature minors," adolescents who understand risks and benefits of Rx and its alternatives.

HISTORY

■ Focus adolescent health Hx on
  • social and emotional development;
  • physical development and health habits;
  • sexual development;
  • family functioning;
  • school performance.

PHYSICAL EXAM

■ Measure and plot on standard growth chart adolescent's height and weight.
■ Determine patient's BMI.
■ Document BP measurement at every annual visit.
■ Evaluate for scoliosis. Look for evidence of physical abuse.
■ Examine teeth for cavities, malocclusion, gingivitis, and congenital dental anomalies.
■ Determine Tanner stage or sexual maturity rating. For girls, provide instruction in breast self-exam and inspect external genitalia.
■ Perform pelvic exam with Pap smear annually for sexually active girls or those aged ≥18.
■ Examine boys for gynecomastia and hernias.
■ Check testicles for abnormal masses or congenital anomalies (at high risk for testicular cancer are boys with Hx of undescended or single testicle).
■ Check skin for acne.

LAB STUDIES

■ Perform random cholesterol determination if positive family Hx for early cardiovascular disease or hyperlipidemia or if unsure of family Hx.
■ Obtain screening hematocrit in girls with heavy menses, weight loss, or eating disorders, or who are extremely athletic.
■ Plant tuberculin skin test if at increased risk for exposure to TB (homeless, Hx of incarceration, immigrant status, HIV infection, living with HIV-infected person, and illicit drug use).

- Test for TB once between age 11–16 if no TB risk factors (see Tuberculosis).
- Screen for STDs (see Cervical Cancer; Chlamydial Infection; Syphilis; Urethritis in Men; Vaginal Discharge) if sexually active.
  - For girls: test during each annual pelvic exam and include cervical culture for gonorrhea, immunologic testing of cervical fluid for chlamydial infection, serologic testing for syphilis, visual inspection of genitalia, and Pap smear for HPV.
  - For boys: check urine DNA or leukocyte esterase for gonorrhea and Chlamydia, perform serologic testing for syphilis, and inspect genitalia for human papillomavirus.
  - Offer HIV testing to those with IV drug use, previous STD, blood transfusion before 1985, exchange of sex for money or drugs, homelessness, >1 sexual partner in last 6 mos, male homosexuality, or sexual partner with any of above risk factors for HIV infection (see HIV-1 Infection).

MANAGEMENT

IMMUNIZATIONS

- Ensure that teenager's immunizations and medical records regarding immunization status are up to date at every clinical encounter (see Immunization).
- Administer tetanus-diphtheria toxoid, MMR vaccine, and hepatitis B vaccine if any recommended doses were missed, undocumented, or given before recommended minimum age.
- Administer tetanus booster by age 11–12.
- For incompletely immunized or unimmunized adolescents (especially newly arrived immigrants), follow Red Book recommendation regarding adolescent immunization schedules.

ANTICIPATORY GUIDANCE

Prevention of Injury and Violence

- Counsel adolescents to use seat belts, and promote use of other safety devices, such as bicycle and motorcycle helmets, protective gear for rollerblading and skateboarding, and appropriate athletic protective devices.
- Ask teenager about access to weapons.

Mental Health

- Screen for depression and suicidal ideation (see Depression).
- Note any risk factors for adolescent depression (poor school performance, family dysfunction, substance abuse, physical or sexual abuse, previous suicide attempts or plans).
- Be aware that vegetative signs of adult depression (sleep disturbance, lack of interest, decreased concentration) can be part of normal adolescent development.
- Keep in mind that adolescent depression may masquerade as vague somatic complaints, such as abdominal pain or headaches.
- Refer immediately for suicidal ideation.
- Obtain mental health consultation for recurrent or serious depression.

NUTRITION AND EXERCISE

- Counsel adolescents about healthful diet, safe weight management, and regular exercise.
- Screen for fad diets, anorexia and bulimia, and use of anabolic steroids by athletes.
- Recommend dietary supplements of calcium (1,000 mg/day) and folic acid (400 mg/day) for girls.

SEXUALITY

- Discuss sex frankly. Explore early adolescents' understanding of sexuality. Discuss responsible sexual behavior, including abstinence.
- Educate about birth control, stressing latex condom use to prevent STDs, especially HIV infection.
- Provide birth control and instructions on appropriate use.

TOBACCO, ALCOHOL, AND OTHER SUBSTANCES

- Ask about smoking and alcohol and other drug use during past 6 mos.
- Educate about harmful effects of substance abuse. Explore family Hx, frequency and amount of use, and circumstances surrounding use.
- Encourage participation in community peer self-help groups.
- Determine social and psychological factors that prompt drug use, and refer to social services and mental health professionals if necessary.

ABUSE

- Screen all adolescents annually for Hx of physical, emotional, and sexual abuse.
- Pursue aggressively any suspicion, asking about circumstances and people involved. Be aware of local reporting requirements to state offices.
- Involve mental health and social services professionals early in all suspected cases of abuse.

SPECIAL ISSUES AND NEED FOR REFERRAL

Scoliosis

- Screen for scoliosis with forward-bend test and visual inspection for rib cage deformation and waistline asymmetry. If positive, obtain "scoliosis plain film series."
- Refer to orthopedic specialist if curvature >15 degrees and spinal growth incomplete (in girls, 18–24 mos after menarche).

Eating Disorders

- See also Eating Disorders.
- Ask about recurrent dieting, body image, interruption of menses, and physical activity.
- Assess for laxative and diuretic use, self-induced vomiting, and starvation.
- Consider eating disorder if weight loss >10% of previous weight or BMI <fifth percentile.
- Rule out other causes of weight loss (hyperthyroidism, inflammatory bowel disease, DM, connective tissue disorders).
- Put together multidisciplinary team for management.

School Failure

■ Check for psychological (depression, anxiety) and physical (hearing, visual) problems, chronic disease (asthma, neurologic dysfunction), learning disorders (attention deficit disorders), drug abuse, limited intellectual ability (developmental delay), and social difficulties (dysfunctional family life, poor peer relations, abuse).

■ Coordinate with parents, teachers, and school counselors. Many school districts are mandated to provide neuropsychological testing to aid in Dx and Rx.

Hypertension

■ Ascertain teenager's BP percentile for age and height. Normal is <ninetieth percentile, high normal is between ninetieth and ninety-fifth, and high (HTN) is SBP or DBP ≥95th percentile on 3 separate occasions.

■ Consider secondary causes of HTN, including renal disease, oral contraception, and use of drugs such as cocaine or steroids (see Hypertension).

■ Focus Hx on growth and development, past illnesses (especially neonatal and as infant), and family Hx.

■ Examine for evidence of end-organ damage.

■ Check urinalysis, BUN, creatinine, electrolytes, and CBC.

■ Consider renal ultrasonography and echocardiography.

Obesity

■ Calculate BMI (see Overweight and Obesity); if between eighty-fifth and ninetieth percentiles, provide diet assessment and counseling.

■ If BMI >ninety-fifth percentile for age and sex, initiate aggressive nutrition counseling and program of diet, exercise, and counseling (see Overweight and Obesity).

Gynecomastia

■ Note that transient enlargement of 1 or both breasts develops during transition from Tanner stage II to stage III and is normal part of puberty.

■ Identify type I idiopathic gynecomastia (usually unilateral, tender; firm mass below areola and type II (more generalized, obese).

■ Reassure that >95% of cases idiopathic and resolve spontaneously, but be alert to pathologic causes (drugs; Klinefelter's syndrome; adrenal, pituitary, and testicular tumors; hypothyroidism; hepatic dysfunction).

■ Note that most idiopathic cases resolve within 2 yrs and require only reassurance and support.

■ Consider pharmacologic Rx (e.g., danazol) or surgical intervention if there is severe psychological difficulty or persistence (see Gynecomastia).

BIBLIOGRAPHY

■ For the current annotated bibliography on adolescents, see the print edition of *Primary Care Medicine*, 4th edition, Chapter 238, or www.LWWmedicine.com.

Alternative Therapies

MANAGEMENT

ECHINACEA FOR UPPER RESPIRATORY INFECTIONS

- Inform patient that best trials have consistently shown nonsignificant decrease of 12–16% in relative risk for respiratory infections.
- Note that substance appears well tolerated but should not be used by persons with autoimmune disease.

GINKGO BILOBA FOR DEMENTIA

- Inform patient that several adequate trials report modest improvement in cognitive function similar to that seen with donepezil in patients with Alzheimer's disease (see Dementia).
- Advise that if taking ginkgo, use only standardized extract containing 24% flavone glycosides and 6% terpene lactones; usual dose is 40 mg tid.
- Avoid use in patients at risk for bleeding, especially those taking warfarin or aspirin; increased risk of cerebral hemorrhage.

KAVA-KAVA FOR ANXIETY

- Note that only 1 adequate trial suggests benefit in generalized anxiety.
- Warn that sedating medications and alcohol may augment effect of kava and that heavy, prolonged use results in dry, yellow scaling of skin; also case reports of dystonic reactions.
- Avoid use in pregnancy and nursing.
- Inform that standard study dose is 100 mg kava (70% kavalactones) tid.

MILK THISTLE FOR HEPATITIS AND CIRRHOSIS

- Note that results are inconclusive; best evidence suggests any benefit limited to alcoholic cirrhosis and disease rated Child's class A.
- Usual dosage is 140 mg tid, standardized to contain 70–80% silymarin.

ST. JOHN'S WORT FOR DEPRESSION

- Note that St. John's wort appears effective in short-term Rx of mild to moderate depression, comparable to low-dose tricyclic antidepressants.
- Inform that adverse effects are generally mild and include GI upset, dizziness, sedation, restlessness, fatigue, and photosensitivity in fair-skinned patients, which can be severe at high doses.
- Advise against use during pregnancy and in combination with other antidepressants.

SAW PALMETTO FOR BENIGN PROSTATIC HYPERPLASIA

- Inform patient that there is modest improvement in BPH symptoms, similar to that achieved with finasteride, and that substance does not affect PSA level; usual dosage, 160 mg bid.
- Note that side effects are few.

VALERIAN FOR INSOMNIA

- Note that only 1 adequate trial supports valerian use and that there are no standardized extracts.
- Advise against use with other sedatives.

BIBLIOGRAPHY

- For the current annotated bibliography on alternative therapies, see the print edition of *Primary Care Medicine*, 4th edition, Chapter 237, or www.LWWmedicine.com.

Index